THIRD EDITION

Hughes, Mansel & Webster's

BENIGN DISORDERS AND DISEASES OF THE BREAST

EDITED BY

R. E. MANSEL CBE MB MS FRCS
Professor of Surgery

D. J. T. WEBSTER MD FRCS
Senior Lecturer and Consultant Surgeon

H. M. SWEETLAND MD FRCS
Reader and Consultant Surgeon

School of Medicine, Cardiff University, Heath Park, Cardiff, UK

WITH THE COLLABORATION OF

L. E. HUGHES MB DS FRCS FRACS Emeritus Professor of Surgery,
Cardiff University, Cardiff, UK

K. GOWER-THOMAS BSC MB BCh FRCR Consultant Radiologist,
Royal Glamorgan Hospital, Llantrisant; Breast Test Wales, Cardiff, UK

D. G. R. EVANS MD FRCP
Professor of Medical Genetics, St Mary's Hospital, Manchester, UK

WITH A FOREWORD BY

H. S. CODY III MD, Attending Surgeon, Breast Service, Départment of Surgery,
Memorial Sloan-Kettering Cancer Center; Professor of Clinical Surgery, The Weill Medical
College of Cornell University, New York, USA

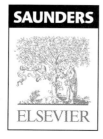

SAUNDERS

ELSEVIER

SAUNDERS

an imprint of Elsevier Limited

First edition 1989 by Baillière Tindall
Second edition 2000 by Harcourt Publishers Limited

ISBN 978-0-7020-2774-1

British Library Cataloguing in Publication Data
A catalogue record for this book is available from the British Library

Library of Congress Cataloging in Publication Data
A catalog record for this book is available from the Library of Congress

Notice
Medical knowledge is constantly changing. Standard safety precautions must be followed, but as new research and clinical experience broaden our knowledge, changes in treatment and drug therapy may become necessary or appropriate. Readers are advised to check the most current product information provided by the manufacturer of each drug to be administered to verify the recommended dose, the method and duration of administration, and contraindications. It is the responsibility of the practitioner, relying on experience and knowledge of the patient, to determine dosages and the best treatment for each individual patient. Neither the Publisher nor the authors assume any liability for any injury and/or damage to persons or property arising from this publication.

The Publisher

ELSEVIER your source for books,
journals and multimedia
in the health sciences
www.elsevierhealth.com

Working together to grow
libraries in developing countries

www.elsevier.com | www.bookaid.org | www.sabre.org

ELSEVIER | BOOK AID International | Sabre Foundation

The publisher's policy is to use paper manufactured from sustainable forests

Printed in China
Last digit is the print number: 9 8 7 6 5 4 3 2 1

THIRD EDITION

Hughes, Mansel & Webster's
BENIGN DISORDERS AND
DISEASES OF THE BREAST

Commissioning Editor: *Michael Houston*

Development Editor: *Alexandra Mortimer*

Editorial Assistant: *Sarah Penny*

Project Manager: *Gail Wright*

Senior Designer: *Sarah Russell*

Cover Designer: *Kirsteen Wright*

Illustration Manager: *Bruce Hogarth*

Marketing Manager: *Brenna Christensen*

Contents

Contents

Contents

Contents

Foreword

Benign breast disease comprises a wide range of conditions which worry patients, which vex physicians, which are vastly more common than breast cancer, and yet which have to date received relatively little attention in the medical literature. It is therefore a particular pleasure for me to introduce the third edition of *Hughes, Mansel & Webster's Benign Disorders and Diseases of the Breast*, a unique and classic work which fully succeeds in addressing this imbalance and builds on the substantial and well-deserved success of the first (1989) and second (2000) editions.

The authors correctly decry the term 'fibrocystic disease', proposing instead that benign breast conditions are not 'disease' *per se*, but are instead minor *aberrations of normal development and involution* ('ANDI'). The ANDI framework, for the first time, puts the study of benign breast disease on a scientific basis which correlates pathogenesis, histology and clinical features. This model is, in my opinion, a robust foundation for further progress in the understanding and treatment of benign breast disease, and deserves much wider recognition, particularly in the US, where it is relatively unknown.

Professor Mansel and his colleagues comprehensively address every aspect of benign breast disease following a format in which all elements (graphics, tables and photographs) work harmoniously to create a whole larger than the sum of its parts. Each chapter heading includes 'key points and new developments' for a quick summary of the contents. As in a Victorian novel, these chapter headings are irresistible and one cannot resist delving into the contents. Throughout, one benefits in equal measure from the authors' scholarship, from their long first-hand experience and from their refreshing practicality in managing benign breast disease.

One highlight of this edition is a remarkable chapter 'History of benign breast disease', which overviews the lives and careers of six great figures (Sir Astley Cooper, Alfred Velpeau, John Birkett, George Cheatle, Joseph Bloodgood and Charles Geschickter), with particular insight into the roles of mentorship, record keeping, acceptance of new technologies, pathologic correlation and the role of international travel and contacts. In an age information technology and instantaneous communication, these elements are more important than ever.

The role of surgery in benign breast disease is changing. Mammography, ultrasound and (increasingly) MRI offer the prospect of earlier cancer diagnosis but bring with them a substantial burden of benign or equivocal findings. Most are amenable to core biopsy but it remains challenging to identify those that do or do not need surgery. Surgical techniques for benign breast conditions may seem simple in concept, but the experienced surgeon will recognize that this simplicity is more apparent than real and that pitfalls abound. In closing, let me enthusiastically recommend the chapter 'Operations'. Here the authors address core biopsy (with and without image guidance) and the full range of surgical procedures for benign breast diseases, presenting a set of 'Important principles' for each. In these lists surgeons in training will recognize a treasury of clinical pearls drawn from the authors' vast hands-on experience, and practising surgeons will recognize their own past surgical misadventures which might have been avoided had these principles been followed. This chapter is a small classic in its own right and should be required reading for all surgeons who treat breast disease, benign or malignant.

Hiram S. Cody III

Preface

It is now 20 years since the first edition of this book and 9 since the second edition. The intervening years have seen advances in imaging technology, understanding of the molecular events leading to disease and drug developments. While most of the focus has been on breast cancer, there have been benefits to an understanding of the changes occurring in the breast from physiology through disorders to diseases.

One of the consequences of an improved understanding of what is happening in the breast and confidence in the ability to diagnose the problem actively has been the disappearance of open surgical diagnostic biopsy and, except for a few areas, surgery for benign conditions. The diagnostic pathway using triple assessment with core needle biopsy is now the standard in most breast clinics; it gives a 99% sensitivity for cancer and dramatically reduces operations for true benign disease.

Much work has been done in identifying patients with an increased risk of developing breast cancer and we have addressed this by including a new chapter on risk of breast cancer written by Professor Gareth Evans of Manchester. Family history is important here but apart from a few cases with atypical epithelial hyperplasia, benign change is not of itself an important determinant. Clinics, however, are dominated by the concern to exclude cancer and to determine future risk.

The imaging chapter has been extensively revised by Kate Gower-Thomas and the xeromammograms have been replaced with modern digital mammograms.

Plastic surgery for both augmentation and reduction is now so well detailed in the plastic surgery literature that we have omitted this chapter; similarly, the chapter on geographical variation has been subsumed into the chapters about individual problems.

Professor Leslie Hughes has provided a fascinating chapter on the lives and influences of some of the great names in the development of our understanding of the changes in the breast.

The ANDI concept provides a framework to enable clinicians to explain to patients the nature of their problem in an easily assimilated way. It is important to emphasise that ANDI is not a diagnosis in itself.

REM, DJTW, HS
January 2009

Acknowledgements

We owe a debt of gratitude to many people who have contributed to work on which this book is based. Foremost are those research fellows who have been responsible for the day-to-day conduct of many studies and clinical trials in this department over the last 30 years: Paul Preece, John Wisbey, Nigel Pashby, Jonathan Pye, Sandeep Kumar, Anurag Srivastava, Barney Harrison, Paul Maddox, Graham Pritchard, Stephen Courtney, Glyn Neades, Richard Cochrane, Eleri Lloyd-Davies, Chris Gateley, Anup Sharma, Eifion Williams, Sumit Goyal, Amit Goyal, Kelvin Gomez, Alok Chaabra and Bedanta Baruah.

We are much indebted to co-operation from the Departments of Radiology – especially Dr Huw Gravelle and Dr Kathleen Lyons, and of Pathology – especially Drs Winsor Fortt and Tony Douglas-Jones. This book could not have been produced without the exceptional service given by the Department of Medical Illustration under Professor R. Marshall and now Professor R. Morton.

The secretarial staff of the University Department of Surgery, both clinical and academic, have facilitated all aspects of the clinical and research work and documentation behind the book, and Mrs Edna Lewis has given many years of voluntary service to the Mastalgia Clinic.

Above all we are grateful to our families who have foregone so much over many years in the cause of research and the writing of this book.

THIS BOOK IS DEDICATED TO

CD Haagensen
Surgeon Pathologist

JD Azzopardi
Surgical Pathologist

Whose meticulous studies have cast so much light on breast disorders, and
whose monographs are quoted so freely in this book

IH Gravelle
Radiologist

Friend, colleague, an imaging pioneer, who enthusiastically joined us in this project to
integrate structure and function in benign disorders of the breast.

CHAPTER 1

Problems of concept and nomenclature of benign disorders of the breast

Key points and new developments

1. Only by taking a historical view of benign disorders of the breast can the confusion persisting until recent decades be understood.

2. In the past, benign conditions (and the patients carrying them) have been regarded as requiring exclusion of cancer or cancer risk, rather than entities requiring management in their own right.

3. Clinical conditions, such as painful nodularity, have been equated with and confused with histological conditions, such as fibrosis or hyperplasia.

4. Most accept that the concepts and terminology of 'fibrocystic disease' and 'fibroadenosis' cannot be justified, but this recognition has so far been matched by masterly inactivity.

5. Accurate and meaningful terminology will be achieved only if those in the field agree on one and accept it and use it. The aberrations of normal development and involution (ANDI) concept and terminology provides a means of achieving this.

The source of the problem

The condition commonly called fibrocystic disease, or fibroadenosis of the breast, has been a clinical problem for centuries, as reflected in writings as early as those of Astley Cooper at the beginning of the nineteenth century. For patients, it causes discomfort and anxiety which varies from nuisance value to serious interference with their quality of life. For clinicians, the condition causes a range of problems of diagnosis, assessment and management which are not always clearly recognized.

Although all clinicians have a concept of what fibrocystic disease represents, it is difficult to define, and none of its protagonists has given a meaningful differentiation between it and normality. One definition[1] is 'palpable lumps in the breast, usually associated with pain and tenderness that fluctuate with the menstrual cycle and become progressively worse until the menopause'. Despite giving a definition, this author, like many before him, states that the term fibrocystic disease has no real meaning and should probably be abandoned. Nevertheless, he also lists the histological features, fibroadenomas, macrocysts, fibrosis, duct dilatation and stasis, periductal round cell infiltrate, fat necrosis, papillomatosis, apocrine metaplasia, sclerosing adenosis and hyperplastic lesions of duct and lobule. This covers the whole range of benign conditions of the breast, and it is clearly inappropriate to equate this histological panorama with a mild, or even severe, degree of painful nodularity.

With such a loose equivalence between clinical and histological detail, it is not surprising that Foote and Stewart wrote in 1945: 'chronic cystic mastitis is so ingrained in the minds of some pathologists that this diagnosis of a locally excised portion of the breast almost amounts to a surgico-pathological reflex'.[2] What is surprising is that pathologists are still the most insistent single group to maintain the use of the term, despite this stinging remark from eminent members of their own discipline.

Greater interest in benign breast disorders in recent years has led to a more precise understanding of the clinical pictures associated with individual elements, and the histological changes of cyclical nodularity are increasingly recognized as lying within the range of histological appearance in the normal breast. Many authors have tried to determine and assess premalignant potential of fibrocystic disease but most attempts have resulted in confusion and frustration. Recent workers, especially Page and co-workers,[3,4] have shown that only a few specific histological patterns have an association with cancer and these show no consistent correlation with the clinical picture which in the past has been ascribed to fibrocystic disease. This poor correlation between histology and clinical symptoms led Love and her co-authors[5] to conclude that fibrocystic disease of the breast is a 'non-disease'. Their arguments are cogent in a histological context by denying the loosely defined cancer risk, but a concept of non-disease does little to help the many women who suffer from a variety of physical symptoms – sometimes of distressing severity. Disorder is a better term than disease because so many of the symptomatic conditions lie within the spectrum of normality. The magnitude of the problem is escalating with the wider concern of women about breast disease and the wider introduction of breast screening programmes.

Benign conditions of the breast have always been neglected in comparison to cancer, despite the fact that only one out of ten patients presenting to a breast clinic suffers from cancer. This is not surprising in view of the emotional implications of breast cancer and its treatment, but it has meant that the study of the benign breast has been undeservedly neglected. Until the 1970s, reported studies were directed largely towards a possible relationship to cancer, rather than towards the basic processes underlying benign conditions.

There has been a noticeable and welcome correction to this neglect in recent years, but already the interest in benign disorders evident for two decades is again on the wane, at a time when advances in molecular biology give promise of understanding the basic physiology of human breast development, function and involution.

This neglect is most evident in standard textbooks (the most recent comprehensive texts on breast disease devote less than 5% of their material to benign conditions) because interest in benign processes can be found when studying historical reference material. Great names in surgery such as Hunter, Astley Cooper, Billroth, Cheatle, Semb, Bloodgood and Atkins appear in the literature. But whereas breast cancer has stimulated a continuous, ongoing body of research – each new project building on the work preceding it – benign disease has been the subject of a relatively small number of isolated and unconnected projects, earlier related work having often been ignored. The sporadic nature of these investigations and the insularity of the resulting publications had led to much confusion which has had more serious consequences than neglect alone.

Consideration of benign breast disorders from a historical point of view provides a clearer understanding of how the present problems have arisen.

History

Sir Astley Cooper was an important early worker in this field. He described many aspects of benign breast disorders as well as malignant disease in his monograph, *Illustrations of Diseases of the Breast*,[6] published in 1829. Among the conditions discussed are cystic disease, pain and fibroadenoma. He distinguished two main groups of patients with mastalgia – those with and those without a palpable tumour, which we might now better define as painful nodularity and non-cyclical breast pain. He also laid much of the basis of the macroscopic anatomy of the breast in his book on the anatomy of diseases of the breast published in 1845. The French surgeon Reclus gave an excellent description of the clinical and pathological aspects of cystic disease in 1893, recognizing both the multiplicity and bilaterality of the cysts.[7]

Many of the current problems in terminology and understanding derive from the publications of German surgeons in the late nineteenth century. Koenig[8] called the disease 'chronic cystic mastitis', because he believed it had an inflammatory basis. At the same time, Schimmelbusch[9] described the same condition, compounding the problem by calling it 'cystadenoma'. Both authors gave the disease inexact names, and both gave incomplete descriptions of the pathology. Certainly they did not recognize the wide range of histological appearances found in these breasts, and they failed to recognize these as merely variants of normal processes within the breast.

There was an early reaction to this confusion. Cabot[10] questioned the inflammatory connotation of the term chronic cystic mastitis and urged more precise terminology, but unfortunately his pleas fell on stony ground. In the 1920s there were major studies by Semb[11] in Norway and Cheatle and Cutler[12] in the UK and their disease descriptions and data are still worth serious study. However, Cheatle and Cutler gave the name 'cystiphorous desquamative epithelial hyperplasia' to the clinical spectrum we have termed aberrations of normal development and involution in Chapter 3 and this can hardly be regarded as helpful. The tendency of the Scandinavians to use Semb's term 'fibroadenomatosis' also caused difficulty because of its confusion with the term fibroadenoma.[11] In spite of detailed investigations, Cheatle and Cutler confused changes of cyclical nodularity with both duct ectasia and fibroadenomas[12] and the term they finally chose – 'mazoplasia' – is hardly evocative in a descriptive sense.

While most workers concentrated on the clinical problems of fibrocystic disease, some gave accurate descriptions of other benign breast conditions. The paper on 'the varicocele tumour' by Bloodgood is a striking account of the clinical and macropathological aspects of duct ectasia and its clinical variants.[13] The accuracy and detail of the observations come as a surprise to those who believe advances in medical understanding are recent.

Special clinics for breast disease set up by Atkins in London and Geschickter in the USA concentrated experience and allowed adequate documentation and assessment of the results of treatment for the first time during the 1940s. Both authors made many contributions to benign breast disorders,[14,15] but suffered equally from the limited knowledge at that time of basic pathology and endocrinology of the breast. They both unfortunately continued the use of the term chronic mastitis. The 50 years since their contributions has seen an increasing momentum in investigation of benign breast conditions. Great benefit has derived from histological study of the normal breast and the development of hormonal estimations using radioimmunoassay. In particular, the autopsy study of Sandison[16] showed that most of the changes previously regarded as disease are so common as to be within the spectrum of normality, and his work stimulated others to define the wide range of histological appearances of the normal breast. For example, Parks[17] studied both surgical and autopsy specimens and showed a gradation between normal lobules and fibroadenomas,

and between involuting lobules and cyst formation. He also showed that papillary epithelial hyperplasia of the terminal ducts is so common in the premenopausal period as to be regarded as normal, and that these lesions regress without treatment after the menopause. In 1961, Oberman and French[18] also stressed the concept of a continuum between normality and benign conditions: 'adenofibromas, fibrocystic disease and intraductal papillomas do not appear to represent distinct entities, but rather form a spectrum of conditions having their basis in an abnormality between hormonal stimulus to the breast, principally estrogen, and stromal and epithelial response'.

These writers have had a profound insight into the concepts discussed in this book, and it is salutary to go back even further. In 1922, McFarland[19] wrote: 'The so-called chronic mastitis is not inflammatory, and is not a pathological entity; it is nothing but a result – or at most a perversion – of involution. The only difficulty lies in clearly defining when the process of involution can be said to become abnormal, when it is so diversified.' The seed scattered by these workers has largely fallen on stony ground.

The present and the future

In the past, each worker has tended to introduce their own terminology for a condition, either to stress a particular aspect they have noted, or through ignorance of work that has gone on perhaps many years before. As an illustration of this, Table 1.1 shows the large number of names that have been associated with just three conditions: so-called fibrocystic disease, duct ectasia and giant fibroadenomas.

This list is by no means comprehensive; some 40 names have been used to describe the variety of conditions covered by the old term, chronic fibrocystic disease, none of which can be considered satisfactory.

Because of their multiplicity and lack of specificity, past terms are better replaced by the use of clinical or histological terms which are specific and accurate in relation to the clinical and/or histological condition to which they refer. Examples of appropriate clinical terms are mastalgia and cyclical nodularity. Examples of appropriate histological terms that have evolved over recent years are sclerosing adenosis and atypical ductal hyperplasia. Terms that accurately reflect both clinical and histological

Table 1.1 Some of the names used for common benign breast disorders

CYCLICAL NODULARITY

Fibrocystic disease

Fibroadenosis

Cystic hyperplasia

Hyperplastic cystic disease

Schimmelbusch's disease

Chronic cystic mastitis

Cystic mastopathy

DUCT ECTASIA/PERIDUCTAL MASTITIS

Plasma cell mastitis

Varicocele tumour

Comedo mastitis

Mastitis obliterans

Secretory disease

GIANT FIBROADENOMATOUS TUMOURS

Giant fibroadenoma

Cystosarcoma phyllodes

Phyllodes tumour

Juvenile fibroadenoma

Serocystic disease of Brodie

counterparts are fibroadenoma, duct papilloma and macrocyst, for example.

When it is desirable to cover the whole range of (unspecified) benign breast disorders, it is appropriate to use a term which, unlike fibrocystic disease, does not imply a disease state, but acknowledges the spectrum of change extending from normality and recognizes that most of the spectrum does not represent disease. We suggest that 'aberrations of normal development and involution' (ANDI) is a term which meets these criteria; it is comprehensive, and meaningful and descriptive in terms of pathogenesis.

Why has it taken so long to reach a reasonable understanding of the processes involved in benign breast conditions? The main stumbling block has been the failure to appreciate the range of basic physiological and structural changes within the normal breast – an organ dynamic throughout the reproductive period of life as it first develops, then undergoes repeated cyclical change and finally involutes. Because it is an organ under systemic hormonal influence, one would expect the breast to be uniform throughout in its appearance and behaviour, but this is not so. Like other endocrine target organs such as the thyroid, it varies greatly from one part to another, and end-organ response must be a factor in this variability. It has been usual practice to concentrate on the local findings as shown by biopsy, at one point in time when the patient presents with a clinical problem, assuming that the particular clinical condition at that time is directly associated with the local radiological and biopsy findings. It is tempting to ignore the findings of Parks and Sandison and others that all these apparently specific findings are frequently found in asymptomatic breasts. So a particular clinical event that leads a patient to biopsy must be assessed against the background of this almost random variation in histological appearance which is a part of normality.

A further source of confusion has arisen from the association of radiological appearances with pathological descriptions, without adequate correlative studies to establish a relationship. An example from recent decades has been the description of radiological density as 'dysplasia' in relation to Wolfe patterns – when detailed study can show that density is unrelated to epithelial dysplasia.[20] The situation was then compounded by using the term 'dysplastic breast' for a radiological pattern, without histological correlation or confirmation. The welfare of the patient with benign breast problems will be best served by abandoning terminology that implies disease, and substituting terminology which reflects the normality of many of the underlying processes, reserving 'disease' for those conditions where clinical morbidity or histological significance warrants such a term. The terminology should come from consideration of the basic physiological and pathological processes that lead a patient to present to a breast clinic.

Perhaps the reason for persisting and increasing confusion is an unwillingness to be sufficiently radical in moving away from ideas that do not fit in with present knowledge. Not only must the concept of fibrocystic disease as a clinical concept or a histopathological entity be done away with, it must be replaced by an accurate terminology consistent with present knowledge. Many breast physicians accept the first half of this statement, but are unwilling to accept the corollary inherent in the second half.

These basic aspects of the non-malignant breast, and the arguments for the aberrations of normal development and involution terminology, are considered in Chapter 4.

REFERENCES

1. Scanlon EF. The early diagnosis of breast cancer. *Cancer* 1981; **48**: 523–526.

2. Foote FW & Stewart FW. Comparative study of cancerous versus noncancerous breast. II. The role of so-called chronic cystic mastitis in mammary carcinogenesis. *Annals of Surgery* 1945; **121**: 197–222.

3. Page DL, Vander-Zwag R, Rogers LW *et al*. Relationship between component parts of fibrocystic disease complex and breast cancer. *Journal of the National Cancer Institute* 1978; **61**: 1055–1063.

4. Page DL & Dupont WD. Anatomic indications (histologic and cytologic) of increased breast cancer risk. *Breast Cancer Research and Treatment* 1993; **28**: 157–162.

5. Love SM, Gelman RS & Silen W. Fibrocystic 'disease' of the breast. A non disease. *New England Journal of Medicine* 1982; **307**: 1010–1014.

6. Cooper A. *Illustrations of Diseases of the Breast*. London: Longmans; 1829.

7. Reclus P. Maladie Kystique De La Mammelle. *La Semaine Medicale* 1893; **13**: 353–354.

8. Koenig P. Mastitis chronica cystica. *Centralblatt für Chirurgie* 1893; **20**: 49–53.

9. Schimmelbusch C. Das Fibroadenom der Mamma. *Archiv für Klinische Chirurgie* 1892; **64**: 102–116.

10. Cabot RC. Irritable breasts, or chronic lobular mastitis. *Boston Medical and Surgical Journal* 1900; **CXLIII**: 555–557.

11. Semb C. Pathologico-anatomical and clinical investigations of fibroadenomatosis cystica mammae. *Acta Chirurgica Scandinavica Supplementum* 1928; **64**(10): 1–484.

12. Cheatle GL & Cutler M. *Tumours of the Breast*. London: Edward Arnold, 1931.

13. Bloodgood JC. The clinical picture of dilated ducts beneath the nipple frequently to be palpated as a doughy, worm-like mass – the varicocele tumour of the breast. *Surgery, Gynecology and Obstetrics* 1923; **26**: 486–495.

14. Atkins HJB. Chronic mastitis. *Lancet* 1938; **i**: 707–712.

15. Geschickter CF. *Diseases of the Breast*, 2nd edn. Philadelphia: JB Lippincott & Co.; 1945.

16. Sandison AT. An autopsy study of the human breast. *National Cancer Institute Monograph No. 8*, US Dept Health, Education and Welfare, 1962.

17. Parks AG. The microanatomy of the breast. *Annals of the Royal College of Surgeons of England* 1959; **25**: 295–311.

18. Oberman HA & French AJ. Chronic fibrocystic disease of the breast. *Surgery, Gynecology and Obstetrics* 1961; **112**: 647–652.

19. McFarland J. Residual lactation acini in the female breasts. Their relationship to chronic cystic mastitis and malignant breasts. *Archives of Surgery* 1922; **5**: 1–64.

20. Mansel RE, Gravelle IH & Hughes LE. The interpretation of mammographic ductal enlargement in cancerous breasts. *British Journal of Surgery* 1979; **66**: 701–702.

CHAPTER 2

History of benign breast disease

Leslie E. Hughes

Introduction

The century and a half from 1800 to 1950 saw a remarkable expansion in the understanding and management of benign breast conditions. Many contributed to this expansion, but six workers have been chosen for this chapter, based on the degree of innovation and the breadth and influence of their work. Of course many others made major contributions, though of less depth and impact. Brodie and Paget of the UK, Semb of Norway, Reclus of France and Schimmelbusch and Billroth of Austro-Germany are examples.

Two other outstanding contributors of the second half of the twentieth century certainly match our chosen six, Cushman D. Haagensen, surgeon pathologist of the USA, and John Azzopardi, surgical pathologist of the UK. As their work overlaps the professional span of many of the present generation of breast specialists, they have been left to future study.

This chapter is not the history of benign conditions of the breast; this is dealt with elsewhere. It is a biographical examination of six great men, with some attempt to discern the social and professional background leading to such major contributions.

Sir Astley Paston Cooper, Bt. FRS DCL GCH. 1768–1841

Cancer of the breast has been recognized and its treatment discussed for many centuries. On the other hand, except perhaps for lactational abscess, benign conditions received little attention, and received no detailed consideration in textbooks until Astley Cooper realized their frequency and significance. The inadequate attention generally given to benign conditions is shown by Lisfranc, who as late as the 1840s was still arguing at the Academie de Medicin in Paris that all breast lumps became malignant.

Evidence that Lisfranc's view was wrong, and details of differentiation of benign from malignant, was first clearly presented by Cooper. Furthermore, he stressed the importance of the non-malignant by devoting Part 1 of his

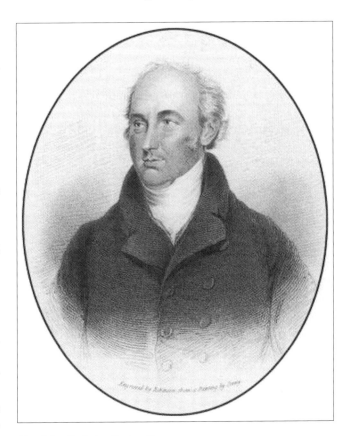

Fig. 2.1 Sir Astley Paston Cooper.

intended two-part book on breast disease to benign conditions. Thus, he presented the first monograph devoted to benign breast disorders in 1829, and this was probably the only such one until the 1980s.[1]

Early life

Astley Cooper enjoyed a good genetic inheritance; his father, a Norfolk vicar, and his mother, a descendant of Isaac Newton, both had considerable literary output, while one uncle and his grandfather were surgeons. Born in 1768, he was one of a family of 10 children, but all five sisters eventually died of tuberculosis.

Educated at home, he was a poor student, showing little interest in study and preferring to roam the countryside and get involved in wild escapades with local youths. In this regard he was remarkably similar to his teacher and guru, John Hunter, and in later life he also resembled Hunter in his passion for research and hard work. Whether these latter attributes were inherent or the result of a direct influence of Hunter, it is difficult to say.

Two incidents helped arouse his interest in surgery. First, his stepbrother was run over by a wagon and died of haemorrhage because no local doctor was willing to come to the accident scene. Second, he observed an operation for stone, performed in a masterly manner in the Norfolk and Norwich Hospital, which 'inspired me with a strong impression of the utility of surgery'.

This led to his apprenticeship at the age of 16 to his uncle, William Cooper, a senior surgeon at Guy's Hospital in London for the usual period of seven years. But Astley Cooper soon transferred his apprenticeship to Henry Cline, a young (34-years-old) surgeon at the closely linked St Thomas's Hospital, with a reputation as an excellent operator and one of the few London surgeons who appreciated John Hunter's teachings. In contrast, William Cooper said he could never understand Hunter's lectures, and usually went to sleep during them. Astley Cooper became a frequent and attentive attender.[2]

He soon exhibited Hunter's passion for acquiring personal knowledge rather than following textbooks, and for experiment and hard work, taking anatomical and pathology specimens to Cline's house for dissection, and was (like Velpeau later) quite heavily involved in the body snatching trade. He used his considerable wealth to placate the municipal worthies unhappy at this practice, as well as supporting the families of some of those imprisoned for the activity.

He soon stood out above his colleagues, and showed an early interest in breast disease from student days. A long convalescence from an attack of typhus gave an opportunity to spend a session in Edinburgh, where his brilliance was recognized and coupled with great popularity. So much did he impress in these ways that an offer was made to make him President of the Royal Medical Society should he return to Edinburgh. At this stage of his life he showed strong support for the revolutionary political developments across the channel in France, tendencies which had an adverse effect when he applied for the vacant consultant post at conservative Guy's when his uncle retired. He was appointed after he renounced all political activity.

With his apprenticeship completed, he married the daughter of a wealthy merchant, so that he never had to work to earn a living. But nevertheless, work he did with a vengeance. With a typical day he would rise at 6 a.m., dissect in his private laboratory for research and to have prepared specimens for his lecture, see non-paying patients before breakfast, then to his consulting rooms (in 1815 his professional income was an incredible £21 000). He would then proceed to Guy's for a ward round with students, seeing every interesting patient and making notes on them, to St Thomas's to lecture, teaching in the dissecting room, followed by private operations, home for dinner followed by 3 hours work in the evening. As his daily activity involved producing dissections for his anatomical lectures and selecting patients for his clinical lectures from those of all surgeons, he had access to a huge body of clinical material, and was able to observe the results of different methods of treatment by different surgeons. This, together with the detailed observation and documentation of his own patients, provided the basis for his teaching and publications.

He was an outstanding operating surgeon, a quality not enjoyed by his two senior surgeon colleagues, who would not operate unless he was available to help.

Cooper's surgical contributions, from advocating catgut 50 years before Lister, to pioneering vascular surgery, are so well known that they need no further recounting. Likewise, his success as a teacher was legendary, with his lectures and ward rounds always crowded with students.

Professional career

Cooper moved rapidly up the professional ladder, and particularly within the Royal College of Surgeons hierarchy, first as anatomy lecturer, then Hunterian Professor of Comparative Anatomy and later President for two terms. Perhaps it was in the organization of the very outmoded College that he was a breath of fresh air and made an outstanding contribution. The younger Fellows of the College were particularly frustrated by outdated attitudes; while senior Council members could enter through the front door; ordinary members had to come through a small back door. Examinations were antiquated and provincial hospitals were not recognized for training. Once elected to Council, the position was held for life.

When some younger fellows were elected to Council, they found Cooper a strong supporter. He was made chairman of a committee which was set up 'to consider the present state of the College', essentially to look at modernization of the College and he was notably successful in introducing many improvements. Placating the elderly College 'establishment' was undoubtedly associated with his popular persona, his high professional standing and his respected judgement. The younger fellows were delighted. The committee was responsible for much modernization: reforming and liberalizing the examination system, ensuring that all members were kept in touch with Council decisions and extending training to provincial hospitals.

Astley Cooper and breast disease

All Cooper's work – lectures, lecture notes and monographs – were based on personal investigation of anatomy, physiology and pathology, followed by personal observation of clinical patients and the results of his treatment. In 1825, he retired from his position as surgeon to Guy's and this gave the time and opportunity to produce his book on breast disease – Part 1 on benign conditions – in 1829 (as well as holding the presidency of the College in 1827). It is a remarkable work for its time, recognizing and giving clear description of much benign pathology and differentiating it from cancer. Likewise, it gives detailed management recommendations, some reflecting the practice of the time, others having a remarkably modern flavour, such as using a lancet to confirm the diagnosis of a simple cyst, a forerunner of the quite recent acceptance of needle aspiration as satisfactory treatment. His description of fibroadenoma and its differentiation from cancer could not be bettered: younger woman, mobile, lobulated, slow growth leading to a stationary phase and finally regression. This appreciation of the limited growth pattern with the possibility of regression

has only been brought back into prominence in the last 20 years of the twentieth century. His illustrations are remarkably accurate – that of cystic disease shows multiple blue domed cysts of varying sizes, preceding Bloodgood by almost 100 years, while his plate of a fibroadenoma shows faithfully the typical lobulation.

Unfortunately, his attention was diverted from Part 2 of his book on breast disease (dealing with carcinoma) to diseases of the testicle and thymus. When he came to take up the subject of breast disease again he realized the fundamental importance of anatomy and physiology, and produced his book *Anatomy of the Breast* in 1840 at the age of 72, dedicated charmingly as follows:

To members of the medical Profession.
I dedicate this work to you for two reasons. First. To express the delight I feel at observing your increased love for the Science of the Profession, and your earnest desire to found your Practice on an intimate knowledge of Anatomy, Physiology and Pathology. Secondly to thank you for your unmeasured kindness and attention to myself during a period of 50 years.[3]

The book contains an amazingly detailed and accurate account of every aspect of anatomy and physiology of the breast at all stages of life, including pregnancy and lactation, and in different races, together with chemical analysis of milk, and injection studies of the mammary glands of a wide variety of animals. Once again, the detail and accuracy of the text and illustrations is amazing. Regrettably, his intention to follow this with Part 2 of his work on (malignant) breast disease was frustrated by failing health and he died a year later, thus depriving surgery of what would have been a remarkable trilogy. This was obviously a disappointment to him, since following a false report in 1835 that he had died of apoplexy, he wrote to his nephew stating that he was still very much alive, that he intended to continue work for a further 13 years (taking him to 80) and then enjoy 20 years of retirement. In fact, he continued operating in spite of severe dyspnoea, so that patients had to be carried downstairs if he was to see them. He performed his last operation on Lady Jersey 2 months before he died.

It is easy to see the basis of his ability, an outstanding intellect, contact with outstanding role models – Hunter in research and Cline in clinical surgery – devotion to personal analysis and recording at experimental and clinical levels, and keeping to his motto, 'first observe and then think'.

John Hunter and Joseph Lister have always been regarded as *the* giants of surgery and rightly so. But considered analysis of Astley Cooper's contributions, experimental, clinical and professional, puts him on a similar level – certainly a charismatic prince among British surgeons, and a pre-eminent investigator of breast disease.

Alfred Velpeau. 1785–1867

Early life

Despite being brought up in a poor, rural environment, Velpeau was blessed with the forenames Alfred Armand Louis Marie. His father was a farrier, and he was expected to take up the same trade. He was given some basic education by the village priest, and became interested in medicine. He fed this interest by buying medical textbooks

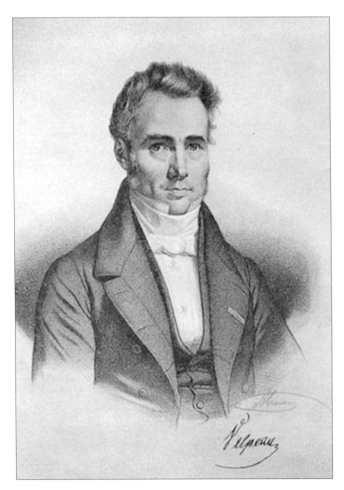

Fig. 2.2 Alfred Velpeau.

with the money accumulated from collecting and selling chestnuts. He used the knowledge gained from these books to attempt the treatment of a sad, depressed young girl with hellebore, a species of *Ranunculus* widespread in southern Europe, used in medicine for its stimulating properties but poisonous in large quantities. He succeeded only in poisoning her.

This proved a turning point in his life; the local physician called in to treat her was so impressed by his medical knowledge and obvious intelligence that he arranged for Velpeau to join in lessons with the children of a local aristocrat. In turn, the two introduced him to the surgeon at the nearby city of Tours. Thus, when Velpeau was 21 years old he came under the influence of Pierre-Fidele Bretonneau, who had recently been appointed as the Head Physician of the hospital.[4]

Bretonneau, although he moved from Paris to the provincial city of Tours, was the outstanding French physician of his time, deeply engrossed in research and study of his patients, as well as research using animals and corpses. He was more interested in these than in publicizing his achievements, which included the recognition and naming of diphtheria, (probably) the first successful tracheostomy for diphtheria and the separation of typhus and typhoid as distinct entities. Indeed, his promulgation of the 'specificity of disease', that different clinical pictures were the end result of different aetiological agents, was a revolutionary concept which was to be fulfilled by the work of Pasteur. He proved to be an outstanding physician and teacher (Trousseau was another of his pupils), and played a pivotal role in training Velpeau in medicine and pathology. Learning pathology necessitated dissection of corpses obtained by body snatching from cemeteries; Velpeau later recounted obtaining 36 necropsies in a few months. As was the case with Astley Cooper, there was some local recognition and tolerance – although Velpeau later said that he still carried lead in his body from having been fired at during these escapades.

At the age of 24 Velpeau was 'Officier de Santé' (surgeon) at the hospital, but Bretonneau was keen to see him undertake formal medical training. So a year later he travelled to Paris and through the support of Bretonneau was given a post at St Louis Hospital, where he earned a small amount teaching younger medical students. He lived under conditions of frugality almost amounting to starvation, yet obtained the anatomy and physiology prizes as well as learning Latin. After 4 years, he was able to graduate with honours, writing his thesis (on chronic and intimate fevers) in Latin under the supervision of Laennec.

Velpeau, the mature surgeon

At 33 he obtained the 'Chirurgical', higher surgical degree, and was appointed surgeon to La Pitié. At 38 he was appointed to the University Chair of Surgery at La Charité which he held for 33 years. On appointment, he wrote to Bretonneau, expressing his gratitude to his patron.

He soon had the largest consulting practice in Paris, and attracted a huge entourage of students and foreign visitors. William Osler describes in detail the experiences of Dr John Bassett, a young Alabama doctor who travelled to Europe in 1836 and spent 3 years in Velpeau's clinic.

His work covered every area of medical practice, and he produced six textbooks, on surgical anatomy, obstetrics, operative medicine, embryology, diseases of the uterus and diseases of the breast. It has been claimed that his publications covered 340 titles and 10 000 pages. Perhaps the very profuseness and breadth of his output may have had a bearing on his work in breast diseases.

At the age of 72, while still totally immersed in his work (he saw his wife, daughter and grandchildren at their country house south of Paris only at the weekend) he caught influenza but refused to lessen his activities. He died a few days after performing his last operation.

Contribution to breast diseases

There can be no doubt that Velpeau had a huge experience of breast disease, that his management commanded much respect amongst his onlookers, and that his publications came to be quoted more than most if not all others, in the literature of the next 50 years, and later in the literature of the history of breast disease. But closer examination suggests part of this may have been more the result of his flamboyance than of making major new contributions.

His book[5] consists of a very large series of case reports, more than 2000 patients treated under his care, put under individual headings and without much in the way of comprehensive classification. In this way it contrasts with the book of our next subject, Birkett. But he does report large numbers of patients, 177 patients with breast abscess for example, and described cases of fistula, both in lactating and non-lactating patients. Perhaps the lesser quality of his treatise may be the result of his wide range of interests and busy lifestyles as hinted at in the preface of his book:

The majority of the cases made use of in this work have been collected under my eyes and by my directions, rather than by me. Four or six young gentlemen have been entrusted with this work year by year; consequently more than 100 medical men have taken part in it. I ought to mention two younger pupils, Messieurs Barbereau and Roby, for the compilation of my statistical tables.

He did not lack confidence, continuing in the preface:

A treatise on diseases of the mamma did not exist in the French language and the articles of Boyer (an 11-volume treatise on surgery by this French surgeon published 40 years earlier) and A. Cooper found in our dictionaries and consecrated to this group of affections could no longer be held to supply the want. The work I now present to the public has as its object to fill up in part this deficiency. It was commenced 30 years ago. It is not the lack of materials which has influenced me (that is to delay writing this book for 30 years) no one I believe has such a mass of material on which to base his opinions. Without neglecting the opinions of my predecessors, I have occasion to remain contented with my own.

It is interesting that the book came out relatively late in his career at the age of 59, and just 4 years after that of Birkett. Could Birkett's publication have stimulated this sudden, rushed book by Velpeau? Could Velpeau have been miffed at losing precedence after this 30 years' gestation period? Some aspects of his preface suggest more than an inkling of this.

I admit that in many parts this work is but a sketch. Engagements of every kind, and the requirements of numerous duties, have prevented my consecrating to its composition all the time necessary.

He was aware of Birkett's book, quoting it a couple of times, but does not give any indication of the groundbreaking nature of the book, nor include it beside the desultory mention of Astley Cooper and Boyer in his preface.

It is clear that the translator of the English edition did not hold Velpeau in the same light as he himself or posterity; he is quite critical in the translator's preface:

It is not for me to express any opinion as to the value of this treatise, but, as a key to certain peculiarities that may strike the reader, it may be observed that M. Velpeau is a great clinical teacher, and as such he appears to exercise a licence in his writings which could pass unnoticed in the lecture theatre, although sure to attract attention in a written document. It will be seen that upon many points of importance I have considered it my duty to express dissent from the claims of priority, which, if allowed would pluck a leaf from the chaplet that adorns the illustrious dead, for the purpose of adding to the reputation, already great, of the author himself. I think the deliberate judgement of any impartial person must be that Sir A. Cooper is not open to the criticisms advanced against him, but that he is fairly entitled to the honours that have usually been accorded to him.[6]

Perhaps this relates particularly to Velpeau's claim to be the first to differentiate benign lumps from cancer: 'I seldom happen to be deceived on this point, as witnessed by many thousands of students and young medical men.' In fact, Astley Cooper had given a much clearer description many years earlier.

Velpeau and the surgical profession

It is perhaps not surprising that Velpeau lacked universal admiration from his contemporaries, and he missed the boat with some other major advances of his time. He remained strongly opposed to anaesthesia throughout his life. 'Avoiding pain is a will-of-the-wisp that is no longer pursued. We must accept that sharp instruments and pain during surgery are two things which will always be linked.'

When Paris surgeon Charles Margault, speaking on diphtheria at the Royal Academy of Medicine in 1830, stressed the importance of early tracheostomy at the time obstruction was first apparent, Velpeau opposed him on the grounds that it might subsequently prove unnecessary, even though Trousseau stated in 1835 that Velpeau had never had a survival from tracheostomy. He took a similar head-in-the-sand attitude to the high rate of wound infection and surgical deaths in Paris hospitals and, when a member of a committee in the 1860s, ruled against the use of alcohol in wounds, despite excellent results reported in relation to compound fractures.

He was equally opposed to the use of the microscope (which he regarded with disdain) in tumour diagnosis, stating that young professionals in Paris, using microscopy, failed to differentiate between two types of tumours 'as different as lipoma and hypertrophy of the tongue'.

Thus, Velpeau was an outstanding, hardworking surgeon of great intellect, but certainly not without fault, and whose lasting reputation for an authoritative contribution to the knowledge of breast disease may have been too highly regarded by posterity. Certainly his work does not show the innovative element so obvious in that of the other five surgeons discussed here.

John Birkett FRCS Fellow of the Linnean Society. 1815–1904

John Birkett, whose surgical career overlapped that of Velpeau although born 30 years earlier, comes down to us as the author of a largely forgotten book on breast disease written in the mid-nineteenth century, and before Velpeau produced a parallel book. It was remarkable, for this time, for the range of conditions covered and the detail in which they are described. In addition, his book is the first to present the varied range of benign conditions in a structured way, all of which is much in advance of his time and of his contemporaries. Yet Birkett has been largely forgotten in the context of breast disease, and also in historical works relating to the College of Surgeons, and receives no mention in Wilks and Bettany's *Biographical History of Guy's Hospital*.

Early life

Born near London in 1815, he received a very wide education at several private schools; among his masters were a Frenchman, a mathematician/astrologer and a Greek scholar. Hence it is not surprising that he moved effortlessly within European surgical societies and translated surgical works from German into English.

At the age of 16 he was apprenticed to Bransby Cooper, the nephew of Astley Cooper and also a surgeon to Guy's Hospital. Birkett was probably one of the last people to follow the tradition of paying an apprenticeship fee of £500 to his master, who expected such a fee in order to enhance his chances of an appointment as surgeon to the hospital when one became vacant. Having been elected assistant surgeon in 1849, he achieved his objective in 1853 when Bransby Cooper retired. During his student training he had attended a course in Paris, and in view of Velpeau's reputation, it seems likely he may have fallen under his influence; if so, we do not know if he was impressed or went away determined to do better!

He early took an interest in histology, and introduced the teaching of histology in Guy's Hospital in 1845. Not surprisingly, he extended this interest to histopathology, and advocated its use in diagnosing cancer at a time when

Velpeau and most other surgeons were disinterested or directly opposed to it.[7]

Birkett and breast disease

In 1848, at the age of 34, he was awarded the Jacksonian Prize of the Royal College of Surgeons for his dissertation on diseases of the mammary gland, and this was published as a monograph entitled *Diseases of the Breast and their Treatment* in 1850.[8] The appearance of his book quickly made him one of the leading authorities on breast disease in Britain. It stood out because of the quality and comprehensiveness of the material and its presentation. For the first time, the dominance of benign conditions in clinical practice, often ignored in favour of cancer, is reflected in 215 pages devoted to benign conditions, and just 42 to cancer. The novelty of these proportions is shown in the extensive bibliography he gives, of 88 publications quoted, almost all relate to cancer. None of the authors discussed in this chapter is now associated with breast disease except Cooper and Brodie.

He states in the preface: 'Opportunities on a large scale have occurred to me through the kindness of many friends and my connection with Guy's Hospital.' He clearly studied clinical aspects in detail and combined this with histological study. He is almost apologetic about the detail given: 'and if I have been rather prolix in my description of their own minute anatomy I trust that the fault may be forgiven'. This detailed personal study contrasts with Velpeau, who used many young surgeons to record his cases, and scorned the use of the microscope. In fact, it seems likely that the publication of his book irked Velpeau by its precedence since Velpeau hurriedly published his own book in 1854, stating that it had been in gestation for 30 years. Although much better known, Velpeau's book compares unfavourably with that of Birkett, who introduced a simple but logical classification which stands out in contrast to previous and contemporary publications:

1. Diseases before puberty
2. Diseases during the establishment of puberty
3. Diseases after the establishment of puberty
   A. During pregnancy, puerperium and lactation
   B. At any period or age after puberty.

Each condition is related to relevant anatomy and physiology, and an accurate clinical description provided, together with useful (if now outmoded) management.

His detailed description of duct ectasia (including museum specimens and his own observations) predates Bloodgood's varicocele tumour by half a century, while a typical mammary fistula and the treatment of fistulae by seton is described.

The plates, for example of duct ectasia and fibroadenoma, show accurate macroscopic and microscopic illustrations ahead of their time. The caption of a duct ectasia illustration is: 'Delineation of a tumour depending on a diseased condition of the ducts – containing solid material consisting of epithelium and oily matter.'

He describes breast cysts in great detail (perhaps not surprising, as one who attended Astley Cooper's lectures) and allocates remarkably prescient significance to the interstitial connective tissue extending right to surround the terminal vesicles, believing it to carry the 'nutrient' serum. Mastalgia and galactorrhea are described in accurate detail.

Birkett's surgical career

He moved up through the Royal College of Surgeons, as lecturer, Hunterian Professor of Anatomy and Pathology, member of Council, member of the Court of Examiners, Vice-President (1875–76) and President 1877.

He is recorded as being a reliable and meticulous surgeon rather than brilliant, and as a slow and uninspiring teacher. Working in pre-Listerian days, he avoided dangerous surgery, abdominal and joint surgery was abhorrent to him, although the results of his breast surgery in particular were regarded as being extremely satisfactory. His patients did well because he did not go to the anatomy room before operating; he kept his hands and his clothes clean and was meticulous in his washing and preparation of the patient both before leaving the ward and in theatre. As he retired in 1875 when aseptic surgery was still in its infancy, it is not surprising that he remained cautious of the serious complications which occurred so often with abdominal surgery.

Like all great men, he had his faults – while President of the College, he spoke out strongly against the admission of women surgeons!

Why was he so successful?

Undoubtedly he was an astute observer; he always made very detailed clinical observations and examinations, and kept meticulous notes of all his patients. His care of patients was equally meticulous, to a degree that caused his students to complain, so he was very much aware of the longer-term outcome of the treatment of the conditions he observed. He was involved in the wider advances in medicine, particularly the application of histology to surgical disease, being a founder member of, frequent contributor to and Vice-President (1860–62) of the Pathological Society of London and the Royal Medical and Surgical Society, and a frequent associate of European surgical societies, including French, German and Danish. His use of the primitive histology available at that time undoubtedly increased his understanding of breast pathology, although microscopy would be taken to a much higher level by the time of Bloodgood, and with the use of whole breast sections by Cheatle. Birkett at this time constituted a pinnacle of accurate clinical observation, analysis and hypothesis; it is unfortunate that much of his pioneering work was subsequently forgotten. In his obituary in the *Lancet*, however, it is stated that 'his success would probably have been greater had he not been of a shy and reserved disposition, totally lacking in the push and go which would have rendered conspicuous, men of far less ability'.

Despite his wide interests in surgery and medical science, he did not confine his interest to these subjects. Other interests included the Worshipful Company of Ironmongers, of which he became Master, expertise in botany and horticulture with frequent visits to Kew and the Alpine region of Switzerland and an enthusiastic walker and map reader, an aspect of his career drawing comment in all his obituaries. He often castigated his younger colleagues for being too ready to use a carriage, and until he reached his eighties, he would frequently walk from home in the West End to Guy's Hospital. He must have passed this on to his children, since two of his sons represented England in international football.

He died following a stroke in his ninetieth year. Four sons and a daughter from his 10 children survived him.

George Lenthal Cheatle. 1865–1951

George Lenthal Cheatle was born on the 13 June 1865, the son of a solicitor, and had an advantaged education typical of many London surgeons. His education at Merchant Taylor's School led on to the medical course at King's College and King's College Hospital. Again, like many London consultants, he pursued his career at the one institution, King's College and the 'old' King's College Hospital in the Strand – anatomy demonstrator,

house surgeon, surgical registrar, demonstrator in surgical pathology and assistant surgeon, this last vacancy arising on the retiral of Lord Lister in 1893 – and finally full surgeon in 1900.

His relationship to Lord Lister was close; he was Lister's last surgical registrar and assistant at Lister's last operation. Cheatle was profoundly influenced by the 'Chief', not only in regard to Lister's surgical knowledge and operative technique, but also by Lister's devotion to research and attention to the most minute of detail. This carried over with Cheatle as nothing less than an obsession. With it went other facets of Lister, his aphorisms, his dress – Cheatle continued to wear morning suit and topcoat long after most of his colleagues had given them up – and his mannerisms; he had Lister's characteristic habit of sighing deeply before answering a question.

It is not surprising that sepsis was the subject of a deep research interest, but although Cheatle was a great advocate of Lister's antiseptic methods, he was flexible in his approach, being the first surgeon at King's to move towards the use of aseptic principles.

Cheatle and breast disease

However, it was in the area of breast disease that he made his greatest contributions – from a combination of insatiable curiosity, hard work to the point of obsession and above all the application of new technology. The technique was whole-organ sections of the breast, cut by his technician on a very large microtome designed by Cheatle himself and capable of cutting sections 10 inches square. His 35-year devotion to this study led to a huge collection of sections of every type of normal breast and breast disease, from which he could readily select examples to support any point he was making.

In this way he was the first to demonstrate conclusively the continuity between Paget's disease and underlying cancer. He also argued conclusively that cells of the lesion now regarded as carcinoma in situ were not precursors of neoplasm, but were malignant cells already. 'From this point of view they are not "pre-cancerous" or "potentially carcinomatous" they are actually in a state of carcinoma.'[9]

Equally, he showed that simple hyperplasia and papillomas were benign, contrary to most views of that time. Whereas many authors equated cysts with dilated ducts, he was convinced they derived from acini. He also recognized the different types of connective tissue related to lobules and periductal tissue – very relevant to present-day understanding of breast pathology – and showed that unsuspected fibroadenomata were present in 25% of 'normal' breasts.

From his studies of serial sections of the whole breast of patients he had examined and followed up, he was able to classify clinical breast disorders in terms of pathology, and correlate pathology with clinical management. This unique work has led to his book with Cutler being described as 'the first modern textbook of mammary pathology'.[9] Perhaps the one downside to all Cheatle's work was the use of very convoluted terminology, such as 'cystipherous degenerative epithelial hyperplasia' which probably inhibited the full recognition of his contributions.

Cheatle's research was interrupted by service in the Boer War and First World War (when he held the rank of Surgeon Rear-Admiral), in both of which he served at home and in the active war front with great distinction. It was also held back by the immense amount of pathological material awaiting analysis, competing with his very onerous duties in the hospital and a very large private practice. His practice was immense; performing 10 radical mastectomies in a week was not unusual, while he put much effort into the planning of the new King's College Hospital and Medical School on Denmark Hill. Some relief came with retiral from his hospital post in 1930, at which time he was able to bring his research work to fruition. This occurred with the publication in 1931, in collaboration with his American radiotherapist colleague Max Cutler (the originator of transillumination as a diagnostic aid in breast disease) of *Tumours of the Breast. Their pathology, symptoms, diagnosis and treatment.*[10]

Cheatle vis-à-vis Bloodgood

It is interesting to see the parallels and the differences between Cheatle's and Bloodgood's work, carried out more or less contemporaneously on opposite sides of the Atlantic. Bloodgood worked in a huge, vibrant, generously funded interactive academic milieu, while Cheatle was a relative loner in terms of his research work, toiling away in a smallish institute, with meagre facilities and little academic buzz. While equally dedicated to breast pathology and disease process, Bloodgood concentrated on frozen sections of small tissue samples to give immediate confirmation or otherwise of his macroscopic diagnosis, and to provide documentary evidence to allow later analysis and correlation with long-term clinical outcome, as well as providing a balm for his itching to know the diagnosis immediately. In contrast, Cheatle

concentrated on the overall picture of the pathological process evolving in the breast, allowing him to trace continuity from normal, through noninvasive cancer cells, to frank malignancy, and also differentiate truly benign lesions from those of greater pathological significance. Yet each in his own way was able to make great contributions to the benefit of women with breast disease. Bloodgood concentrated on the wider picture from immense numbers of cases with long-term follow-up, and took his crusades to the wider medical community, and even more to the public. Cheatle concentrated on much more detailed analysis of pathological processes, and sent his message largely to the medical profession involved with breast disease, although he by no means lacked wider recognition; he received high honours from the governments of France and Italy as well as Britain and the USA.

Cheatle the teacher

Tall, slender and upright, with a winning smile, Cheatle was always popular, but most of all with his students, for he preferred discussing patients or his histological sections with small groups rather than formal lectures. There are many reminiscences of this work from his students and registrars. He had two small laboratories, one at King's and one in his Harley Street home.

He was always happy when his ward round was over, so that he could rush away to the little room in the hospital where was housed the giant microtome of his invention. There his technician would be cutting and staining sections of the whole breast removed at operation. The sections that were ready for examination would be wrapped up in a brown-paper parcel for Cheatle to take home to Harley Street, where in a little room on the first floor, he used to keep them in a state of apparent disarray. There seemed to be thousands of them littering this room, huge plates of glass, 10 inches square. It was fascinating to spend an hour or two with him there, and none would enjoy it more than Cheatle himself.[11]

He was critical of work with which he didn't agree, and took an uncompromising attitude towards his critics. When Geoffrey Keynes gave a Hunterian lecture on chronic mastitis and published the same material simultaneously in two journals, he deflected anticipated criticism with a statement: 'I am aware that at the present time it is considered in some quarters that the only satisfactory way of examining a breast is by means of large scale or "window-frame" sections of the whole gland, and the method I have used has been somewhat contemptuously designated the "cheese-tasting" method.' When one looks at the superficial nature of Keyne's work, with its multiple publications, there is little doubt as to who was contemptuous of his work, and there is no doubt that Cheatle held the high moral ground.

Cheatle's eminence culminated in a prolonged tour of the USA in 1936, lasting 2 years. One surprising feature was the granting of honorary American citizenship for 1 week, to allow him to lecture and operate at the Hines Hospital, in Chicago, an appointment normally allowed only to American citizens. This was possibly an unprecedented concession. How did it come about? Perhaps a clue comes from his book, dedicated to 'Our generous friend the Honourable Lucius Littauer'. Littauer was the son of a Jewish immigrant who joined his father's glove-making business after graduating from Harvard. (He is also reputed to have been the first ever coach in American college football history when he coached the Harvard team.) He grew the leather glove business into the largest in the USA, and became one of the great American philanthropists. Later a Republican member of Senate, he was one of the most valued and trusted personal advisers of Franklin D. Roosevelt – probably the route to Cheatle's award.

Cheatle's wife was equally welcome as she travelled with him, a tireless charity worker and an excellent speaker with a mastery of prose similar to that of her cousin, Robert Louis Stevenson; it is recorded that her 'histrionic gifts' were well known in both the UK and the USA.

Cheatle died on 2 January 1951.

Joseph Colt Bloodgood. 1867–1935

If Astley Cooper had a profound effect on the practice of the whole subject of surgery in the UK, Bloodgood was to have a profound effect in the USA on two particular aspects, the interaction of surgery with pathology (particularly the relation of benign and malignant breast conditions) and the interaction of cancer surgery with public health. Along with Cheatle, Bloodgood stands at a turning point in surgical history, because the development of microscopy meant they could combine expertise in the cellular understanding of disease and the macroscopic understanding of disease which comes from the practice of surgery.

He had outstanding mentors, first Osler then Halsted in clinical surgery and Halsted and Welch in histopathol-

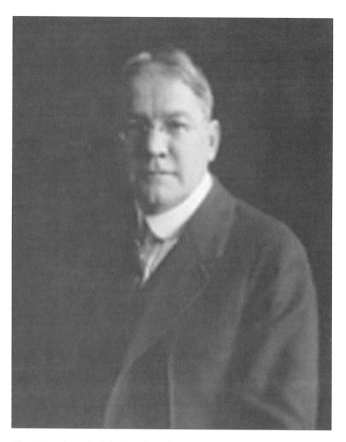

Fig. 2.3 Joseph Colt Bloodgood. (From the Alan Mason Chesney Archives of the Johns Hopkins Medical Institutions, with permission.)

ogy. Again, he was extremely hard working, and a meticulous recorder of patient detail. In addition, he was very popular with everyone, especially students, who called him 'old bloody'. Paradoxically, it is also claimed that he was well known for his lack of organization!

Early life and formative years

Joseph Colt Bloodgood was born into a distinguished Milwaukee law family in 1867, and took a science degree in histology and embryology, during which he learned to make histological sections. He took his medical degree at the University of Philadelphia and, caught in the fire of enthusiasm about the opening of the new hospital in Baltimore so richly endowed by the Quaker wholesale grocer Johns Hopkins, joined Halsted's resident staff (his fourth and youngest resident) at Johns Hopkins in 1892. Halsted was not initially very impressed with Bloodgood, and appointed him as resident only after the intervention of William Osler. Both Halsted and Bloodgood had worked with Osler, the latter when resident at the Philadelphia Children's Hospital. He obviously impressed, for after 6 months Halsted sent him on a years' tour of Europe. He visited widely, to see all the major European surgical centres, as well as centres with an interest in pathology, visiting von Recklinghausen and spending time in Vienna where Billroth was one of the great surgical pathologists. He returned home with a frozen section microtome, 'which allowed us to see the sections more quickly after the operation to satisfy our curiosity'. After moving through the residency programme he became Halsted's chief assistant in 1897 with special responsibility for organizing a Department of Surgical Pathology and the teaching of the subject. He also played a major role in collecting and collating material for Halsted's studies, who wrote: 'It affords me the greatest pleasure to express anew my obligation to Dr. Bloodgood for his efficiency and inexhaustible zeal in collating facts year after year'. His early studies included a review of Halsted's inguinal hernia cases (459) and radical mastectomies (232). Bloodgood was assisting Halsted during a particularly difficult operation when Halsted said, 'You know Bloodgood, you will never be as good a surgeon as I.' Bloodgood, visibly shaken, asked why. 'Because, dear sir,' replied Halsted, 'you do not have a Bloodgood.'[12]

Although he could be a speedy and skilful operator, operations tended to be slow and tedious, because Bloodgood would take numerous tissues for frozen section, and leave the theatre in the middle of the operation to review the prepared slides, as well as leaving an operation to take part in another operation proceeding in an adjacent theatre.

He was passionate about maintaining the highest standards in surgery, and was the first surgeon to insist that rubber gloves be worn by all members of the operating team at all operations.

Surgical pathology was initiated and practised within Departments of Surgery in most institutions at this time, academic pathologists on the whole being interested only in research based on material from autopsy studies. This practice had continued from the birth of pathology in renaissance Italy in the fifteenth century, when physicians started performing autopsies on their patients who died without obvious cause. The surgical pathology department was the first speciality initiated by Halsted within his Department of Surgery. Halsted was himself a surgical pathologist, having worked with Welch, the first Professor of Pathology at Johns Hopkins. Halsted described in detail the techniques of fixation, etcetera when making slides. He insisted all specimens should be kept complete

with orientating ligature. 'One person should be responsible for the preservation of breast material from first to last' – and it was obvious that this should be the surgeon. Shortly after Bloodgood's appointment as resident, Halsted suggested he undertake the pathological study of all tumours and other tissues removed at operation. Perhaps Halsted was influenced by Howard Kelly's adjacent Department of Gynaecology, which was prominent in gynaecological pathology and already studied all surgical specimens.

Deliberately or fortuitously, Halsted arranged for the laboratory to be set up across the hall from Welch's laboratory. Welch and Bloodgood became close friends and informally exchanged information on problem cases.

In 1906, Bloodgood became Chief Surgeon to St. Agnes Hospital, Baltimore, while maintaining his role as Clinical Professor of Surgery in charge of Surgical Pathology at Johns Hopkins.

Only at the age of 41 did Bloodgood have time to marry, Edith Holt, daughter of a publishing magnate, a perfect hostess noted for her philanthropy and charitable work, particularly on behalf of the blind.

Bloodgood died of heart disease on 2 October 1935.

Bloodgood and breast surgery

His interests gradually concentrated on breast disease (and on bone tumours).

He soon began to make good use of the massive databases he had accumulated on behalf of Halsted and in relation to his own practice, correlating clinical features with macroscopic and histological findings and long-term outcome. By 1923, he could refer to 33 000 patients with these data recorded in the surgical pathological laboratory. A detailed, systematic, correlative study on this scale was unique for that time, and hence a great advance on the much more limited contributions of Cooper, Birkett and Velpeau. One incident underlines the value of this collection of cases. When William Osler left Johns Hopkins to take up the Regius Chair of Medicine in Oxford, he was asked to write an article for Keen's 'New System of Surgery' on abdominal tumours. He wrote to his colleague C.P. Howard, in Baltimore, 'ask Bloodgood if you could not look over his list'.

In breast disease he was the first to give a credible account of the malignant potential of benign breast conditions and stress that mastectomy was not necessary in most. Before him, many surgeons regarded 'chronic cystic disease' as premalignant and hence as requiring mastectomy, particularly in young women, presumably because of their long life expectancy. In a stunning 97-page paper in the *Archives of Surgery* in 1921, he set out in great detail the clinical, macroscopic and histological features of 'chronic cystic disease', based on 350 cases personally studied in his laboratory. A majority of these had undergone mastectomy by other surgeons, so he was able to study individual benign conditions in relation to the total breast histology.[13]

He recognized the problem of borderline conditions (a term he used – and probably introduced – for lesions about which 'both the surgeon and pathologist are in doubt'), submitting 60 such lesions to a group of pathologists and showing how they were unable to agree on whether the lesions were benign or malignant.

He emphasized the benign nature of duct papilloma, something pathologists and surgeons contested for another 50 years, and gave a comprehensive account, both clinical and pathological, of duct ectasia and periductal mastitis based on 41 cases. However, he quotes no previous literature on the subject and doesn't mention Birkett's excellent clinicopathological description based on a smaller number of cases.

Whether or not he knew of Cooper's and Birkett's work, he expanded and built on their more limited clinical and pathological accounts by adding greater numbers and detailed histological correlations. So comprehensive were his clinical descriptions, for example of duct ectasia, that he was called the 'Hippocrates' of benign breast disease. One interesting feature of Bloodgood's publications on breast disease is the lack of reference to relevant work by other authors. He does not seem to mention Birkett's book anywhere, although he does cite Velpeau's book occasionally, describing him as a good macroscopic surgical pathologist but an inexperienced histologist. Perhaps he considered that his combination of macroscopic, histological and clinical data with prolonged follow-up eclipsed all previous work. In his most seminal papers, the only references given are to his own publications, and these are freely given! Perhaps this is why not everyone could resist taking a gentle 'dig' at him. Sir Lenthal Cheatle wrote in a letter to Sir Harold Stiles in Edinburgh in 1932, 'I expect Bloodgood will annex your letter, I have noticed he collects a great deal of information of which he makes no particular use.'

It is not clear whether he visited the UK during his year-long European tour of 'the surgical clinics of most of the countries in Europe', although in view of his admiration of Lister and the Edinburgh school, it is likely he would have done so. He had a penchant for descriptive names that stuck; as well as the blue domed cyst (although this had been described by Astley Cooper) and the varicocele tumour, he was the first to use the term comedo cancer for obvious reason.

He published some 80 papers on breast disease, while the index of his publications, including those in the lay press and public education pamphlets, runs to 50 pages.

Bloodgood as a surgical oncologist

The value of his papers owes much to his attention to detail. Even when his records exceeded 30 000 cases, he insisted on annual or semiannual letters to both patient and referring physician, funded by a research fund he set up in his own name.

He dictated elaborate operative notes to his secretary at St. Agnes Hospital and then telephoned equally detailed notes to Johns Hopkins. Five copies had to be made, two of which remained in the Surgical Pathology Laboratory at Johns Hopkins. Likewise, duplicates were kept of all correspondence.

Bloodgood became an excellent microscopist, and was also known as 'the doctor with a microscope'. When other surgeons had doubt as to the nature of the pathology on their slides, they always said, 'send it to Bloodgood'. He was convinced that cancer developed in abnormal tissue rather than ab initio – and thus laid the basis for diagnosis, assessment and management of hyperplasias and carcinoma in situ. Perhaps he got some of his ideas from Cheatle, who was demonstrating these concepts so clearly with his whole-organ sections.

He was an advocate of biopsy of clinical lesions before malignancy became obvious, and as a skilled microscopist he appreciated the presence of borderline lesions and the difficulties of interpretation. But his careful study of so many specimens, and prolonged follow-up, allowed him to make much progress in defining benign, premalignant and malignant processes. Thus, his insistence in his later years on biopsy before radical surgery, and diagnosing and treating premalignant lesions, and forceful advocacy to the surgical profession, was pivotal in allowing preventive surgery for many, while avoiding unnecessary mastectomies in young women.

He was the first consistent advocate of the use of frozen section routinely in surgical diagnosis, although earlier he was reluctant to rely on a frozen section diagnosis, proclaiming in 1904 'Bloodgood's Law' in relation to tumours 'the lynch law is a far better procedure than due process', implying it is better to risk an unnecessary operation than miss a malignancy. At this time he used frozen section mainly for investigation, teaching and to get a quick satisfaction of his curiosity. But his attitude was to undergo total transformation, by 1927 becoming a fervent advocate, and recommending that every surgical theatre in the country should have frozen section facilities available. He was very effective in popularizing the procedure, not only because of his surgical stature, but because of his previous opposition. His change of heart is not altogether surprising; there were many frozen section misdiagnoses in 1904, and by 1927 women were presenting earlier with less obvious lesions.

He was one of the first surgeons to see the benefit of irradiation for cancer, trying to decide whether to give it pre- or postoperatively for breast cancer.

As a surgical oncologist, Bloodgood's contribution to bone tumours, his second great interest, was also great. He was a key figure in setting up the first bone tumour registry, and made a great advance in the management of giant cell tumour of bone. His was the first scientific analysis to show giant cell tumours to be benign, and showed that they could be adequately managed by curettage. He advocated at least 6 years' follow-up to define efficacy of treatment, leading to a management programme which could be confidently recommended, and which in many ways remains unchanged today.

In 1929, Francis Garvan, a chemical industrialist, gave $60 000 to enlarge the Surgical Pathology Laboratory and train young surgical pathologists, setting up the Garvan Research Institute. In return, Bloodgood was to experiment with new chemical dyes for use in frozen section diagnosis. This institute was to provide the milieu for the next progressive step in the investigation of breast disease under Geschickter.

Bloodgood the public educator

Bloodgood believed passionately that better cancer control would come from public education. He believed his greatest contribution was his conclusion that cancer usually developed in a focus of abnormal tissue already having undergone a still noninvasive change, thus opening the possibility of detection and pre-empting frank malignant change. He took this message to the public, speaking at meetings for lay people, and advocating (often in newspapers) periodic examinations of

apparently normal individuals to detect precancerous lesions, such as of the uterine cervix. This caused great antipathy among some of his younger colleagues, who felt he was only trying to increase his private practice; they even tried unsuccessfully to have him expelled from the local medical and surgical society. Both Bloodgood and Howard Kelly (the eminent gynaecologist) received harsh treatment at Johns Hopkins in their later years, and this is now considered a very dark blemish on the otherwise outstanding record of a great medical institution.

His zealousness for communicating with the public led him to be the first physician to give radio talks on cancer prevention sponsored by the Federal Government, and led to a major role in establishing the American Society for the Prevention of Cancer.

Some of his newspaper headlines were:

Wants tax to push medical research (*NY Times* 1928)
Education saves lives (*The Democrat* 1929)
The use of tobacco may induce cancer (*NY Times* 1930)
Says people need women physicians (*NY Times* 1934)

Bloodgood the teacher

We have already seen that Bloodgood had a very great influence as an educator of the surgery and pathology worlds and the public. Equally profound was his influence on medical students and surgical residents. Bloodgood saw the problem of limited exposure for medical students to less common conditions when depending on out-patient clinic teaching, so in 1903 presented his answer in a paper to the American Surgical Association. He described his practice of giving systematic instruction in surgical diseases using museum specimens with associated pamphlets setting out the clinical and histological features relating to the specimen. He further pre-empted by a century the current 'fashion' of surgeons (and plastic surgeons in particular!) to use simultaneous projectors, but not just two projectors for Bloodgood! He would use four lantern projectors and screens to show the patient, X-ray, gross specimen and histology simultaneously. Soon he began courses of study in surgical pathology for medical students and residents, as well as outside surgeons, which he pursued until his death.

His entire team had to present themselves at his laboratory on Sunday mornings, when they would go over histories and specimens of cases being prepared for publication, with his technician cutting further frozen sections from formalin-fixed specimens to confirm the conclusions. Such sessions often lasted from 10 a.m. to 4 p.m. On Sunday evenings he would dictate publications to his secretary, reputedly while Mrs Bloodgood sat quietly by mending socks. 'One of us (a resident) had to be present with the histories and tabulations from the laboratory records.'[14]

He kept abreast of surgical literature, not only of the English-speaking world but French and German as well. This was possible because his secretary, Herman Shapiro, was fluent in both. Shapiro would collect articles from the library, shut himself with Bloodgood in the laboratory, and translate line-by-line as Bloodgood made notes. He spent every working hour in his laboratory, teaching undergraduates or postgraduates, and analysing and recording material. He scorned wasting time driving, so used his wife as a chauffeur, with his personal secretary in the back seat of the car taking notes or dictation while travelling between hospital and consulting rooms or clinic.

While in the early years he was said to be a tyrant, like most of his colleagues at Johns Hopkins including Harvey Cushing, Geschickter, who worked with him for 10 years in his later life, said, he 'never heard him utter a harsh or profane word, and certainly in later life he was exceptionally kind, hospitable and generous to a fault'.

Charles F. Geschickter. 1901– ?

Charles Freeman Geschickter holds an interesting place in the history of benign breast disease. He appears to be the first investigator to pursue large and integrated studies into the physiological basis and hormonal therapy of benign breast conditions, particularly mastodynia. His life story is of interest, too, in that he fades from a position of considerable prominence in its first half to a state of virtual oblivion in the second. A biographical sketch by his oncology colleague Dr Murray Copeland,[15] covering the first section of his life, appeared in 1959, along with many important contributions to the medical literature up to that time. Thereafter, he virtually disappears from website search engines, apart from a monograph on the kidney in 1973, and many references to a 1977 Senate enquiry into postwar covert research for the CIA.

Early life

He was born on 8 January 1901 in Washington DC of a father who had a wide variety of interests including cabinet making and the fur trade, with an entrepreneurial trait suggested by his penchant toward amateur inventions and mechanical devices. Geschickter also showed early entrepreneurial activity, partly financing his education by his own endeavours, starting with delivery of baseball scores to cigar stores at the age of 10. Raising money was something he did throughout his life, for the Geschickter Foundation was a successful private charitable fund set up to support his work at the Georgetown University and was still in existence in the 1970s.

His achievements in early adult life already marked him out as a person of exceptional ability. He worked as an engineer while at college, but moved to postgraduate study in educational psychology, a field in which he was very successful, being awarded MA and MS degrees. This lead to a scholarship in the subject in a prestigious unit at Columbia University. Although after this he was diverted into medicine, psychology was presumably an influence carried on into later life in his CIA connections.

His move to medicine came via an interest in zoology, and a special letter of recommendation from the Professor of Zoology at George Washington University led to his later admission as an extra student to an already full class at Johns Hopkins in 1923. Here Bloodgood noted Geschickter's enthusiasm and analytical mind during the surgical pathology element in the third year of the medical course. He invited Geschickter to work on multiple myeloma, fitting in with Bloodgood's second major interest – bone tumours. Geschickter in turn invited a classmate, Murray Copeland, to work with him. Later they were to cooperate extensively in the Departments of Pathology and Oncology at Georgetown University. They were obviously a powerful team, for this led to their widely acclaimed book on tumours of bone published in 1931.

After internship, Bloodgood invited both to return to work in his surgical pathology laboratory studying bone tumours, where Dean Lewis, head of surgery at Johns Hopkins, was also impressed by them and arranged surgical fellowships for both at the Mayo Clinic in 1929.

After only a few months at the Mayo, Bloodgood sent an urgent call to Geschickter to come back and work in the recently created Garvan Cancer Research Laboratory, to which he acceded. He was first sent to Europe, where he visited many of the leading pathology centres including Warburg's biochemistry unit in Berlin. Henceforward, his interest would lie more in pathology and basic cancer research than surgery, yet his publications show that he retained an active interest in clinical problems, both medical and surgical. Thus, he became a pathologist with a clinician element grafted on, contrasting with Bloodgood, a clinical surgeon with a pathology element grafted on.

Contributions to breast disease

When Bloodgood died in 1935, Geschickter took over the running of the Garvan laboratory, where he had access to all the past data on breast disease, and was also pathologist to St. Agnes Hospital, Baltimore. From his publications, he must have continued to see patients to a degree which must have been exceptional for a pathologist, as well as carrying out pioneering research into hormone therapy and the hormonal basis of breast disease. This led to a seminal text on breast disease.[16] Although a single-author work (apart from a chapter on surgery for cancer by Copeland) he does not hesitate to give a full discussion of clinical management, much apparently from personal experience.

The following appears in the preface to the first edition:

> *In addition to the patients seen in practice and in the surgical wards of Dr. Dean Lewis at the Johns Hopkins Hospital, a study has been made of the cases histories, specimens and follow-up studies recorded in the surgical pathological laboratory of Johns Hopkins. This library of data to which Dr. Bloodgood and his predecessors, Halsted and Welch, so largely contributed, has been analysed and presented in tabular form.*

It is a landmark publication, much the most comprehensive book on breast disease up to that time. Half (400 pages) is devoted to benign conditions, including 100 pages on anatomy and endocrine physiology, and half to cancer, including 100 pages of experimental studies. It is equally unique in its follow-up data, much more comprehensive than others of this time. He later reports (together with Murray Copeland) follow-up of at least 5 years of 310 patients with mastodynia, the first comprehensive study of this symptom, and 445 patients with cystic disease. (It contrasts with contemporaneous books, such as that published by Fitzwilliam in London only 20 years earlier. Although 270 of 430 pages in this book deal with benign conditions, it is basically a collection of anecdotal case reports.) On the other hand, Geschickter's book does not rival Cheatle's with its detailed histological study of the genesis of breast neoplasia. Geschickter was more of

an endocrine and biochemical investigator, reflected in his studies of oestrogen, testosterone, prolactin and progesterone in relation to breast physiology and benign and malignant disease. We have little indication of his clinical practice. He must have seen many patients with breast disease through the Garvan Institute, drawn perhaps from the Department of Surgery. It is also recorded that he saw many patients, mainly with cancer and 'unusual conditions', in his private rooms. It is not clear whether he performed surgery, but probably not as he did not complete his surgical training.

Life after Johns Hopkins

After a period of service during the Second World War as Head of Pathology at the Bethesda Naval Hospital, he was appointed in 1946 to the Chair of Pathology at Georgetown University, and Director of The Clinical Research Unit, allowing further patient interaction. In the early years at Georgetown, he was again noted for new ideas, including being the first to use EDTA in clinical medicine. The chemical had been patented in Germany in 1935 as a means of removing calcium in the textile industry, but its possible clinical value was not capitalized upon until Geschickter and Rubin did so. He was also a popular teacher; in his pen portrait in 1959, Copeland wrote, 'Dr. Geschickter's witticisms, clarity of expression, provocative ideas and wealth of information hold students in rapt attention and make him popular with the student body.'[15]

A remarkable aspect of the post-1950 period is the apparent disappearance of Geschickter from professional life, at least as recorded in the medical press, and in marked contrast to his prolific period at the Garvan Institute. In the same 1959 pen portrait, Copeland refers to him as 'quietly working on a new book on pathology, shortly to be published'. As far as the author can determine, this publication did not eventuate.

In the 1970s, a Senate investigation into CIA activities in the postwar period was carried out, looking particularly at covert research into defensive measures against drugs and techniques used in interrogation and brainwashing. The CIA provided funding towards financing a research building at Georgetown Medical Center channelled through Geschickter's private foundation. In return, they were to receive access to human patients and volunteers for experimental studies, particularly using radioisotope techniques with which Geschickter was a recognized authority. Though there are a number of reports of both animal and human experiments relating to these funds detailed in various publications, Georgetown University claimed to have no knowledge of these activities.[17]

The findings of the Senate investigation were given extensive coverage in the New York and Washington press, and perhaps explain the low (or absent) profile of Geschickter in the later decades of his life. This blackout extends even to the apparent absence of a death or funeral notice in the Washington press, although he was still alive at the time of his wife's funeral notice in 1979. The only picture of his later professional life seems to come from comments of some colleagues in the newspaper reports of his CIA activities in 1977. They describe him as very bright, very generous and responsible, while also being quiet, reserved and keeping pretty much to himself. He is recorded as running a private clinic in which he saw 'many very grateful patients, mainly with cancer and unusual conditions, managed with unusual treatments'.

It is unfortunate that one so obviously gifted should have had his academic contributions apparently curtailed in this way. It is possible that he was diverted along lines which interested the CIA by his early productive studies in educational psychology, to which they would seem to be more closely related than to surgery or pathology. It is regrettable that a curtain seems to have been drawn over his career at Georgetown University, with enquiries from a number of the usual biographical sources proving unproductive.

Geschickter benefited from having an outstanding mentor in Bloodgood, and from his expertise and innate entrepreneurial abilities being recognized at different stages of his career by people as widely different as a zoologist, a psychologist and surgeons, all added to a keen mind and investigative entrepreneurial ability. This led to the exploitation of evolving physiological and biochemical investigative techniques and consequent therapeutic studies which constituted a sea-change in direction from the clinicopathological studies of his predecessors into benign breast disorders.

An analysis of the contributions of these six men

These men were all obviously highly intelligent and talented. Are there other similarities between the six men which might indicate how and why they came to make such significant contributions? It is easy to identify some features common to most if not all.

Mentors

Each of the six had outstanding mentors who were themselves innovators, devoted and even addicted to research (Fig. 2.4). Hunter and Lister were legendary as fathers of surgical research; Bretonneau stood out for his epidemiological and animal and cadaver studies. Astley Cooper dissected throughout his life. Halsted was a constant researcher, performing 90 experiments on 68 dogs in a single study to determine the effectiveness of gradual arterial occlusion proximal to an aneurysm.

With the possible exception of Birkett, the master–pupil interaction was early, close and profound. They passed on this personal and intense commitment to research to their pupils to varying degrees; with Astley Cooper (anatomy and physiology), Cheatle (histopathology), Bloodgood (records and follow-up) and Geschickter (endocrine and biochemistry) research was a passion.

Mentors sometimes had wider influences: Bloodgood could not find time to marry until he was 41, Halsted married at 38, Osler at 43, and Welch remained a bachelor until he died at 85.

Record keeping and hard work

All were notable for detailed clinical study and personal meticulous note keeping of their patients' condition and outcome. This was the dominant basis of Birkett's and Bloodgood's contributions; only Velpeau delegated this to many young surgeons working with him. All men worked extremely hard and for long hours. When one considers their busy clinical practices, demanding teaching commitments, time taken by slow transport (or walking!) it is surprising how much was achieved in taking knowledge forward. It is clear that they devoted long hours to their profession; Astley Cooper's daily routine (in winter as well as summer) extended from 6 a.m. to 10 p.m., while Bloodgood had his wife drive him between hospitals so he could dictate to his secretary during the journey.

Acceptance of new technology

Birkett embraced microscopy from its earliest times. John Hughes Bennett, the Scottish histologist and physician, published his important ground-breaking article on a comparison of benign and malignant cells in cytological scrapings only in 1845;[18] Birkett started teaching histology in 1846. Bloodgood was early in the use of frozen

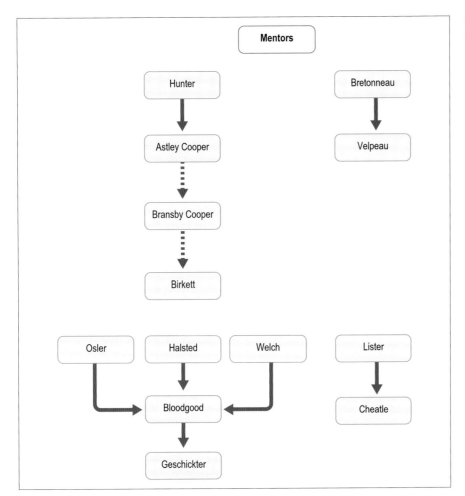

Fig. 2.4 The influence of mentors on professional achievement.

section, seen on his European trip, as an adjunct to macroscopic diagnosis, and later came round to insist on its use as essential to the diagnosis of cancer. He also seized on the role of the developing media in promulgating knowledge to the wider public. Cheatle took histology further by building his own sledge microtome to study whole-organ sections. Geschickter embraced advances in biochemistry and endocrinology to open up new aspects of breast disease. Velpeau was an odd-man-out, campaigning against a number of crucial developments, including the use of microscopy and anaesthesia, throughout his career.

Dedication to pathology

Perhaps their dedication to pathology and fascination with disease process, in addition to the straightforward clinical work practised by their colleagues, was related to the absence at that time of pure pathologists with interest

in surgery, so they were coming afresh to new fields. The first paper on breast disease by a nonsurgical pathologist only appeared in 1911, from William McCarthy, from the Mayo Clinic,[19] while Cheatle and Cutler's book, described as the *first* textbook of surgical pathology, was the work of two practising clinicians. Prior to the nineteenth century, academic pathologists had little interest in the operating theatre, and so it was left to surgical departments to develop the discipline of surgical pathology, notably Bloodgood at the Johns Hopkins, and Warren at the Massachusetts General. The lack of knowledge of the pathology of surgical conditions, the need for accurate diagnosis, and the development of new technology must have acted as a stimulus to surgeons to take up the technology.

International travel and contacts

The mentors of Bloodgood and Geschickter sent them on trips around Europe at an early stage of their career, so that they were able to see the latest developments in European centres. (Welch, Halsted and Osler had already done so.) These international links were maintained, so that they remained in contact with new developments. Their subsequent careers show that this travel at an early stage had a profound effect on their later work.

Birkett (and Bloodgood's secretary) were familiar with European languages, and Cheatle maintained strong links with European and American surgery. Such contacts would not be remarkable today, and were not exceptional then, but they would have required much more effort without modern means of communication.

While such attributes would be seen in the work of many of their contemporaries, it is clear from studying their lives that they far excelled most of their colleagues in these ways. In particular, the progression from clinical recording to macroscopic and then increasingly sophisticated microscopic pathology, with systematic and disciplined record keeping, was undoubtedly responsible for much of the progress made. These techniques brought understanding of breast surgery to a peak in the 1950s, which has only since been advanced by small increments. There is no doubt that the recent advances of molecular biology are throwing completely new light on the subject, but whether it will remain possible for individual workers to combine all these attributes remains to be seen. Five of our 'giants' were primarily surgeons, *surgeon* pathologists, Geschickter provided the link to *surgical* pathologists by progressing from his early surgical interest to a full-time pathologist still within a surgical department, and finally into a pathology department with a biochemical flavour, albeit still with a clinical interest.

It remains to be seen whether there will be further evolution into surgeon–pathologist–molecular biologist without losing the unique insights provided by extensive clinical surgical experience. Such an unlikely combination, should it occur, would be likely to lead to contributions to match any of the above.

REFERENCES

1. Cooper A. *Illustrations of Diseases of the Breast.* Part I. London. Longman, Rees, Orme, Brown and Green; 1829.
2. Brock RC. *The Life and Work of Astley Cooper.* Edinburgh: Livingstone; 1952.
3. Cooper A. *On the Anatomy of the Breast.* London: Longman, Orme, Green, Brown and Longman; 1940.
4. Dunn PM. Dr Alfred Velpeau of Tours: the umbilical cord and birth asphyxia. *Archives of Diseases of Childhood, Foetal Neonatal Edition* 2005; **90:** F184–186.
5. Velpeau AALM. Maladies du Sein. Paris; Masson: 1854.
6. Velpeau AA. *A Treatise on Cancer of the Breast and Mammary Region.* London: Henry Renshaw; 1856 (English translation).
7. Obituary. *Lancet* 1904; **ii:** 182–184.
8. Birkett J. *The Diseases of the Breast and Their Treatment.* London: Longman, Brown, Green and Longman; 1850.
9. Koerner FC. A brief historical perspective on the pathology of the breast: from Cheatle to Azzopardi and beyond. *Seminars in Diagnostic Pathology* 2004; **21:** 3–9.
10. Cheatle GL, Cutler M. *Tumours of the Breast. Their Pathology, Diagnosis and Treatment.* London: Edward Arnold; 1931.
11. Obituary. *Lancet* 1951; **i:** 115–116.
12. Marmon LM, Mandal A, Goodman D *et al.* The life of Joseph Colt Bloodgood MD. *Public Surgeon Surg Gynec Obstet* 1993; **177:** 193–200.
13. Bloodgood JC. The pathology of chronic cystic mastitis of the female breast. *Archives of Surgery* 1921; **3:** 445–542.
14. Geschickter CF. Joseph Colt Bloodgood. Biographic sketch. *Clinical Orthopaedics and Related Research* 1956; **7:** 3–8.
15. Copeland MM. Charles F Geschickter. *The Bulletin – Georgetown University Medical Center* 1959; **XII:** 163–165.
16. Geschickter CF. *Diseases of the Breast, Diagnosis, Pathology and Treatment.* 2nd edn. Philadelphia: JB Lippincott; 1945.
17. *The Washington Post.* 3 August 1977 and 7 August 1977.
18. Bennett JH. Introductory address to a course of lectures on histology and the use of the microscope. *Lancet* 1845; **i:** 517–522.
19. Rosai J (ed.). *Guiding the Surgeon's Hand. The History of American Surgical Pathology.* Washington: American Registry of Pathology; 1997.

Breast anatomy and physiology

Development

The prepubertal breast is identical in both sexes and consists of a number of small ducts embedded in a collagenous stroma. The ducts develop in utero from an ectodermal mammary ridge which invades the epidermis at the seventh embryonic week and progresses to a budding stage at the twelfth week. The classical view has been that the mammary ridge extends from the base of the upper limb bud to the base of the lower limb bud (Fig. 3.1).

This view arose from theories derived from comparative anatomy, and is not supported by studies of human embryos, which show that the mammary ridge extends only over the axillopectoral area. (Pathology in the groin mimicking mammary disease mostly arises from mammary-like anogenital glands (MLG), which are normal constituents of the vulva and perianal region.

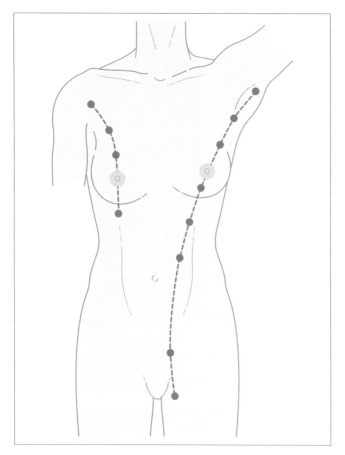

Fig. 3.1 The classical (patient's left side) and modern views of the extent of the fetal mammary ridge. It is now accepted that the ridge does not normally extend as far as the abdomen in the human (right side). Hence in practical terms accessory nipples or breasts are found only along the proximal half of this line (see Ch. 15).

They are considered to be related to eccrine and apocrine glands, and to be the source of mammary-like pathology in this region, such as lactating glands, fibroadenoma, extramammary Paget's disease, etc.[1])

Already by the 12-mm stage the mammary ridge is shortening and migrating dorsoventrally, so by the 14-mm stage it is found only as an elevated nipple primordium on the ventral wall of the thorax.[2] The epithelial bud then branches and canalizes between weeks 13 and 20 to form the 5–9 major ducts found in the adult breast.[3] The major ducts at this stage only have small vesicles at the distal ends and no lobular development is visible. The increasing development of the fetal breast parenchyma induces considerable growth and specialization of the surrounding stroma. A comprehensive three-layer vascular network forms at the 9–10-week budding stage and eventually produces a cylindrical vascular envelope around each of the major ducts.[4] From the tenth week in utero to birth a series of developments occur. Ingrowth of connective tissue gives rise to partitions between each of the end vesicles (primitive alveoli) and acts as a framework for the adult segmental pattern. Specialized fat cells also invade the matrices between the blood vessels and fibrous septae. Externally the nipple is small and flattened, although rudimentary sebaceous glands and Montgomery's tubercles are present. The circular interlacing smooth muscle fibres that give the nipple its erectile properties are already developed at this stage.

All the above changes are completed by the time of birth. At this time, transient secretory changes occur in the newborn breast which give rise to the clinical entities of 'witches' milk' or 'neonatal mastitis'. In late pregnancy the high levels of luteal and placental hormones in the mother's blood cross the placenta into the fetal circulation and cause stimulation of the fetal breast. This primes the primitive fetal end vesicles for milk production in an analogous fashion to the adult female breast in late pregnancy. Birth inevitably causes separation of the maternal and fetal circulations, resulting in a rapid fall in circulating sex steroids in the baby's blood, whereas prolactin secretion is maintained by the baby's pituitary. These conditions correspond once more to the maternal situation and result in secretion of colostrum which can be expressed from the nipple in 80–90% of newborn breasts of either sex. The newborn prolactin levels then decline and the secretion dries up over the next few weeks. Thus, the secretion of colostrum and the swelling of the newborn breast are both normal physiological events and should not be considered as due to disease unless they become persistent.

Detailed histological information has been given about the state of the breast during this neonatal period and the first 2 years of life.[5] The pattern is identical in males and females. Three morphological degrees of development are seen, varying from minimal blunt budding to fully developed lobules equivalent to the type 1 virginal lobule described in the adult by Russo and Russo (see below). Five functional stages are described which are seen as a continuum, proliferation proceeding to active secretory epithelium followed by apocrine metaplasia, formation of microcysts and involution. Embryonic fat is sometimes seen as well-defined islands surrounded by fibrous tissue. The morphology of the myoepithelial cells varies, apparently in tandem with the functional activity of the underlying epithelial cells. The intralobular stroma also shows changes, being very loose and vascular during the secretory stage, and more dense, less cellular and vascular during the involutional stage. All these changes are remarkably similar to those seen during adult reproductive life.

Changes at puberty

The next steps in development are activated at puberty in the female and follow the well-ordered sequence described by Marshall and Tanner[6] and Zacharias et al.[7] (Fig. 3.2).

The first change (at about the age of 10 years) is growth of the mammary tissue beneath the areola with enlargement of the areolar area producing the characteristic swelling known as the breast bud or mound. This development is often asymmetrical. At 12 years the nipple begins to grow outwards and the breast elevation increases, but there is no distinct separation between nipple and areola. Between the ages of 14 and 15, increasing subareolar growth leads to elevation of the areola above the breast outline giving the 'secondary mound'. The familiar shape of the adult resting breast is then attained by a recession in the level of the areola to that of the surrounding breast, leaving the nipple projecting.

The exact physiological mechanisms that trigger and control the changes of puberty are not fully understood but the primary event in the initiation of puberty is the increasing secretion of follicle-stimulating hormone (FSH) and luteinizing hormone (LH) from the anterior pituitary in response to increasing stimulation by the hypothalamus. Detectable levels of FSH and LH are found

in prepubertal children showing that some hypothalamic activity is present even in young children. As maturation proceeds, this hypothalamic activity increases progressively between the ages of 8 and 18, and during these years sexual development can be shown to correlate with plasma oestradiol levels. This is probably due to a change in frequency of the pulsatile secretion of the gonadotrophin-releasing factors.[8] The increased FSH/LH causes activation of primordial ovarian follicles and secretion of oestrogen which is responsible for the first stages of breast development. Oestrogen, predominant during the anovulatory cycles typical of the first years, induces duct sprouting and branching but lobular development at this stage consists only of small buds. Adult levels of progesterone are required for further development of the lobular component at puberty as well as during the menstrual cycle and pregnancy.[9] Oestrogen also induces connective tissue and vascular growth which is required for the support of the new ducts; the connective tissue in turn stimulates fat deposition. When ovulating cycles begin, luteal function improves, and the increased output of progesterone balances the oestrogen and results in differentiation of the terminal ductular buds to produce adult lobules. These differential growth patterns associated with the two major ovarian steroids have been studied principally in animals,[10,11] but appear to be true also for the human. While it is generally accepted that progesterone is important for lobuloalveolar development at puberty, during menstrual cyclical changes and during pregnancy, details of the underlying mechanisms remain unclear. It is still uncertain whether the action on cell proliferation is direct via progesterone receptor, or by some other progesterone-related factor. Insulin, growth hormone, corticosteroids and prolactin are also required for optimal growth of the breast but only play minor roles.

Adult anatomy

The adult female breasts lie on each side of the anterior thorax with their bases extending from about the second to the sixth ribs. Medially, the breasts reach the sternal edge and laterally the midaxillary line and extend up into the axilla via a pyramidal-shaped axillary tail (Fig. 3.3). In the midclavicular line the breast extends from the second to the sixth rib.

The breast lies on a substantial layer of fascia overlying the pectoralis major muscle superomedially, the serratus anterior muscle in the lower outer one-third, and the

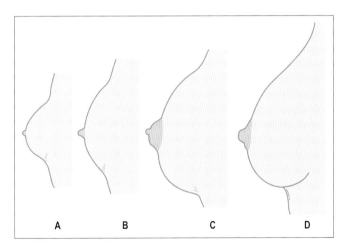

Fig. 3.2 The stages of breast development at puberty.
(**A**) Breast bud elevation; (**B**) growth and protrusion of the nipple; (**C**) elevation of the secondary areolar mound; (**D**) regression of the areolar mound to the level of the general breast contour.

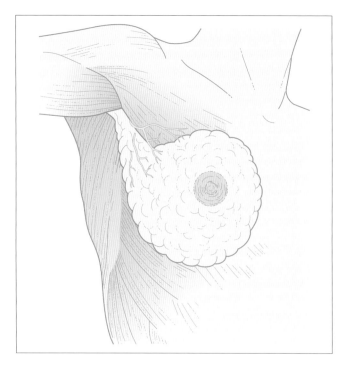

Fig. 3.3 The gross anatomy of the breast. The upper two-thirds lie on the pectoralis major and the lower one-third on the serratus anterior. Note the prolongation of the upper outer quadrant into the axilla. Breast tissue extends much more widely than shown here in a significant minority of women.

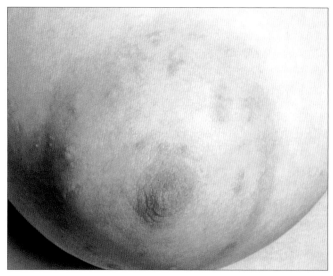

Fig. 3.4 The normal nipple and areola. The pinker areolar skin is clearly demarcated from the surrounding breast skin and shows several small nodules which mark the openings of Montgomery's tubercles.

anterior rectus sheath in the lower medial area. Duct injection under pressure to distend terminal ductules shows that duct-containing breast tissue often extends more widely than this – to the midline, and well up into the axilla.[12] Breast tissue extends below the costal margin in 15% of cases, and beyond the anterior border of latissimus dorsi in 2%. Ductal elements also extend very close to the skin. This wide extension explains the difficulty of removing all breast tissue by subcutaneous mastectomy and is important for matching the contralateral breasts in cosmetic and reconstructive surgery. Considerable asymmetry is frequently found among normal women, and the patient may not be aware of it, or may accept it as a normal variant. One half of women have a volume difference of 10% between left and right breasts, and a quarter have a 20% difference.[13] The left breast is usually the larger.

Westreich[14] has reviewed the anthropomorphic measurements of the 'aesthetically perfect' breast, important in assessing the need for and results of reconstructive and cosmetic surgery. This paper provides a simple protocol for measurement of the breast and its landmarks in relation to fixed skeletal points. The precise position of the nipple areolar complex varies widely with the fat content of the breast and the age of the woman. In the nulliparous breast, it lies between 19 and 21 cm from the suprasternal notch measured diagonally.

The amount of fat within the breast varies widely, as would be expected. The intimacy with which it is mixed with glandular tissue also varies, and is important in relation to the use of liposuction as an adjuvant to reduction mammoplasty. The question has been studied quantitatively in material removed during reduction procedures.[15] The proportion of the breast mass constituted by fat varied from 2% to 78%, with a mean in this group of patients of 48%. Breast fat increases with age, body mass and total breast volume, but this is not absolute; fat can predominate over glandular tissue in young women as well. The amount of fatty tissue in the breast is well imaged by magnetic resonance imaging (MRI).[16]

The nipple extends about 5–10 mm above the level of the areolar skin and is covered with rugose skin which is variably pigmented (Fig. 3.4). Microscopic examination shows that the nipple is composed of the terminal ducts with a supporting stroma of smooth muscle that are mainly arranged in a circular fashion (Sappey's muscle) while a few are arranged radially (Myerholtz muscle). Contraction of the circular muscle causes nipple projection; contraction of the radial fibres causes retraction.

The surface of the areola shows a number of small protuberances. These are the openings of modified large sebaceous glands called Montgomery's glands, which lubricate the areolar skin during suckling. Montgomery originally described his tubercle as a combined sebaceous unit and mammary lactiferous gland, and this has been confirmed by Smith et al.[17] The sebaceous gland produces the palpable lump. The lactiferous duct opens into the sebaceous duct close to the areola, or occasionally directly onto the areola alongside. The lactiferous gland lies deeper in the breast, can produce milk and is subject to the development of typical breast pathology (see Fig. 12.11).

Apocrine sweat glands occur in the nipple and areola, but are not reported elsewhere in the skin of the breast. This is surprising, since hidradenitis suppurativa is rare in the areolar region (contrary to early reports which apparently confused periareolar fistula with hidradenitis) but not uncommonly affects peripheral skin of the breast, especially in the submammary region. This confusion is compounded by the imperfect correlation of hidradenitis with apocrine glands.

The adult ductolobar system

The breast consists of lobes separated from each other by fascial envelopes – usually stated to be 15–20 in number, but in reality, more of the order of 7–8. The higher number comes from looking at transverse sections of the nipple, but is in conflict with the clinical experience that excision of a ductolobar unit appears to remove far more than one-twentieth of the breast. The reason for the difference is largely explained by two papers. Koenecke[18] in 1934 examined in detail the breast of a woman who died after childbirth. He showed that about half the ducts radiating from the nipple (and seen histologically in cross-section) are rudimentary, and do not drain a functional lobe. They extend only to 3–4 branchings, and do not form lobular structures. Koenecke believed that 95% of breast function is provided by about seven fully developed duct systems. Moffatt and Going[19] used computer modelling software to reconstruct a three-dimensional model of the breast of a young woman from 2-mm slices examined in detail. The amount of work involved was such that only 10 duct territories, those in the centre of the breast, were covered. They showed that each duct drains its own territory, but the territories vary greatly in extent and shape; the volume of individual lobes varied by a factor of 20–30 times. Interlocked like a three-dimensional jigsaw, the transverse sectional outline of individual lobes was also variable, convex, concavo-convex, flattened or biconcave. Most lobes do not conform to the pear-shaped structure usually illustrated in operative diagrams of segmental excisions. The shapes suggest contact inhibition between adjacent ducts as they develop their individual territories. Some lobes have a long duct before branching, so that they have a deep territory close to the pectoral fascia, others branch very early, or have a series of lobules leaving the duct by short extralobular ducts. Love and Barsky[3] have confirmed these findings using several different methods to assess the nipple ducts.

Each lobe is drained by a ductal system from which a lactiferous sinus (5–8 mm in diameter when distended) opens on the nipple, and each lactiferous sinus receives a lobar duct 2 mm or less in diameter. Within the lobe are up to 40 (or more) lobules, the 'definitive' anatomical and functional entity. A lobule is 2–3 mm in diameter and may be visible to the naked eye. Each lobule contains 10–100 alveoli (or acini), the basic secretory unit. Some prefer to reserve the terms alveolus or acinus for the pregnant/lactating breast only, using the term ductule or ductulo-tubule for the non-pregnant state.

The lobar structure based on an individual duct system is more important than previously recognized, since it is the anatomic–pathological entity requiring excision of some multifocal papillary conditions, particularly in the elderly, and possibly the important macroentity (in contrast to the microentity of the terminal ductal lobular unit [TDLU]) in some cases of ductal carcinoma in situ (DCIS).

Vascular anatomy

The blood supply is from the axillary artery via its thoracoacromial, lateral thoracic and subscapular arteries, and from the subclavian artery via the internal thoracic (mammary) artery. The internal thoracic artery supplies three large anterior perforating branches through the second, third and fourth intercostal spaces. Perforating branches from the anterior intercostal arteries also come through these spaces more laterally. The veins form a rich subareolar plexus and drain to the intercostal and axillary veins and to the internal thoracic veins.

The detailed vascular anatomy of the breast[20] is important in more extensive procedures for benign conditions, particularly in relation to avoiding nipple and areolar necrosis.

Lymphatics of the breast

The lymphatic drainage of the breast is of great importance in the spread of malignant disease of the breast but of lesser importance in benign breast disease. Several lymphatic plexi issue from the parenchymal portion of the breast and the subareolar region and drain to the regional lymph nodes, the majority of which lie within the axilla. Most of the lymph from each breast passes into the ipsilateral axillary nodes along a chain which begins at the anterior axillary (pectoral) nodes and continues into the central axillary and apical node groups. Further drainage occurs into the subscapular and interpectoral node groups. A small amount of lymph drains across to the opposite breast and also downwards into the rectus sheath. Some of the medial part of the breast is drained by lymphatics which accompany the perforating internal thoracic vessels and drain into the internal thoracic group of nodes in the thorax and on into the mediastinal nodes. The older accounts of breast lymphatics derived from dissection studies have been clarified. Our understanding of the lymphatic drainage has been modified by the experience of sentinel node biopsy.[21]

Nerve supply

The innervation of the breast is principally by somatic sensory nerves and autonomic nerves accompanying the blood vessels. In general, the areola and nipple are richly supplied by somatic sensory nerves while the breast parenchyma is mostly supplied by autonomic supply which appears to be solely sympathetic. No parasympathetic activity has been demonstrated in the breast.[22] Detailed histological examination has failed to show any direct neural end-terminal connections with breast ductular cells or myoepithelial cells, suggesting that the principal control mechanisms of secretion and milk ejection are humoral rather than nervous mechanisms. It is interesting that the areolar epidermis is relatively poorly innervated whereas the nipple and lactiferous ducts are richly innervated; these findings are supported by the clinical findings of poor appreciation of light touch and two-point discrimination over the areola. The rich nipple innervation is thought to be the basis of the well-known suckling reflex whereby a neural afferent pathway causes rapid release of both adenohypophyseal prolactin and neurohypophyseal oxytocin on suckling.

The somatic sensory nerve supply is via the supraclavicular nerves (C3, C4) superiorly and laterally from the lateral branches of the thoracic intercostal nerves (third to fourth). The medial aspects of the breast receive supply from the anterior branches of the thoracic intercostal nerves which penetrate the pectoralis major to reach the breast skin. A major supply of the upper outer quadrant of the breast is via the intercostobrachial nerve (C8, T1) which gives a large branch to the breast as it traverses the axilla.

The detailed nerve supply to the nipple is important in operations in this region, and has been reinvestigated.[23,24] The subareolar nerve plexus receives branches on the lateral side from the third to the fifth intercostal nerves, and on the medial side from the second to the fifth intercostal nerves. This supply is quite variable, and may differ on the two sides of the same patient, but the majority supply comes from the third and fourth nerves.

Fascia of the breast

The fascial framework of the breast is important in relation to clinical manifestations of disease and surgical technique. Because the breast develops as a skin appendage, it does so within the superficial fascia, such that the superficial part of the superficial fascia forms an anterior boundary and the deep layer of the superficial fascia forms a posterior boundary. In between, condensation of this interlobar fascia gives rise to the pyramidal-shaped ligaments of Cooper, called suspensory ligaments because they provide a supporting framework to the breast lobes. They are best developed in the upper part of the breast and are connected to both pectoral fascia and skin by fibrous extensions. In spite of these fibrous extensions, the superficial layer of superficial fascia gives a plane of dissection between the skin and breast. (The small subcutaneous fat lobules are readily differentiated from the much larger mammary fat lobules.) Likewise, the retromammary space provides a ready plane of dissection between the deep layer of superficial fascia and the deep fascia of pectoralis major and serratus anterior. This structural fascial support is so intimately connected to interlobular and intralobular fascia with their enclosed ductal units, that no ready plane of dissection exists within the breast substance and all surgery must be carried out by sharp dissection. The skin overlying the breast has been shown to vary in thickness from 0.8 mm to 3 mm on mammograms of normal breasts and tends to decrease with increasing breast size.[25]

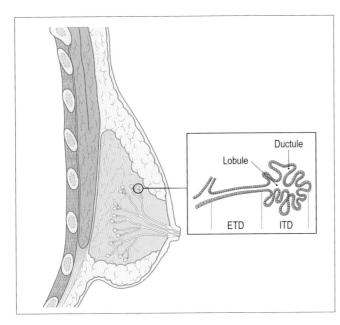

Fig. 3.5 Cross-section of the breast to show the ductal and lobuloalveolar structure. The expanded diagram shows the schematic structure of the TDLU. ETD, extralobular terminal ductule; ITD, intralobular terminal ductule.

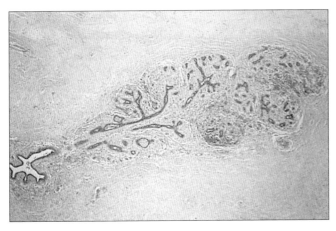

Fig. 3.6 Histological section showing a TDLU adjacent to a major duct, the latter showing typical infolding. The pale and loose intralobular connective tissue contrasts with the denser collagenous interlobular stroma.

Microscopic anatomy

The terminal ductal lobular unit

The adult resting breast has a branching major duct system leading to the terminal ductal lobular units (TDLUs) (Figs 3.5 and 3.6).

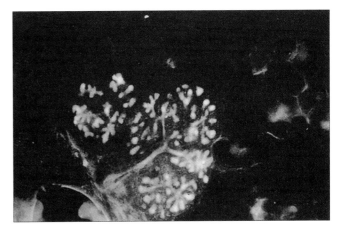

Fig. 3.7 Microradiograph of breast tissue showing a small duct branching into ductules and lobules.

The entity of the TDLU, described in detail by Wellings et al.[26] and comprising extra- and intralobular terminal ducts and the lobules arising from the intralobular terminal ductule (ITD), is an important entity in the origin of much breast disease, benign as well as malignant. The treelike branching structure of breast ductules is very nicely shown by the technique of microradiography, which has been developed in Cardiff, UK, for small pieces of breast tissue (Fig. 3.7).

Lobular development during reproductive life

Four types of lobules, representing progressive stages of lobular development from lobular bud to complete differentiation, have been recognized in the human breast.[27] Type I lobules are the most undifferentiated, budlike structure; type II are more complex, with a higher number of ductules per lobule. Further progression to types III and IV is seen especially during pregnancy and lactation. Type I is seen at the menarche consisting of about 10 alveolar buds clustered around a terminal duct. Types II and III consist of increasing ductules around the duct, and type IV has fully developed acini.[28] The average number of components per lobule increases from type I to type IV with mean figures of 11, 47, 81 and 180, respectively. After weaning, there is an abundance of type III, which are more differentiated, have a low oestrogen receptor content and low proliferative activity. In nulliparous women, type I is the most frequent found at all ages, while type III is the most frequent found in parous women. Type I has a high content of oestrogen receptors and a high rate of cellular proliferation.

Type I is considered to be the site of development of ductal carcinoma in situ, and type II of lobular carcinoma. Type III is thought to originate adenomas, fibroadenomas, sclerosing adenosis and cysts. Types I and II lobules have proved to be more reactive to chemical carcinogens in vitro than type III.

Changes in lobule number and structure with age have been studied in detail.[29] The largest number of lobular units occurs in the third decade, and decreases rapidly thereafter until the sixth decade, with a parallel decrease in size of the lobules. The greatest proportion is seen in the upper quadrants a decade earlier than in the lower quadrants, and the upper outer quadrant shows a surprising second peak in the fifth decade, in contrast with the steady decline in the others.

The epithelial cells

The ductal and alveolar epithelium are similar in structure and consist of two layers of cells, the basal cells being cuboidal and the surface cells being cylindrical with their long axes at right angles to the duct wall. Surrounding the ductal and alveolar walls is a discontinuous fenestrated layer of contractile myoepithelial cells. The myoepithelial cells contract in response to oxytocin stimulation and are responsible for the ejection of milk from the expanded TDLU of pregnancy into the larger ducts.

Light microscopy has shown some variation in the epithelial cells and two main cell types have been described by Bassler.[30] The more numerous basal cells have a light cytoplasm and were called clear basal B cells by Bassler, who thought they might function as stem cells for differentiation into myoepithelial cells or the second cell type (A cells). The darker A cells are luminal cells and have an eosinophilic cytoplasm packed with ribosomes which are responsible for the darker appearance under the microscope. Bassler postulated that the dark A cells develop from the clear B cells under the influence of oestrogen and migrate towards the luminal surface where they engage in secretory activity. A number of dark cells show regressive changes and are then shed as cellular debris into the lumen. Some dark A cells which have large membrane-bound vesicles containing lipid have been described as 'foam cells'; these may represent phagocytic histiocytes.[31]

Ultrastructural studies show that breast epithelial cells have well-developed luminal microvilli and complex interdigitating basal laminae with prominent desmosomes at intercellular boundaries. Cytoplasmic densities have been shown to vary in the same way as observed in light microscopy, in that a population of pale and dark cells can be identified.[32,33] As might be expected, myoepithelial cells contain well-marked contractile myofilaments and cilia running parallel to the long axis of the cell. Myoepithelial cells are closely related to the basement membranes of the luminal epithelial cells and to the basal lamina, to which they are attached by numerous hemidesmosomes. Ultrastructural studies have revealed the unsuspected complexity of the epithelial–stromal junction (ESJ), which is the crucial interface across which all nutrients must pass to reach the breast ductal cells.[32,34] The ESJ consists of a complex intertwining of fibroblasts, elastic fibres and endothelium and it is possible that the cause for some of the puzzling aspects of benign breast disease may lie in disorders of this region. It is also the area at which much of the paracrine and autocrine activity associated with growth factors occurs, as discussed below.

Work from Coombes's unit suggests that major advances in producing experimental models to understand lobular development and growth will soon be made with the human breast.[35] Having developed techniques for separating epithelial and myoepithelial cells from normal breast lobules, they have been able to identify some of their nutritional requirements and growth characteristics. This has allowed them to put the two cells together again and form typical two-cell-layer alveolar structures.

The basement membrane

The increasing knowledge of the activities of the basement membrane constitutes an exciting element of breast physiology and pathology. A complex, lattice-like structure lying between the epithelium and stroma, it clearly influences both.[36] It is a dynamic structure, with both lysis and resynthesis going on to give constant remodelling. Principal constituents include collagens, fibronectins and proteoglycans. Enzymes capable of degrading the basement membrane may be found in stromal cells, myoepithelial cells and blood vessels. Contact with adjacent epithelial cells determines their polarity, contributes to their differentiation and helps control their secretory functions. At the same time, the epithelial cells are capable of stimulating the formation of a basement membrane.

The breast stroma

The importance of the stroma in general organ development was illustrated graphically by the mouse experiments of Kratochwil.[37] He showed that mouse mammary epithelium grown in organ culture grew normally when co-cultured with mammary stroma, but developed salivary morphology and invasive properties when co-cultured with salivary stroma. Much work in murine culture systems has defined aspects of this interaction. Macromolecules, such as collagen and proteoglycans produced by fibroblasts, influence many aspects of epithelial cell behaviour – from proliferation to cell division and motility. Conversely, epithelial cells have similar effects on fibroblasts, including deposition and resorption of matrix molecules and structures. While these experimental systems are far removed from the human breast in vivo, it is likely that the general principles will be found to be similar as more sophisticated techniques are brought to bear on human studies, and in particular on the interaction of epithelium and stroma within the lobule. Indeed, Ferguson and co-workers have been able to demonstrate changes in the lobular extracellular matrix at different times of the menstrual cycle: interlobular fibroblasts showing characteristics of 'fetal' fibroblasts, intralobular fibroblasts showing the characteristics of 'adult' fibroblasts, and fetal fibroblasts showing enhanced migratory function compared to adult fibroblasts.[38]

Careful histological study by Parks has shown the heterogeneity of connective tissue in the breast.[39] The intralobular and periductal connective tissue is probably as important in physiological terms as the interlobular Cooper's ligaments in structural terms, although only recently is our knowledge of the physiology of the lobular stroma extending beyond the rudimentary. The segmental and interlobular fascia is dense and reticular, while the periductal and intralobular stroma is much looser – a contrast between loose and dense reminiscent of the papillary and reticular layers of the dermis, the tissue from which the breast arises.

The interlobular fascia often shows a large amount of fatty infiltration, especially in the larger breast. Further differences can be detected between periductal and lobular stroma. Periductal connective tissue is found as a cuff of loose stroma around the ducts in which the lymphatic vessels run. It is more cellular (fibrocytes) than the supporting fibrous tissue and contains a considerable amount of elastic tissue, which tends to increase with age and parity. The lobular stroma is even more loose, more vascular, more cellular and markedly mucoid – a structure which facilitates expansion of the developing acini in pregnancy. Biochemical studies[40] have shown that the distribution of a cell-surface enzyme called dipeptidyl

peptidase IV provides a clear delineation of two functionally distinct populations of breast fibroblasts: those of the intralobular stroma and those of the interlobular stroma. This is a striking confirmation of the difference suspected from conventional histology.

Similarly, fetal antigen 2 (FA2) is present in the intralobular stroma as a broad band around acini, but is not found in the interlobular stroma.[41] The lobule contains no elastic tissue and this fact is helpful to the pathologist in differentiating lesions arising from the lobule from those arising from ducts. Lobular stroma, and probably periductal stroma, is under hormonal influence, but little is known about the detailed hormonal responsiveness of this tissue.

Durnberger et al.[42] have shown that the differentiation of the mammary epithelial bud in the male fetal rodent occurs in response to a transient increase in testosterone secretion which does not affect the mammary ductular epithelium directly but is mediated by the surrounding stromal fibroblasts. Work from our laboratories has shown that human breast fibroblasts are highly stimulatory to human breast cancer cells in an in vivo nude mouse xenograft model.[43] These experiments point to a major regulatory role for breast fibroblasts in epithelial cell growth, while other work points to a possibility that breast epithelial cells may influence the stroma, particularly intralobular stroma.

McCune et al.[44] have demonstrated three transforming growth factor (TGF)-β isotopes lying intracellularly in most active epithelial cells, but not within stromal cells. At the same time, a technique which demonstrates the same isotopes in extracellular conformation stained normal intralobular stroma, and particularly the stroma of active fibroadenomas, lesions believed to develop from lobules. This indicates a possible paracrine and autocrine interaction between TGF-β from epithelial cells and the surrounding intralobular stroma as a control mechanism in mammary development and the pathogenesis of disease. Similar findings relate to immunoreactive endothelin-1, which is found only in mammary epithelial cells, but with cell-surface receptors found only on fibroblasts – a possible mechanism by which epithelial cells may influence stromal cells, as discussed in Chapter 7.

The long-term administration of androgens to female-to-male transexuals has provided a clinical experimental system.[45] When administered to hormonally normal women, the main effect on the breast has been a marked hyalinization of both intralobular and extralobular stroma, with especially marked periductal fibrosis. This is accompanied by atrophy of ductal epithelium and marked decrease in ducts and lobules. A similar effect has been reported in mice.

The cellular changes in the stroma during progression from the benign breast to malignancy have been reviewed.[46]

Biochemical control of breast epithelium

The breast tissues are under a complex system of control by systemic factors, particularly hormones acting through their respective receptors, and a number of local factors. These include paracrine hormones, released by one type of cell to influence adjacent cells of similar or differing function; juxtacrine factors, situated on the surface of the producing cell to influence adjacent cells by direct contact; and autocrine hormones, which act on the same cell by intracellular or surface receptors. All interact, as the systemic hormones also act, by influencing the locally derived factors – cell adhesion-related proteins as well as autocrine and paracrine hormones – to produce signal pathways that finally result in cell regulation and stimulation.

Studies of the molecular mechanisms controlling breast epithelium have concentrated on cancer cells; only recently has the situation in the normal breast been studied. The growth factor receptor EGF-R and the oncogene product C-erbB-2 are involved in the control of proliferation and probably differentiation of breast epithelial cells, although their precise role in the normal breast is unclear.[47] EGF-R is found mainly in the stroma (periductal and perilobular fibroblasts), myoepithelial cells and to a lesser extent basal epithelial cells, whereas C-erbB-2 expression is exclusively epithelial, mainly on the inner layer of epithelial cells of duct and lobule. Some heterogeneity of staining from one lobule to another in the same biopsy was found in this study, although both were more strongly expressed in the luteal phase.[47]

C-erbB-2 appears to be negatively related to proliferation of mammary epithelium and positively related to differentiation. The predominant distribution of expression of EGF-R suggests a paracrine pathway between stromal, myoepithelial and basal epithelial cells, influencing the basal epithelial cells which are proliferating. Some of the more superficial cells which fail to express EGF-R could still be cells which produce, or are stimulated by, epithelial growth factor (EGF) or transforming growth factor (TGF)-α, since ligand binding can lead to a decrease in receptor levels by internalization or degradation. TGF-α is a member of the EGF family which binds to EGF-R, and has been detected in normal breast cells.

Until recently, the only function of oxytocin in the breast was thought to be related to lactation. The discovery that oxytocin receptors are widely distributed in the brain and that some are strongly influenced by steroids such as oestrogen, progesterone and testosterone has led to more detailed study of the breast. The mammary gland, and especially the nipple, is richly innervated with peptidergic nerve fibres with receptors to which oxytocin can bind. Oxytocin functions are thought to be very wide, perhaps even being responsible for the anxiolytic effect of breastfeeding, since oxytocin levels vary inversely with anxiety and aggression.[48]

There is increasing evidence in animals that oxytocin is related to differentiation of myoepithelial cells, and now a similar function has been demonstrated in humans. Oxytocin receptors (OT-R) can be found in myoepithelial cells of normal ductules, in benign hyperplastic lesions and some cancer cells, and are abundant in sclerosing adenosis.[49] OT-R-positive cells in hyperplasias are likely to be myoepithelial rather than classical epithelial cells, and there is evidence that this is so. Epithelial and myoepithelial cells differ markedly in the production and response to growth factors[50] in that myoepithelial cells produce basic fibroblast growth factor (FGF)-2, which in turn affects the proliferation and survival of epithelial cells.

Much interest has also been shown recently in the fact that prostate-specific antigen (PSA) can be found in many breast conditions, such as in cyst fluid or nipple secretions. Yu et al.[51] have shown that it can often be demonstrated in normal breast tissues (33% of samples), benign breast disease (65%) and cancers (28%). The highest levels were found in fibroadenomas. Parathyroid-like peptide (PLP), structurally homologous to parathyroid hormone but of uncertain function, is another substance recognized in breast cancers, and now found with more sophisticated tests to be in the cytoplasm of normal and benign proliferative breast epithelial cells; it is increased in lactation and benign adenosis or ductal hyperplasia, and decreased in atrophic lobules. Its association with calcification in cancers suggests that it may play a local role in calcium metabolism in the normal breast.

Hepatocyte growth factor/scatter factor is present in benign, lactating and malignant breast epithelium, and an autocrine loop action in proliferating epithelium has been suggested.

Peptide growth factors such as EGF and TGF-α can be obtained from breast fluid aspirated from the nipple. Individual women secrete consistent and individually distinct levels, which in some cases can be correlated with circulating hormone levels.[52]

Cyclical changes in breast epithelium

Physiological control of ovarian function

Ovarian function is increasingly recognized as much more complicated than earlier conventional concepts. Ovarian activity is under the control of the pituitary gonadotrophins FSH and LH. The latter is secreted in pulsatile fashion under control of gonadotrophin-releasing hormone (GnRH), but modulated by a negative feedback effect of oestradiol and progesterone, and responding to a positive feedback in midcycle leading to the LH surge responsible for ovulation. FSH control is more complicated since it is partly under the control of GnRH, but partly independent of this. As well as the negative feedback from oestradiol and progesterone, there is a further negative feedback from inhibins and a positive stimulating effect of activins. Inhibins are dimeric glycoprotein hormones from the ovary suppressing FSH by a direct effect on the pituitary; activins are dimers which act mainly at a local level in paracrine or autocrine fashion. Activins are in turn activated by follistatin, an activin-binding third gonadal peptide.[53]

The breast during the menstrual cycle

Each breast cell has a finite lifespan before progressing to mitosis or apoptosis. The balance between mitosis and apoptosis is obviously of great importance in many aspects of breast functioning. Oestrogen tends to cause mitosis in ductular and alveolar cells, and during the follicular phase there is a modest increase in mitoses in the ductular cells, little in those of the alveoli.

Progestogens have a biphasic effect, at first stimulating mitosis with movement from G_1 phase to S phase, but then slowing down mitotic activity by arresting the cells in early G_1 phase. Progestogens also induce cytoplasmic changes conducive to lactation, with accumulation of fluid, protein and electrolyte. Hence, administration of progesterone in clinically moderate dosage will give full, tender breasts for a few weeks, but these symptoms will ease as apoptosis exceeds mitosis in the alveolar cells.

Anderson and co-workers[54] have quantified the incidence of mitosis and apoptosis morphologically in relation to the stage of the menstrual cycle. Both processes reach a peak incidence towards the end of the cycle and during menstruation, but with a statistically significant difference of 3 days between the two peaks – day 25 for mitosis and day 28 for apoptosis. This is the mirror image of the changes in the endometrium, when maximal mitosis occurs in the first half of the cycle. The results did not vary with parity, history of contraceptive pill use or with the presence of a fibroadenoma, and the changes observed in the cells of the lobules were also seen in the cells of the adjacent ductules. The cyclical nature of the changes was most marked in younger women; indeed there was no cyclical pattern for apoptosis in the 35–45-year age group. This may reflect the involutional changes usually detectable throughout this age period. Likewise there is a trend towards a decreased incidence of mitosis, but a more significant decrease in apoptosis with increasing age, shown as a loss of the late cycle peak. This more marked decrease in apoptosis than mitosis in the 35–45 group could also be responsible for some of the involutional changes of ANDI.

There was a consistent finding of a higher rate of apoptosis in the right breast than the left. It is interesting to speculate that this lower level of natural cell death on the left may be related to the higher incidence of many disease conditions found in this breast.

Russo et al.[55] used DNA-labelling techniques to measure cell proliferation in normal breast tissue adjacent to biopsies. The DNA-labelling index and the growth fraction were always greatest in the terminal ductule of the TDLU, less in the alveolus and still less in the ducts (0.74 vs 0.22 vs 0.04). This decreased with age, but even in the older patients the index was greatest in the terminal ductule (0.33 vs 0.08 vs 0.04). There is increasing evidence that mitogenic factors other than the sex hormones influence these cells; EGF is one candidate.

These and similar studies have helped to clarify the previous conflicting evidence regarding cyclical changes in breast epithelium, while animal studies are also producing new insights. For instance, a fatty acid-binding protein, mammary-derived growth inhibitor, can be shown to act locally in the mouse to inhibit growth of ductal epithelioid cells, produce no effect on the stroma and stimulate the development of lobuloalveolar structures.

In the human, Haagensen[56] emphatically stated that he was unable to confirm any cyclical variation in the number of acini per lobule, despite a search for the purported specific changes.

Anderson et al. have summarized the situation at present.[57] Both epithelial and stromal cells show cyclical changes reflecting menstrual hormone fluctuations. Epithelial proliferation peaks in the midluteal phase and is followed by increased apoptosis. There is a dissociation between steroid receptor expression and cell proliferation. Oestrogen receptor (ER)-positive cells are distributed evenly throughout the lobule, and 96% of ER-positive cells are also progesterone receptor (PR)-positive. Since the proliferating cells are usually ER- and PR-negative, it is likely that oestrogen has its main proliferating effect via adjacent ER-positive cells acting in paracrine fashion. Oral contraceptives prolong the length but not the magnitude of cellular proliferation and the degree of fluctuation becomes much less in older women.

Despite the conflicting evidence of histological change, there is clearly documented evidence that breast volume measured by water displacement methods increases during the luteal phase of the cycle and falls at menstruation.[58] Fowler et al.[59] in their MRI study of menstrual breast change established that much of the increased volume was due to water retention but some was due to stromal or epithelial changes. These changes are noticed by a large number of women and may be explained by vascular or lymphatic changes without requiring obvious changes in breast histology, although cellular proliferation in the lobules is believed to contribute to breast swelling. Mammary bloodflow shows a cyclical increase, an oestrogen effect, maximal for 3–4 days before menstruation, and this plays a part in the increased breast volume and discomfort typical of this period.

Matrix metalloproteinases play an important role in such basic functions as proliferation, differentiation and apoptosis[60] under the regulation of reproductive hormones.

Breast size correlates (in epidemiological terms) with height, weight and body mass index. However, current use of the oral contraceptive pill causes independently an increase in breast size which overrides this association.[61]

As a sexually responsive organ, the breast shows vascular engorgement and enlargement following sexual arousal, with nipple congestion and erection, followed by detumescence. In a similar manner to increased vascularity in the pelvic organs, these changes may be associated with discomfort that may become a cause for clinical presentation.

Changes during pregnancy and lactation

Anatomy

The greatly increased levels of luteal and placental sex steroids, with the addition of placental lactogen and chorionic gonadotrophin in pregnancy, cause a remarkable increase in lobuloalveolar growth. Prolactin levels also increase progressively throughout pregnancy but this hormone appears to be mainly concerned with milk production at the end of pregnancy after the preceding hormones have primed the breast by inducing marked proliferative changes. The chronological changes are shown in Table 3.1.

Histologically, the most remarkable features are the great predominance of dilated alveoli and the conversion of the resting two-layer epithelium to a monolayer within the alveoli (Fig. 3.8).

The large ducts maintain their two-layer configuration.

Physiology

Basal prolactin levels increase from the non-pregnant level of 10 ng/mL to peak values of over 200 ng/mL at week 40, postpartum prolactin levels fall over the next 4 weeks to around 20 ng/mL but are immediately elevated to about 10 times basal levels on suckling the infant. Although, as previously described, some colostral secretion is visible in the breast before term, the process of

Table 3.1 Changes in the breast during pregnancy

Week	Change
0	Resting breast approx. 200 g in weight
1–4	Ductular sprouting/lobular formation
5–8	Breast enlarges/vascular engorgement/areolar pigmentation/predominant lobular formation
12	Large alveoli with single epithelial cell layer Beginning of colostrum formation
>20	Alveolar dilatation/colostrum formation New capillary formation/myoepithelial cell hypertrophy
Term	180% increase of mammary bloodflow Weight approx. 400 g Fat droplet accumulation in alveolar cells

After Vorherr.[62]

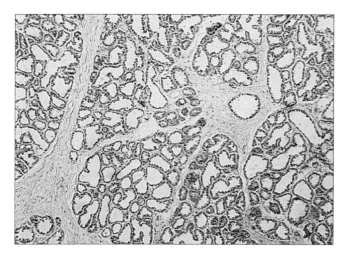

Fig. 3.8 Histological section (H&E) of lactating breast showing grossly dilated acini lined by a low cuboidal epithelium. Note the high ratio of epithelium to stroma.

milk production proper begins 2–5 days after birth. The change from colostrum to milk is caused by high levels of prolactin maintained against a rapidly falling level of ovarian and placental sex steroids.

Prolactin is the primary stimulant for galactopoiesis and has been shown to have a variety of actions on breast tissue, which would contribute to milk production.[62] The increased mitosis required for alveolar growth and early colostrum production is stimulated primarily by ovarian and placental sex steroids, placental lactogen, cortisol and growth hormone, with the placenta supplying the bulk of the sex steroids and lactogenic factors. Although some milk protein and fat synthesis is seen from midpregnancy onwards, the full lactogenic stimulation of prolactin is inhibited by the high levels of circulating sex steroids. Birth and the consequent loss of the placenta reverse the inhibition and full milk production then begins. The predominant role of prolactin in lactopoiesis is illustrated by the fact that ovariectomized women and animals can successfully breastfeed.

Established lactation

Once established, lactation will continue almost indefinitely, provided the milk is regularly removed from the breast. After 48 hours of milk stagnation, milk synthesis begins to fall rapidly.[63,64]

During milk secretion, alveolar cells change shape and histological appearance. During active lactation, the upper part of the cell breaks away or is extruded and the cell changes from a columnar shape to a low cuboidal shape.

Thus, milk secretion is an apocrine- and merocrine-type secretion as only part of the cell is lost. The fat globules in milk are surrounded by a membrane which is presumably derived from the luminal cell membrane of the alveolar cell. Following secretion, resynthesis of milk proteins such as lactalbumin and casein and milk fats occurs and the cell begins to elongate. Prolactin is the primary stimulant for lactose synthesis by stimulation of lactose synthetase and protein synthesis by stimulation of nuclear RNA polymerase. Lactose synthesis takes place in the Golgi apparatus and the cell becomes large and swollen with secretory products.[65,66] Secretion then takes place with fats and protein being excreted by apocrine secretion, lactose by merocrine secretion and inorganic ions by a combination of active transport and diffusion. The cycle of extrusion and resynthesis then restarts.

The active transport processes across the luminal cell (the blood–milk barrier) are of considerable interest as recent studies of cyst fluids suggest that different morphological types of epithelium may differ in the handling of ions.[67] Umemura and colleagues have carried out a histochemical study to define the cell kinetics and functional morphology of the lactating breast. They have defined four types of lobules: type I, prelactating; type II, lactating; type III, early regression; and type IV, advanced regression.[68]

Postlactational involution

Postlactational involution starts on weaning and is initiated by local mechanical factors causing alveolar distension and capillary obstruction. The one-layer secretory alveolar cells regress and reform the two-layered epithelium characteristic of the resting breast. This process is facilitated by cell death and phagocytosis performed by invasion of the alveoli by histiocytes. A lymphocytic infiltrate is also characteristic, but connective tissue regression is limited. The branching alveolar structures become fewer in number but the ductular structure remains mostly intact. This is the fundamental difference between postlactational and postmenopausal involution; in the latter both lobules and ductules are reduced in number. The ducts become smaller although some secretion persists in the duct lumen in the postlactational breast and can be aspirated or expressed from the nipple in most parous women.[69] Much work in rodents is currently in progress identifying the precise hormonal and biochemical substances and mechanisms responsible for this remarkable involution. In time, this will undoubtedly throw light on the human process.

Postmenopausal involution

Physiological control

Follicle-stimulating hormone (FSH) levels rise progressively from the age of 30 to the menopause, while levels of oestradiol and LH remain relatively constant during this period. This rise in FSH in the presence of a maintained oestradiol may be due to a fall in inhibins, produced by the granulosa cells of the ovary. With this change from the age of 30, it is not surprising that the involutional structural changes of ANDI may be seen in the breast long before the menopause. Oestradiol levels fluctuate widely in individuals at the time of the menopause, and very high levels in some women may be responsible for the breast tenderness that is sometimes seen at this time. Surprisingly, tissue steroid levels show little difference in premenopausal and postmenopausal women, despite the differences in circulating levels.

In postmenopausal women, continuous oestrogen administration may stimulate ductal cell proliferation, leading to breast fullness with discomfort and paraesthesiae of the nipple, but these changes do not persist. However, administration of combined oestrogen/progesterone supplementation may give more marked and persisting fullness and tenderness.

Histological changes

The process of postmenopausal involution can be divided into a preclimacteric phase starting at about the age of 35 and a postmenopausal phase starting at the time of the menopause. The predominant feature is regression of the glandular epithelium and adjacent connective tissue with gradual replacement by fat. In the preclimacteric phase there is a gradual loss of lobules and infiltration by round cells and the specialized loose connective tissue around the lobules changes into dense collagen. In the post-menopausal phase, the typical outline of a lobule is lost and is replaced by dense collagen containing a compressed epithelial remnant. Lobular involution may proceed to formation of microcysts which may be mistaken for cystic disease microscopically. The essential difference between the two conditions is the preservation of the specialized lobular stroma in the former.[70] Stromal changes dominate and fat deposition accelerates and connective tissue regression is marked. The end result is that the branching major duct system is visible, but very few lobules can be seen and these are embedded in dense fibrotic capsules unlike the loose stroma surrounding the lobules in the breasts of younger women. Some lobules may develop into microcysts by dilatation, possibly due to obstruction of the terminal ductule, and interlobular connective tissue is greatly reduced. Externally, these changes produce the shrunken, pendulous breast of the old woman and, when mammography is performed, are responsible for the good contrast of parenchyma to fat obtained on mammograms of the older breast. Variations of this process are responsible for many of the clinical presentations and histological appearances of benign breast disease and are discussed fully in the next chapter.

REFERENCES

1. Van der Putte SC. Mammary-like glands of the vulva and their disorders. *International Journal of Gynecological Pathology* 1994; **13**: 150–160.
2. Hughes ESR. The development of the mammary gland. *Annals of the Royal College of Surgeons of England* 1950; **6**: 99–119.
3. Love SM, Barsky SH. Anatomy of the nipple and breast ducts revisited. *Cancer* 2004; **101**: 1947–1957.
4. Dabelow A. Die Milchdruse In: Bagman W (ed.) *Handbuch der mikroskopischen Anatomie des Merchen.* vol 3, part 3, *Haut und Sininesorgane.* Berlin: Springer-Verlag; 1957:277–485.
5. Anbazhagan R, Bartek J, Monaghan P et al. Growth and development of the human breast. *American Journal of Anatomy* 1991; **192**: 407–417.
6. Marshall WA & Tanner JM. Variations in pattern of pubertal changes in girls. *Archives of Diseases of Childhood* 1969; **44**: 291–303.
7. Zacharias L, Wurtman RJ & Schatzoff M. Sexual maturation in contemporary American girls. *American Journal of Obstetrics and Gynecology* 1970; **108**: 833–846.
8. Wildt L, Marshall G & Knobil E. Experimental induction of puberty in the infantile female rhesus monkey. *Science* 1980; **207**: 1373–1375.
9. Graham JD & Clarke CL. Physiological action of progesterone in target tissues. *Endocrine Reviews* 1997; **18**: 502–519.
10. Topper YJ & Freeman CS. Multiple hormone interactions in the developmental biology of the mammary gland. *Physiological Reviews* 1980; **60**: 1049–1106.

11. Davies RL, Flores NA & Pye JK. Developments in contact X-ray microscopy in biomedical research. *Journal of Microscopy* 1985; **138**(Part 3): 293–300.

12. Hicken NF. Mastectomy: a clinical pathologic study demonstrating why most mastectomies result in incomplete removal of the mammary gland. *Archives of Surgery* 1940; **40**: 6–12.

13. Loughry CW, Sheffer DB, Price TE *et al.* Breast volume measurement in 598 women using biostereometric analysis. *Annals of Plastic Surgery* 1989; **22**: 380–385.

14. Westreich M. Anthropomorphic breast measurement: protocol and results in 50 women with aesthetically perfect breasts and clinical application. *Plastic and Reconstructive Surgery* 1997; **100**: 468–479.

15. Lejour M. Evaluation of fat in the breast tissue removed by vertical mammaplasty. *Plastic and Reconstructive Surgery* 1997; **99**: 386–393.

16. Boston RC, Schnall MD, Englander SA *et al.* Estimation of the content of fat and parenchyma in breast tissue using MRI T1 histograms and phantoms. *Magnetic Resonance Imaging* 2005; **23**: 591–599.

17. Smith DM, Peters TE & Donegan WL. Montgomery's areolar tubercle. *Archives of Pathology and Laboratory Medicine* 1982; **106**: 60–63.

18. Koenecke IA. An anatomical study of the mammary gland twenty four hours postpartum. *American Journal of Obstetrics and Gynecology* 1934; **27**: 584–592.

19. Moffatt DF & Going JJ. Three dimensional anatomy of complete duct systems in human breast – pathological and developmental implications. *Journal of Clinical Pathology* 1996; **49**: 48–52.

20. Maliniac JW. Arterial blood supply of the breast. *Archives of Surgery* 1943, **47**: 329–343.

21. Suami H, Pan WR, Mann GB *et al.* The lymphatic anatomy of the breast and its implications for sentinel lymph node biopsy: a human cadaver study. *Annals of Surgical Oncology* 2008; **15**: 863–871.

22. Vorherr H. *The Breast: Morphology, Physiology and Lactation.* New York: Academic Press; 1974.

23. Sarhadi NS, Dunn JS, Lee FD *et al.* An anatomical study of the nerve supply of the breast, including the nipple and areola. *British Journal of Plastic Surgery* 1996; **49**: 156–164.

24. Jaspars JJP, Posma AN, Van Immerseel AAH *et al.* The cutaneous innervation of the female breast and nipple areola complex: implications for surgery. *British Journal of Plastic Surgery* 1997; **50**: 49–59.

25. Wilkson SA, Adams EJ & Tucker AK. Patterns of breast skin thickness in normal mammograms. *Clinical Radiology* 1982; **33**: 691–693.

26. Wellings SR, Jensen HM & Marcum RG. An atlas of sub-gross pathology of the human breast with reference to possible pre-cancerous lesions. *Journal of National Cancer Institute* 1975; **55**: 231–273.

27. Russo J & Russo IH. Toward a physiological approach to breast cancer prevention. *Cancer Epidemiology, Biomarkers and Prevention* 1994; **3**: 353–364.

28. Russo J & Russo IH. Development of the human mammary gland. In: Neville MC & Daniel CW (eds). *The Mammary Gland.* New York: Plenum; 1987.

29. Hutson SW, Cowen PN & Bird CC. Morphometric studies of age related changes in normal human breast and their significance for evolution of mammary cancer. *Journal of Clinical Pathology* 1985; **38**: 281–287.

30. Bassler R. The morphology of hormone-induced structural changes in the female breast. *Current Topics in Pathology* 1970; **53**: 1–89.

31. Toker C. Observations on the ultrastructure of a mammary ductule. *Journal of Ultrastructure Research* 1967; **21**: 9–25.

32. Stirling JW & Chandler JA. The fine structure of the normal, resting terminal ductal-lobular unit of the female breast. *Virchows Archiv. A, Pathological Anatomy and Histopathology* 1976; **372**: 205–226.

33. Ahmed A. In: *Atlas of the Ultrastructure of Human Breast Diseases.* Edinburgh: Churchill Livingstone; 1978:1–26.

34. Stirling JW & Chandler JA. The fine structure of ducts and subareolar ducts in the resting gland of the female breast. *Virchows Archiv. A, Pathological Anatomy and Histopathology* 1977; **373**: 119–132.

35. Gomm JJ, Coope RC, Browne PJ *et al.* Separate breast epithelial and myo-epithelial cells have different growth factor requirements in vitro but can reconstitute normal breast lobulo-alveolar structure. *Journal of Cellular Physiology* 1997; **171**: 11–19.

36. Fu HL, Moss J, Shore I *et al.* Ultrastructural localization of laminin and type IV collagen in normal human breast. *Ultrastruct Pathology* 2002; **26**: 77–80.

37. Kratochwil K. Organ specificity in mesenchymal induction demonstrated in the embryonic development of the mammary gland of the mouse. *Developmental Biology* 1969; **20**: 46–71.

38. Ferguson JE, Schor AM, Howell A *et al.* Changes in the extracellular matrix of the human breast during the menstrual cycle. *Cell Tissue Research* 1992; **268**: 167–177.

39. Parks AG. The micro-anatomy of the breast. *Annals of the Royal College of Surgeons* 1959; **25**: 295–311.

40. Atherton AJ, Monaghan P, Warburton MJ *et al.* Dipeptidyl peptidase IV expression identifies a functional sub-population of breast fibroblasts. *International Journal of Cancer* 1992; **50**: 15–19.

41. Rassmussen HB, Teisner B, Andersen J *et al.* Fetal antigen-2 in the stromal reaction induced by breast carcinoma. *APMIS* 1992; **100**: 39–47.

42. Durnberger H, Heuberger B, Schwartz P *et al.* Mesenchyme-mediated effects of testosterone on embryonic mammary epithelium. *Cancer Research* 1978; **38**: 4066–4070.

43. Horgan K, Jones DL & Mansel RE. Mitogenicity of human fibroblasts in vivo for human breast cancer cells. *British Journal of Surgery* 1987; **74**: 227–229.

44. McCune BK, Mullin BR, Flanders KC *et al.* Localisation of transforming growth factor-beta isotypes in lesions of the human breast. *Human Pathology* 1992; **23**: 13–20.

45. Sapino A, Pietribiasi F, Godan A *et al.* Effect of long-term administration of androgens on breast tissue of female to male transexuals. *Annals of the New York Academy of Sciences* 1990; **586**: 143–145.

46. Ronnov-Jessen L, Petersen OW & Bissell MJ. Cellular changes involved in conversion of normal to malignant breast: importance of the stromal reaction. *Physiological Reviews* 1996; **76**: 69–125.

47. Gompel A, Martin A, Simon P *et al.* Epidermal growth factor receptor and C-erb-2 expression in normal breast tissue during the menstrual cycle. *Breast Cancer Research and Treatment* 1996; **38**: 227–235.

48. Uvnas-Moberg K & Eriksson M. Breast feeding: physiological, endocrine and behavioural adaptations caused by oxytocin and local neurogenic activity in the nipple and mammary gland. *Acta Paediatrica* 1996; **85**: 525–530.

49. Bussolati G, Cassoni P, Ghisolfi G *et al.* Immunolocalisation and gene expression of oxytocin receptors in cancerous and non-neoplastic tissues of the breast. *American Journal of Pathology* 1996; **148**: 1895–1903.

50. Coombes RC, Bullweza L & Gomm JJ. The role of myo-epithelial derived growth factors in the human breast. *Endocrine-Related Cancer* 1997; **4**: 35–43.

51. Yu H, Diamandis EP & Levesque M *et al.* Prostate specific antigen in breast cancer, benign breast disease and normal breast tissue. *Breast Cancer Research and Treatment* 1996; **40**: 171–178.

52. Gann P, Chatterton R, Vogelsong K *et al.* Mitogenic growth factors in breast fluid obtained from healthy women. *Cancer Endocrinology, Biomarkers and Prevention* 1997; **6**: 421–428.

53. Burger HG. The menopausal transmission. *Baillière's Clinical Obstetrics and Gynaecology* 1996; **10**: 347–359.

54. Anderson TJ, Ferguson DJP & Raab GM. Cell turnover in the 'resting' human breast – influence of parity, contraceptive pill, age and laterality. *British Journal of Cancer* 1982; **46**: 376–382.

55. Russo J, Calaf G, Roi L *et al.* Influence of gland age and topography on cell kinetics of normal breast tissue. *Journal of the National Cancer Institute* 1987; **78**: 413–418.

56. Haagensen CD. *Diseases of the Breast.* 3rd edn. Philadelphia: Saunders; 1986:50–54.

57. Anderson E, Clarke RB & Howell A. Change in the human breast throughout the menstrual cycle: relevance to breast carcinogenesis. *Endocrine-Related Cancer* 1997; **4**: 23–34.

58. Milligan D, Drife JO & Short RV. Changes in breast volume during normal menstrual cycle and after oral contraceptives. *British Medical Journal* 1975; **iv**: 494–496.

59. Fowler PA, Casey CE, Cameron GG *et al.* Cyclic changes in composition and volume of the breast during the menstrual cycle, measured by magnetic resonance imaging. *British Journal of Obstetrics and Gynaecology* 1990; **97**: 595–602.

60. Hulboy DL, Rudolph LA & Matrisian LM. Matrix metalloproteinases as mediators of reproductive function. *Molecular Human Reproduction* 1997; **3**: 27–45.

61. Jernstrom H & Olsson H. Breast size in relation to hormone levels, body constitution and oral contraceptive use in healthy nulligravid women aged 19–25 years. *American Journal of Epidemiology* 1997; **145**: 571–580.

62. Vorherr H. Puerperium: maternal involutional changes and lactation. In: Posinsky JJ (ed.) *Davis' Gynecology and Obstetrics*, vol I, chap 20. New York: Harper; 1972:1–46.

63. Cowie AT. Induction and suppression of lactation in animals. *Proceedings of the Royal Society of Medicine* 1972; **65**: 1084–1085.

64. Zilliacus H. Physiologie und Pathologie des Wockenbettes. In: Kasero O *et al.* (eds). *Gynakologie und Geburtshilfe*, vol II. Stuttgart: Thième; 1967:966–997.

65. Turkington RW. Measurement of prolactin activity in human serum by the induction of specific milk proteins in mammary gland in vitro. *Journal of Clinical Endocrinology and Metabolism* 1971; **33**: 210–216.

66. Turkington RW, Brew K, Vanaman TC *et al.* The hormonal control of lactose synthetase in the developing mouse mammary gland. *Journal of Biological Chemistry* 1968; **243**: 3382–3387.

67. Dixon JM, Miller WR, Scott WN *et al.* The morphological basis of human cyst populations. *British Journal of Surgery* 1983; **70**: 604–606.

68. Umemura S, Osamura RY & Tsutsumi Y. Cell renewal and functional morphology of the human lactating breast. *Pathology International* 1996; **46**: 105–121.

69. Petrakis NL. Physiologic, biochemical and cytologic aspects of nipple aspirate fluid. *Breast Cancer Research and Treatment* 1985; **8**: 7–19.

70. Azzopardi JG. Problems in breast pathology. In: Bennington JL (ed.). *Major Problems in Pathology*, vol II, Chap 2. London: WB Saunders; 1979:8–22.

Aberrations of normal development and involution (ANDI): a concept of benign breast disorders based on pathogenesis

Key points and new developments

1. Terminology in benign breast disease has been confused by a multiplicity of terms which do not relate accurately to clinical or histological patterns, and which are not based on sound concepts of pathogenesis.

2. Most benign breast disorders derive from minor aberrations of the normal processes of development, cyclical activity and involution.

3. The ANDI classification allows precise definition of an individual patient problem in terms of pathogenesis, histology and clinical significance.

4. ANDI replaces the conventional view of 'normal' and 'disease' with a spectrum ranging from normal, through slight abnormality (aberration), to disease.

5. Recent developments in molecular biology give support to, and provide possible mechanisms for, the concept.

Introduction

The aberrations of normal development and involution (ANDI) classification of benign breast disorders[1] provides an overall framework for benign conditions of the breast, encompassing both pathogenesis and degree of abnormality. It was developed because the concepts used in teaching about, and managing, benign conditions of the breast (particularly 'fibrocystic disease') have been bedevilled by obscurities and inaccuracy. This is in marked contrast with breast cancer, where there is a clearly defined framework. A patient with cancer is investigated along two directions – a 'longitudinal' direction which will assess the tumour in temporal terms, in situ or invasive, size and extent of primary tumour, presence or absence of lymph node involvement and systemic spread; and a 'horizontal' direction assessing biology, histological type (e.g. lobular, ductal or other), grading, hormone receptor/growth factor status, etc. This will allow a patient to be placed within this well-recognized and well-defined

framework, with a management policy appropriate to her individual status.

The situation with benign conditions has been different until recently. A large number of clinical and histological conditions, such as fibroadenoma, duct papilloma, subareolar abscess and nipple discharge right through to the ubiquitous fibrocystic disease have been seen as individual and unrelated entities in terms of pathogenesis and management. Alternatively, some workers equated the whole range of benign breast disease with fibrocystic disease and tried to push all its manifestations into this one ill-defined complex, with even greater confusion. There was no overall framework for benign disorders into which an individual condition could be placed for assessment and management. Thus, historically, patients with breast cancer have been managed more logically, consistently, comprehensively and with more conviction than those with benign breast disease.

The ANDI classification, also a bidirectional framework, provides a means to reverse this disparity (Table

4.1), and is based on the fact that most benign breast conditions arise from normal physiological processes.

The horizontal assessment defines the position along a spectrum from normality, through mild abnormality ('aberration') through to severe abnormality ('disease'). The vertical component defines the pathogenesis of the condition, for almost all conditions are related to the three different phases of activity in the breast during reproductive life. Together, the two provide a comprehensive framework, into which can be fitted most aspects of benign breast disorders, in terms of concept, pathogenesis and severity (Table 4.2).

The basic principles underlying the ANDI classification are set out in Table 4.3.

Since the ANDI concept was first proposed in 1979, and published in 1987, a great deal of new information, relating both to physiology and to pathology, has come forward, providing a surprising degree of support to those elements of the concept which were speculative at that time. The ANDI classification was accepted and recommended by an international multidisciplinary working party in 1992.[2]

The ANDI framework is consonant with and builds on work of many earlier workers, extending back as far as 1922.[3] Yet its postulates are in total contrast to the widely accepted concepts of fibrocystic disease, and hence it is necessary to present the background, rationale and supporting material in some detail.

Table 4.1 The basic bidirectional framework of the ANDI classification

	Horizontal – Spectrum of severity
	Normal Aberration Disease
Vertical – Pathogenesis based on reproductive period	
Development	(15–25 years)
Cyclical activity	(25–45 years)
Involution	(35–55 years)

Table 4.3 The principles underlying the ANDI concept

1	Most benign disorders are related to normal processes of reproductive life.
2	There is a spectrum that ranges from normal to aberration, and occasionally to disease.
3	The definition of normal and abnormal is pragmatic.
4	The ANDI concept embraces all aspects: symptoms, signs, histology and physiology.

Table 4.2 Classification of the more important conditions of BBD into ANDI and non-ANDI

Stage		**Main clinical presentations**	
	Normal process	**Aberration**	**Disease**
Early reproductive (15–25 years)	Lobular development	Fibroadenoma	Giant fibroadenoma
	Stromal development	Adolescent hypertrophy	Gigantomastia
	Nipple eversion	Nipple inversion	Subareolar abscess/mammary duct fistula
Mature reproductive (25–40 years)	Cyclical changes of menstruation	Cyclical mastalgia Nodularity	Incapacitating mastalgia
	Epithelial hyperplasia of pregnancy	Bloody nipple discharge	
Involution (35–55 years)	Lobular involution	Macrocysts Sclerosing lesions	
	Duct involution – dilatation – sclerosis	Duct ectasia Nipple retraction	Periductal mastitis/abscess
	Epithelial turnover	Simple epithelial hyperplasia	With atypia
Non-ANDI	Conditions of well-defined aetiology, such as fat necrosis, lactational abscess, etc., together with extrinsic precipitating factors such as smoking and oro-nipple contact in severe nonpuerperal abscess.		

Recognition of the normality of much benign breast 'disease'

In the 1950s, a number of seminal studies demonstrated that the histological changes of fibrocystic disease are widely distributed in patients who had not claimed to be symptomatic or demonstrated overt disease. Parks[4] showed, from studies of both surgical and autopsy specimens, a complete gradation between normal histology and disease; for example, between developing lobules and fibroadenomas, and between involuting lobules and macroscopic cysts. He also showed that epithelial hyperplasia is so common around the menopause as to be normal and that these lesions, so often in the past regarded as indicative of cancer risk, could regress without treatment.

Extensive autopsy studies over the past 50 years have shown that most of the benign changes previously considered as disease are so common that they must be regarded as lying within the spectrum of normality. For example, a study of 200 breasts at autopsy from 100 postmenopausal patients (mean age 62 years) without clinical breast disease, confirmed earlier studies and showed changes of 'fibrocystic condition' (normal to aberration) in 54% of cases, with only 46% histologically normal. Hyperplasia with severe atypia (disease) was seen in only 3% of patients.[5]

Mastalgia provides an example of horizontal assessment. Studies in Cardiff, UK, over the past 20 years have shown the high incidence of painful nodularity: two-thirds of a population of working women will experience mastalgia. The clinical significance of mastalgia was quantified in the Cardiff Mastalgia Clinic through accurate classification and assessment of impact on patients' lives by visual linear analogue scales and breast pain charts. This has demonstrated that much breast pain can be considered as 'normal', some is sufficiently troublesome to warrant attention and can be regarded as a 'disorder', but in a minority pain is sufficiently severe as to be a major interference with quality of life and to be regarded as disease.

Individual conditions can also be put into a longitudinal grouping related to the three main phases of breast activity during reproductive life, since these conditions can be recognized as arising from aberrations of normal processes within the breast.

While the changes of ANDI, both clinical (painful nodularity) and histological ('fibroadenosis'), are now recognized as part of a spectrum extending from normality and probably arising from minor hormonal abnormalities, no specific aetiological factors have been identified, except for those of altered prolactin secretion and possibly changes in fatty acid intake. Nor is there any good evidence as to whether the condition has always occurred with the same frequency. One study of women of all age groups showed fewer histological changes of ANDI than were reported in the 1950s and 1960s.[6] While microcysts were seen in most breasts, and duct ectasia in one-third, both conditions showed a uniform age spread. In contrast, epithelial hyperplasia and sclerosed lobules were uncommon, and no case of premalignant hyperplasia was seen. Only further work will show whether this is a genuine epidemiological trend, since population (autopsy) studies common 40 years ago have in general been replaced by more detailed study and follow-up of biopsy material. There is some evidence of changing incidence patterns in non-Western populations as social and dietary conditions change, as discussed in Chapter 7.

Problems with the conventional view of benign breast disease

When problems are defined, solutions are more easily found. Even just recognizing the problems goes a long way towards resolving them. We see four main problems in the classical approach to benign breast disease:

- Nomenclature
- The borderline between normal and abnormal
- Correlation of clinical symptoms and signs with histological changes
- The assessment of premalignant potential.

Nomenclature

As discussed in Chapter 1, the situation has been beset by multiple loose terminology. Each worker in the past has tended to introduce his or her own terminology, reflecting personal ideas of disease and its underlying pathology, without linking it to earlier studies. At first, the terms were mainly clinical, e.g. 'chronic mastitis', but later reflected biopsy appearance, e.g. 'fibrocystic disease', of symptomatic lesions without appreciating the range of histological appearance in patients without symptoms. This leads on to the second problem.

The borderline between normal and abnormal – what determines normality or abnormality?

Many organs under endocrine control show a wide range of appearances associated with cyclical or pulsed hormonal secretion. This is especially true in females, where cyclical changes are set against a background of the broader changes of development and involution at the extremes of reproductive life, and particularly so in the breast. Most of these cyclical changes show a spectrum which on occasions may extend outside the normal range. Clearly, it is important to try to define the point, even if blurred, at which normality crosses the line to abnormality.

A number of factors must be assessed in deciding where the boundary of normality lies, including incidence, clinical impact and histology. Macrocysts are an example of the importance of incidence; they are common and commonly multiple, while microcysts are found in almost all breasts if looked for carefully enough. Clearly, microcysts must be regarded as normal, and macrocysts – with an incidence of perhaps 10% of all women – are at most an aberration of normality and cannot be considered as disease.

The importance of clinical impact can be illustrated by mastalgia. A large proportion of women experience premenstrual discomfort for a few days; this causes little interference with quality of life, and can be considered as normal. However, when pain persists for 3 out of 4 weeks of the cycle and is of great severity, it must be looked at in a different light. This is quite uncommon, and the clinical impact can be quite severe; hence, it can be regarded as an aberration of normality and, perhaps in the most extreme cases, as disease.

Histological appearances have given particular difficulty in this area; even minimal degrees of hyperplasia have been regarded as carrying cancer risk in the past, but recently the high incidence of simple hyperplasias in normal women has caused a reassessment of significance. A number of pathologists, and Page and co-workers in particular,[7] have defined and categorized histological patterns and their significance with considerable precision. This has allowed hyperplasias to be placed in three broad groups: normal (no increased cancer risk), slightly increased risk (equivalent to aberration) and high cancer risk.

Benign breast conditions cannot always be categorized as definitively normal or abnormal using these three criteria because there is usually a spectrum of severity. However, it is possible, using considerations such as these, to assess where an individual patient lies along this spectrum, so that an appropriate management policy can be determined.

Correlation of clinical symptoms and signs with histological changes

In the past, a patient with a local clinical abnormality such as an area of painful nodularity has been subjected to biopsy and the histological changes correlated with that clinical nodule. This ignores the fact that the classic changes of 'fibrocystic disease', including fibrosis, adenosis, cyst formation and lymphocytic infiltration, may be seen in the asymptomatic breast, and ignores the dynamic changes within the breast from month to month. Thus, a second biopsy from a clinically identical area a few centimetres away might show different histological changes, as might a biopsy a few months later. One study provides interesting confirmation of this heterogeneity of response within different areas of the breast. Normal volunteers given defined oral contraceptives showed diverse histological changes on biopsy, often with secretory and involutional changes coexisting in different parts of the same breast.[8]

The histology of a clinical lesion must be assessed against the broad spectrum of histological change which might be seen within a 'normal' breast, symptomatic or not. Failure to do so leads to confusion of significance; painful nodularity, a clinical condition which has no distinct radiological or pathological counterpart, has been called fibroadenosis, and correlated with cancer risk.

Only lesions which are both definite clinical and pathological entities, e.g. a macrocyst, can be assessed from both points of view. Terms such as fibroadenosis or fibrocystic disease are misleading, because they imply that these histological patterns are abnormal and that they correlate with clinical conditions. Histological changes are best described by a general term such as ANDI, which correctly indicates pathogenesis without using misleading specific terms, or by the specific individual histological elements present in the biopsy material.

The assessment of premalignant potential

This aspect has understandably dominated the efforts of breast surgeon and pathologist alike. Both have been frustrated by the three factors discussed above and it is not surprising that attempts to assess premalignant potential of fibrocystic disease have given almost infinitely variable results from one study to another. Confusion of nomenclature is particularly great when discussing the epithelial hyperplasias. Because of their precancerous association, the use of different terms in different countries has led to serious misunderstanding, compounded by failure to define the borderline between normal and abnormal. Only recently has this problem been addressed in a uniform and structured manner, as with the work of Page discussed above.[9]

Where do the answers to these problems lie? Firstly, in defining the range of normality, both in terms of clinical symptoms and signs, and of histological appearance. Secondly, recognizing that breast problems may be clinical, physiological or histological, and each problem may sometimes reflect only one of these three: sometimes more than one. Thirdly, by providing a comprehensive framework within which individual clinical or histological situations can be placed so that they are seen within an overall context. This must allow precise placement of a problem within the overall clinicopathological framework of benign breast disease and also encompasses the decision whether an individual clinical situation lies towards the normal or abnormal end of the spectrum of a particular process.

The physiological processes underlying the ANDI concept

The physiology of the breast has been described in detail in Chapter 3, but the broad outline is important in understanding ANDI. The main processes are related to hormonal effects on the breast during reproductive life, in the three phases of development, cyclical change and involution. As these three stages are of increasing complexity, it is not surprising that the processes go wrong more often during the long period of cyclical activity than during development, and even more commonly in the long and complex process of involution. Consideration of the impact of these hormonal events on lobules, ducts and stroma sets the scene for an understanding of the clinical conditions which arise from them.

Pathogenesis, clinical presentation and management of benign breast disorders are set out in this chapter only in conceptual terms. The details of clinical features, pathology and management are given in the rest of the book. We hope readers will persevere with the concepts of this chapter; we believe it makes detailed assessment and management of individual clinical problems so much easier.

Hormone-controlled processes of the breast

Breast development

The premenarchal breast consists of a few ducts only. The striking feature of the perimenarchal development of the breast is the addition of lobular structures to the already developing duct system. The lobules develop particularly during early reproductive life at 15–25 years of age. At first, 'primitive' type 1 lobules of Russo and Russo (Ch. 3), they are gradually replaced by more mature and less active lobules during the cyclical period, and especially with pregnancy. This explains the frequency of fibroadenoma during early and midreproductive life, for it is a condition analogous to gross hypertrophy of a lobule. Until the age of about 35 years, the luteal phase is also associated with enhanced acinar sprouting from the ductules.

A distinctive element of the lobule is its highly specialized connective tissue, and the close interaction between epithelium and connective tissue separated only by a basement membrane. This lobular connective tissue is pale and loose (Fig. 4.1) with mononuclear infiltrate and differs notably from the much less interesting and urbane interlobular fibrous stroma (see Ch. 3).

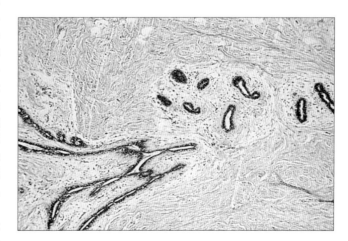

Fig. 4.1 The perimenarchal breast showing early lobular development. The pale, loose lobular connective tissue contrasts with the denser interlobular fibrous stroma.

Cyclical change

Both epithelial and stromal elements of the lobule are under hormonal control and there is evidence that the two work in tandem. In fact, normality seems to be very much dependent on a normal, balanced relationship between both elements. The details of the interaction of hormones and growth factors on epithelium, myoepithelium, basement membrane and stroma are now being elucidated (as discussed in Ch. 3) and give an inkling of the mechanisms underlying this relationship. It is likely that interference with these close relationships is responsible for many of the conditions that are often included under the term 'benign breast disease'. The changes occurring with each menstrual cycle have been summarized by Vorherr,[10] and expanded with more recent studies which demonstrate a peak of mitosis in the late cycle followed by apoptosis (see Ch. 3). They provide a potent opportunity for minor upsets to occur with repetitive cyclical changes.

These cyclical changes are associated with clinical symptoms of heaviness and fullness that are not associated with consistent histological change, but for which a hormonal basis is being elucidated through recent studies. A correlation with prolactin secretion in response to pituitary stimulation, and particularly with bioactive forms of prolactin,[11] brings new supportive evidence not available until recently. This illustrates the need to consider physiological aspects as equal to, or more important than, structural changes in assessing benign disorders. Superimposed on the cyclical changes are the much more radical effects of pregnancy and lactation. With the repeated development and involutional changes of menstruation and pregnancy occurring throughout 40 years of reproductive life, there is abundant opportunity for minor aberrations to occur.

When one studies a section of normal breast from a patient who has no breast complaint or overt clinical disease on examination, the striking feature is the wide spectrum of histological appearance. Figure 4.2 is from an asymptomatic patient in her thirties, and within a small area may be seen well-developed lobules, poorly developed lobules, dilated ducts and normal ducts, lobule-deficient fibrous tissue and fatty tissue.

These normal appearances provide the elements 'fibrosis' and 'adenosis' that have been documented as the histological appearance of biopsies taken from patients with nodular breasts. It has not always been appreciated that the same changes may be evident elsewhere in the same breast, where there is no clinical complaint.

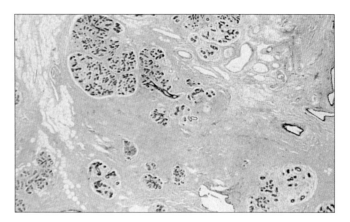

Fig. 4.2 Section from a normal asymptomatic breast. It shows a wide variety of histological appearances, the changes commonly ascribed to 'fibrocystic disease'.

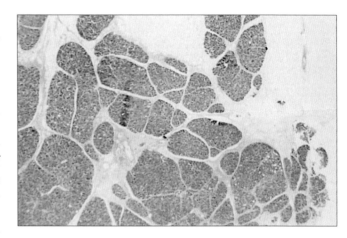

Fig. 4.3 A section of normal pregnant breast, showing extreme, uniform lobular development.

The variability of appearance within the normal breast is illustrated following pregnancy. Under the intense hormonal stimulation associated with pregnancy, a uniform pattern of lobular development and maturation is seen (Fig. 4.3), but postlactational involution is patchy (Fig. 4.4).

With such variable involution following the total stimulation of pregnancy, it is not surprising that the more minor cyclical changes with menstruation can, compounded over a long period, produce marked differences in the structure and appearance of various areas of the breast tissue on a purely random basis.

Breast involution

Involution starts quite early and changes are obvious by 35 years of age and often earlier. Thus, cyclical change

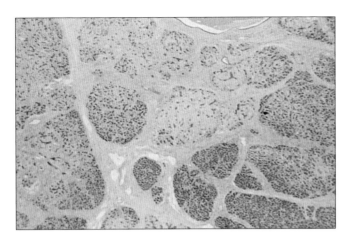

Fig. 4.4 Histological section from a postlactational breast. Involution is patchy, varying from marked to negligible.

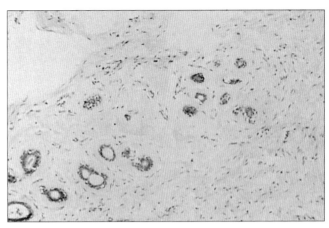

Fig. 4.6 A section of postmenopausal breast, showing advanced lobular involution.

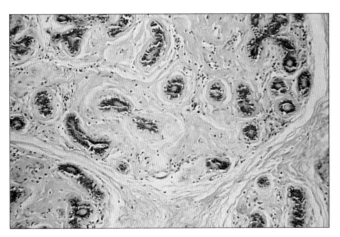

Fig. 4.5 Section from a normal involuting breast. The orderly regression of both epithelial and stromal elements of the lobule is obvious. The lobular stroma has been replaced by fibrous tissue, and there is little residual epithelial tissue.

and involution run in tandem for 20 years or more, increasing the chance of aberration of normality, as reflected in the high frequency of presentation to a breast clinic during this period. The involution affects the lobules particularly and is much dependent on the relationship between the epithelium and specialized stroma of the lobule. In Figure 4.5, which shows an involuting breast, an orderly regression of lobules and surrounding fibrous tissue can be clearly seen.

During this process of lobular involution, the loose hormone-responsive intralobular connective tissue is replaced by the more standard interlobular type of fibrous tissue. If this replacement is well coordinated with the regression of epithelial tissue, the uniform picture of

involution shown in Figure 4.5 is seen. Eventually, by the time the menopause has been reached and passed, involution is extensive (Fig. 4.6) with only a few ducts remaining, and few if any lobular structures.

But it does not always happen in that way, and minor aberrations of this process are very common during a period of fluctuating involution extending over 20 years. It appears that normal epithelial involution of the lobule is dependent on the continuing presence of the specialized stroma around it. Should the stroma disappear too early, the epithelial acini remain and may form microcysts. The exact mechanism is not known, but one finding is that the structural protein fodrin (expressed in normal breast epithelium) is not expressed in micro- or macrocysts,[12] although it is not certain whether this is a primary or secondary phenomenon. Microcysts are obviously a prime target for macroscopic cyst formation if pressure disparity occurs between secretion and drainage, as might occur with obstruction of the draining ductule. Microcyst formation is very common in normal breasts (Fig. 4.7), as demonstrated by Parks,[4] and, in this process of cystic lobular involution, microcysts may appear even though there is still specialized stroma present.

Presumably, this arises from minor obstruction to the duct by kinking or compression from fibrous tissue, or perhaps by vigorous secretion from still active epithelial tissue. (It is interesting that the lobular vein exits from the lobule alongside the ductule, so venous compression readily occurs.)

Recent work has shown that there is continual turnover of fluid within cysts, but, paradoxically, that particular molecules (e.g. hormones) may persist in a cyst for

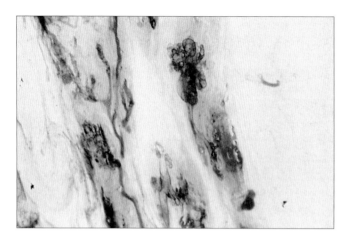

Fig. 4.7 Involuting breast showing microcystic lobular change (thick section technique).

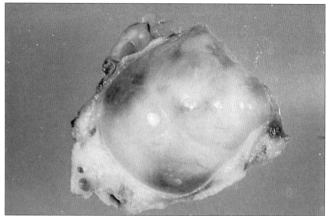

Fig. 4.9 In a fully developed macrocyst, the bands in the wall reflect the origin from gross distension of a number of acini (ductules) within a single lobule.

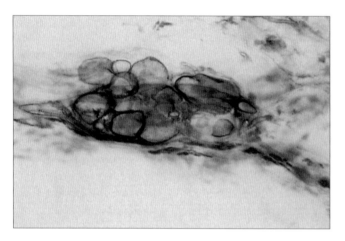

Fig. 4.8 A further stage in the evolution from microcystic involution to macrocyst formation.

months or even years (see Ch. 10). As long as some of the specialized stroma remains, the lobule can still involute normally in spite of these microcysts, but should the specialized stroma disappear early then further cystic change is likely (Fig. 4.8).

Mechanical duct obstruction leading to macrocysts (Fig. 4.9) is almost bound to occur in a proportion of lobules, because there are many possible mechanisms: from internal blockage by epithelial cells or debris, through simple kinking and angulation, to strangulation by the surrounding maturing fibrous tissue.

Recent work on the neonatal breast is of great interest, since it shows that the involution which occurs in the first year of life following withdrawal of maternal hormones follows an identical pattern to that seen over 20 years of adult involution, even to microcyst formation as the stroma reverts to the banal interlobular form. It is now known that the number of ovarian follicles decreases progressively from the age of 35 years, so there is a progressive withdrawal of hormonal stimulation over the full period in which these involutional changes and aberrations occur.

Thus, three periods occur and overlap: lobule development at 15–25 years, cyclical change at 15–50 years and involution at 35–55 years. Each period has its own clinical presentations, but overlapping and interacting processes also lead to complex clinical situations. The introduction of hormone replacement therapy has complicated the situation by extending these changes beyond the menopause. Thus, benign disorders expected to resolve at the menopause may persist, or even arise de novo.

A framework based on pathogenesis

Table 4.2 sets out a classification of the more important clinical benign breast disorders that make up the main constituents of ANDI. An important point of the classification is the replacement of the term disease by disorders in the interpretation of benign breast disorders (BBDs). This does not mean that there is no benign breast disease, but recognizes that most breast complaints are due to disorders based on the normal processes of development, cyclical change and involution, and lie towards the normal or aberration end of the spectrum, with only a few severe enough to be placed at the disease end. The concept that conditions such as fibroadenoma and duct ectasia lie within the normal or minor aberration range is foreign to conventional teaching in pathology and surgery. Hence, we give the reason in some detail.

Reasons for including various benign breast disorders as part of ANDI

Disorders of development

Fibroadenoma

Since it can be shown that fibroadenomas arise from lobules, it is not surprising that these are seen predominantly in women in the 15–25 age group, even though they may not be diagnosed until later, when postpregnancy or involutional changes facilitate clinical recognition in the softer, drooping, involutional breast, or ultrasound demonstrates impalpable lesions.

What is the evidence to support the contention that fibroadenoma should be placed in the benign breast disorder side of ANDI rather than regarded as a neoplasm? Parks[4] showed that hyperplastic lobules, histologically identical to clinical fibroadenomas, are present so commonly as to be regarded as normal; they can probably be found in all breasts if they are sought sufficiently carefully. A full spectrum can be found between these hyperplastic lobules and clinical fibroadenomas, which do not show the inexorable growth typical of true neoplasms. They usually grow to 1 or 2 cm in diameter and then stay constant in size. They show hormonal dependence similar to normal lobules by lactating during pregnancy (Fig.

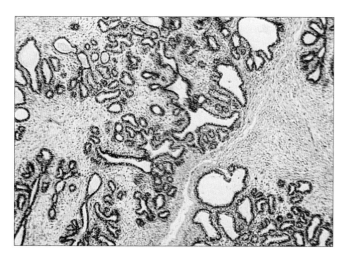

Fig. 4.10 A fibroadenoma removed in the postpartum period. It shows lactation similar to the normal breast, indicating that fibroadenomas respond readily to normal physiological stimuli.

4.10) and will involute, to be replaced by hyaline connective tissue in concert with the rest of the breast in the perimenopausal period.

These hormonal responses are much more complete than those usually seen in benign tumours. Rarely, a fibroadenoma will continue to grow to a size of 3 cm, although this is sufficiently common to be regarded as within the normal spectrum. Growth beyond 5 cm is sufficiently uncommon in Western populations as to justify being regarded as a disease, known as giant fibroadenoma. Similarly, a multiple fibroadenoma (five or more lesions in one breast) is so uncommon in Western populations, and its implications so uncertain, as also to justify being considered a disease. Thus, fibroadenoma fits well into the ANDI classification: small fibroadenomas are normal, clinical fibroadenomas are a mild aberration of the normal processes, and giant and multiple fibroadenomas are placed to the disease end of the spectrum.

Good evidence can be put forward to support this view that fibroadenoma should not be regarded as a neoplasm, as discussed in Chapter 7. All the cellular elements of fibroadenoma are normal on conventional and electron microscopy, and epithelium and myoepithelium maintain a normal relationship,[13] while molecular biology studies have shown that fibroadenomas are polyclonal in keeping with hyperplasia, in contrast to phyllodes tumours which are monoclonal in keeping with a neoplastic condition.

Adolescent hypertrophy

This condition is associated with gross stromal hyperplasia at the time of breast development. The aetiology is unknown, and this is not surprising because so little is known about the control of breast stroma, important though this is. Nevertheless, it is likely that there is a hormonal basis to the condition, a view supported by recent reports that danazol (an antigonadotrophin) may have a beneficial effect. The continuous spectrum from a small breast through to massive hyperplasia fits the horizontal element of the ANDI concept, with excessively large breasts an aberration, and the extreme hyperplasia of gigantomastia placed at the disease end.

Disorders of cyclical change

Mastalgia and nodularity

Premenstrual enlargement and postmenstrual involution of the breast occurring with each cycle is so commonly associated with discomfort and nodularity as to lie firmly within the spectrum of normality. We have used the term 'cyclical pronounced mastalgia' or 'severe painful nodularity' to differentiate the clinical disorder from the more common physiological discomfort and lumpiness. A duration of painful nodularity of more than 1 week of the cycle is a useful definition for differentiation from normal discomfort, and the severity of the pain can be quantified with a pain chart. This is a more pragmatic approach than the inaccurate histological concepts of fibrocystic disease, or the concept of 'non-disease'[14] which is unhelpful to those unfortunate women who suffer from its more severe manifestations. While no histological basis has been defined for these changes, the objection of such women to the concept of non-disease is supported by hormone studies,[11] which show an underlying physiological abnormality demonstrated by excess prolactin release from the pituitary following stimulation of the hypothalamic–pituitary axis.

These findings stress the importance of taking a broad view of benign breast disorders, avoiding undue emphasis on non-specific histological changes and giving due attention to significant physiological changes. It is likely that subtle stromal and epithelial changes accompany physiological variations in more severe cases of cyclical nodularity and mastalgia, but more sensitive techniques may be necessary to demonstrate them. Oedema, stromal or lobular, can be demonstrated in the late cycle, but at present good evidence correlating this with clinical symptoms is lacking.

Painful nodularity of the predominantly cyclical phase of reproductive life (20–35 years) merges into and overlaps those symptoms which are more typically part of the involutional phase, especially cyst formation and sclerosing adenosis. While all have been lumped together as fibrocystic disease (or fibroadenosis) in the past, the clinical problems and management differ.

Disorders of involution

Since the process of involution extends over 20 years of monthly cycles of mitosis and apoptosis, it is not surprising that a number of aberrations should arise involving different elements of the normal breast. As discussed below, the evidence favours an aberration of normal processes for most of these. It is interesting that the incidence of these changes is similar in a number of races with widely differing cancer incidences,[15] supporting the 'normal' view against the 'precancerous' view.

Cyst formation

The desirable integrated involution of stroma and epithelium outlined earlier in this chapter is not always seen, and minor aberrations of the process are understandably common during a period of fluctuating involution extending over 20 years. The exact mechanism of this involution is not well understood,[16] but it appears that the normal epithelial involution of the lobule is dependent on the continuing presence of the specialized stroma around it. If the stroma disappears too early, the epithelial acini remain and may form microcysts, setting the pattern for macrocyst development by obstruction of the efferent ductule as discussed above. This concept of the macrocyst as being an involutional aberration (and hence part of ANDI), rather than a disease, fits in with its common occurrence and the fact that it is so frequently multiple and subclinical.

The fact that macrocysts appear to develop in two directions – apocrine and non-apocrine cysts[17] – is something which is as yet poorly understood, but the evidence is strong that both develop from a common origin of microcystic involution.[18]

Sclerosing adenosis

This condition may be considered as an aberration of either the cyclical or the involutional phase of breast activity because it can show histological changes which are both proliferative and involutional. This illustrates the complexity on the one hand, but the simplicity of concept on the other, of regarding these as aberrations of so many interacting normal processes. Considering the complex interrelationship of stromal fibrosis and epithelial regression occurring during involution, superimposed on cyclical changes of ductal sprouting, it is not surprising that this complex picture, in which epithelial acini are strangled and distorted by fibrous tissue, should arise. It is surprising that it does not occur more commonly.

Duct ectasia and periductal mastitis

The second major group of benign breast disorders consists of those associated with duct ectasia and periductal mastitis. The pathogenesis of duct ectasia is obscure. The classic theory, proposed by Haagensen,[19] regards duct ectasia (dilated ducts) as being the primary event leading to stagnation of secretion, epithelial ulceration and leakage of duct secretions containing chemically irritant fatty acids into periductal tissue to give a chemical inflammatory process. This secondary inflammation is then seen as leading to periductal fibrosis, with subsequent fibrous contraction and nipple retraction.

An alternative theory sees the primary process as periductal mastitis, perhaps on an autoimmune basis, leading to weakening of the muscle layer of the ducts and secondary dilatation. It is likely that both processes may occur separately or in conjunction, thus explaining the wide spectrum of clinical behaviour in this condition. Both duct dilatation and duct sclerosis may represent an aberration of involution. Periductal fibrosis can occur in the absence of duct ectasia or of inflammation[20] and probably represents part of the normal involutional process. Duct ectasia is so common in the postmenopausal breast that it must be regarded as part of the normal ageing process.

The wide variety of clinical symptoms associated with this condition – nipple discharge, nipple retraction, inflammatory masses and abscesses (sterile or bacterial) – can best be explained and understood by accepting more than one process in the pathogenesis. Duct ectasia appears to be a simple involutional process in the elderly, and congenital inversion of the nipple is an aberration of nipple eversion during breast development. Both are aberrations of ANDI, which may progress to disease, as discussed fully in Chapter 11. Nonbacterial periductal inflammation is multifactorial, due to smoking in some cases, idiopathic and possibly involutional in others. The fact that some aspects of this complex condition are clearly parts of ANDI, some parts probably are not, and others are of unknown cause at present, illustrates the view that the ANDI concept should be utilized where it is appropriate, but that those aspects where an association is not obvious can be left outside until the pathogenesis has been clearly established.

Epithelial hyperplasias

The third element of the benign breast disorder complex, epithelial hyperplasias, has given rise to most confusion and problems in management. Many people would see this lying firmly on the side of disease rather than disorder, but a number of studies have shown that this is not so with simple hyperplasias. Parks[4] showed that lobular and intraductal papillary hyperplasia is common in the premenopausal period and tends to regress spontaneously after the menopause, and hence should be regarded as an aberration of normal involution. Kramer and Rush[21]

found in their autopsy study that 59% of women over the age of 70 exhibited some degree of epithelial hyperplasia. Sloss et al.[22] concluded from their autopsy study that 'the mere presence of blunt duct adenosis, apocrine epithelium and intraductal epithelial hyperplasia in the breast of women is insufficient to warrant such tissue being called disease'.

Hence the simple epithelial hyperplasias may be placed firmly within the concept of benign breast disorder. However, careful studies by Page et al.[7] and Wellings et al.[23] have shown that the other ends of the spectrum – atypical lobular hyperplasia and atypical ductal hyperplasia – particularly as seen in the terminal ductal lobular unit (TDLU), are sufficiently commonly associated with malignancy as to be regarded as associated or premalignant conditions. Hence, epithelial hyperplasias with marked atypia belong firmly under the column of BBD.

There is at present insufficient evidence to allow a firm opinion as to whether conditions placed under the benign breast disorder column present a continuous spectrum, with the implication that the 'disorders' move to 'diseases'. They may be entirely separate processes and certainly, at the present time, no such progression of hyperplasias to cancer in situ should be assumed; it should be left as an open question.

An extension of the concept of ANDI to include most benign breast disorders?

Since the conceptual thinking prior to ANDI was encompassed in the chronic mastitis/fibroadenosis/fibrocystic disease attitude to BBD, it is not surprising that ANDI is equated sometimes with these conditions and used as a synonym for painful nodularity. This is restrictive, as it has been shown that a majority of benign breast disorders lie within the concept, some clearly do not and some remain inconclusive.[24] Our current view of the classification of all benign disorders is shown in Table 4.2. Most conditions are regarded as part of ANDI, and the old term 'fibroadenosis' is designated 'painful nodularity of ANDI'.

Some of the less common benign breast disorders also fit well into the concept of aberrations of normality and it is useful to consider the arguments for including them within this framework. Briefly, these arguments are as follows:

- *Nipple inversion*: This is an aberration of development of the terminal ducts, preventing the normal protrusion of ducts and areola.
- *Mammary duct fistula*: Nipple inversion predisposes to terminal duct obstruction, leading to recurrent subareolar abscess and mammary duct fistula, the usual form of periductal mastitis seen in younger women. Extraneous factors such as smoking and oro-nipple contact interact with the processes of ANDI.
- *Epithelial hyperplasia of pregnancy*: Marked hyperplasia of the duct epithelium occurs in pregnancy, and the papillary projections sometimes give rise to bilateral bloody nipple discharge, a condition which is always benign when occurring in pregnancy.
- *Benign duct papilloma*: This is a common condition during the period of cyclical activity and shows minimal if any malignant potential. It is reasonable to regard it as an aberration of cyclical epithelial activity.
- *Adenosis*: For similar reasons it might be considered logical to extend the concept of aberration of normality to encompass adenosis as a manifestation of involution.

Implications for the management of benign breast disorders

It follows from the foregoing that most of the conditions listed under benign breast disorders can be regarded as minor aberrations of normality and hence do not demand active specific treatment. This being the case, any active management of these conditions should be based on considerations such as accurate diagnosis, patient concern and interference with quality of life. No treatment is required based solely on inherent pathological significance until the disease end of the spectrum is reached. This concept of management is outlined here and details of management are given in the appropriate chapters.

Adolescent hypertrophy

In its more severe forms, treatment is indicated because of psychological and physical morbidity from the size and weight of the breast. It is the degree of this morbidity that determines treatment with hormonal or surgical therapy.

Fibroadenoma

The concept of fibroadenoma being a part of ANDI and not a neoplasm has been one of the conceptual changes behind us moving gradually from active to conservative management over the past 20 years. The results from many centres now justify this approach, as discussed in Chapter 7.

Inverted nipple

This is the failure of development of major ducts, and treatment short of severing the ducts is unlikely to give a long-term satisfactory result. Hence, treatment is related to the patient's view of the cosmetic deformity, and recommended only after recognizing the uncertain long-term results of minor surgical procedures for this condition, and the consequences of total duct division for cosmesis and lactation if the defect is to undergo total correction.

Likewise, recurrent subareolar abscess associated with nipple inversion will require eradication of the sump-like dilated duct underlying the recurrent infection.

Cyclical mastalgia and nodularity

It is generally accepted that these manifestations are physiological, and that most cases can be treated by adequate reassurance. But the view that the most severe cases, those lasting perhaps 2 weeks or more of the menstrual cycle, interfere so much with the quality of life as to merit consideration as disease is confirmed by the high incidence of hormonal abnormalities in these patients. It is unhelpful to tell the patient that she has a non-disease if her symptoms interfere with her quality of life. Rather, the severity of her mastalgia should be assessed objectively with pain charts so that her condition can be placed on the normal–aberration–disease scale and appropriate management instituted. There is equally strong evidence that most cases are not psychologically based, and hence endocrine-related treatment is appropriate in those cases severe enough to warrant therapy.[25]

Cysts

Macrocysts and microcysts are so common as to need no active treatment other than that required to allow diagnosis and allay patient concern. It is now well established by practice that simple cysts are satisfactorily treated by aspiration, a policy that might have been predicted from the ANDI concept. The recent differentiation of cysts into apocrine and non-apocrine[17] does not at present alter this conservative therapeutic approach, because any breast cancer risk is a general one, and not related to the individual cyst. Likewise, since the condition is a minor aberration of a normal process, excision is not required for multiple or recurrent cysts, except in the presence of a bloody aspirate or a residual lump, both requiring exclusion of coexisting cancer.

Sclerosing adenosis

This condition causes diagnostic problems to surgeons, radiologists and histopathologists and sometimes problems to the patient in the form of a lump or pain. It requires no treatment other than careful exclusion of cancer, although it sometimes requires symptomatic treatment for pain.

Postmenopausal nipple retraction

The only importance of this is to recognize that it may be caused by the simple involutional process of periductal fibrosis. It requires no active management other than exclusion of cancer. In our experience, nipple retraction is more commonly due to ductal fibrosis than to cancer, and fortunately the diagnosis is easily made in older patients because the postmenopausal breast lends itself to accurate mammography.

Duct ectasia/periductal mastitis complex

The symptoms of this condition that can be categorized under the aberration column cause little clinical upset and require no therapy other than reassurance for opaque, non-bloody discharge.

Rarely, the discharge may be sufficiently profuse to cause social embarrassment. In this case, after a pituitary adenoma has been excluded, the patient may be treated in mechanical fashion by a total duct excision. This approach is rarely necessary, but it again demonstrates the value of assessing the impact of symptoms on quality of life to place them appropriately along the spectrum of severity.

Management of blood-related discharge is directed towards excluding more serious pathology.

Epithelial hyperplasias

Epithelial hyperplasias without atypia usually found as a chance histological finding fall somewhere between normality and an aberration in significance. With atypical hyperplasias, the emphasis moves towards the disease state, and special consideration should be given to assessment of cancer risk, as defined particularly by Page and Dupont.[9]

Aberration to disease?

The ANDI concept is based on the progression from normal to aberration to disease. Sound evidence for the progression from normal to aberration exists, as discussed in the section on fibroadenoma. However, no evidence exists for or against the supposition that giant fibroadenomas arise from the continued progression of small fibroadenomas, i.e. that aberration progresses to disease. It is possible that giant fibroadenoma is a separate condition de novo, or an added factor may lead to progression from a 'standard' fibroadenoma. There is certainly evidence from molecular biology that a change from polyclonality occurs with phyllodes tumours, although it is not clear whether this is a secondary change in a fibroadenoma, or is present in a phyllodes tumour de novo (see Ch. 7).

Likewise, it is likely that normal epithelium and apocrine changes form a continuum with simple hyperplasias, but there is less evidence to support the direct progression from the latter to atypical hyperplasias or carcinoma in situ. Thus, on the basis of present evidence we do not know whether disease in this case is a progression from aberration or whether disease and aberration are two separate conditions.

This is one of the most interesting areas of benign breast disorders, and new evidence is starting to provide answers to some of these questions. For instance, simple fibroadenoma is classified as an aberration, but multiple fibroadenomas are sufficiently rare and troublesome to be classified as disease. It has recently been found that transplant patients on ciclosporin have an increased incidence of multiple fibroadenomas, giving a new insight into progression from aberration to disease. Cigarette smoking has a similar significance for duct ectasia/periductal mastitis, and it is likely that the various factors that lead to atypical hyperplasias will become elucidated in the near future.

The time is approaching when we are likely to have much greater insight into these questions. Meanwhile, this does not compromise the utility of the ANDI classification in helping understand benign breast disorders, and the concepts are sufficiently flexible to allow us to incorporate new information as it becomes available. The past 10 years have seen the concept strengthened and refined by new knowledge.

Recent developments having a bearing on the ANDI concept

Apocrine metaplasia

Apocrine metaplasia has a particular interest in that it is a frequent finding in ANDI, suggesting normality, yet carrying a slight but definite increase in cancer risk. For that reason, there is much interest in possible mechanisms for indicating cancer risk, and which might throw light on the evolution from normal to aberration to disease.

Haagensen[26] suggested three possible mechanisms by which apocrine metaplasia might relate to cancer:

- Apocrine metaplasia is a precursor to malignant transformation.
- Apocrine metaplasia may result from a response to the same stimulus as can cause cancer.
- Apocrine metaplasia might itself have a higher propensity for malignant change.

Kumar and colleagues[27] demonstrated by an immunohistochemical technique that cells of apocrine metaplasia have very high levels of prolactin not seen in normal ductal cells, blunt duct adenosis, lobules or fibroadenoma. Tschugguel et al.[28] found that apocrine metaplastic cells demonstrate endothelial calcium-dependent nitric oxide synthase, unlike other cells of benign breast disorders, suggesting that the vascular effects of nitric oxide might play a part in progression to malignant change. A study of fetal breast tissue has made the situation even more complex.[29] Epithelial cells bearing a biochemical marker for apocrine cells (anti-GCDFP-15 monoclonal antibody) were found in some duct cells of fetal breasts, and in lobules of adult breasts, although no cells with histological or ultrastructural apocrine features were found. This suggests that apocrine cells appear when some unknown stimulus causes apocrine precursor cells to take on the typical morphology.

Cyst formation and duct ectasia

These processes have largely eluded research efforts into pathogenesis, although the absence of fodrin in the wall of cysts may be important.[12] Animal experiments are notoriously irrelevant to human breast disease, although the action of keratinocyte growth factor (KGF-7) commands some interest in such an otherwise sterile field. Yi et al.[30] have shown that this stromal cell-derived paracrine mediator for epithelial proliferation causes hyperplastic changes in ducts in rats similar to ANDI. In mice it causes dilatation of ducts along much of their length (duct ectasia?), and when given together with exogenous oestrogen and progesterone, it produces numerous end-buds with a picture resembling the histological changes of ANDI.

Fibroadenoma and hyperplasias

It seems likely that an imbalance between cell proliferation and apoptosis may be involved in the development of ANDI conditions, as breast tissues under hormonal control undergo continuing remodelling, involving a balance between quiescence, proliferation and apoptosis. Evidence supporting this is becoming available: Ferrieres et al.[31] found that bcl-2 levels in normal ducts and lobules varied with the menstrual cycle, being higher in the follicular than luteal phases, with high progesterone levels apparently suppressing bcl-2 activity. Levels of bcl-2 were higher and the progesterone effect absent in fibroadenomas, giving a possible mechanism for excessive lobular growth in this condition. There is also evidence for a role for matrix metalloproteinases in this hormone control of reproductive organs.[32]

Allan et al. studied apoptosis in normal epithelial cells adjacent to pathology (fibroadenoma, fibrocystic disease and cancer), and found reduced apoptosis in the case of the latter two.[33] They suggest that this reduced apoptosis may be the cause of cellular build-up in ANDI, although an alternative is that the pathological tissue could affect apoptosis by a (secondary) paracrine mechanism.

Loss of heterozygosity (LOH) is an indicator of a clonal, neoplastic condition rather than a simple hyperplasia. Lakhani et al. have shown that LOH is a feature of atypical ductal hyperplasia (ADH) as well as ductal and lobular carcinoma in situ (DCIS and LCIS), suggesting that the essential step towards malignancy (aberration to disease) has already taken place at the stage of ADH. They have recently shown[34] evidence of LOH in some cases of ductal hyperplasia without atypia, but not in apocrine cysts or benign papillomas. The cases showing LOH could not be distinguished morphologically from those without. This would suggest that progression from aberration to disease may occur early in some cases of hyperplasia without atypia, presumably those that will progress to more severe pathology, or that these cases may be different ab initio. However, other workers[35] have found differing results, emphasizing the preliminary nature of these approaches.

These findings as yet raise as many questions as they answer, but they do hold out hope that similar techniques may soon give a much deeper understanding of the mechanisms of ANDI, and of the relationship between aberration and disease.

REFERENCES

1. Hughes LE, Mansel RE & Webster DJTW. Aberrations of normal development and involution (ANDI): a new perspective on pathogenesis and nomenclature of benign breast disorders. *Lancet* 1987; **2**: 1316–1319.

2. Hughes LE, Smallwood J & Dixon JM. Nomenclature of benign breast disorders: report of a working party on the rationalisation of concepts and terminology of benign breast conditions. *The Breast* 1992; **1**: 15–17.

3. McFarland J. Residual lactation acini in the female breast. Their relationship to chronic cystic mastitis and malignant breasts. *Archives of Surgery* 1922; **5**: 1–64.

4. Parks AG. The microanatomy of the breast. *Annals of the Royal College of Surgeons of England* 1959; **25**: 295–311.

5. Sarnelli R & Squartini F. Fibrocystic condition and 'at risk' lesions in asymptomatic breasts: a morphological study of postmenopausal women. *Clinical and Experimental Obstetrics and Gynecology* 1991; **18**: 271–279.

6. Hutson SW, Cowen PN & Bird CC. Morphometric studies of age related changes in normal human breast and their significance for evolution of mammary cancer. *Journal of Clinical Pathology* 1985; **38**: 281–287.

7. Page DL, Vander-Zwag R, Roger LW *et al.* Relationship between component parts of fibrocystic disease complex and breast cancer. *Journal of the National Cancer Institute* 1978; **61**: 1055–1063.

8. DiLieto A, De Rosa G, Albano G *et al.* Desogestrone versus gestodene in oral contraceptives: influence on the clinical and histomorphological features of BBD. *European Journal of Obstetrics, Gynecology, and Reproductive Biology* 1994; **55**: 71–83.

9. Page DL & Dupont WD. Anatomic indicators (histologic and cytologic) of increased breast cancer risk. *Breast Cancer Research and Treatment* 1993; **28**: 157–162.

10. Vorherr H. *The Breast. Morphology, Physiology and Lactation.* New York: Academic Press; 1974.

11. Kumar S, Mansel RE, Hughes LE *et al.* Prediction of response to endocrine therapy in pronounced cyclical mastalgia, using dynamic tests of prolactin release. *Clinical Endocrinology* 1985; **23**: 699–704.

12. Simpson JF & Page DL. Loss of expression of fodrin (a structural protein) in cystic changes in the human breast. *Laboratory Investigation* 1993; **68**: 537–540.

13. Archer F & Omar N. The fine structure of fibroadenoma of the human breast. *Journal of Pathology* 1969; **99**: 113–117.

14. Love SM, Gelman RS & Silen W. Fibrocystic 'disease' of the breast – a non disease. *New England Journal of Medicine* 1982; **307**: 1010–1014.

15. Bartow SA, Pathak DR, Black WC *et al.* Prevalence of benign, atypical and malignant breast lesions in populations at different risk of breast cancer. *Cancer* 1987; **60**: 2751–2760.

16. Azzopardi JG. *Problems in Breast Pathology.* London: WB Saunders; 1979.

17. Miller WR, Dixon JM, Scott WN *et al.* Classification of human breast cysts according to electrolyte and androgen conjugate composition. *Clinical Oncology* 1983; **9**: 227–232.

18. Dixon JM, Scott WN & Miller WR. An analysis of the content and morphology of human breast microcysts. *European Journal of Surgical Oncology* 1985; **11**: 151–154.

19. Haagensen CD. Mammary duct ectasia – a disease that may simulate carcinoma. *Cancer* 1951; **4**: 749–761.

20. Davies JD. Inflammatory damage to ducts in mammary dysplasia: a cause of duct obliteration. *Journal of Pathology* 1975; **117**: 47–54.

21. Kramer WM & Rush BF. Mammary duct proliferation in the elderly – a histological study. *Cancer* 1973; **31**: 130–137.

22. Sloss PT, Bennett WA & Clagett OT. Incidence in normal breasts of features associated with chronic cystic mastitis. *American Journal of Pathology* 1957; **33**: 1181–1191.

23. Wellings SR, Jensen HM & Marcum RG. An atlas of subgross pathology of the human breast with reference to possible pre-cancerous lesions. *Journal of the National Cancer Institute* 1975; **55**: 231–273.

24. Hughes LE. Classification of benign breast disorders. *British Medical Bulletin* 1991; **47**: 251–257.

25. Pye JK, Mansel RE & Hughes LE. Clinical experience of drug treatments for mastalgia. *Lancet* 1985; **ii**: 373–377.

26. Haagensen DE Jr. Is cystic disease related to cancer? *American Journal of Surgical Pathology* 1991; **15**: 687–694.

27. Kumar S, Mansel RE & Jasani B. Presence and possible significance of immunohistochemically demonstrable prolactin in breast apocrine metaplasia. *British Journal of Cancer* 1987; **55**: 307–309.

28. Tschugguel W, Knogler W, Czerwenka K *et al.* Presence of endothelial calcium-dependent nitric oxide synthase in breast apocrine metaplasia. *British Journal of Cancer* 1996; **74**: 1423–1426.

29. Viacava P, Naccarato AG & Bevilacqua G. Apocrine metaplasia of the breast: does it result from metaplasia? *Virchows Archiv. A, Pathological Anatomy and Histopathology* 1997; **431**: 205–209.

30. Yi ES, Bedoya AA, Lee H *et al.* Keratinocyte growth factor causes cystic dilatation of the mammary glands in mice. *American Journal of Pathology* 1994; **145**: 1015–1022.

31. Ferrieres G, Cuny M, Simony-Lafontaine J *et al.* Variation of bcl-2 expression in breast ducts and lobules in relation to plasma progesterone levels: overexpression and absence of variation in fibroadenomas. *Journal of Pathology* 1997; **183**: 204–211.

32. Hulboy DL, Rudolph LA & Matrisian LM. Matrix metalloproteinases as mediators of reproductive function. *Molecular Human Reproduction* 1997; **3**: 27–45.

33. Allan DJ, Howell A, Roberts SA *et al.* Reduction in apoptosis relative to mitosis in histologically normal epithelium accompanies fibrocystic change and carcinoma in the premenopausal breast. *Journal of Pathology* 1992; **167**: 25–32.

34. Lakhani SR, Slack DN, Hamoudi RA *et al.* Detection of loss of heterozygosity (LOH) indicates that mammary hyperplasia of usual type is a clonal, neoplastic proliferation. *Journal of Pathology* 1996; **178**(Suppl): 5A.

35. Kasami M, Vnencak-Jones CL, Manning S *et al.* Loss of heterozygosity and microsatellite instability in breast hyperplasia. *American Journal of Pathology* 1997; **150**: 1925–1932.

CHAPTER 5

The approach to diagnosis and assessment of breast lumps

Key points and new developments

1. Triple assessment – clinical examination, imaging and pathology – is the standard approach to all breast lumps.

2. Examination, ultrasound and core biopsy should normally be available at the first visit.

3. A standard sequence should be followed to exclude normal structures and differentiate normal nodularity from a dominant lump.

4. A clear discharge policy is desirable to prevent clinics being overwhelmed by patients without serious disease.

5. Ultrasound is important in differentiating a discrete lump from general nodularity, in locating deep-seated cysts and in ensuring accurate targeting for core biopsy and cytology specimens.

6. Guidelines regarding staffing and organization of breast clinics have been drawn up in the UK to ensure efficient handling of patients by appropriately experienced staff.

PART 1: The differential diagnosis and clinical assessment of breast lumps

Although imaging and wide-bore needle biopsy, the second and third aspects of triple assessment, are of increasing importance in reaching a rapid, accurate diagnosis of a breast lump, clinical assessment is still of great value in ensuring that these are used to best advantage. It is also important to be aware of the many minor and less common abnormalities which may simulate a pathological breast lump; this awareness may save the patient much unnecessary investigation.

It is fortunate that, although there are many causes of lumps in the breast (Table 5.1), a few diagnoses cover the large majority.

There are two major problems of diagnosis: first to decide whether the lump is within or outside the spec-

trum of normality and, secondly, if abnormal, whether it is benign or malignant.

In the past, there has been a tendency to biopsy all breast lumps irrespective of their characteristics. This results in a large number of biopsies. In one series,[1] 75% of benign biopsies showed tissues which could be regarded as normal. Because benign lumps need just as careful assessment as malignant ones and in an effort to avoid unnecessary biopsies and, in particular, repeated unnecessary biopsies, the practice of triple assessment has been widely accepted, as set out in this chapter. The introduction of cytology into the breast clinic in one study reduced the overall open biopsy rate by half, and the rate for benign masses by two-thirds.[2] Improved biopsy

Table 5.1 Causes of lumps in the breast

Type	Cause	Frequency of presentation
Normal structures	Normal nodularity	Common
	Prominent fat lobule	Less common
	Prominent rib	Less common
	Intramammary lymph node	Rare
	Edge of biopsy wound	Less common
	Accessory breast	Rare
ANDI	Fibroadenoma	Common
	Cyclical nodularity	Common
	Cyst	Common
	Galactocele	Rare
	Sclerosing adenosis	Less common
	Stromal fibrosis	Rare
Inflammatory	Chronic infective abscess	Rare
	Fat necrosis	Rare
	Foreign body granuloma	Rare
	Mondor's disease	Rare
Benign tumours	Duct papilloma	Less common
	Giant fibroadenoma	Rare
	Lipoma	Rare
	Granular cell myoblastoma	Rare
Intermediate tumours	Phyllodes tumour	Rare
	Carcinoma in situ	Less common
Malignant	Primary tumour	Common
	Secondary tumour	Rare
Lesions of the nipple and areola	Squamous papilloma	Less common
	Leiomyoma	Rare
	Retention cyst	Rare
	Papillary adenoma	Rare
Lesions of the skin	Sebaceous cyst	Less common
	Hydradenitis	Rare
	Benign and malignant skin tumours	Rare

techniques mean that open biopsy is now performed infrequently.

Clinical assessment of a breast lump

History

The history is particularly important in the assessment of breast lumps, especially in relation to the duration of the mass, fluctuation in size with the menstrual cycle and any associated pain. Each must be considered in association with the overall clinical picture and no one feature should be allowed to dominate clinical thinking. In the past, it has been widely thought that a small, painful lump is not malignant; however, pain can be the primary presentation of cancer in around 6% of cases,[3] although it should be noted that the pain indicative of cancer differs in characteristics from that of cyclical mastalgia (see Ch. 8).

Inspection

Detailed and systematic examination is of great importance, particularly in elucidating the early signs of malignancy. These are well known, but two of them, skin attachment and nipple inversion, can sometimes be caused by benign conditions.

Cancer is the likely diagnosis when nipple retraction is associated with a lump, but two benign lumps may also cause nipple retraction. A chronic abscess associated with periductal mastitis may cause retraction by a combination of shortening of the ducts and areola oedema. A large cyst or fibroadenoma arising centrally among the major ducts can cause relative shortening by displacement and so give rise to apparent nipple retraction (Fig. 5.1).

The same mechanism can operate with skin attachment. Haagensen[4] called this false retraction. Large cysts or fibroadenomas can displace Cooper's ligaments and give rise to apparent skin fixity and distortion, while a chronic abscess associated with periductal mastitis will lead to actual skin attachment, oedema and sometimes 'peau d'orange'. Mondor's disease may also give rise to the appearance of skin retraction (see Fig. 17.10). It is therefore necessary to obtain cytological or histological confirmation in all cases of suspected malignancy.

Palpation

History before palpation remains important, because of the increasing use of devices which can confound breast examination, ranging from augmentation prostheses to pacemakers. The patient may forget to mention it, or may assume that the physician will recognize it.

Consistency, surface characteristics and mobility in relation to surrounding tissues are each important in diagnosing benign lesions. A fibroadenoma has a characteristic rubbery consistency, a smooth or lobulated surface and a considerable degree of mobility within the breast. This combination of characteristics provides an

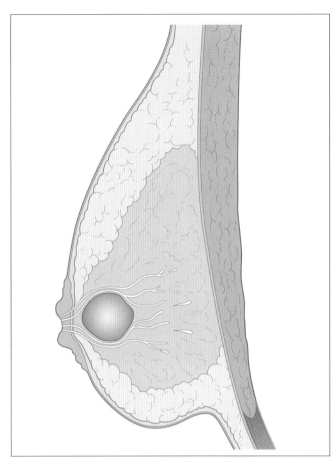

Fig. 5.1 A large benign cyst may stretch and distort main ducts or Cooper's ligaments, leading to 'pseudoretraction' of skin or nipple.

unequivocal clinical diagnosis. This classic pattern is usual in young girls, but in older women a fibroadenoma may not have its characteristic features if surrounded by involutional changes.

While palpation of a moderately tense cyst is equally characteristic, the clinical findings vary depending on the degree of intracystic tension, which may vary from normal tissue tension to a hardness which exceeds that of cancer. Thus, cysts are commonly misdiagnosed. They may be missed completely because they are soft; but in other cases cancer is confidently diagnosed because the cyst is so hard. The surface of a cyst is usually smooth, but a large cyst may be lobulated and occasionally a group of small cysts will feel nodular so as to simulate a fibroadenoma.

Assessment of the mobility of a breast lump within the surrounding tissue provides diagnostic information; as illustrated in Figure 5.2, there are three degrees of mobility of a lump in relation to the surrounding breast tissue.

A fibroadenoma has no attachment to a surrounding capsule except for a single stalk, so it is very mobile. The wall of a cyst is confluent with the fibrous breast stroma; hence the surrounding parenchyma can be felt to move with the cyst, giving it an intermediate degree of mobility. At the other extreme, an infiltrating cancer fixes the surrounding breast tissue so that the affected quadrant of the breast moves with the mass. But, occasionally, a very large

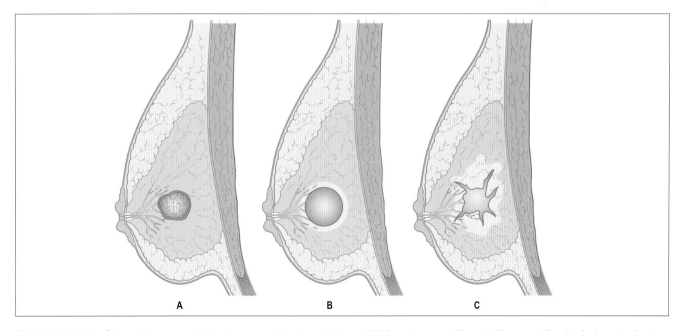

A   B   C

Fig. 5.2 Mobility of breast lumps in relation to surrounding breast tissue. (**A**) Fibroadenoma; (**B**) cyst; (**C**) cancer. The shaded area indicates the amount of breast tissue 'moving' with the lump.

cyst or benign tumour will have a similar effect by stretch-fixation of Cooper's ligaments so that the quadrant of the breast moves with the lump.

Palpation is even more important for ill-defined lumps. By far the commonest problem in breast assessment is to decide whether an area which feels abnormal to the patient is truly abnormal, or whether it is part of general nodularity of the breast. This arises particularly when a woman's attention is drawn to the upper outer quadrant of the breast by premenstrual pain or tenderness. Careful assessment to determine the pattern of nodularity in both breasts is essential. One breast should be compared with the other. It is surprising how often an apparent single mass is found to be bilateral and symmetrical when the mirror image sections of the breast are examined together. In this situation, ultrasound is invaluable in deciding if a true discrete abnormality is present or whether the palpable abnormality is simply glandular breast tissue. If an abnormal area is noted on ultrasound it can be sampled histologically under ultrasound guidance.

A complete physical examination, including axillary and supraclavicular fossa palpation, is important in all breast disease, but rarely provides discriminatory diagnostic information with benign conditions.

Assessment of nodularity

Normal nodularity or a dominant lump?

The commonest presenting lump in women during the reproductive period is normal breast nodularity, or the cyclical nodularity of aberrations of normal development and involution (ANDI), felt in the upper outer quadrant and axillary tail of the breast.

To decide whether a mass is dominant or merely part of normal or cyclical nodularity is critical in order for an early carcinoma not to be missed. Assessment is essentially clinical in young women, supplemented by ultrasound, with or without core needle histology. In an older woman (>35 years) where there is doubt as to whether or not a dominant mass is present, mammography and ultrasound are indicated.

To avoid unnecessary biopsy, a well-defined approach must be taken to determine whether a mass is dominant and persistent. If a single examination is inconclusive, the following sequence is useful:

- Examine both breasts.
- Confirm or refute a localized abnormality by ultrasound examination.

- Use wide-bore needle biopsy for histology if necessary.
- If there is any inconsistency in the results, review the patient 2 months later. If doubt still persists or any of the triple assessment tests are discordant, repeat biopsy should be performed.

Clinical findings are recorded on a scale of 1 to 5. If full assessment shows nothing more than general nodularity that is deemed to be within normal limits (P2), reassurance and explanation of the physiological basis of the nodularity is adequate treatment. Specific treatment is only required when pain is the major symptom; this is dealt with in the section on breast pain (see Ch. 8).

Particular notice should be taken of a patient who is certain that she can feel an abnormality in her breast, especially if she is over the age of 40. A woman may feel an abnormality some time before her medical attendant is able to do so, and the older the patient, the more likely she is to be right. Such a patient should be subjected to a full triple assessment and, if no abnormality is found on examination or investigation, she should be reviewed in 2–4 months.

Assessment of a discrete or dominant mass

Having decided that a lump is not just part of normal nodularity, the physical characteristics should be carefully assessed to make a specific diagnosis. If the clinical features are definitely those of a normal structure and this is confirmed by triple assessment, surgical biopsy can be avoided. Nevertheless, the emphasis must always be on repeat assessment and ultimately excisional biopsy if doubt persists regarding the diagnosis of any persisting dominant mass in a woman of cancer age group or where one of the elements of the triple assessment is discordant.

Features of individual lesions

Normal structures

Prominent fat lobule

Fat lobules are often easily palpable and one may become more prominent than another. This is seen most frequently along the inferior margin of the breast or over the axillary tail. The superficial nature of the lesion, its site, soft, smooth consistency and softness to a needle point will usually allow a confident diagnosis. Ultrasound also clearly shows the fat lobules as characteristic fat pockets.

Prominent rib

It is not uncommon for a patient, usually young, to present with a 'breast lump' which appears to be normal breast tissue over a normal prominent rib or costochondral junction. Sometimes the rib is asymmetrical, but more often it is identical to the opposite side and it is difficult to know why the patient has suddenly become aware of it. Ultrasound of the area of patient concern can be reassuring.

Intramammary lymph node

Intramammary lymph nodes are usually confined to the axillary tail of the breast and are impalpable because they are small and embedded in the breast stroma. Sometimes lymph nodes in the outer quadrant of the breast proper may enlarge sufficiently to be palpable. Although they feel cystic, they are slightly elongated and peripheral to the breast area. They have a soft feel to a needle point and have a characteristic appearance on mammography and ultrasound, being smooth ovoid lesions, sometimes with a notch along one margin. Lymphocytes are found on cytology, which can be guided by ultrasound for small mobile nodes. It is usually possible to make a diagnosis and to avoid surgery.

Accessory breasts

Accessory breasts occur under the anterior axillary fold, are usually bilateral and come to notice during pregnancy or if the patient gains weight. They may be affected by the full range of breast pathology, including nodularity, or cysts of ANDI, fibroadenoma, carcinoma, etc. The condition is described more fully in Chapter 15.

Edge of a previous biopsy wound

Patients may present complaining of a 'lump' at the site of a previous scar which is due to the persisting edge of a defect in the breast which sometimes occurs after a large amount of tissue has been removed. These are seen less often now that nonsurgical methods of diagnosis have improved and better localization allows smaller biopsies to be taken for diagnostic purposes if open biopsy is required. They are most common deep to the nipple/areola, and the most important aspect is awareness.

Masses due to ANDI

Fibroadenoma

In its classic form, this tumour is the most easily diagnosed breast lump. When it occurs in the age group of 15–25 years it is rubbery, firm, smooth or lobulated and extremely mobile. Clinical diagnosis is usually accurate but ultrasound and histology (fine needle aspiration cytology [FNAC] or core needle biopsy) is essential in all patients, even in this age group. While cytology could be used for women younger than 25 years, fibroadenoma is one of the lesions that are well known to cause difficulties in cytopathological diagnosis and therefore a core biopsy is preferable if possible.

Fibroadenomas are also commonly seen in later life when the diagnosis is much more difficult. The patient has now reached the cancer age group, so definite exclusion of malignancy is mandatory. The fibroadenoma is caught up in the involutional fibrosis of the breast, so that it loses its characteristic smoothness and mobility; it requires full assessment as for any other dominant lump, by clinical assessment, mammography and needle biopsy. Calcified and noncalcified fibroadenomas are often seen on screening mammograms.

The clinical and radiological similarities between fibroadenoma, cyst and some circumscribed cancers (especially medullary cancer) should be remembered. Where an otherwise typical fibroadenoma is softer than expected, a phyllodes tumour should be suspected (see Ch. 7).

Cyclical nodularity ('fibroadenosis')

The problem of cyclical nodularity has already been discussed – the discrimination between general nodularity and a prominent mass in an individual patient. The problem becomes worse as normal nodularity moves across the spectrum to the more severe cyclical nodularity of ANDI.

Perhaps the most interesting aspect of this problem is why some patients with cyclical nodularity develop a dominant lump. In many cases, cyst formation or localized adenosis with or without fibrosis may underlie the mass, but in other cases, histological findings are no different from the adjacent clinically unremarkable breast. Exaggerated local end-organ response to hormonal stimulation seems the most likely cause.

The recognition of the basic normality of cyclical nodularity as a part of ANDI should be extended to histological assessment.

Cysts

A cyst is the commonest discrete mass found in patients presenting to a breast clinic. It has been estimated that about 1 in 10 of all women will develop a symptomatic breast cyst during their reproductive life, and recurrent or multiple cysts are common.

Clinical diagnosis is surprisingly uncertain; variation in size, variation in shape, multiplicity and variation in consistency due to intracystic pressure mean that cysts can as easily be missed completely as confidently diagnosed as cancer. Fortunately, a definite diagnosis is made by a typical appearance on ultrasound and simple needle aspiration which is done clinically or under ultrasound guidance.

Galactocele

Galactocele presents in the same way as a cyst, some time after parturition. It is managed in the same way as other cysts, and is discussed more fully in Chapter 10.

Sclerosing adenosis

Sclerosing adenosis presents most commonly as a radiological abnormality, a chance histological finding or as a cause of mastalgia. When it presents as a lump, it is dealt with as any dominant mass, and requires no specific treatment (see Ch. 9).

The remaining lesions listed in Table 5.1 present in more specific fashion than the manifestations of ANDI and are dealt with in the appropriate sections of this text.

Isolated axillary masses

The possibility of benign axillary pathology mimicking cancer should be remembered. Reactive lymphadenopathy and ANDI in axillary accessory breast tissue are two conditions which may mimic secondary cancer, and both illustrate the importance of separate assessment of axillary masses.

The commonest cause of a clinically significant axillary mass is occult malignancy, either from the breast (often ipsi- or contralateral) or other sites of carcinoma or lymphoid malignancy. Benign causes include reactive lymphadenopathy (temporary or associated with conditions such as rheumatoid arthritis), lipoma or accessory breast tissue containing any pathology (including manifesta-

tions of ANDI) that may be seen in the breast itself.[5] Isolated axillary masses are subjected to the same triple assessment as breast lumps.

Follow-up after assessment and/or benign breast biopsy

A clearly defined discharge policy is particularly important in busy breast clinics because routine follow-up of patients presenting with breast lumps is not necessary once a definite diagnosis has been made.

- Patients over the age of 50 should be encouraged to attend the regular NHS Breast Screening Programme (NHSBSP).
- Most patients should be discharged at the first clinic visit, but if there are any equivocal results or diagnostic uncertainty persists, the patient is best managed by reassessment after 2 months.

All results of triple assessment should be reviewed at a regular multidisciplinary meeting which includes radiologists, pathologists and surgeons discussing all patients who have had biopsies.

Most benign breast lumps are not now excised, unless the diagnosis has not been confirmed.

Management of recurrent lumps following biopsy

Many breast lumps, such as fibroadenoma, cysts and nodularity, are prone to be multiple over a period of time. However, a new lump may be cancer, so any new lump must be reassessed in the same way as the original lump.

When a lump appears in the region of a previous biopsy it must also be reassessed completely but a number of additional factors need consideration.

Recurrent fibroadenoma may represent inadequate removal of the stalk or involvement of adjacent lobules. Phyllodes tumours are also known to recur locally and the original sections should be checked to be certain that fibroadenoma remains the correct diagnosis.

Recurrent cysts are common and require no treatment other than reaspiration provided the rules governing aspiration are adhered to (Chapter 10).

The breast parenchyma may fail to heal following a biopsy, leaving a palpable dip with a prominent edge in the breast tissue which is frequently mistaken for a new mass.

Breast masses related to different life periods

Breast masses in adolescence

A number of papers have reported studies of breast tumours in adolescence (Table 5.2).

Stone et al.[6] in 1977 reported on 143 masses presenting between the ages of 10 and 20. The incidence increased steadily throughout the decade with a marked predominance in 16 to 20-year-olds: 70% were fibroadenomas, 6% cysts and 12% 'hyperplasias', presumably nodularity of ANDI. Other diagnoses were seen in only one or two cases.

A second study[7] of 74 cases in a paediatric population (to 18 years) gives a similar distribution and includes prepubertal asymmetrical development of the nipple bud. This is much the commonest swelling of the early part of adolescence. Recognition is vital, because ill-advised biopsy will lead to amastia. A further paper on clinicopathological correlation in the adolescent group[8] showed that 12% of referrals and 3% of histological specimens came from this age group. Among 151 histological specimens were 114 fibroadenomas, 3 duct papillomas, 4 cysts and 4 cases of duct ectasia. Foxcroft et al. in 2001[9] showed that of 634 referrals (age 9–19 years), 619 had an ultrasound for assessment of which 59% had no abnormality, but the commonest abnormality was a fibroadenoma. A similar study in 2006[10] showed that adolescents accounted for 1.35% of referrals to a breast clinic but 30% reported a family history of breast cancer and 35% were using the oral contraceptive.

Concern has been expressed that fibroadenoma in this age group must be removed because of the possibility of cancer. Cancer in adolescence is exceedingly rare and a review of case reports and the authors' experience show that a mistaken diagnosis of fibroadenoma has usually been made because of the age group, not because of typical physical signs of fibroadenoma. Thus, masses with rapid growth, recent nipple retraction, surrounding tissue and lymph node involvement have been diagnosed as fibroadenoma. The risk of cancer can, for practical purposes, be ignored in an adolescent with a lump showing the typical features of the common fibroadenoma. The commonest metastatic tumour in this age group is rhabdomyosarcoma.

Lumps in the male breast in adolescence are less common. One series[6] reported cases over a 15-year period. All were due to gynaecomastia. Unlike girls, there is a marked peak incidence at the age of 13 or 14. Gynaecomastia is much more common than this series would suggest but the authors have seen no other cause for breast mass in an adolescent male (see Ch. 16). Inflammatory masses in human immunodeficiency virus (HIV)-positive males have been reported.

Breast problems associated with pregnancy and lactation

The enlarging breast of pregnancy typically obscures any underlying pathology, while the softness and dependency of the postlactational breast may reveal pre-existing pathology; hamartoma is a typical example. The conditions that appear in association with pregnancy are listed in Table 5.3.

Fibroadenoma may increase in size quite markedly in early pregnancy, but this is not normally associated with

Table 5.2 Summary of breast masses found during adolescence (10–20 years)

	Breast mass	Frequency of presentation
Male	Gynaecomastia	Common
Female	Premenarchal development of breast bud	Common
	Fibroadenoma	Common
	Cyst	Rare
	Giant fibroadenoma	Rare
	Phyllodes tumour	Rare
	Adenocarcinoma	Very rare
	Metastatic tumour	Very rare
Nipple and areola	Retention cysts	Uncommon
	Inversion	Uncommon
	Molluscum contagiosum	Rare
	Leiomyoma	Rare
Other conditions	Duct papilloma	Rare
	Subareolar abscess (periductal mastitis)	Uncommon
	Virginal hypertrophy	Uncommon
	Nipple discharge from Montgomery's tubercle	Rare

Table 5.3 Breast problems during pregnancy and lactation

	Frequency of presentation
Mass	
Enlargement of axillary breast	Uncommon
Enlarging fibroadenoma	Rare
Gigantomastia	Rare
Mastitis/abscess	Common
Galactocele	Uncommon
Other conditions	
Blood-stained nipple discharge	Uncommon

increased malignancy. Pregnancy may precipitate some cases of the very rare condition of gigantomastia due to multiple fibroadenoma (see Ch. 7).

Operations on the breast during this period may cause problems; damage to the ducts in late pregnancy or the puerperium may give milk fistula, while pregnancy occur-ring within a year of total duct excision may cause marked breast engorgement.

Breast lumps in older women

The incidence and nature of benign breast lumps in older women (more than 55 years) differ from those of the reproductive period. In a comprehensive study, Devitt[11] reviewed 581 women in this age group presenting with benign breast disorders. The commonest presentation was with non-specific nodularity, 25% associated with pain. Eight per cent had simple cysts, most under the age of 60, and there was a significant relationship to use of postmenopausal hormone replacement therapy. Eight patients had fibroadenomas, four of which were calcified. Thus, a similar range of benign breast lumps is seen in the older woman, but characterized by a much lower incidence and a much lower frequency compared to cancer than that seen during reproductive life.

PART 2: Triple assessment and organization of the breast clinic

In the past, clinical assessment was not only the mainstay of diagnosis of breast lumps, but usually the only assessment prior to surgical excision, frozen section and possible mastectomy. The three modalities of clinical assessment, imaging and pathological examination, known as triple assessment, are now standard practice.

Since clinical examination alone is relatively inaccurate for diagnosing cancerous masses and has limited repro-ducibility (only 73% accuracy in one series of malignant lumps examined by four surgeons[12]) it becomes manda-tory to image and sample pathologically any suspicious area in the breast. In women below 35 years the imaging should be by ultrasound, with a combination of mam-mography and ultrasound in older women.

Ultrasound is now a major technique used as part of triple assessment for the examination of solid lumps and as a guide for accurate cytological and histological sam-pling of solid lesions. Specialist breast units base their diagnostic practices on standard triple assessment and the most accurate results are obtained when the information provided by each individual test is put together to ensure consistency between tests. A review has shown a 99% predictive value for the diagnosis of benign breast changes if all three components of the triple assessment are found to be benign.[13]

Fine needle aspiration cytology

Fine needle aspiration cytology (FNAC) is now being superseded by core needle biopsy but it can have a role for assessing very small, mobile fibroadenomas which cannot be biopsied safely by wide-bore needle techniques. The technique is important in taking a specimen for cyto-logical study (see Ch. 18) and appropriate equipment should always be available. The diagnostic smear is either sent dry or in formalin, depending on preference of the local pathology laboratory. Cytological examination of cyst fluid is unnecessary unless the fluid is blood stained or a residual mass is seen on ultrasound imaging.

FNAC results are reported on a consistent grading scale from 1 to 5 as shown in Table 5.4.

Table 5.4 Results of fine needle aspiration cytology (FNAC)

C1	Inadequate	Acellular or sparsely cellular or poorly preserved smear
C2	Benign	Adequately cellular with unequivocal benign epithelial cells
C3	Probably benign	Adequately cellular with mainly benign cells present but some mild atypia present
C4	Suspicious/ probably malignant	Some features of malignancy in a low cellularity sample or highly cellular with some atypical cells present
C5	Malignant	Frankly malignant cells present Cells showing lack of cohesion with large nuclear to cytoplasmic ratios and nuclear variability Severe nuclear pleomorphism

Similar grading systems are applied to imaging and clinical examination results which then allow a shorthand description of triple assessment. For example, a young woman with a fibroadenoma which is classically palpable as a breast 'mouse', and with a typical ultrasound image and typical benign cytology, would be graded P2 U2 C2. A frank carcinoma would be P5 M5 C5.

The use of this shorthand coding allows immediate identification at a multidisciplinary group meeting and can indicate discordant results between the different modalities, thus giving a higher rate of overall diagnostic accuracy after further or repeated investigations for suspicious results. It is not an infrequent experience that the multidisciplinary discussion and scoring system allows a small and difficult cancer to be diagnosed by highlighting one of the modalities in a way which might be missed in a routine paper report sent to the clinician from the laboratory.

FNAC has an accuracy of around 99% when carried out by experienced aspirators and read by an expert cytopathologist.[14] In one series of 1104 cases with a false-positive rate of 0.4%, the benign conditions which led to a false-positive diagnosis were postradiation changes, granulomatous mastitis and fibroadenoma.[15] Maygarden and colleagues reviewed the cytological features of 265 benign masses, and discussed those features which are helpful in cytological diagnosis of benign conditions, and those benign conditions which can be diagnosed by cytology.[16]

The technique has a lower accuracy in benign lesions but this is mainly due to the higher rate of acellular smears produced on aspiration of benign lesions. Specimens from masses arising during pregnancy and lactation require assessment that takes into account the specific cellular changes in the breast at this time.[17]

FNAC has the advantage of being ready for interpretation by an expert cytopathologist within a short time, so it is useful for 'one-stop clinics' and for the diagnosis of benign lesions.

Limitations and complications

Fine needle aspiration is generally considered to be an innocuous procedure, in spite of occasional local complications such as pneumothorax (see Ch. 18). However, it may also cause local tissue trauma which may interfere with definitive histology of a small lesion. Lee and colleagues[18] studied 184 definitive specimens with a history of preceding fine needle aspiration and were able to find definitely attributable changes in 17 (9.3%). Changes included near-total destruction of the lesion from haemorrhage or infarction, and one of benign papilloma cells implanted in surrounding fibrogranulation tissue causing diagnostic problems.

Mammography should ideally be performed before fine needle aspiration. In a study of 52 women, repeat mammography was performed within 5 days of FNAC; in three cases significant differences were seen (probably due to haematoma) although the diagnosis was not changed in any case.[19] However, when a mass has been assessed by sonography and FNAC or core biopsy, mammography is normally being used to assess the rest of the breast, rather than the mass in question. If this is the case, it can proceed provided the radiologist is informed. A study assessed the effect of FNAC prior to or after ultrasound and showed that there was no difference in diagnostic accuracy or effect on patient management.[20]

The presence of a prosthesis should be excluded in every case, so that ultrasound-guided fine needle aspiration can be performed.[21]

Ultrasound in triple assessment

Ultrasound has several uses in the triple assessment setting. The main uses are to clarify the presence or not of a discrete abnormality within a vague palpable area or an asymmetric density on mammograms. It is of no value as a routine screen of the whole of a breast without any palpable abnormality. It is useful for differentiating deep cysts from nodularity and allows accurate aspiration of those cysts.

Ultrasound can be used to direct a core needle biopsy or FNAC to ensure that lesions are properly and accurately sampled.

Ideally, ultrasound is performed in the clinic by a radiological member of the team with a special interest in breast disease or by a breast surgeon who has been trained in ultrasound techniques. Colour Doppler ultrasonography has been used to differentiate benign from malignant masses.[22] It can also be used to highlight the presence of a blood vessel before a biopsy is taken.

Wide-bore needle biopsy

The use of wide-bore needle biopsy (WBN) has increased dramatically (see Ch. 18). This technique has two major advantages over FNAC. First, it supplies a histological section and so the pathologist only requires histology skills. Secondly, since histology is evaluated, the technique can make a definitive diagnosis for benign problems and differentiate between in situ and invasive breast cancer. Malignant specimens can be further assessed for oestrogen receptor, progesterone receptor status and HER-2 status.

The original wide-bore needles, such as the Tru Cut®, were actuated manually and rather cumbersome. The early needles often produced poor cores from benign breast lesions and were painful for patients. The introduction of spring-loaded 'guns' with rapid firing of needles produce much better cores and, as the needles cut quickly, they are less painful. Using a gun, a 14-gauge needle will cut through even the toughest breast tissue and has the added bonus that it is easily visible on ultrasound. McMahon and colleagues found such a gun to give a higher success rate with less pain than the older types of needles.[23]

The disadvantage of a core biopsy is that the tissue sample is not ready for interpretation for at least 24 hours and a diagnosis cannot be made in clinic. The use of touch imprint cytology is a method that can be used to complement core needle biopsy in order to provide immediate and reliable cytological diagnosis of symptomatic breast disease.[24,25]

Mammotome or vacuum-assisted biopsy

A further development from wide-bore needle biopsy is a mammotome or vacuum-assisted biopsy which uses a wider-bore needle (11-gauge) and can be used for diagnostic purposes and treatment, as it takes larger and multiple cores of tissue. It can be guided by ultrasound or stereotactic methods. It is commonly used for the further assessment of impalpable lesions and in particular for areas of microcalcification.[26] It has been shown to improve the preoperative diagnosis rate and reduce the need for diagnostic excision biopsies.[27] In some centres it is used to remove and therefore treat benign lesions such as fibroadenomas.[28,29] The procedure is accurate and well tolerated.[29] Complications of the procedure are few but include haematomas which can usually be managed conservatively.[28]

Organization of clinics

In order to deliver high-quality triple diagnosis all three elements of clinical examination, imaging and cytology have to be present. Traditionally, these were performed by the surgeon or gynaecologist (in some European countries) but it was unusual to find all three skills in one individual. Thus, it was common for the symptomatic patient to be referred first to the surgeon who then arranged the other investigations. In the past the three elements were often separated in time but this practice came under criticism by patients and the lay media.

As a result of several high-profile media features in the early 1990s which demonstrated wide variations in the efficacy and speed of breast diagnosis, several groups of breast specialists set up working parties to define good practice in breast clinics. In 1994, a working party of the British Breast Group published a document calling for the establishment of multidisciplinary breast specialist units with a core staff of a surgeon, radiologist, pathologist, oncologist and breast care nurse and with a specified caseload of breast referrals, giving a minimum of 50 new breast cancers annually.[30] This was based on the service that had developed within the NHS Breast Screening Service since it had been established in 1989.

This report was followed by a major report published in 1995 by the Breast Surgeons Group of the British Association of Surgical Oncologists (BASO), which laid down guidelines for the management of symptomatic referrals to breast specialists.[31] This report defined both the core multidisciplinary team and the facilities that should be available for rapid and accurate diagnosis of breast lumps (Tables 5.5 and 5.6). Revised versions appeared in 1998 and 2005.[32]

Both reports endorsed the widespread use of triple assessment with mandatory case conferences on a regular basis to discuss the final diagnosis prior to discharge from the clinic or therapeutic surgery, as appropriate. The advantages of this close cooperation would be a high rate of preoperative diagnosis of breast cancer and a concomitant fall in the number of open surgical biopsies for both benign and malignant problems. The cost effectiveness

and accuracy of triple assessment had been confirmed in two US studies.[33,34]

These arrangements were endorsed by the National Health Service Executive in the UK in a report of good practice published in 1996 – 'Improving Outcomes'[35] with central funding support. Similar media and patient pressures occurred in the USA where additional funding was also provided.

In developing this service it was proposed that there should be 'one-stop' clinics for women with suspected breast cancer, with all tests performed at one visit with a view to results being given on the same day. One clinic found that this was impossible, as up to one-third of referrals to the clinic were inappropriate and this therefore had an effect on the patients who had significant symptoms.[36] Most clinics found that it was cost-effective for benign problems but most patients with cancer needed to return at a later date for further tests.[37] Dey et al. assessed the cost and anxiety state of women referred to a one-stop clinic compared with a normal breast clinic and found that although the anxiety level of women attending the one-stop clinic was lower after 24 hours it was no different at 3 weeks or 3 months, but the cost was significantly increased.[38]

In 1998, the 'two-week wait' directive was introduced in the UK. The Health Service Circular[39] guaranteed that 'everyone with suspected breast cancer will be able to see a specialist within 2 weeks of their GP deciding that they need to be seen urgently'. This allowed GPs, rather than specialists, to prioritize referrals and several studies showed that after introduction of this policy in the UK, there was an increase in the number of 'urgent' referrals, a decrease in cancer detection rate and an increase in waiting time for patients not deemed 'urgent' by their GP.[40,41] To try to improve the accuracy of referrals, guidelines for referral[42] and proformas for referral are used by many clinics with variable effect.[43,44] Referrals to breast clinics are often influenced by external unpredictable factors such as a celebrity diagnosed with breast cancer.[45]

In 2002, a second edition of 'Improving Outcomes in Breast Cancer'[46] was published which provided further guidance on the organization of breast clinics, the provision of services for women at increased risk of breast cancer, patients with breast cancer, follow-up, palliative care, use of guidelines and protocols. It also highlighted that all breast units should keep accurate records for data analysis and audit purposes.

Table 5.5 Composition of a breast unit recommended by the BASO Guidelines[29]

Each member should have a special interest in breast disease:
  Surgeon
  Radiologist
  Pathologist
  Clinical oncologist
  Medical oncologist
  Nurse specialist

Table 5.6 Breast clinic diagnostic services recommended by the BASO Guidelines[29]

1	The breast clinic should diagnose more than 50 cancers per year
2	Diagnosis should be based on triple assessment
3	Mandatory multidisciplinary review sessions should be carried out
4	The majority of patients without cancer should receive all diagnostic tests at first visit
5	Patients without cancer should be given a diagnosis at first visit
6	Patients with newly diagnosed cancer will usually be given the diagnosis at a second visit
7	A breast care nurse should be present with the surgeon when this occurs, and the patient should be encouraged to bring a partner or friend when the results are being discussed
8	Patients should not receive abnormal results by telephone or letter

In an effort to try to improve the efficiency of breast clinics many units are training people to have several skills. Surgeons who read symptomatic mammograms are improving the sensitivity[47] and surgeons who perform ultrasounds make accurate diagnoses and the ultrasound is a useful adjunct to clinical assessment[48] However, one of the most important ways of ensuring the multidisciplinary team is effective and efficient is by good communication within the team.[49]

A recent review of the 'two-week wait' analyzed referrals between 1999 and 2005.[50] It found that there was a 9% increase in the number of referrals but the percentage of patients diagnosed with cancer in the 'two-week wait' group decreased from 12.2% in 1999 to 7.7% in 2005, while the number of cancers in the 'routine' group increased from 2.5% to 5.3%. Waiting times for routine referrals have therefore increased with time.

The organization of clinics needs to be kept under review in order to provide an efficient service to make a rapid diagnosis for the increasing number of 'worried' women who present to symptomatic breast clinics.

Medico-legal issues

Breast surgeons are increasingly being sued for missing breast cancers, leading to a delay in diagnosis and consequent claims for morbidity and worsening of prognosis. The commonest and most expensive actions relate to failure to diagnose breast cancer in young women who present with typical symptoms of benign breast change as described in this text, and develop breast cancer at a later date at the same site where the previous signs or symptoms were noted. Since no test or combination of tests have a 100% sensitivity in the diagnosis of breast cancer, it follows that even if all tests are performed and read accurately, some breast cancers may still not be diagnosed at the first attendance. It also means that if a cancer is missed, it does not necessarily imply negligent treatment provided the appropriate tests have been carried out and interpreted correctly.

In the law of England and Wales there are absolute requirements that must be met if any action for medical negligence is to succeed. Firstly, the doctor must have a duty of care for the patient and this is usually established by the fact that the GP has referred the patient to the surgeon/breast physician for an opinion. Secondly, it must be established that the doctor has given treatment below the standard that no equivalent competent doctor would have given (referred to as the Bolam test, after a landmark legal case). As breast surgery becomes more specialized, it becomes harder to define the average or equivalent practitioner, particularly as many of the traditional surgical roles in diagnosis are being undertaken by a range of doctors, nurses and others. Thirdly, if the treatment or management is found to be deficient (legal liability is established), the patient has to prove that some measurable loss has been suffered as a result of the negligent treatment (legal causation), either financial or physical losses such as worsened prognosis or unnecessary operations or treatment. If there is no measurable or provable loss, the claimant's case will fail completely.

The commonest legal actions result from failure to diagnose a lump/nodularity as breast cancer, usually due to the fact that the physical signs on palpation do not impress the clinician sufficiently to suggest a reasonable probability of cancer, and as a result no investigations are performed and the patient is discharged. This is particularly true of the young patient where cancer is less likely, and mammograms are not routinely performed. Also, these patients obtain the highest financial settlements, as they have major commitments to dependants and would probably have lived a long life if the cancer had not intervened. In general, clinical palpation has a sensitivity for cancer around 60%, and mammography of around 90%. Other less common reasons for failure to diagnose are misreading of mammograms and pathology, where there is evidence of abnormality on review of the tests by a third party (usually the claimant's medical expert).

In order to minimize the risk of missing a cancer, a full triple assessment should be carried out as described in this chapter, for all cases of definite lumps and suspicious nodularity, regardless of the age of the patient. After a thorough triple assessment has been performed, all results should be carefully discussed in the multidisciplinary team, making sure that all the results are concordant if a decision is made not to excise the index lesion. Any discordant result should mandate repeat investigations (e.g. FNA or core biopsy), or a definitive excision of the index lesion should be carried out, if doubt remains. All of the history, examinations and investigations should be recorded in detail, preferably on a computer-based proforma, so that nothing is omitted, as many legal actions succeed on the basis that the clinician has made such poor notes that no defence is possible. It should be remembered that most actions take place years after the events and recall will not be sufficient to mount a reasonable defence.

REFERENCES

1. Cox PJ, Li MKW & Ellis H. Spectrum of breast disease in outpatient surgical practise. *Journal of the Royal Society of Medicine* 1982; **75**: 857–859.

2. Dixon JM, Clarke PJ, Crucioli V *et al*. Reduction of the surgical excision rate in benign breast disease using fine needle aspiration cytology with immediate reporting. *British Journal of Surgery* 1987; **74**: 1014–1016.

3. Preece PE, Baum M, Mansel RE *et al*. Importance of mastalgia in operable breast cancer. *British Medical Journal* 1982; **284**: 1299–1300.

4. Haagensen CD. *Diseases of the Breast*. Philadelphia: WB Saunders; 1986:252.

5. Moreira De AJ, Cosiski MHR, Filho JM *et al*. Differential diagnosis of axillary masses. *Tumori* 1996; **82**: 596–599.

6. Stone AM, Shenker RI & McCarthy K. Adolescent breast masses. *American Journal of Surgery* 1977; **134**: 275–277.

7. West KW, Rescorla FJ, Scherer LR *et al*. Diagnosis and treatment of symptomatic breast masses in the paediatric population. *Journal of Paediatric Surgery* 1995; **30**: 182–187.

8. Sandison AT & Walker JC. Diseases of the adolescent female breast. A clinico-pathological study. *British Journal of Surgery* 1968; **55**: 443–448.

9. Foxcroft LM, Evans EB, Hirst C *et al*. Presentation and diagnosis of adolescent breast disease. *Breast* 2001; **10**: 399–404

10. Ravichandran D & Naz S. A study of children and adolescents referred to a rapid diagnosis breast clinic. *European Journal of Paediatric Surgery* 2006; **16**: 303–306.

11. Devitt JE. Benign disorders of the breast in older women. *Surgery, Gynecology and Obstetrics* 1986; **162**: 340–342.

12. Boyd NF, Sutherland HJ, Fish EB *et al*. Prospective evaluation of physical examination of the breast. *American Journal of Surgery* 1981; **142**: 331.

13. Layfield LJ, Glasgow BJ & Cramer H. Fine needle aspiration in the management of breast masses. *Pathology Annual* 1989; **24**: 23.

14. Barrows GM, Anderson TJ, Lamb J *et al*. Fine needle aspiration of breast cancer: relationship of clinical factors to cytology results in 689 primary malignancies. *Cancer* 1986; **58**: 1493–1498.

15. Jatoi I & Trott PA. False positive reporting in breast fine-needle aspiration cytology: incidence and causes. *Breast* 1996; **5**: 270–273.

16. Maygarden SJ, Novotny DB, Johnson DE *et al*. Subclassification of benign breast disease by fine needle aspiration cytology. *Acta Cytologica* 1994; **38**: 115–129.

17. Finley JL, Silverman JF & Lannin DR. Fine needle aspiration cytology of breast masses in pregnant and lactating women. *Diagnostic Cytopathology* 1989; **5**: 255–259.

18. Lee KC, Chan JKC & Ho LC. Histologic changes in the breast after fine needle aspiration. *American Journal of Surgical Pathology* 1994; **18**: 1039–1047.

19. Horobin JM, Matthews BM, Preece PE *et al*. Effect of fine needle aspiration on subsequent mammograms. *British Journal of Surgery* 1992; **79**: 52–54.

20. Laws SA, McMara IR, Cheetham JE *et al*. Fine needle aspiration cytology prior to breast ultrasonography does not alter ultrasound diagnostic accuracy or patient management. *Breast* 2002; **11**: 320–323.

21. Fornage BD, Sneige N & Singletary SE. Masses in breasts with implants: diagnosis with U-S guided fine needle aspiration biopsy. *Radiology* 1994; **191**: 339–342.

22. Holcombe C, Pugh N, Lyons K *et al*. Blood flow in breast cancer and fibroadenoma estimated by colour flow ultrasonography. *British Journal of Surgery* 1995; **82**: 787–788.

23. McMahon AJ, Lutfy AM, Matthew A *et al*. Needle core biopsy of the breast with a spring-loaded device. *British Journal of Surgery* 1992; **79**: 1042.

24. Klevesath MB, Godwin RJ, Bannon R *et al*. Touch imprint cytology on core needle biopsy specimens: a useful method for immediate reporting of symptomatic breast lesions. *European Journal of Surgical Oncology* 2005; **31**: 490–494.

25. Qureshi NA, Beresford A, Sami S *et al*. Imprint cytology of needle core biopsy specimens of breast lesions: is it a useful adjunct to rapid assessment breast clinics? *Breast* 2007; **16**: 81–85.

26. Kettritz U, Morack G & Decker T. Sterotactic vacuum-assisted breast biopsies in 500 women with microcalcifications: radiological and pathological correlations. *European Journal of Radiology* 2005; **55**: 270–276.

27. Dhillon MS, Bradley SA & England DW. Mammotome biopsy: impact on preoperative diagnosis and rate. *Clinical Radiology* 2006; **61**: 276–281.

28. Mathew J, Crawford DJ, Lwin M *et al*. Ultrasound-guided vacuum assisted excision in the diagnosis and treatment of clinically benign breast lesions. *Annals of the Royal College of Surgeons of England* 2007; **89**: 494–495.

29. Plantade R, Hammou JC, Gerard F *et al*. Ultrasound-guided vacuum assisted biopsy: review of 382 cases. *Journal of Radiology* 2005; **86**: 1003–1015.

30. British Breast Group. Working Report. *Breast*; 1994 Supplement.

31. BASO Guidelines for surgeons in the management of symptomatic breast disease in the United Kingdom. *European Journal of Surgical Oncology* 1995; **21**: S1–S13.

32. BASO Guidelines for surgeons in the management of symptomatic breast disease in the United Kingdom – 1998 revision. The BASO Breast Specialty Group. *European Journal of Surgical Oncology* 2005; **31**: S1–S21.

33. Schmidt WA, Wachtel MS, Jones MK *et al.* The triple test: a cost effective diagnostic tool. *Laboratory Medicine* 1994; **25**: 715–719.

34. Vetto J, Pommier R, Schmidt W *et al.* Use of the triple test for palpable breast lesions yields high diagnostic accuracy and cost savings. *American Journal of Surgery* 1995; **169**: 519–522.

35. NHS Management Executive. *Improving Outcomes in Breast Cancer.* EL (96)15, July. London: Department of Health, 1996.

36. Patel RS, Smith DC & Reid I. One stop breast clinics – victims of their own success? A prospective audit of referrals to a specialist breast clinic. *European Journal of Surgical Oncology* 2000; **26**: 452–454.

37. Chan SY, Berry MG, Engledow AH *et al.* Audit of a one-stop breast clinic – revisited. *Breast Cancer* 2000; **7**: 191–194.

38. Dey P, Bundred N, Gibbs A *et al.* Costs and benefits of a one-stop clinic compared with a dedicated breast clinic: randomized controlled trial. *British Medical Journal* 2002; **324**: 507.

39. NHS Executive. *Manual of Cancer Service Standards.* Department of Health 2000.

40. Khawaja AR & Allan SM. Has the breast cancer 'two-week wait' guarantee for assessment made any difference? *European Journal of Surgical Oncology* 2000; **26**: 536–539.

41. Cant PJ & Yu DS. Impact of the '2-week wait' directive for suspected breast cancer on service provision in a symptomatic breast clinic. *British Journal of Surgery* 2000; **87**: 1082–1086.

42. Austoker J, Mansel R, Baum M *et al.* Guidelines for referral of patients with breast problems. *Cancer Research Campaign and NHSBSP.* 1995.

43. Cochrane RA, Davies EL, Singhal H *et al.* The national referral guidelines have cut down inappropriate referrals in the under 50s. *European Journal of Surgical Oncology* 1999; **25**: 251–254.

44. Imkampe A, Bendall S & Chainakwalam C. Two week rule: has prioritization of breast referrals by general practitioners improved? *Breast* 2006; **15**: 654–658.

45. Twine C, Barthelmes L & Gateley CA. Kylie Minogue's breast cancer: effects on referrals to a rapid access breast clinic in the UK. *Breast* 2006; **15**: 667–669.

46. National Institute of Clinical Excellence. *Improving Outcomes in Breast Cancer.* NICE. 2002.

47. Rao MC, Griffiths CD & Griffiths AB. Can breast surgeons read mammograms of symptomatic patients in the one stop breast clinic? *Annals of the Royal College of Surgeons of England* 2001; **83**: 108–109.

48. Whitehouse PA, Baber Y, Brown G *et al.* The use of ultrasound by breast surgeons in outpatients: an accurate extension of clinical diagnosis. *European Journal of Surgical Oncology* 2001; **27**: 611–616.

49. West N. The importance of communication within the multidisciplinary team. *Advances in Breast Cancer* 2006; **3**: 3–5.

50. Potter S, Govndarajuku S, Shere M *et al.* Referral patterns, cancer diagnoses and waiting times after introduction of two week wait rule for breast cancer: prospective cohort study. *British Medical Journal* 2007; **335**: 288–290.

CHAPTER 6

Imaging of the breast

Kate Grower-Thomas

Key points and new developments

1. Digital enhancement of mammographic images have allowed more detailed examination of dense breasts in young women and those on hormone replacement therapy.

2. Ultrasound is an essential component in the evaluation of patients with breast symptoms.

3. Image-guided diagnosis allows confident therapeutic decisions to be made.

4. Cyclical changes can modify the appearance of MRI images.

5. Optimal use of imaging facilities requires close cooperation of clinician, radiologist and pathologist best done at multidisciplinary meetings.

Introduction

Despite the fact that the breast has low inherent contrast, being comprised of soft tissue structures such as fat and gland, there are various ways in which its internal architecture may be visualized with modern imaging, thereby giving valuable information about its structure and any abnormal features. In this chapter all the current methods of breast imaging will be discussed.

Although imaging of the breast has been developed with a view to improving the accuracy of diagnosing malignancy, useful information about benign changes in the breast may be obtained. The current useful investigations are X-ray mammography, ultrasound and magnetic resonance imaging. Thermography and diaphanoscopy are of historical interest but are not sufficiently sensitive for diagnosis. The latter technique may be of value in assessing breast density.[1]

Breast density

The density of breast tissue is variable between women and at different stages of their lives. The epithelial and stromal elements of breast tissue respond to circulating oestrogen and progesterone levels. This is typically denser and more difficult to interpret in younger women. Other women may also have dense breasts before the menopause and/or when on hormone replacement therapy. Following menopause the breast tissue involutes, with the glandular structures becoming increasingly of fatty density with time. There are generally considered to be four mammographic parenchymal patterns, depending on the amount of dense glandular tissue present, as described by Wolfe.[2] Women with the two higher breast density patterns (P2 or dysplastic) have a significantly increased risk of breast carcinoma.[3]

Mammography

The earliest report of mammography was by Salomon in 1913 although it was not until the 1960s that it developed a place in the routine management of breast disease.[4] Improvements in technology have allowed increasing detail to be shown while reducing the exposure to radiation.

Film screen mammography (Fig. 6.1) is the gold standard breast imaging modality. The breast is placed on the Bucky plate and a compression paddle is applied to compress the breast down to a thickness of a few centimetres, thereby also reducing movement and improving contrast, resulting in a superior image. A high-quality film is placed into a cassette containing intensifying screens and the cassette is put into the Bucky tray. The breast is exposed to the X-ray beam and the image is recorded on the film, which is then processed.

The more recent film screen mammography units have the capability to predetermine the optimal exposure for each particular breast, thus reducing unnecessary radiation and improving the image. The upper limit of dose per breast is 2.6 mGy. A denser and bigger breast may receive a higher dose.

The images obtained are of very high quality; a detail of at least 11–12 line pairs per millimetre is obtainable.

The breast may be positioned in different ways for mammography; the standard series would be a mediolateral oblique and a craniocaudal view of each breast (Fig. 6.2). Other views are reserved for the assessment of particular mammographic abnormalities. These would include the lateral projection and extended views more laterally or medially in the craniocaudal plane. The mammographer is skilled in obtaining the appropriate view to aid the radiologist. In addition, the use of a smaller compression paddle aids in determining whether a lesion is real or purely a summation shadow of the gland tissue. Magnification images (Fig. 6.3) for areas of microcalcification are valuable in discerning whether or not the lesion requires biopsy.

Digital and computerized mammography

Increasingly, radiology departments are moving from the older technology of film screen mammography (FSM), which has limitations with breast contrast, to computerized (CR) or digital (DR or FFD, [full field digital]) technology.[5] These are able to optimize subtle differences in

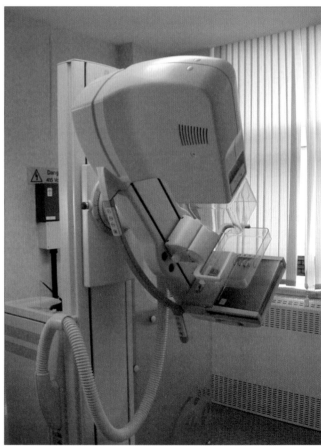

Fig. 6.2 Position of mammography unit for right mediolateral oblique view.

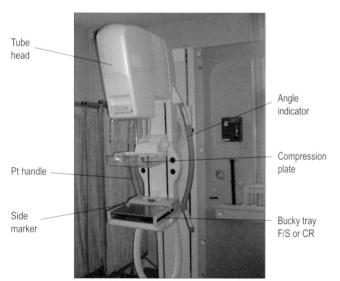

Tube head

Pt handle

Side marker

Angle indicator

Compression plate

Bucky tray F/S or CR

Fig. 6.1 A typical mammography unit.

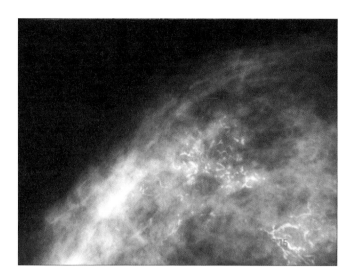

Fig. 6.3 Magnification view of benign ductal calcification.

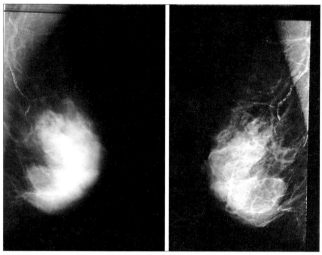

Fig. 6.4 Comparison of film screen (*left*) and digital mammography (*right*) of the same breast.

the inherently low contrast within the intermediate densities of breast structures. Digital systems are increasingly showing increased performance as compared to film/screen combinations and at lower radiation doses. Exposure using X radiation is still required but minimizing radiation dose is important; the ALARA principle, 'as low as reasonably achievable', applies.

With CR, the image is recorded on a reusable filmless cassette which is processed and the image is recorded electronically, having been scanned by a laser reader to form a digital image. With DR, the image is transmitted automatically to the work station without the need for a cassette. The images are viewed on a computer screen (soft copy reporting) and no film is produced, unless required, when a laser printer is used.

These new techniques enable images to be viewed utilizing the hospital picture archiving and communications system (PACS), in the out-patient clinic, theatre, at the multidisciplinary meeting, etc., without the images getting lost or needing to be copied. Also, film storage is no longer needed; the images are instead stored electronically and they will not deteriorate with age as do film images. These electronic images may be manipulated on the computer screen, thereby negating the need for extra-conventional views, e.g. magnification images. Digital mammography is particularly useful for women with dense breasts, such as younger women (Fig. 6.4). The newer digital mammography units use multiple charge couple devices arranged in an array. X-ray photons are converted into a signal through either a two-dimensional amorphous silicon read-out matrix or a caesium iodide

needle-structured scintillator. There are now several different units on the market. Images obtained this way are available instantly, thereby removing the inevitable wait required for film developing with conventional film screen mammography. Other advantages include a greater dynamic range, so that different window widths and levels are available, meaning fewer additional supplementary images are required. Edge enhancement and other postprocessing options are used, which may aid in the visualization and interpretation of microcalcification. The images may be transferred using teleradiography to a radiologist for reporting remotely or for a second opinion.

Digital radiography is significantly more expensive than FSM, both in capital and maintenance cost, and with only limited savings to be made from film costs or storage. Overall, the costs are currently at least twice that for conventional mammography. This needs to be balanced against increased patient throughput, fewer repeats and fewer extra films being required. The computer monitors required to read these high-quality images need a very high resolution.

Tomosynthesis

Digital mammography and computer manipulation of images lends itself to further techniques, for example tomosynthesis.[6] This developing technique involves sequentially moving the X-ray tube over the breast at the area of concern, in an arc above the detector, obtaining multiple images. Image reconstruction enables the reader to visualize true abnormalities more clearly in plane within the breast tissue using three-dimensional imaging whilst reducing the inherent noise of surrounding tissues.

Digital mammography also lends itself to subtraction techniques which may be utilized for newer applications using contrast enhanced breast tomosynthesis, which is still experimental and whose application will be mainly in malignant disease.

Computer-aided detection

Technologies are now available which can 'read' and mark digital mammography images to highlight areas of concern, thereby acting as a 'prompt' tool for the reader to analyse. Ideally, it should detect significant abnormalities and have a high specificity and sensitivity for carcinoma detection, which is its main use. Computer-aided detection (CAD) is particularly good at identifying suspicious calcification, but not so good at asymmetric densities. The sensitivity of the device is set at such a level so as to not give an excessive number of prompts. It can also be used to 'read' mammographic films that have been 'digitized', i.e. converted into a digital format. This technology is expensive and not yet widely available in the UK.

Ductography

Ductography, involving cannulation of a discharging duct, is of historical interest. The technique has been superseded by ultrasound, magnetic resonance imaging and endoscopic ductography.

Unwanted effects of mammography

The compression required to produce optimum images is considerable and many patients find this an uncomfortable experience. In patients with painful breasts it may limit the examination. Occasionally nipple discharge is elicited and cysts may very rarely rupture during the compression.

Much debate has centred on the risk of radiation-induced cancers.[7] The low doses now used make this risk acceptable but multiple mammograms may increase the risk. The usually quoted risk of radiation-induced breast cancer is about 3×10^{-5} per mSv. This risk is so low that it is not clinically detectable although the risk is thought to be higher in young women, particularly in their teens, when the breast tissue is more radiosensitive. Women with Li-Fraumeni syndrome are also susceptible to radiation-induced cancer.

Breast ultrasound

Ultrasound imaging of the breast was first described in 1951.[8] The advent of new technologies has given improved inherent tissue contrast and reduced ultrasound artefacts that previously degraded the image. Modern equipment incorporates a real-time, high-frequency (7.5–13 MHz) hand-held linear probe with adjustable focus.

Ultrasound is the primary examination of choice in women under the age of 35 years, children and in male patients. It is the imaging modality most dependant on the operator's skill and technique, both of which require optimal attention to detail. A typical fibroadenoma is shown in Figure 6.5. The operator should have an excellent knowledge of mammography, especially when attempting to locate an abnormality noted on mammography.

The patient should be positioned lying on a couch, with the head raised a little using a pillow. The position of the breast lesion under scrutiny influences the final position of the patient. If the lesion is in the medial half of the breast then the patient lies supine; if the lesion is in the lateral half of the breast, then, particularly if the breast is large, the patient might be better positioned in the anterior oblique so that the breast falls medially. The patient's arm is placed behind her head and the examination commences. The aim is to immobilize the breast,

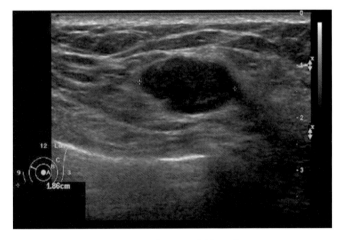

Fig. 6.5 Ultrasound image of a typical fibroadenoma.

fixing it to the chest wall to reduce movement and spread the tissue.

The area of concern should be palpated, allowing the patient the opportunity to indicate where she localizes her abnormality. This gives the operator extra information gained by palpating the area before commencing the scan.

The ultrasound probe should be covered with a small amount of acoustic gel. This may be covered with a disposable latex sheath. This keeps the probe clean and is mandatory when interventional procedures are performed to prevent contamination. The sheath is then also coated with gel. The hand not holding the probe, or that of an assistant, can also be used to further immobilize the tissue under examination, particularly in the large ptotic breast. The probe itself can also be used to further compress the tissue, without hurting the patient.

Scanning should be performed in two orthogonal plains, i.e. longitudinally and transversely. Some operators also scan in a radial fashion, particularly if the lesion is adjacent to the areola. Lesions which are superficial or under the nipple–areola complex may be very difficult to image adequately with ultrasound. The use of a block of stand-off gel can prove to be invaluable (Fig. 6.6). This also needs to be liberally smeared with acoustic gel and applied to the patient's breast. The ultrasound probe then scans through the gel block. The depth and focal zone positions of the ultrasound beam need to be adjusted accordingly.

If any suspicious lesion is identified, it is good practice to scan the patient's axilla too, in order to find abnormal lymphadenopathy. Abnormal nodes may then be needled to confirm possible malignancy, thereby negating the need for surgical sentinel node procedure in some patients.

Breast magnetic resonance imaging

Magnetic resonance imaging (MRI) is the newest of the breast imaging modalities frequently used (Fig. 6.7). The earliest reports date from the mid-1980s.[9] Rapid developments in the technology of this technique together with the development of dedicated breast coils now permit the production of high-quality images. A useful review of magnetic resonance imaging in breast disease is that of Van Goethem et al.[10]

A high magnetic field strength (typically 1.5 Tesla or above) and radiofrequency pulses are needed in order to obtain images. MRI utilizes the properties of the hydrogen atom, which is in high concentration in biological tissues. The protons are manipulated so that they emit an electromagnetic signal recorded as an induced voltage which is detected in receiver coils and converted into a visual image. The time taken for the signal to rise and fall are the T1 and T2 relaxation times. Due to the properties of different tissues, e.g. fat, blood, fluid, tumour and their water content, these vary, thus resulting in a picture. Gadolinium contrast enhancement (Fig. 6.8) is used in patients with malignant disease. This works by altering the relaxation times of certain tissues thereby making tumour foci more readily visible.

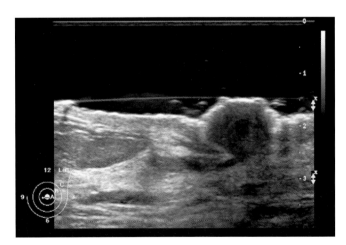

Fig. 6.6 Ultrasound image using stand-off gel to better delineate the subareolar structures.

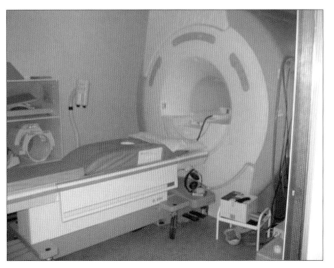

Fig. 6.7 MRI scanner showing the breast coil (pink cushion).

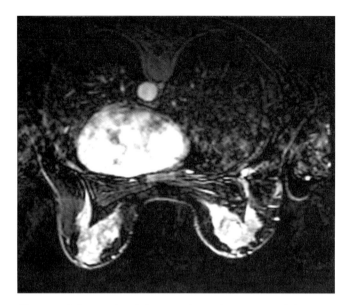

Fig. 6.8 Subtracted gadolinium enhanced MRI image of the breasts.

A patient undergoing breast MRI is required to lie prone on the MRI couch with the breasts dangling into a special device, the surface coil. Padding is placed around the breasts to reduce movement. The position is uncomfortable, particularly as it must be maintained for long periods in order to reduce movement artefacts during imaging, particularly important in subtracted contrast enhanced sequences.

The premenopausal breast is subject to cyclical changes in hormonal levels that alter the uptake of contrast. This must be borne in mind when scheduling and interpreting the examination. Ideally, the scan should occur during days 6 to 16 of the cycle. It may be performed following needle biopsy as long as no significant haematoma develops, but recent open surgery will result in spurious results. Scans should ideally be deferred for up to 6 months as wound healing may make images more difficult to interpret, similarly with radiation, which should be delayed a little longer.

The majority of patients undergoing breast MRI in the UK are those in whom malignancy is suspected or confirmed. It does, however, have a use in those post-treatment patients in whom a new area of concern is identified, which could be post-treatment fibrosis or recurrent tumour.

MRI is useful in the augmented breast with silicone or saline/silicone implants when rupture or other complication is suspected. Contrast enhancement is not needed, only the inherent differences in the implant components. Particular sequences are used to maximize these properties. Implant contraction, silicone leaks, bleeds and siliconoma are readily recognized. The techniques are now sufficiently refined that the nature of material used in augmentation mammoplasty can be elucidated.[11]

When a lesion is identified on MRI and not visible using other modalities, then MRI-guided biopsy may be required. This is not currently a widely available technique in the UK, but some manufacturers produce non-ferromagnetic equipment (usually an alloy containing nickel and titanium, or ceramic needles) suitable for use in the MRI environment. It is likely that with further developments in MRI technology, particularly the development of real-time imaging, that this will be more readily available in the future.

Biopsy techniques

There are several ways in which imaging can aid in the percutaneous biopsy of lesions identified on ultrasound or mammography. These include fine needle aspiration (FNA), wide-bore core needle biopsy (WBN) and mammotomy. FNA produces an aspirate of cells which is smeared onto a slide, fixed and presented to the pathologist. WBN obtains small cores (18, 16 or 14 French) of the tissue using a cutting needle, either using a disposable needle with a spring-loaded mechanism or a needle inserted into a spring-loaded gun device. This tissue is placed into formalin and sent to the histopathologist. Mammotomy uses a wider-bore needle (8 or 11 French) and requires suction to retrieve the specimen and aspirate any bleeding produced. All these procedures are well tolerated. Local anaesthetic is administered as a routine for WBN and mammotomy. Figure 6.9 illustrates the commonly used types of biopsy needle.

These techniques may be employed using mammography or ultrasound as the imaging guide. Ultrasound has the advantage of being able to use real-time imaging (Figs 6.10 and 6.11), Mammography may require the use of special stereotactic techniques (Fig. 6.12).

FNA has been largely superseded by the histological techniques but is still invaluable in giving rapid answers in the clinic situation and in patients taking anticoagulants. The tissue retrieved using the other methods needs more lengthy preparation prior to definitive results being available, but more useful information about the tissue is obtained.

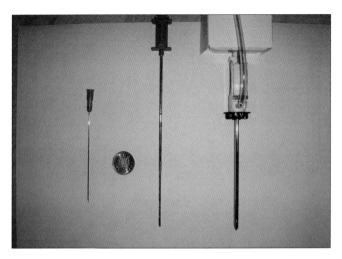

Fig. 6.9 21 French FNA needle, 14 French wide-bore core needle and 11 French Mammotome™ needle.

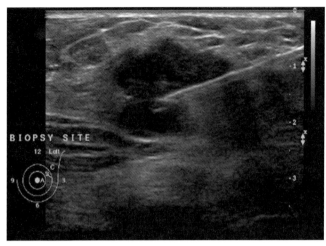

Fig. 6.11 Ultrasound image showing needle within the lesion for biopsy.

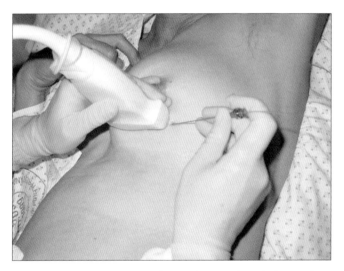

Fig. 6.10 Patient positioning for an ultrasound-guided procedure.

Prone table

Although mammographic-guided mammotomy may be performed with the patient seated in a mammography chair, ideally a prone table should be used. Here, the patient lies prone with the relevant breast protruding through a hole in the table top. Prone tables (Fig. 6.13) are advantageous for several reasons, particularly as the patient is more comfortable. Also the breast hangs freely and lesions against the chest wall are more easily accessible. In addition, the patient is unable to see the procedure and less likely to faint as a result. The operator performing the procedure is seated beneath the table, and the biopsy probe is held in a stand.

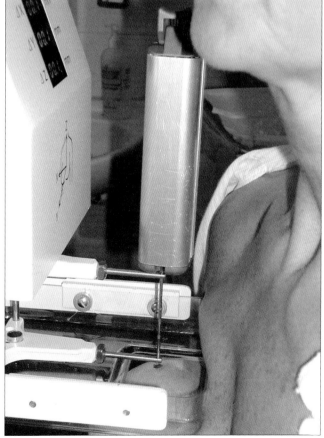

Fig. 6.12 Patient undergoing stereotactic needle biopsy.

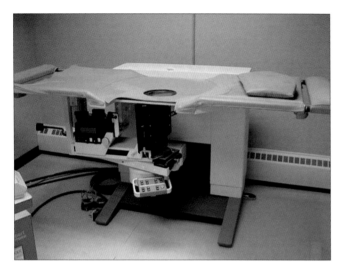

Fig. 6.13 Prone table for stereotactic biopsy.

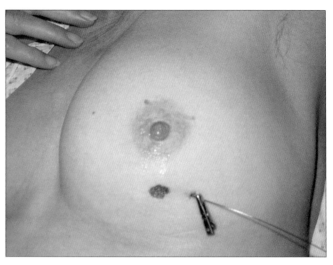

Fig. 6.14 Patient with guide wire in position prior to surgery.

Mammotomy, as well as being invaluable in retrieving microcalcifications for analysis, may be used to percutaneously excise fibroadenomata or gynaecomastia using a hand-held mammotomy device under ultrasound guidance.

Markers

When small foci of calcification are biopsied percutaneously, the sample may remove all of the calcium. Small MRI-safe metal markers are now available which are deployed at the site of the lesion during the image-guided biopsy. They frequently also contain a gel mark which is sonovisible for several weeks before being resorbed. These serve as a reference point to mark the site of the original abnormality so that if the lesion proves to be malignant, the surrounding area can be accurately identified and subsequently excised. It would normally be localized prior to surgical removal.

Specimen radiography

Core biopsy specimens targeting foci of calcification may be radiographed to confirm the retrieval of calcium prior to ending the procedure. The tissue is placed in special specimen containers or plastic clips. Conventional magnification images may be performed. More recently, dedicated digital cabinets which give instant images have speeded up the process, giving high-quality, detailed images. These are also very useful in the operating theatre

where the surgeon can confirm removal of a particular abnormality.

Radiographic imaging of excision specimens serves two purposes. It confirms for both the surgeon and the radiologist that the lesion localized has been excised. It may also be used to help localize the lesion within the specimen for the pathologist to block. In addition, the specimen may be further sliced and labelled, then radiographed prior to blocks being taken. This aids in identifying within which level the lesion is located, which may save pathological time.

Breast localization techniques

The localization of impalpable abnormalities in the breast prior to their surgical excision has become a widespread practice secondary to the mammographic screening programme that identifies significant numbers of impalpable tumours (Figs 6.14–6.16). Some benign lesions such as radial scars may also require excision, as they are also usually impalpable.

There are various methods by which a lesion can be identified to aid the surgeon. Some lesions may be palpable to the patient, but only just so by the surgeon, necessitating skin marking using a felt pen mark. This is best performed using ultrasound guidance. Indeed, felt pen marking of ultrasound-visible lesions, directly anterior to the area of concern, is good practice, whether

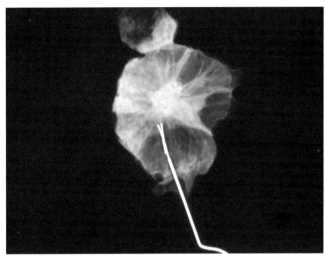

Fig. 6.16 Excised specimen confirming removal.

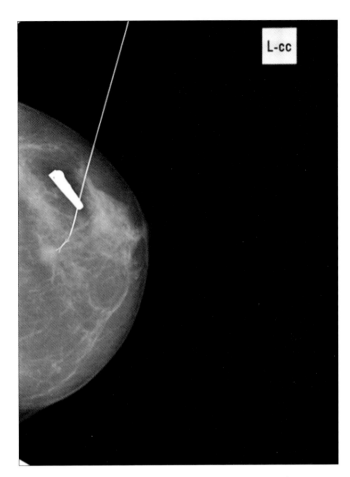

Fig. 6.15 Craniocaudal view of X Reidy wire position adjacent to breast lesion.

a marking wire is used or not, giving the surgeon more information regarding the lesion position.

If the lesion is sonographically visible, then it may be easily marked with a guide wire. There are several available commercially, with either hooks or barbs to anchor into the breast tissue, so as not to move prior to the surgery. These are preloaded into a needle, which is then placed into or adjacent to the lesion under ultrasound guidance, depending on local preference. Either way, the marker should not be further than 1 cm away from its target.

Other lesions, in particular calcifications, for example in ductal carcinoma in situ, may be difficult to visualize with ultrasound, despite new technology. These are located using other techniques of which there are primarily three; stereotaxis, perforated plate and measurement.

If stereotaxis is available, this is a useful and accurate method of localization. With the patient sitting in a mammography chair, a stereotactic film pair is obtained in whichever plane is preferred, depending on the site of the

lesion and local preference. For example, a lesion in the lower outer quadrant might be best targeted via the lateral approach, rather than by traversing the breast from top to bottom using the craniocaudal (CC) plane.

The site for marking is determined using either algorithmic or, more commonly, digital estimation. The depth of the wire location (Z axis), however, should be about minus 10 mm so as to traverse the lesion and not fall short of it when the breast is uncompressed.

Alternatively, a perforated plate may be used to localize. This has the disadvantage of not being able to accurately estimate the depth of penetration required, particularly in the nonskilled operator. This may necessitate several needle positions and films before an accurate point is reached.

The third method for sonoinvisible lesions is to use a measurement method. This requires measurements to be transferred from the mammograms onto the patient's skin using a pen and ruler. The site of the lesion is measured using the nipple as the reference point from the CC and the lateral films. True measurements are taken for the distances posterior to and to the side of the nipple (lateral or medial) on the CC view, then on the lateral view, the distance posterior to the nipple. The vertical measurement is halved. These distances are transferred onto the skin and the wire is placed accordingly to target the lesion. Check mammograms confirm the needle position prior to deployment.

As with all localizations, a specimen radiograph is essential to confirm the lesion has been appropriately excised surgically, prior to reversal of anaesthesia (Fig. 6.16).

REFERENCES

1. Simlick MK & Lilge L. Optical transillumination spectroscopy to quantify parenchymal tissue density: an indicator of breast cancer risk. *British Journal of Radiology* 2005; **78**: 1009–1017.

2. Wolfe JN. Breast patterns as an index of risk of malignancy for developing breast cancer *American Journal of Roentgenology* 1976; **126**: 1130–1139.

3. Boyd NF, Guo H, Martin LJ *et al.* Mammographic density and the risk and detection of breast cancer. *N Eng J Med* 2007; **356**: 227–236.

4. Gold RH. The evolution of mammography. *Radiological Clinics of North America* 1992; **30**; 1–19.

5. Fischer U, Hermann KP & Baum F. Digital mammography: current state and future aspects. *European Radiology* 2006; **16**: 38–44.

6. Smith A. Contrast-enhanced breast tomosynthesis: a promising tool for identifying breast cancer. *HIRE* 2006; **1**: 25–26.

7. Byrne C, Schairer C, Wolfe J *et al.* Mammographic features and breast cancer risk: effects with time, age, and menopause status. *Journal of the National Cancer Institute* 1995; **87**: 1622–1629.

8. Wild JJ, & Neal D. Use of high frequency ultrasound waves for detecting changes in texture of living tissues. *Lancet* 1951; **1**: 655–657.

9. El Yousef SJ, Alfidi RJ, Duchesneau RH *et al.* Initial experience with nuclear magnetic resonance (NMR) imaging of the human breast. *Journal of Computer Assisted Tomography* 1983; **7**: 215–218.

10. Van Goethem M, Tjalma W, Schelfout K *et al.* Magnetic resonance imaging in breast cancer. *European Journal of Surgical Oncology* 2006; **32**: 901–910.

11. Kawahara S, Hyakusoka H, Ogawa R *et al.* Clinical imaging diagnosis of implant materials for breast augmentation. *Annals of Plastic Surgery* 2006; **57**: 6–12.

CHAPTER 7

Fibroadenoma and related tumours

Key points and new developments

1. Mixed stromal and epithelial tumours fall into two main types: fibroadenoma (simplex) and phyllodes tumour. These are differentiated by the cellularity and activity of the stromal element.

2. Behaviour is determined by the stroma, with the age of the patient a second important element. The obsolescent term 'cystosarcoma phyllodes' should be abandoned since many are not cystic and most are benign.

3. Fibroadenoma arises from a lobule, probably as the result of increased sensitivity to oestrogen.

4. Molecular biology is providing interesting insights into possible mechanisms. For example, fibroadenomas show the *bcl-2* gene, which delays apoptotic cell death in similar situations.

5. Most fibroadenomas do not show progressive growth, but the growth phase is followed by a static phase in about 80%, regression in about 15% and progression in only 5–10%.

6. Fibroadenomas can be treated conservatively provided diagnosis is confident and the patient compliant; routine excision is no longer appropriate.

7. Triple assessment is by clinical examination, ultrasound and pathology, with fine needle aspiration cytology (FNAC) or core needle biopsy.

8. Fibroadenomas carry a small risk of increased future breast cancer, seen mainly in cases showing a complex histology. The risk is sufficient to be of biological interest, but not to influence management. Molecular biological studies have supported the clinical view that most fibroadenomas have no increased risk of malignancy but genetic changes are apparent in large fibroadenomas and phyllodes tumours.

9. Up to four fibroadenomas in one breast, and fibroadenomas up to 4 cm in diameter, are not uncommon. Appropriate definition for multiple fibroadenomas is thus five or more in one breast and for giant fibroadenoma is a diameter >5 cm.

10. Giant fibroadenoma and phyllodes tumour in adolescence usually behave in a benign fashion, managed by enucleation without reconstruction.

11. Phyllodes tumours in adults have a high local recurrence rate unless the initial excision is adequate, i.e. 1 cm clearance. Hence, the diagnosis should be made by core needle biopsy before surgery, to ensure an adequate primary excision.

12. Pseudoangiomatous hyperplasia (PASH) should be regarded as a fibroadenoma variant.

Terminology

The World Health Organization has simply defined a fibroadenoma as 'a discrete benign tumour showing evidence of connective tissue and epithelial proliferation'.[1] It has long been recorded and recognized as an entity and as a benign tumour; in the early nineteenth century Sir Astley Cooper used the term 'chronic mammary tumour'. In its classic form, fibroadenoma is one of the commonest, best-recognized and most easily managed conditions, yet paradoxically fibroadenomas which are not entirely typical have given rise to more confusion than most breast conditions. This is due to the use of a plethora of terms to describe the more exuberant forms of tumour (in either a histological or clinical sense). Indeed, it is the confusion caused by clinical variants (those of large size or rapid growth) or histological variants (hypercellularity or atypia) which has been the root of the problem.

Now there is a better understanding of the wide spectrum of histological appearances and disease behaviour with mixed epithelial and connective tissue proliferation; but the benefits of this better understanding can only be gained by insisting on precise terminology.

The fibrous stromal element of these tumours is the key to classification and behaviour, with any epithelial variant being treated as a secondary problem. Thus, on the basis of the stromal element, the tumours fall into two main groups: fibroadenoma and phyllodes tumour, with a few less common and less important variants. The term 'fibroadenoma' is used for all such tumours in which the fibrous stroma is of low cellularity and regular cytology. It covers tumours of all sizes, because their behaviour is basically similar, i.e. uniformly benign, whatever the size. The group of tumours where the stroma shows markedly increased cellularity and atypia is termed 'phyllodes tumour' (cystosarcoma phyllodes in older terminology).

It is stressed that this diagnosis is made on histological grounds, not size. Thus, while most phyllodes tumours are large, the term should also be applied to small tumours if they show the appropriate histological changes in the stroma. Most phyllodes tumours also behave in a benign fashion, although showing a tendency to local recurrence. But there is a spectrum of clinical behaviour as well as of histological atypia, and an occasional case will be frankly malignant and may metastasize. Similarly, there is a spectrum of genetic changes that reflect this.

In summary, fibroadenoma is common, usually small but sometimes large, and for practical purposes always benign. Phyllodes tumour is uncommon, usually large but sometimes small, usually benign but occasionally malignant. The two lesions cannot be distinguished clinically and not always on macroscopic section. Both occur throughout reproductive life; fibroadenoma presents predominantly in the first half, phyllodes tumour more commonly in the second.

Age is an added and important factor in two respects. Tumours of adolescence usually behave in benign fashion irrespective of histology. Tumours of the perimenopausal period, which recur, may then behave in more serious fashion, even if histologically they look benign at the first presentation.

Fibroadenoma simplex

This tumour usually appears in young women as a rubbery-firm, smooth, very mobile mass. These features – and in particular its striking mobility – are so characteristic that a confident diagnosis can be made in most cases in young women. The term 'simplex' differentiates the common, everyday fibroadenoma from the 'complex' fibroadenomas recently delineated, and from multiple and giant fibroadenomas falling outside the range of the simple lesion. The overall incidence is highest in the mid-thirties and early forties, but in this age group diagnosis is more common from imaging or by pathology, and physical signs are less characteristic.

Age and natural history

Clinically, the lesion is predominantly a tumour of young women. This would be expected from its lobular origin, for the time of greatest lobular development is the first years after the menarche. Yet studies have always shown the median age of diagnosis as about 30 years. This seems older than clinical experience suggests but is confirmed in a Cardiff, UK, series (Fig. 7.1).

The older patients are diagnosed in the pathology department, not in the clinic, and this can be explained

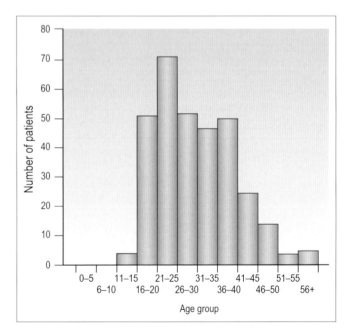

Fig. 7.1 The age at presentation with fibroadenoma – Cardiff patients. (Reproduced from Foster et al.[30] by courtesy of the *Journal of the Royal College of Surgeons of Edinburgh*.)

by the differing physical characteristics of fibroadenomas in different age groups. Lesions with classic physical signs (discrete, smooth, mobile) appear in the 16–25-year age group, being noticed accidentally whilst bathing or dressing. In the older age group the classic clinical symptoms may be obscured by coexisting involutional changes and the histological diagnosis may come as a surprise following tissue diagnosis of a clinical dominant mass, which lacks the notable discreteness and mobility of fibroadenoma in the younger girl.

Widespread use of ultrasound confirms that subclinical fibroadenoma is common throughout reproductive life.

Many fibroadenomas will not be felt in the young, firm breast and, if left alone, will remain static or gradually increase in size until 1–3 cm in diameter, taking 1–5 years to do so. During the growth phase, the tumour doubles in size in 6–12 months[2] and is then likely to remain static for the rest of the patient's life or gradually decrease in size. A fibroadenoma may become clinically apparent in the third or fourth decade as the tumour enlarges or the breast becomes softer or more pendulous after childbirth.

A more detailed knowledge of the natural history has come from a number of prospective studies where patients have been followed during conservative management. In the first major study, Dent and Cant[3] followed 63 young women in Capetown with a clinical and cytological diagnosis of fibroadenoma. They found that 31% of 201 lumps disappeared and a further 12% became smaller over 13–24 months' observation, 25% remained static and 32% grew. Regression was slightly more likely with single than multiple lesions. In a study from Edinburgh,[4] 201 patients less than 40 years old were offered conservative management after fibroadenoma diagnosed clinically was confirmed by ultrasound and cytology. The diagnosis was confirmed histologically in all 17 patients opting for surgery, confirming the accuracy of the triple diagnostic assessment. Two-thirds of the tumours were <2 cm in diameter, and one-third were 2–4 cm. Objective assessment of tumour size was obtained by ultrasound measurement. During follow-up, 13% resolved and 85% were unchanged; 2% increased in size and were removed, all four were simple fibroadenomas on histology. Thus, it may be accepted that most fibroadenomas remain static over several years following diagnosis, a few regress and a very small number grow. Indeed, Takei et al.[5] were able to derive an equation that predicted the rate (0.34 mm annual decrease) at which fibroadenomas, in Japanese women, changed size between the ages of 20 and 40.

To investigate why most fibroadenomas stop growing in this way, Meyer measured cell proliferation in normal breast epithelium, fibroadenomas and epithelial hyperplasias[6] and found that epithelial cells from fibroadenomas differed from the other two. They showed less variation in mitotic rate during the menstrual cycle, and the mitotic rate decreased with age. This may explain why growth stops.

Incidence

It is difficult to give an accurate assessment of the incidence and prevalence of fibroadenoma, although it is thought to be about 10%. In symptomatic clinics the ratio of fibroadenoma to cancer is about 1:4.[2] The advent of screening and the use of ultrasound and mammography in the clinic has shown that small asymptomatic fibroadenomas are common. New fibroadenomas appearing after the first screening round are associated with hormone replacement therapy. Fibroadenomas are more common on the left side (Fig. 7.2).

Geographical variation

Fibroadenoma makes up such a large proportion of benign breast disorders in India and Africa that an excess in these populations could be considered likely. However, there are no population-based figures to support this. In one study from Africa[7] fibroadenoma comprised 55% of all benign breast disorders, which is much higher than general experience in Western populations. The reported incidences in Chinese women[8] seem lower than those in African women and the fibroadenoma proportion of benign breast disorders in India is falling dramatically as painful nodularity becomes more obtrusive.[9] Onuigbo[10]

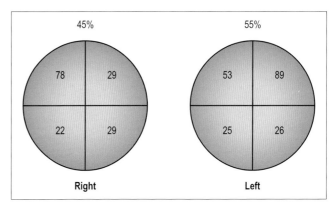

Fig. 7.2 Distribution of fibroadenomas in breast quadrants – Cardiff series.

considered that the increasing frequency of fibroadenoma in Africa between the 1970s and the 1990s, coupled with the lack of delay and smallness of the lesions, was due more to awareness of breast disease than any increase in the condition.

In a comparison of the incidence of benign lesions in three ethnic groups with widely differing breast cancer incidence (Anglo-Americans, Hispanics and American Indians), the incidence of fibroadenoma was similar in all three groups, unlike the incidence of severe hyperplasia, which differs in these three groups.[11] Thus, the incidence of simple fibroadenomas appears to be fairly constant across many ethnic groups, a pattern which differs from that of hyperplasias, which are more common in Western populations, and giant fibroadenoma, which is more common in non-Western populations.

In conclusion, it seems that the different reported incidences of fibroadenomas in populations are more to do with healthcare provision that any real ethnic differences.

Giant fibroadenoma

Onukak and Cederquist[12] found that 29% of fibroadenomas exceeded 6 cm in diameter, similar to the 30% reported from Uganda, and qualifying for designation as giant fibroadenoma. In contrast, only 4% of fibroadenomas exceeded 5 cm (and that included pregnancy, lactating adenomas, etc.) in an Indian/African population in South Africa. Although this latter figure is probably higher than in the UK, it is not markedly so. The high figures in Nigeria and Uganda are dramatically different to those reported in Western series, so probably represent a true excess, and a similar pattern is reported anecdotally from the West Indies.

Phyllodes tumour is particularly interesting, with evidence that the incidence varies considerably, and without obvious reason. There are considerable differences between different areas in Nigeria and India, which are probably significant, even allowing for variation among pathologists regarding diagnostic criteria. Perhaps the absence of virginal hypertrophy (usually seen particularly in black girls) in the series from northern Nigeria where phyllodes tumour was also absent reflects a lack in this area of some agent stimulatory to breast tissue.

Pathogenesis

We have already discussed in general terms in Chapters 1 and 4 our reasons for regarding fibroadenoma as part of aberrations of normal development and involution (ANDI), an aberration of normal lobular development rather than a neoplasm. There is good histological evidence that these tumours develop from the breast lobule; for example, elastic tissue is present in ducts but is not present in normal lobules, and elastic tissue is not seen in fibroadenomas.[13] The lobular origin explains many features of fibroadenoma, for instance, why most arise in young women at the time of maximal lobular development and why the stroma forms such a major element in fibroadenomas. This is derived from the hormone-dependent stroma of the lobule and not the simple fibrous stroma of the breast parenchyma. It also explains why many of the (very rare) cases of cancer arising in a fibroadenoma are of the more 'benign' type – lobular carcinoma in situ (LCIS).

This concept is supported by the work of Archer and Omar, who found that all the cellular elements of fibroadenoma are normal on conventional histology and electron microscopy.[14] Epithelial and myoepithelial cells maintain a normal relationship. The tumour bulk is due to an increase in fibroblasts, fibrocytes and collagen, and all show normal characteristics.[15,16] Noguchi and co-workers[15,16] have shown that common fibroadenomas are polyclonal, indicating that they are hyperplasia rather than neoplasia. This is in contrast to fibroadenomas in patients who subsequently developed recurrence in the form of phyllodes tumours, which were found to be monoclonal. The polyclonality of fibroadenomas is seen in both epithelial and stromal elements. The monoclonality of the phyllodes tumour applies only to the stromal element, the epithelial cells remaining polyclonal. These workers suggest that all fibroadenomas begin as polyclonal lesions, but with phyllodes tumours a monoclonal change occurs in the stromal element at an early stage. (If the stroma was monoclonal de novo, the phyllodes tumour would be expected to consist of stroma only; this situation is found in the rare pulmonary metastases.) This view has been challenged by Sawyer et al.[17] who found changes in both the epithelial and stromal elements of phyllodes tumours.

Steroid receptors have been studied in fibroadenoma.[18] Oestrogen and progesterone receptors can be demonstrated in relatively low concentrations in both cytoplasm and nucleus. These receptors are more easily demonstrated in fibroadenoma than in other ANDI conditions. Higher levels of oestrogen receptor appear to be associated with epithelial proliferation, and lower levels with stromal cell proliferation.[19] These workers found that progesterone receptors are less related to cellularity, and the overall conclusion was that hormone dependence of fibroadenomas diminishes rapidly as the lesions develop, a further possible explanation for the plateauing in the growth curve.

The aetiology of fibroadenoma is not known, but the fact that lobular proliferation is a response to oestrogen stimulation suggests that it may arise as the result of a lobule becoming unusually responsive to oestrogen. It grows both by proliferation of the lobule and also involvement of adjacent lobules, a fact of relevance to the significant recurrence rate after removal. It is interesting that four fibroadenomas and one phyllodes tumour reported in males from the Armed Forces Institute all occurred in patients with gynaecomastia, who had unusually developed lobule formation.[20] The development of lobules in males apparently requires a greater degree of oestrogenic stimulation than that which commonly induces gynaecomastia.

One interesting hypothesis relates to the finding of increased levels of the *bcl-2* gene in the epithelial cells of fibroadenomas.[21,22] The gene occurs in a number of tissues and tumours, where it acts to extend cell life by preventing the onset of apoptosis. Thus, failure of cell loss by apoptosis could be important in the development of fibroadenoma, although it is surprising that the gene was found only in the epithelial cells, and not in the stromal cells.

The widespread use of the contraceptive pill in young women makes it difficult to obtain accurate data on its role in pathogenesis. There is no evidence that the use of the contraceptive pill increases the risk of developing fibroadenoma and the epidemiological data available suggest that it may be associated with a decreased incidence. A majority of studies show that the risk of developing fibroadenoma is more than halved among those taking the contraceptive pill, particularly long-term users. The epidemiological studies suggest that it is the progestogen element of the combined preparation that is protective.

In this regard, the study by Canny et al.[23] is particularly interesting because all ages were investigated in a large case-control study, and differing effects were seen. Women less than 45 years showed a decreased incidence of fibroadenoma (OR = 0.57) in association with oral contraceptive use, while those over 45 showed an increased incidence (OR = 1.65 but not significant). The difference may be associated with the age at which oral contraceptive use was started, different formulations or other unknown

reasons. Women over 45 taking hormone replacement therapy (HRT) had a much increased incidence (OR = 2.83 but not significant due to small numbers); all patients were on oestrogen alone. No fibroadenoma was seen in seven controls taking a combined pill, again consistent with progesterone being protective.

Cigarette smoking appears to be protective with regard to fibroadenoma. In a study from Canada[24] the reduced risk 0.49 (0.28–0.98) was greatest in current active smokers but there was a less marked effect on previous smokers. Baildam et al.[25] drew attention to the relationship of fibroadenoma to ciclosporin A used in transplant patients. Son et al.[26] found that 2% of transplant patients developed fibroadenoma-like lesions that tended to be larger, multiple and some with worrying histological features. These fibroadenomata also had atypical ultrasound features. Although the mechanism is not clear, it is considered to be hormonal. Serum follicle-stimulating hormone (FSH) levels were significantly lower, and prolactin and oestradiol levels tended to be higher in patients with fibroadenoma. Such a hormonal effect could be a direct effect of ciclosporin, or a secondary one. In some patients, regression of the lesions had been seen after changing their immunosuppression from ciclosporin to tacrolimus.[27]

Koerner and O'Connell[28] have taken an opposing view to the ANDI hypothesis and regard fibroadenoma as a neoplasm, largely on the grounds that a human adenovirus 9 may induce a similar lesion in rats. However, the observed transition from fibroadenomatoid hyperplasia, fibroadenoma simplex to larger fibroadenomas and phyllodes tumours together with the observed genetic changes lend support to our hypothesis.

Pathology

The macroscopic appearance of fibroadenoma is of a sharply demarcated rounded or bosselated tumour with a white, glistening, bulging surface on section (contrasting with the convex cut surface of a cancer). The surface is irregular due to the epithelial-lined clefts which break up the uniformity. It is easily enucleated from its pseudocapsule of compressed breast tissue to which it is attached by a well-defined stalk. If the surface is brownish, phyllodes tumour should be considered.

The histological appearance is very characteristic, consisting of a combination of loose pale stroma and duct-like structures lined by regular epithelial cells. There is a tendency for this to follow one of two broad patterns, to which Cheatle[29] gave the terms 'pericanalicular' and 'intracanalicular'. In the pericanalicular pattern the epithelial structures are abundant, with the appearance of stroma surrounding circular ducts (Fig. 7.3a). In the intracanalicular form (Fig. 7.3b), the preponderance of stroma tends to push into elongated epithelial-lined clefts, so that the epithelial clefts now appear to surround islands of stroma. It is now recognized that both patterns are often seen in a single fibroadenoma, and there is no useful purpose in maintaining the differentiation. Varying degrees of epithelial hyperplasia are common and reflected in cytology specimens.

Fibroadenomatoid hyperplasia is a histological pattern of 'microfibroadenomas' occurring as ill-defined areas in the breast, in contrast to the well-defined discrete clinical fibroadenoma. They are best regarded as one part of the spectrum of lobular overgrowth correlating with a spectrum of clinical presentations. While most fibroadenomas in young women are well demarcated and mobile, other areas of lobular overgrowth may be less well demarcated and may even be multicentric; others are no more than a histological finding.

The tissues of a fibroadenoma will respond to external influences in a manner similar to normal breast lobules. Thus, they will undergo hyperplastic changes during pregnancy, secrete milk during lactation and involute at the menopause. The hyperplastic changes during pregnancy may outgrow the blood supply, leading to infarction.

It is important to recognize the wide variety of histological changes that may be seen in typical fibroadenomas compared to fewer variations in clinical behaviour. Such histological changes include apocrine and squamous metaplasia, neither of which is significant (except

possibly in relation to future cancer risk, as discussed further below). Marked hyperplasia of epithelial elements is also common but does not reflect aggressive behaviour. However, such florid epithelial changes cause trouble to cytologists, and benign fibroadenoma is an important cause of false-positive diagnosis of cancer on cytology in all but the most experienced hands.

Clinical features

Common clinical presentations

Differing clinical presentations are seen in young girls, during later reproductive life and in postmenopausal women. The clinical features of fibroadenoma are so characteristic in a young woman that the diagnosis can be made with a degree of confidence equalled only by that of a cyst after aspiration. The features are not so characteristic in older women, where the diagnosis should be made with care. In the young woman, fibroadenoma is a smooth, round or lobulated, firm discrete swelling with high mobility, giving rise to the term 'breast mouse'. The degree of mobility is truly remarkable, and the diagnosis should be circumspect when a lesser degree of mobility can be demonstrated. One exception to this rule is a fibroadenoma arising behind the nipple, where the surrounding ducts will limit its mobility. (It is not always recognized that there is much lobular tissue behind the areola in many women, explaining the findings that cysts and fibroadenomas, both of lobular derivation, are sometimes found behind the nipple.) The extreme mobility of the tumour in young women is due to encapsulation (Fig. 7.4) and to the softness and pliability of breast stroma in this age group. This also explains why fibroadenomas may appear on palpation to be much more superficial in the breast than their true position, a fact which should lead a surgeon to ensure that adequate facilities are available before embarking on the removal of a fibroadenoma under local anaesthetic.

The classic picture is not so obvious in older women, where involutional fibrotic changes surrounding the tumour will decrease its mobility. In this age group, fibroadenoma often masquerades as a dominant mass of ANDI ('fibroadenosis'), the diagnosis only made on tissue examination (Fig. 7.5). The physical signs of cancer and fibroadenoma may then come much closer together and fibroadenoma should not be diagnosed clinically in this age group until cancer has been excluded unequivocally.

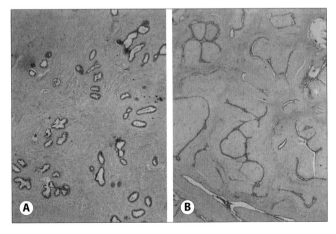

Fig. 7.3 The histological patterns of pericanalicular (**A**) and intracanalicular (**B**) fibroadenomas.

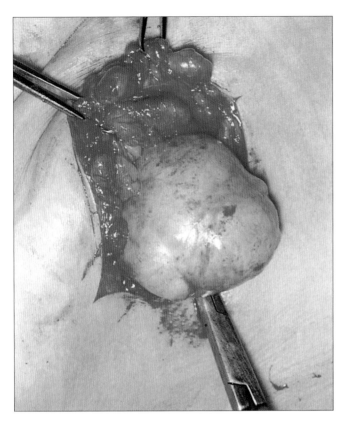

Fig. 7.4 The typical fibroadenoma of adolescent girls has a well-defined capsule, giving the tumour great mobility.

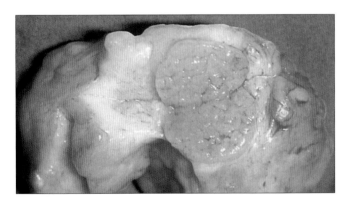

Fig. 7.5 A fibroadenoma in a 35-year-old patient. The typical clinical features were obscured by the involutional changes in the surrounding breast tissue.

A fibroadenoma is sometimes discovered in an elderly woman as a small, stony, hard, discrete mass, still moderately mobile. At this age the physical characteristics are again so precise that a clinical diagnosis can often be made with confidence. However, it can readily be (and must be) confirmed by mammography that the stony-

hard consistency is due to calcification. It is a reasonable assumption that small fibroadenomas discovered in the late reproductive or postmenopausal periods arose many years earlier, remained static, and are then discovered only as a result of involutional changes allowing them to be palpated more readily. Such lesions are not uncommonly seen in breast screening mammography.

Less common presentations

Very small superficial nodules of fibroadenomatous tissue, 3–4 mm in diameter, are sometimes seen in young women, and often remain unchanged for many years. These are felt only because of their superficial position; similar small static lesions deep in the breast are likely to be present much more frequently than clinically recognized, as borne out by histological study of whole breast sections. Cheatle[29] found small fibroadenomas in 25% of normal breasts.

Increase in size, sometimes marked, is sometimes seen during pregnancy. This may be associated with the general glandular hyperplasia seen in pregnancy, due to infarction or due to stromal hyperplasia.

A few fibroadenomas first become obvious as discrete masses in the late years of reproductive life. These may show a remarkable propensity for growth, rapidly reaching a large size. They have the gross and histological features of a simple fibroadenoma and behave in a benign fashion (but see pp. 97–98). It is interesting that similar rapid growth of a fibroadenoma is also seen in the 13–18-year age group, so that 'giant' fibroadenomas tend to have a bimodal distribution at the extremes of reproductive life (Fig. 7.6).

In the series reported by Foster et al.[30] four of the five fibroadenomas in the 11–15-year age group were more than 4 cm in diameter, as were about 15% of those between 16 and 25 years. Large tumours are seen less commonly in the next decade but reappear in smaller numbers around the menopause. Even less commonly, they may first present during early pregnancy. While giant fibroadenomas in both adolescent and menopausal age groups are uncommon, giant tumours are more common at adolescence than at the menopause.

The infrequency of fibroadenoma after the menopause suggests that they involute with perimenopausal breast involution. During this process they may calcify. Devitt[31] reported a series of 4379 women over 55 years who presented with a breast complaint. Only eight had fibroadenomas, and four of these were calcified. Similarly

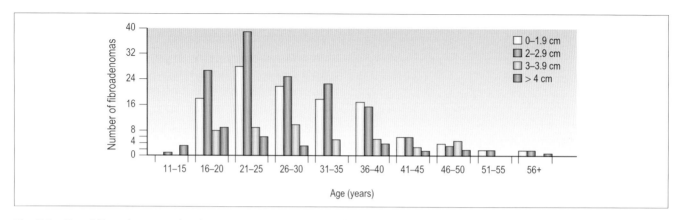

Fig. 7.6 Size of fibroadenomas related to age at presentation. Large fibroadenomas tend to occur at the extremes of reproductive life. (Reproduced from Foster et al.[30] by courtesy of the *Journal of the Royal College of Surgeons of Edinburgh*.)

Sandison[32] found an incidence of only 0.5% in his post mortem study. This situation is changing with widespread use of hormone replacement therapy. Occult fibroadenoma in postmenopausal women may be seen to increase in size on imaging when the patients are given unopposed oestrogen as HRT.[33,34]

Thus, simple fibroadenomas fall into four main groups:

- The small, static fibroadenomas of 3–4 mm palpable in the superficial breast
- The commonest type, which reaches a diameter of 1–3 cm before becoming static; this type comprises 80% of all fibroadenomas and hence must be regarded as the 'norm'
- The very few giant fibroadenomas of adolescence and the perimenopausal age; these groups are discussed later
- Fibroadenomas in the 4–5 cm group, which are larger than average but not in the 'giant' range; these comprise about 10% of the total and are distributed fairly evenly over the age range, but form a higher proportion in the perimenarchal and perimenopausal age groups.

Foster et al.[30] investigated whether these larger tumours constitute a different group in terms of histology or behaviour by comparing the cellularity of fibroadenomas of different size groupings. Stromal cells were counted by grey level analysis from a computer-linked TV image. They found no relationship between stromal cellularity and size of fibroadenomas, but cellularity was related to the age of the patient. The mean cell count in patients younger than 20 years was almost double that of older patients, although there was a second lesser increase in stromal cellularity just before the menopause, which might be explained by the stimulation of unopposed oestrogen at this time. Thus, larger tumours did not appear to be related to cellularity and there is no obvious reason at present why some fibroadenomas should grow to a larger size than average. There is also no reason to treat these larger fibroadenomas differently, nor in our series did they have a particular tendency to recur or to be multiple. Similarly, when Noguchi and co-workers identified fibroadenomas which later recurred as phyllodes tumours, the original fibroadenomas had not shown any peculiarity in relation to size or multiplicity.[16]

Special investigations

Mammography

Mammography is best avoided in younger women, both on grounds of poor diagnostic yield in the dense breast of this age and because of the radiation risk. Certainly, it is not indicated in the diagnosis of fibroadenoma under the age of 35.

In the older patient, fibroadenoma can be seen as a solitary smooth lesion, of similar density to the surrounding breast tissue when small, and more dense when large. When small, it may be difficult to detect, except as a smooth border outlined by the mammary fat. It may be surrounded by a halo of compressed fat, when the diagnosis is easier. In the postmenopausal period, at least half of all fibroadenomas will show typical stippled ('popcorn') calcification, similar to that seen in a uterine fibroid.

Ultrasonography

The ultrasonic features of fibroadenoma (Fig. 7.7) include a round or oval sharp contour, weak internal echoes in a uniform distribution and intermediate attenuation (see also Ch. 6). Ultrasound does not always distinguish these from other masses with certainty. Claims that Duplex spectral Doppler, and more recently colour Doppler, will reliably differentiate from cancer have not been confirmed.[35,36]

Cytology

The typical cytological appearance of fibroadenoma can be recognized by experienced cytologists. Aspirates vary greatly in cellularity, from scanty to an abundance of epithelial and stromal cells. The epithelium forms broad sheets that are uniform, equally spaced and cohesive.

Cohesive cells typically show branching epithelial structures resembling 'antler horns' and 'bare' nuclei are evident (Fig. 7.8). In less experienced hands, the hyperplastic epithelium typical of fibroadenoma may suggest a malign significance which is not justified by behaviour. Indeed, fibroadenomas are the main cause of false-positive cytology reports. In practice, FNAC has now been largely superseded by core needle biopsy.

Management

The management of fibroadenoma has become much more conservative since the first edition of this text. In part, this is due to the acceptance of fibroadenoma as part of ANDI and an appreciation of its natural history. Also, many patients now prefer to avoid surgery if at all possible. It remains a fundamental tenet of treatment that the patient should be fully informed so that she can make an appropriate decision for herself. It is our policy to offer excision for fibroadenomas over 3 cm in diameter. This is because it is in this group that atypical fibroadenomas will be found most frequently. This approach presupposes that a tissue diagnosis with a core biopsy has been obtained. The evidence that fibroadenomas may be treated conservatively at any age comes from the studies of Wilkinson and Forrest[37] and Dixon and colleagues[38] who undertook studies where all fibroadenomas in patients under the age of 35 were observed, provided cytology was negative. This carried some risk of missing cancers as these studies preceded the widespread use of image-guided core needle biopsy. Cant et al.[39] considered the same question, and concluded that a conservative policy is safe in women under the age of 25 years, although they found that 'a majority would prefer excision'.

The safety of conservation has been assessed in a prospective study[38] in which the criteria for conservation were age <40 years and a clinical diagnosis confirmed by cytology and ultrasound (and mammography if >35 years). Ninety per cent of patients opted for conservation and were monitored regularly; excision was advised if the volume increased by 20%, as occurred in 8% of the patients. Patients were discharged after 2 years if the lesion remained static or regressed. No mass under observation proved to be a cancer, and the authors regard the

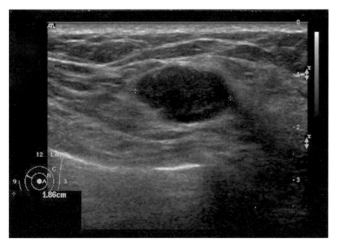

Fig. 7.7 Sonogram of small fibroadenoma: well-defined, slightly lobulated hypoechoic nodule.

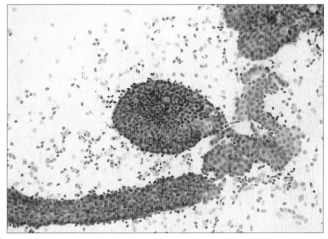

Fig. 7.8 Cytology preparation from a fibroadenoma, showing sheets of cohesive epithelial cells against a background of 'bare' nuclei.

criteria as defining a safe policy. Provision of histology by core needle biopsy can further increase safety. However, some reservations must remain because of the limited follow-up, and 20% of patients defaulted from observation before reaching that point.

Provided a formal triple assessment has been performed, a conservative approach is appropriate if that it is acceptable to the patient. Different groups interpret patient acceptance in different ways. Dixon and colleagues[38] claim 90% acceptance, in spite of 20% of the patients defaulting. Cant et al.[39] found that 73% of patients requested operation. Counselling techniques undoubtedly influence patients' preferences and a confident clinician will lead most women to accept conservation. It is also easy to underestimate the ongoing concern experienced by some women who continue to palpate a lump in their breast over years, during repeated campaigns counselling them not to ignore breast lumps.

How can one summarize to give a reasonable, pragmatic policy? Certainly, many fewer fibroadenomas need be removed than was previously the case, but it would be wrong to insist on a rigid conservative policy for all.

The approach to patients with fibroadenoma will depend on the demonstrated accuracy of triple assessment in the individual clinic, and the enthusiasm with which the patient accepts conservative management. If there is doubt regarding the nature of the presumed fibroadenoma it is easy to perform ultrasound-guided wide-bore core biopsy which will give a definitive histological diagnosis. A minority of patients may prefer a definitive minor procedure under local anaesthesia to the concern of carrying a breast lump. Others will welcome the option of avoiding surgery. Since most patients with a lump attend in order to obtain a definitive exclusion of cancer, they should be allowed to express their own views freely.

Surgical treatment

The classic surgical treatment is to excise the fibroadenoma though a small incision over the fibroadenoma. For those within 3 cm of the nipple a periareolar incision is appropriate. Although some surgeons do this procedure under a local anaesthetic, for deep-seated lesions a general anaesthetic is appropriate. Minimally invasive techniques have been described, and of these the vacuum assisted core biopsy technique is most widely available. Iwuagwu and Drew[40] have reviewed the role of ultrasound-guided, vacuum-assisted excision of fibroadenoma. This technique seems established but alternative

techniques such as laser ablation and cryosurgery still require formal evaluation. There is a danger that lesions that could otherwise be left untreated will be removed: minimally invasive techniques should not lead to a change in indications for removal. Although usually straightforward, it is impossible to be certain that it has all been removed and post-treatment bruising is almost inevitable. The same comments apply to laser ablation[41] and cryotherapy.[42]

Hormonal therapy

There has been a tendency on the European continent to treat fibroadenomas, along with other breast masses, by hormonal therapy, using tamoxifen, danazol and progestogens among others. It is difficult to assess results because of the lack of histological diagnosis or long-term follow-up. Viviani et al.[43] reported the results of treating 62 premenopausal women with varying doses of tamoxifen for 50 days. Patients taking 20 mg per day showed a significant size reduction; as the fibroadenomas were removed at the end of the observation period, no information on the subsequent changes in the lesions are available. The breast cancer prevention trials, IBIS and the NSABP prevention trial, will give an opportunity to follow the effect of tamoxifen on benign lesions in the breast. Tan-Chiu et al.[44] reported on the NSABP findings. They derived relative risk factors for a number of benign breast conditions including fibroadenoma based on histological material obtained during the observation period of the trial. The relative risk reduction for fibroadenoma was 0.77, 95% CI 0.56–1.07. Most of the risk reduction was confined to women under 50 years of age.

We have not followed this practice because of the uncertain long-term effects of hormonal manipulation, especially with tamoxifen, in young women.

Recurrence after surgery

New fibroadenomas which appear after removal of a previous tumour are often referred to as recurrent tumours, but this is a loose term and covers at least three groups.

Recurrence at the site of previous removal may represent incomplete removal, or adjacent lobules undergoing the same process. Some surgeons believe that removing the base of the 'stalk' lessens the risk of recurrence and this seems a reasonable step to take.

Newly noted tumours in the same or opposite breast represent the multiplicity of fibroadenomas often seen on careful histological examination of 'normal' breasts. Clinical experience suggests that multiple fibroadenomas may be occurring more frequently in recent years, although there are few firm data to support this.

It is not unknown for the original tumour to be missed and an adjacent area of nodularity excised, particularly if the operation is not carried out by the surgeon who examined the patient before operation. It is important that the surgeon is familiar with the site and characteristics of the lesion before the patient goes to theatre. Ultrasound localization will help in difficult cases.

In the Cardiff series of 322 patients, 23 patients are known to have developed a further fibroadenoma during follow-up, with an interval of 1–6 years (mean 2.6 years), 16 in the same breast and seven in the opposite. Of the 16 'recurrent' tumours in the same breast, nine were at the same site and seven elsewhere. Recurrence at the same site was not related to the size of the fibroadenoma, or to use of the contraceptive pill. Two of these patients have developed a carcinoma during the follow-up period, neither at the site of the fibroadenoma. During the same period, seven cases of phyllodes tumour were also treated; one recurred after an interval of 8 years.

Local recurrence of fibroadenoma is best excised because of the small risk of a more active tumour.

New tumours elsewhere in the breast are managed on the same principles as for the original tumour. The very rare syndrome of very large numbers of fibroadenomas (i.e. more than five in a single breast) needs to be managed on an individual basis, as discussed below.

Variations in histological appearance of fibroadenoma

Pregnancy

Fibroadenomas frequently show increase in size during pregnancy and secretory changes during lactation, and may show involution after parturition. Moran[45] described 10 cases removed during pregnancy. Azzopardi[13] described cases showing similar secretory changes to those of lactation in patients receiving large doses of progestogens.

Infarction

Infarction is a complication most commonly seen during pregnancy and lactation. It is usually asymptomatic, but may lead to an increase in size, raising the spectre of lac-

tational cancer. Unrecognized infarction may well be the cause of the calcified fibroadenomas characteristically seen in the elderly patient. The frequency of infarcted fibroadenoma is difficult to assess. In his histological analysis of 530 fibroadenomas teenage girls from south West Nigeria Onuigbo[10] found five (0.9%) infarcted.

Sclerosing adenosis

This may occur in a fibroadenoma and present some difficulty in histological assessment, but has no other implications for clinical management, except that it is one of the signs of a 'complex' fibroadenoma carrying a slight increased risk of future breast cancer.[46]

Myxoid fibroadenoma

Myxoid change may occur in any fibroadenoma, but a special, hereditary condition in which fibroadenomas may be associated with myxomas of the heart and skin has been described (Carney syndrome).[47] It is important to recognize this condition because of the dangers of atrial myxoma; about 25% of patients present first with the breast lesions.

Juvenile fibroadenoma

Ashikari et al.[48] studied 181 fibroadenomas in adolescent females and picked out 12 which they regarded as being floridly glandular and with a more cellular stroma. They gave these the name of 'juvenile fibroadenoma', but there is no uniformity of opinion among pathologists as to the specificity of this subgroup and it remains to be determined whether the histological picture they describe has a special clinical significance. The term is best avoided in favour of the clinical term of giant fibroadenoma of adolescence, which is considered on page 95.

Adenoma of the breast

There has long been argument as to whether or not a true adenoma of the breast exists, or whether these tumours just represent epithelial dominance in a fibroadenoma. More recently, it has been accepted as a distinct entity.[49] Tubular adenoma is a benign, circumscribed, 2–3 cm brownish-yellow tumour occurring mainly in young women. Histologically, it shows closely packed tubules of uniform, benign, two-layer epithelium. These lesions may also lactate in association with pregnancy.

Fibroadenoma with multinucleated stromal giant cells

Fibroadenoma with multinucleated stromal giant cells (MSGCs) may be found in otherwise unremarkable breast tissue, but Powell et al.[50] report 11 cases of fibroepithelial tumours containing these cells. They conclude that the presence of MSGCs, whether in simple fibroadenoma or in phyllodes tumour, does not affect behaviour. The tumours should be assessed on the normal criteria applied to the stroma, ignoring the MSGCs.

Cancer and fibroadenoma

There are three clinical aspects of the relationship of fibroadenoma and malignancy which require consideration: the association of cancer with a fibroadenoma, the incidence of subsequent breast cancer in patients with a fibroadenoma and the possible progression of fibroadenoma to phyllodes tumour. Consideration also needs to be given to molecular changes within a fibroadenoma that may predispose to carcinoma.

Cancer in a fibroadenoma

The common presence of epithelial hyperplasia in fibroadenomas, which is of no serious import, has led to overdiagnosis of cancer in the past. Cancer is rare; Haagensen[2] found only two true cases in the Columbia records over a 45-year period, both of which were LCIS. He points out that many of the reported cases are cancer adjacent to a fibroadenoma, multifocal cancer also involving a fibroadenoma, or low-grade lobular neoplasia of questionable malignancy. LCIS has classically been regarded as the common type, as would be expected from the lobular origin of fibroadenoma, but a series of 105 cases found equal frequencies of lobular and ductal carcinoma in situ (95% of cases were in situ cancer).[51] The mean age of the patients was 44 years, and the clinical characteristics usually did not differ from those without cancer. In the rare cases with invasive cancer, carcinoma in situ is usually present also, suggesting this as the origin of the invasive cancer.

Haagensen[2] reports two cases of LCIS treated conservatively, i.e. by local excision, without further trouble. In the series reported by Diaz and colleagues[51] only one of 26 patients treated conservatively for in situ cancer developed ipsilateral invasive cancer and the prognosis for all patients treated conservatively or by mastectomy was excellent. If LCIS is found in a fibroadenoma after enucleation, it would seem prudent to do a further local excision to determine whether the carcinoma is present in the surrounding breast and then treat it accordingly.

Ductal carcinoma often occurs in association with fibroadenoma rather than confined to it, and takes two forms: (1) direct infiltration from an adjacent cancer and (2) cancerization of the fibroadenoma by a tumour growing along the duct into the epithelial clefts, a process analogous to the cancerization of lobules by duct cancer. In either case, the fibroadenoma should be ignored in deciding on a treatment policy for the cancer.

Fibroadenoma and subsequent cancer risk

There are two avenues of investigation that may be used to assess the subsequent risk of breast cancer in patients with fibroadenoma: epidemiological studies and studies of genetic changes in patients with fibroadenoma.

Epidemiological studies

El-Wakeel and Umpleby[52] have provided a systematic overview of the epidemiological papers. They found seven assessable cohort and case-control studies. Overall, the relative risk lies in the range 1.48–1.7 for those without hyperplasia and 3.47–3.7 for those with hyperplasia. They were unable to determine whether excising the lesion altered this risk. The most compelling of the single studies is that of Dupont et al.[46] who reported a large retrospective study of this question. Patients with a complex fibroadenoma and a family history of breast cancer had a relative risk of 3–4 times higher than those without. This relative risk persisted for decades after diagnosis. Complex fibroadenoma was defined as those showing cysts, sclerosing adenosis, epithelial calcifications or papillary apocrine change. Patients with a complex fibroadenoma often carried similar changes in the surrounding breast tissue if this was included in the specimen. Since a fibroadenoma carries the same lobular elements as the normal breast, which is under the same influences, it is not surprising that a fibroadenoma should sometimes show the same changes, and carry the same significance. The histological association of carcinoma with phyllodes tumour is similar to fibroadenoma: a predominance of LCIS, and occasionally involvement of the lesion from adjacent cancer. There is some evidence for an increased incidence of related breast carcinoma, simultaneous or subsequent, in patients with phyllodes tumour and this is an added reason for careful long-term follow-up of such patients.

At present, the bulk of evidence indicates an increased incidence of breast cancer to a degree which is of biological interest, but not sufficient to alter management. The definition of a significant subgroup by confirmation of the work of Dupont and colleagues should be a priority for further research.

Genetic changes

A number of studies have investigated genetic changes in fibroadenoma and compared them to changes in breast cancers. For example, Sucic et al.[53] examined COX expression, using an immunocytological technique in fine needle aspirates. They found COX expression raised in carcinoma (8/9), fibroadenoma (3/9), but not in patients with fibrocystic disease, findings which suggest some overlap between fibroadenoma and breast cancer at the cellular level.

Studies of EGFR (epidermal growth factor receptor) show a closer relationship between fibroadenoma and normal breast than between fibroadenoma and breast cancer.[54] Study of the expression levels of NM23-H1 messenger RNA in fibroadenoma leads to a similar conclusion.[55]

Several studies have reported abnormalities of P53 in patients with fibroadenoma. These have been correlated with stromal changes and are more common as the lesion becomes more cellular and certainly more so in phyllodes tumours.[56] Amiel et al.[57] have reviewed the chromosomal aberrations found in fibroadenomas and in general they do not mirror those seen in breast cancer. The group in Dijon have failed to demonstrate any correlation between benign breast change and the molecular and genetic abnormalities associated with breast cancer.[58,59] They failed to confirm the findings of Tibiletti et al.[60] who found that there was a common cytogenic deletion of 6q in both fibroadenoma and carcinomas and who considered this deletion to occur in the epithelial component of the fibroadenomas.

The evidence suggests that for most fibroadenomas there is no increased risk of developing breast cancer. Some of the complex lesions do, however, have molecular changes that reflect those seen in some breast cancers. These findings are consonant with the risk profile derived from the epidemiological studies. Cericatto et al.[22] have confirmed the previously described increase in bcl-2 gene, but in addition increased ERα but normal c-myc in small fibroadenomata but with increased expression in tumours over 3 cm. Similarly, Tse et al.[61] have shown that CD10 expression is normal in fibroadenoma but raised in phyllodes tumours.

On the basis of both epidemiological studies and the molecular changes most patients with fibroadenoma can therefore be reassured that their risk is no greater than the general population; for a small number of women with complex lesions and those at the phyllodes end of the stromal spectrum a small relative risk persists.

Multiple fibroadenomas

Fibroadenomas are often multiple to the extent of three or even four developing concurrently or successively in both breasts. This is sufficiently common to be regarded as part of the 'normal spectrum', so that a pragmatic definition of multiple fibroadenomas as a separate entity would be five or more separate lesions in an individual breast. Haagensen[2] reported an incidence of more than one tumour of 16% among both white and black patients in his series, and points out that this is a minimal figure because the patients are not followed long term.

Our experience in Cardiff is similar. Seven per cent of patients had 2–4 tumours on presentation, and 7% had a further fibroadenoma either before or after the diagnosis for this survey.[30] One-third of the metachronous tumours occurred in the same quadrant as the first fibroadenoma, with an average time of 4 years to the second presentation. The mean age of these patients was 4 years less than those with single tumours. All these figures must be regarded as understatements, because complete follow-up of patients is very difficult in this age group and many tumours undoubtedly go unnoticed. It has been suggested that multiple fibroadenomas are more common in non-white populations. While we have seen this in a very small number of such cases there are few hard data to quantify this.

Multiple fibroadenomas as a distinct entity

If a cut-off point of more than five fibroadenomas in one breast is used to define a specific entity, such an entity is very uncommon in white populations in Western countries, although much higher numbers of fibroadenomas are sometimes reported in black and Oriental populations. In spite of this general perception of a high frequency in black and Oriental patients, attempts to obtain hard confirmatory data from those working among such populations has proved unrewarding. Otu[62] reported 8% fibroadenomas as multiple in Nigeria, a figure similar to the 7% reported in Cardiff, although the actual numbers in each case are not given. Personal enquiries we have made from West Africa, India, China and the West Indies suggest that the situation does not differ greatly from that seen in Western populations, with most cases of multiplicity falling into the 2–4 range (and some cases being small numbers of giant fibroadenomas rather than more than five). Such cases as have been reported tend to have a familial basis, and are not associated with the contraceptive pill.[2,63] An exception to this is South Africa: Cant and Dent have provided us with unpublished data from their clinic where 11 patients aged 15–29 had more than five fibroadenomas in one breast out of a total of approximately 350 non-white patients with fibroadenoma. This would suggest an increased incidence in their population. None had been on the contraceptive pill before developing a fibroadenoma.

Individual patients may show bizarre features. One 28-year-old Indian woman from Trinidad has had a total of 200 fibroadenomas removed over 6 years from the left breast and 10 (6 years earlier) from the right breast. They continue to form in the left breast, but not in the right. The patient's sister had a smaller (normal range) of fibroadenomas. As this surgeon has seen three cases of multiple fibroadenomas, it would seem possible that this condition is also more common in the West Indies.[63]

The situation in white populations in Western countries is poorly documented. Williamson et al. from Cardiff[64] reported a single case, and proposed that a register of such cases should be set up. Only two further cases were submitted in response to this request, one in Britain and one in Australia. A follow-up is available on all three patients. They were fully described in the second edition of this text. Interestingly, the fibroadenomas associated with ciclosporin are often multiple: 10 of 13 in the series reported by Baildam et al.[25]

Multiple giant fibroadenomas

This is a rare condition which combines features of both multiple and giant fibroadenomas (Figs 7.9 and 7.10).[65] It occurs mainly in young adolescents, usually black, girls. Growth of the masses is rapid during adolescence, but

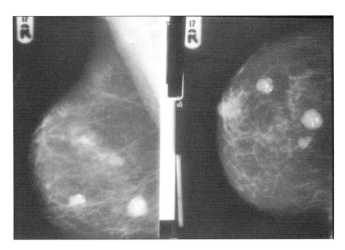

Fig. 7.9 Multiple fibroadenomata on mammography; several well-defined dense nodules with classical early 'popcorn-like' calcification.

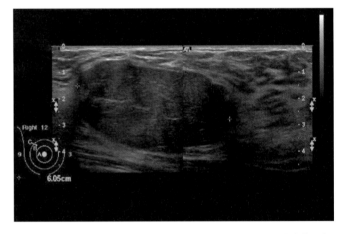

Fig. 7.10 Ultrasound image of giant fibroadenoma; well-defined, slightly hypoechoic mass.

slows during adult life. It is usually bilateral, but can be unilateral.[66] Rapid enlargement of multiple giant fibroadenomas may be one of the causes of gigantism of pregnancy.[67]

Any form of conservative management is problematical because of the high incidence of new lesions during the active growth phase. Management should be individualized on the basis of the extent of morbidity, with initial policy concentrating on attempts to conserve breast tissue by enucleating individual lesions.[68] However, in general, it is inevitable that some will need mastectomy to obtain reasonable symptomatic control.

Giant fibroadenoma

Giant fibroadenoma is predominantly a condition of the extremes of reproductive life, the first 5 years after the menarche and a decade before the menopause, and occurs when a fibroadenoma keeps growing beyond the usual 1–3 cm diameter. Fibroadenoma is designated 'giant' on the basis of its clinical size alone. This is a matter of definition which has varied widely in the past, some authors suggesting a weight of 500 g, some a diameter of 5 cm and others a 10-cm diameter. In practice, most tumours are closer to 10 cm than 5 cm and sudden growth in size is a dominant feature of adolescent tumours. Since the great majority of common fibroadenomas reach only 2–3 cm in size, greater than 5 cm seems a reasonable definition to pick out this group, particularly when associated with rapid growth. Ashikari et al.[48] combined cellularity of the stroma with size but this is confusing. Size and histology are better kept separate, because clinical behaviour in young girls does not parallel histological appearance. Giant fibroadenomas should be considered in relation to age: adolescent or perimenopausal.

Nomenclature

The nomenclature and definition used for this disorder are often confused due to the loose employment of three terms: giant and/or juvenile fibroadenoma, cystosarcoma phyllodes and sarcoma. Haagensen[2] set out clearly the histological features of the main groups, showing that giant fibroadenoma, phyllodes tumour and sarcoma should be defined on histological features only. His classification has been endorsed by Azzopardi[13] with a significant modification, that the term 'cystosarcoma' be dropped because these tumours are so rarely malignant.

This view is now generally accepted and three terms are used for breast tumours with a conspicuous stromal element:

1. fibroadenoma
2. phyllodes tumour and sarcoma
3. 'pure' sarcoma of the breast.

Phyllodes tumour carries a benign connotation but phyllodes sarcoma is malignant, the differentiation being made on the degree of cytological aberration; both are tumours showing a combination of stromal and epithelial tissues. The term 'phyllodes sarcoma' should be used sparingly, taking cognizance of the benign behaviour of most phyllodes tumours, especially in the young. Pure sarcoma is a tumour of connective tissue only. It behaves in a much more malignant fashion than phyllodes sarcoma, and is outside the scope of this text.

The entity of 'juvenile fibroadenoma' is not easily defined. The term has usually been used to designate a fibroadenoma in adolescence which grows rapidly and often reaches a large size, but some authors (e.g. Ashikari et al.[48]) describe histological features which they feel are specific to a subgroup of fibroadenomas in this age group. However, as discussed above, this histological specificity is not generally accepted and there is at present no agreement that juvenile fibroadenoma is a distinct histological group. There is no advantage to the term over a simple classification on the basis of size alone.

Giant fibroadenoma of adolescence[69]

This is a rare but important condition where an unusually large fibroadenoma occurs at or within a few years of puberty. It may be defined more precisely as a fibroadenoma-like tumour greater than 5 cm in diameter and presenting between the ages of 11 and 20 years. The importance of the group lies in the presentation and management. At presentation, the diagnostic problems range from failure to detect an abnormality to confusion with malignancy or virginal hypertrophy. Management has been obscured by unnecessary confusion with other related clinicopathological entities, including phyllodes tumour, and particularly the fibroadenomatous tumours seen later in life.

Giant fibroadenomas in this age group may be associated with multiple fibroadenomas, but usually only one enlarges to a great degree. Nambiar and Kannan-Kutty[70] regarded giant fibroadenoma as a more or less distinct clinicopathological variant, but our own studies show no great difference (apart from size) in disease behaviour or cellularity when compared with smaller fibroadenomas.[30] It is important that this condition be recognized as benign and that it be separated from phyllodes tumour or phyllodes sarcoma.

Nambiar and Kannan-Kutty[70] reported 25 cases and found a further 61 in the literature. They reported no recurrence or distant metastases, but their own 25 patients were all Chinese, Malays or Indians. Haagensen reports seven cases, of which five were in black patients. Cases reported from Hong Kong do not show great differences between Chinese and white patients. We have treated four patients aged 14–16 and one aged 18,[69] all white.

An extreme form of single giant fibroadenoma is also occasionally seen in pregnancy as one form of gigantomastia.

Clinical features

Although the clinical features of giant fibroadenoma of adolescence are varied, there is a remarkable overall similarity in the features described in all publications on this subject. Onset at or soon after puberty, sudden growth, prominent veins and occasional skin ulceration due to pressure are typical. Patients frequently report cyclical changes in the affected breast with premenstrual pain and increased breast size and tension during menstruation. The growths are unilateral, but it is not uncommon for a fibroadenoma of conventional size to present at the same time or later in the opposite breast.

It might be thought that a giant tumour would be diagnosed without difficulty, but this is not always the case. It often occurs at the time of rapid breast development and the mass is obscured by this development. If the consistency of the mass is similar to that of normal breast it may be regarded merely as asymmetry of the breasts (Fig. 7.11).

In other cases it may be clear that there is a well-defined mass, firmer than the rest of the breast (Figs 7.12 and 7.13).

In the third group, malignancy is simulated by such rapid growth that there are large dilated veins present over the mass (Fig. 7.14). Pressure necrosis of the overlying skin may occur, so that carcinoma or sarcoma is diagnosed.

Pathology

A wide spectrum of changes in both epithelial and connective tissue elements is found in these tumours. The epithelial element may show varying degrees of hyperplasia, while the stroma varies from fibrous to cellular, with

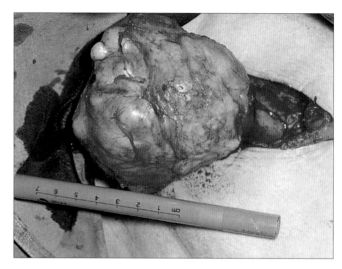

Fig. 7.12 An 8-cm fibroadenoma at operation.

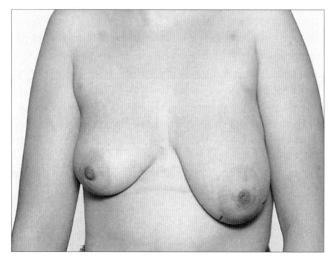

Fig. 7.11 Eighteen-year-old patient presenting with recent breast asymmetry. She was unaware of the presence of a large discrete mass in the left breast.

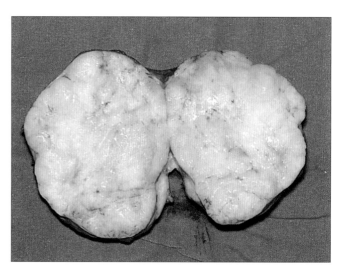

Fig. 7.13 Macroscopic cut surface of tumour seen in Figure 7.12.

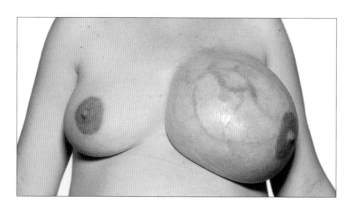

Fig. 7.14 Benign giant fibroadenoma of adolescence. Rapid growth, vascularity and pressure skin necrosis raised the question of malignancy.

or without mitotic activity, and thus may embrace the spectrum of phyllodes tumour. However, significant cellular atypia is not a feature, and this is important. In our experience, a number of cases have been referred with cytology or histology reports where the pathologist has considered the appearance as sufficiently worrying to recommend wide excision or mastectomy. Where such a report is given in an adolescent patient, further opinions should be sought from pathologists of great experience as these tumours act in a clinically benign fashion, even though clinical and histological features at first sight may suggest malignancy.[13]

The aetiology is obscure, and although a hormonal basis would be expected, there is little direct evidence to support this. There is no clear relationship to the contraceptive pill, with none of the Durban patients taking it.[71]

Management

Age is of great importance in assessing giant breast tumours; for practical purposes these lesions in adolescence are always benign. Our small series of six cases[69] showed no recurrence, and the literature supports the view that in white adolescent patients, discrete giant tumours, which contain both epithelial and connective tissue elements, have a uniformly benign clinical behaviour even though they may have a wide spectrum of histological appearances.[72] Some of the tumours in our series had a typical fibroadenoma appearance on histology; others had an appearance indistinguishable from benign phyllodes tumour. There do not appear to have been any

reports of local recurrence or malignancy in such tumours in white patients of this age group, and age takes precedence over histological assessment in adolescence.

It is reasonable to treat these lesions, on the basis of clinical diagnosis, by enucleation. Mammography and biopsy do not influence the treatment and may even lead to a false diagnosis of malignancy and consideration of unnecessarily radical treatment. Clearly, a different attitude will be taken to tumours in patients over the age of 20, and perhaps young patients of non-white races, although the available evidence from black and Indian patients suggests that malignancy is rare in these groups.[70,71]

Giant fibroadenomas tend to be deeper in the breast than is clinically apparent and, for this reason, are best approached from behind through a submammary incision (the Gaillard Thomas approach; see Ch. 18). This gives an excellent cosmetic result, and with negligible damage to breast ductal tissue. With large tumours, the remaining breast exists only as a compressed rim around the periphery, but this may be expected to expand and lead to a breast of roughly normal size and contour (Figs 7.15 and 7.16).

Simple mastectomy as recommended and practised in the case reported by Holbrook and Ramsay[73] is certainly to be condemned. Complex reconstructive procedures, such as the insertion of a de-epithelialized flap and silicone prosthesis as recommended by Hoffman,[74] reduction mammoplasty[75] or insertion of a tissue expander[76] are also inappropriate. Such approaches ignore the fact that the compressed breast tissue rapidly returns to normal after removal of the fibroadenoma, a process that might well be inhibited by an implant. Even closure of the cavities by sutures is unnecessary and may lead to breast distortion. Any reconstructive approach should be left until full spontaneous recovery has occurred, since this may be expected with considerable confidence.[69,71]

Giant breast tumours of the perimenopausal period

Giant tumours of the breast show a second peak of incidence in the pre- and perimenopausal period. Such tumours need careful clinical and histological assessment to put them in one of five categories:

- giant fibroadenoma
- recurrent and progressive fibroadenoma

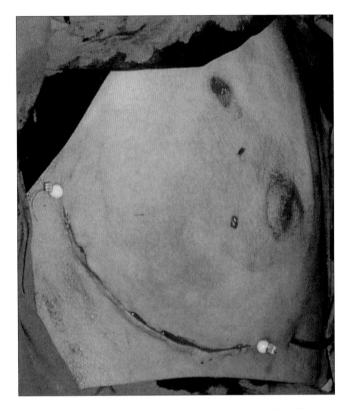

Fig. 7.15 The tumour has been enucleated via a Gaillard-Thomas (lateral) approach, leaving only a thin rim of compressed breast tissue. At the end of the operation the chest wall was flat.

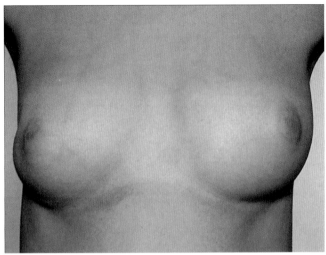

Fig. 7.16 One year later, the breast has regained almost normal size.

- phyllodes tumour and phyllodes sarcoma
- pure sarcoma
- carcinoma.

The last two are outside the scope of this text.

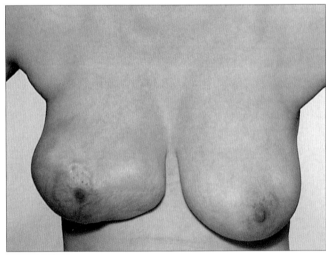

Fig. 7.17 Recurrent giant fibroadenoma of the perimenopausal period.

Giant fibroadenoma

A large tumour which clearly has the histological features of a benign fibroadenoma will usually behave in a benign fashion. It may be treated as a fibroadenoma of normal type in younger age groups, although it may not enucleate because of associated involutional fibrosis in the surrounding breast. In this age group they may recur (Fig. 7.17).

Fibroadenomatoid hyperplasia

This is a condition in which the breast contains multiple foci that are histologically identical to fibroadenoma, but not necessarily well defined from the surrounding breast. The spectrum extends from a minor histological finding, where fibroadenoma and 'fibroadenosis' overlap, to multiple distinct areas of considerable size. Hanson et al. found it in 11% of consecutive breast biopsies[77] and considered it to be a benign condition requiring histological diagnosis, without having any clinical significance. Such a histological finding is not uncommon in core breast biopsies performed for what is apparently nodular breast change. It is this merging from fibroadomatoid hyperplasia to fibroadenoma that contributes to our view that fibroadenoma may be regarded as part of ANDI. A bilateral variant has been described in a male with bilateral gynaecomastia following prolonged treatment with digoxin and spironolactone.[78]

Phyllodes tumour and phyllodes sarcoma (cystosarcoma phyllodes)

Although phyllodes tumour and phyllodes sarcoma are dealt with under the heading of giant breast tumours of the perimenopausal period, this is only because they are seen most commonly in this form and at this stage of life. Tumours can occur in any age group, as may tumours as small as a centimetre or so across. The pathology and management of these smaller tumours are similar to the more classic presentation discussed here.

This is a tumour with a dramatic clinical picture and aggressive histological features, so it is not surprising that it has received attention beyond any it deserves in view of its predominantly benign behaviour. It was Johann Muller who first gave it the name 'cystosarcoma phyllodes' in 1838, because it is often cystic and classically has leaf-like projections into it. While these terms were accurately descriptive, the term 'sarcoma' is not justified in a majority of cases, hence the suggestion that the term 'phyllodes tumour' be substituted, with the term 'phyllodes sarcoma' restricted to the small proportion that justify this designation on histological grounds or by clinical behaviour. This is another condition where confusion reigns, and much of the blame must again be directed against imprecise terminology. Since the tumour may be neither cystic nor sarcomatous, 'cystosarcoma' should be abandoned in favour of phyllodes tumour (benign) or phyllodes sarcoma (malignant). This case is well argued by Azzopardi.[13] Phyllodes tumour is distinct from giant fibroadenoma both macroscopically and histologically, but it must be reiterated that the diagnosis is a histological one and may apply to any size of tumour. The histological features may be seen in small as well as large tumours. Likewise, it is the pathologist who should decide (on histological grounds) whether the term 'sarcoma' is justified. To diagnose the tumour, both epithelial and fibrous stromal elements must be present, with the stroma showing cellularity, irregularity, hyperchromatism and significant mitosis. Stromal changes are patchy, so many sections need to be studied in the assessment of a large tumour. Contrasting histological pictures of fibroadenoma and phyllodes tumour are shown in Figures 7.18 and 7.19.

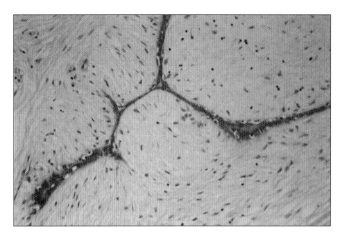

Fig. 7.18 Giant fibroadenoma – microscopic, hypocellular stroma.

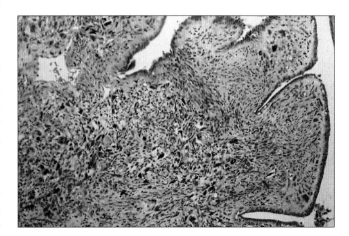

Fig. 7.19 Phyllodes tumour – cellular stroma with marked pleomorphism.

The stroma is notably more cellular than in a fibroadenoma, and is dominant in relation to the epithelial component. The stroma is concentrated around the epithelial clefts. An excellent description of the histological details assessed by the pathologist is provided by Azzopardi.[13] The typical macroscopic appearances of giant fibroadenoma and phyllodes tumour are contrasted in Figures 7.13 and 7.21.

Aetiology

Phyllodes tumour is clearly related to fibroadenoma in some cases, because patients may develop both lesions and histological features of both lesions may be seen in the same tumour. However, whether phyllodes tumour develops from a fibroadenoma or both develop simultaneously, or whether phyllodes tumour may arise de novo, is not clear. Noguchi and colleagues[16] have studied this question by clonal analysis in three cases where fibroadenoma and phyllodes tumour were obtained sequentially from the same patients. In each case, both tumours were monoclonal and demonstrated the same inactivated allele. They argue cogently that the phyllodes tumour had the same origin as the fibroadenomas, so that certain fibroadenomas can progress to phyllodes tumours.

An intriguing study by Yamashita et al.[79] looking at immunoreactive endothelin-1 (irET-1), exemplifies the manner in which modern science is elucidating mechanisms that will obviously prove to be important in understanding both normal breast function and pathology, while allowing a shift in emphasis from rodent models to human study. Tissue levels of irET-1 were measured in extracts from four phyllodes tumours and 14 fibroadenomas. Immunoreactive endothelin-1 was demonstrable in all cases, but levels were very much higher in phyllodes tumour than in fibroadenoma. Endothelin-1 is primarily a potent vasoconstrictor, but has many other functions. It causes a modest stimulation of breast fibroblast DNA, but can combine with insulin-like growth factor-1 (IGF-1) to produce potent stimulation. ET-1 is not present in normal breast epithelial cells, but specific ET-1 receptors are present on the surface of normal stromal cells. ET-1 receptors are found on the cell surface of phyllodes tumour stromal cells but immunoreactive cells were found within the epithelial cells but not the stromal cells, suggesting that ET-1 is synthesized by the epithelial cells of phyllodes tumours. Hence, this provides a possible paracrine mechanism for the stimulation of rapid stromal growth often seen with phyllodes tumours.

What is important is that phyllodes tumour should not be confused with pure sarcoma (without any epithelial element) for these have a greater degree of malignancy and lumping the two together can obscure the essentially benign nature of many phyllodes tumours. Immunocytochemistry and electron microscopy show that the stromal cells in both benign and malignant phyllodes tumour are a mixture of fibroblasts and myofibroblasts.[80]

These techniques allow differentiation from leiomyosarcoma and myoepitheliomas, which can mimic phyllodes tumours but behave differently.

Clinical features

Haagensen[2] reports approximately one phyllodes tumour to every 40 fibroadenomas. Our own hospital experience is similar; seven phyllodes tumours were diagnosed during one period when 332 fibroadenomas were treated.

The age distribution is broad, being from 10 to 90 in Haagensen's series of 84 patients, but with a majority between 35 and 55 years. Bilateral tumours are very rare, although an unusual case of three separate tumours in bilateral axillary ectopic breast tissue as well as a normal breast has been reported.[81] Phyllodes tumour is rare in patients before the age of 20, when it appears to behave in a particularly benign fashion, regardless of the histological features.[82] It has also been described in mammary-like glands in the vulva, in the male breast and in the prostate and seminal vesicle.

Most tumours grow rapidly to a large size before the patient presents, but the tumours are not fixed in the sense of a large carcinoma. This is because they are not particularly invasive; the bulk of the tumour may occupy much of the breast, or the whole of it, and produce pressure ulceration of the skin, but still show some mobility on the chest wall (Fig. 7.20).

The tumours are usually softer than fibroadenomas, grossly bosselated and the skin over them shows large, dilated veins. The axillary lymph nodes are not usually involved; a reasonable estimate of the incidence in the malignant subgroup is 10%, so overall the figure is very low.

On section, the tumour is well defined, but histologically may show limited invasion of the pseudocapsule of compressed breast tissue, accounting for the tendency to local recurrence. On cut surface, it has a moist, necrotic, characteristically brownish appearance (Fig. 7.21), sometimes with obvious mucoid, haemorrhagic or necrotic areas, and a softer consistency than a fibroadenoma.

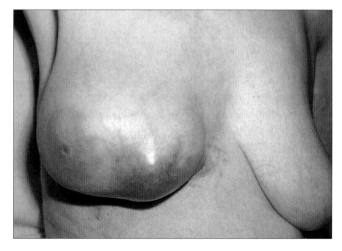

Fig. 7.20 Phyllodes tumour in a middle-aged woman. Pressure has led to thinning of the overlying skin.

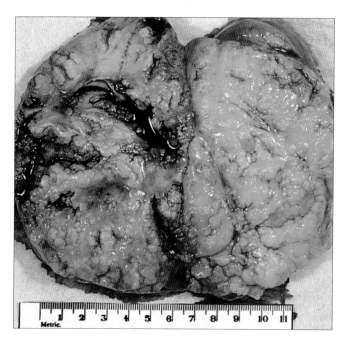

Fig. 7.21 Giant phyllodes tumour – macroscopic brown, irregular, cellular, leaflike masses, necrosis and haemorrhage.

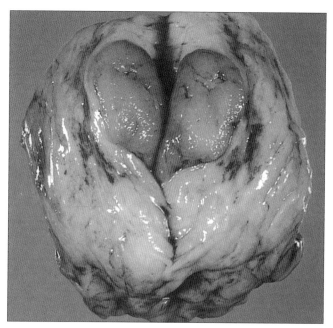

Fig. 7.22 Small benign phyllodes tumour. Note similarity to Figure 7.5, but with distinct brownish colour.

The brown colour is notable even with smaller tumours (Fig. 7.22) and should alert the surgeon to this diagnosis.

Behaviour

While phyllodes tumour shows a distinct tendency to recur locally if excised by a close margin, local or distant metastasis is uncommon. In fact, those tumours assessed as benign after comprehensive histological study can be expected to have an excellent prognosis, especially if treated initially by complete excision. Those which are histologically malignant (phyllodes sarcoma) are unpredictable in behaviour. A single-centre study of 32 cases provides a fair indication of behaviour.[82] Benign tumours showed no recurrence if completely excised, but half (6 of 13) incompletely excised recurred locally. No recurrence was seen after complete excision of four borderline and four malignant tumours, but incomplete excision of a malignant tumour led to uncontrolled chest wall disease. A report from Portsmouth[83] reported on 29 cases of benign phyllodes tumour and had one recurrence at 25 months in a patient with clear resection margins. Interestingly, 12 of these patients had positive resection margins without a recurrence. The median follow-up, however, was only 35 months and it will be interesting to see if further recurrences develop in the next few years.

In Treves and Sunderland's study[84] of 77 cases, 50% of those classified as malignant metastasized. It is difficult to predict behaviour on histological grounds. It is generally felt that mitotic rate is the best guide, although far from uniformly predictive. A mitotic rate less than 4 per 10 high power fields (HPFs) carried an excellent prognosis, 5–9/10 HPF is intermediate and more than 10/10 HPF carries a worse prognosis. Small tumours (less than 4 cm in diameter) have an excellent prognosis, and a 'pushing' margin is favourable. There are some indications that the behaviour of phyllodes tumours can be anticipated by the genetic changes identified by molecular biology.[85]

The overall favourable prognosis is shown by Haagensen's series, in which only four out of the 84 patients are known to have metastasized. While we have seen local recurrence in patients, none has as yet metastasized. A series of 66 cases from the Mayo Clinic[86] confirms that most behave as low-grade, nonmetastasizing tumours, but neither histological evaluation nor DNA analysis by flow cytometry gives a reliable assessment of behaviour in an individual tumour.

Treatment

Age is important in the management of these lesions. Under the age of 20, they may be treated by enucleation since they almost invariably behave in a benign fashion. The situation is less clear-cut in older patients. Few surgeons have sufficient experience to be dogmatic about management. Haagensen reports one of the largest series,[2] and recommends wide local excision as the primary approach to treatment of benign phyllodes tumours. He had a local recurrence rate of 28% among 43 patients treated by local excision, with a minimum 10-year follow-up. But only three of the recurrences required secondary mastectomy, and none has died from the tumour. Only 1 in 21 patients treated by mastectomy (simple or radical) developed local recurrence; this was a phyllodes sarcoma which rapidly produced both local and systematic metastases. Higher recurrence rates for benign than malignant phyllodes tumour have been reported in a number of series, reflecting a more casual surgical approach for the tumours considered less serious.

It is clear that incomplete excision is the main determinant of recurrence in benign and intermediate lesions. Why are high recurrences reported from most series when this is so well demonstrated? There are two main reasons: the failure to anticipate the possibility of a phyllodes tumour and the failure to define a technique which will ensure complete excision. The first can be met only by a high level of suspicion, and triple assessment of all masses before surgery. It is particularly important to avoid excision biopsy as a diagnostic procedure because it is almost impossible to effect a defined excision margin of a biopsy cavity, whereas this is easily done as a primary procedure while the tumour is still in situ. For this reason, histological diagnosis should be made by core needle biopsy.

Complete macroscopic excision, with a suggested margin of 1 cm, can be ensured by appropriate technique. With the usual technique of excision while applying traction to the mass, it is easy to dissect too close to the tumour at some point of the dissection. A reliable way to avoid this is for the surgeon to place the left fingers on the mass, and dissect outside the fingers, with traction only on the surrounding breast tissue. The inherent reluctance to cut one's own finger will ensure a full centimetre clearance around the whole circumference of the tumour!

For small lesions where the diagnosis is suggested by triple assessment or macroscopic appearance (soft, brown, fleshy appearance), the tumour should be excised with a 1-cm margin of normal breast tissue. If histology is benign, this would be sufficient treatment, with a quadrantic excision for intermediate lesions. Where the diagnosis is first recognized on histological examination of an excision biopsy specimen, quadrantic excision of the scar is recommended as a means of ensuring adequate local clearance. For large lesions and recurrent lesions, a good clearance inevitably involves near total mastectomy and we prefer simple mastectomy, with immediate reconstruction should the patient wish it. Mastectomy is a small price to pay for freedom from local recurrence, and reconstruction can readily lessen the price. We are reinforced in this policy by the fact that the stroma sometimes shows increased malignancy with recurrence.

Zurrida and colleagues take a more conservative approach,[87] recommending a 'wait and see' policy after a phyllodes tumour is first diagnosed after excision, provided it is assessed as benign on histology. This is on the basis that only 10% of such cases recurred in their series. However, this figure is lower than other series, and the avoidance of unnecessary surgery has to be set against the psychological stress to the patient of frequent follow-up, knowing that she has had a suboptimal procedure, and the small but definite risk of developing a more malignant recurrence. Clearly, the optimal management is to make a preoperative diagnosis and ensure total excision at the primary operation.

Pseudoangiomatous hyperplasia

There are several reasons for considering pseudoangiomatous hyperplasia (PASH) as a variant of fibroadenoma and thus as part of the ANDI spectrum. Clinically, mammographically and sonographically it simulates a fibroadenoma (see Fig. 7.23). On macroscopic examination, the mass is well circumscribed with a firm greyish-white cut surface so that it resembles a fibroadenoma. Histologically, it shows a fibrotic stroma with interconnecting slit-like spaces. The cytology of the accompanying spindle cells varies from bland to plump, proliferative looking cells. This curious lesion was described during Rosen's careful analysis of vascular tumours of the breast in the mid-1980s published as a series of papers in the *American Journal of Surgical Pathology*.[88] The clinical lesions are uncommon but a careful study of 200 consecutive breast specimens showed that 23% had at least one microscopic focus of PASH, none suspected clinically.[89]

This condition is a benign stromal tumour that simulates a vascular lesion and must be differentiated histo-

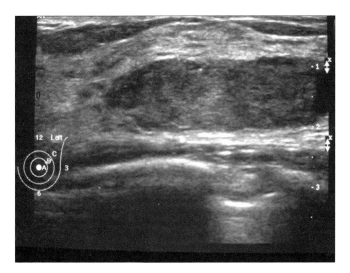

Fig. 7.23 Sonogram of small fibroadenoma: well-defined, slightly lobulated hypoechoic nodule.

logically from an angiosarcoma. It is seen most often as an incidental histological lesion at one end of its spectrum but at the other end can present as a clinical lump occupying the whole breast. It does not appear to change into angiosarcoma. Rosen believes the lesions most probably arise from the effect of endogenous or exogenous hormones on myofibroblasts.[90] Powell et al. reviewed 40 cases, palpable clinically in 39, with an age range from 14 to 67, and a mean in the fourth decade.[90]

The similarity to fibroadenoma is also evident at the molecular level since both express CD34 and bcl-2.[91] Anderson et al.[92] demonstrated that these lesions expressed progesterone receptors and consider progesterone stimulation as an aetiological factor. Zanella et al. showed that two of 14 lesions expressed both oestrogen and progesterone receptors.[93] These authors also noted associated glandular hyperplasia and considered PASH a focal form of breast stimulation.

Simple excision is adequate for the lesions, as well as for the uncommon recurrences, which may occur in the same or contralateral breast. One incompletely excised lesion regressed spontaneously. Salvador et al.[94] have suggested that no treatment beyond observation is necessary. Given the putative endocrine cause for this lesion it is not surprising that tamoxifen has been used although there is no large study to confirm its usefulness.

REFERENCES

1. World Health Organization. *Histological Typing of Breast Tumours,* 2nd edn. Geneva: WHO; 1981.

2. Haagensen CD. *Diseases of the Breast,* 3rd edn. Philadelphia: WB Saunders; 1986.

3. Dent DM & Cant PJ. Fibroadenoma. *World Journal of Surgery* 1989; **13**: 706–710.

4. Dobie V, Walsh J, Lamb J et al. Natural history of fibroadenoma of the breast. In: Mansel RE (ed.) *Recent Developments in the Study of Benign Breast Disease.* London: Parthenon; 1994:75–81.

5. Takei H, Iino Y, Horiguchi J et al. Natural history of fibroadenomas based on the correlation between size and patient age. *Japanese Journal of Clinical Oncology* 1999; **29**: 8–10.

6. Meyer JS. Proliferation in normal breast ducts, fibroadenomas and other ductal hyperplasias measured by nuclear labelling with tritiated thymidine. *Human Pathology* 1977; **8**: 67–81.

7. Ihekwaba FN. Benign breast disease in Nigerian women: a study of 657 patients. *Journal of the Royal College of Surgeons of Edinburgh* 1994; **39**: 280–283.

8. Algaratnam TT & Wong J. Benign breast disease in non-Western populations. *World Journal of Surgery* 1989; **13**: 343–345.

9. Khanna S, Arrya NC & Khanna NN. Spectrum of benign breast disease. *Indian Journal of Surgery* 1988; **50**: 169.

10. Onuigbo W. Breast fibroadenoma in teenage females. *Turkish Journal of Pediatics* 2003; **45**: 326–328.

11. Barton SA, Pathak DR, Black WC et al. Prevalence of benign, atypical and malignant breast lesions in populations at different risk of breast cancer. *Cancer* 1987; **60**: 2751–2760.

12. Onukak EE & Cederquist RA. Benign breast disease in Northern Nigeria. *World Journal of Surgery* 1989; **13**: 750–752.

13. Azzopardi JG. *Problems in Breast Pathology.* London: WB Saunders; 1979.

14. Archer F & Omar M. The fine structure of fibroadenoma of the human breast. *Journal of Pathology* 1969; **99**: 113–117.

15. Noguchi S, Motomura K, Inaji H et al. Clonal analysis of fibroadenoma and phyllodes tumour by means of polymerase chain reaction. *Cancer Research* 1993; **53**: 4071–4074.

16. Noguchi S, Yokouchi H, Aihara T et al. Progression of fibroadenoma to phyllodes tumour demonstrated by clonal analysis. *Cancer* 1995: **76**: 1779–1785.

17. Sawyer EJ, Hanby AM, Poulsom R et al. Beta-catenin abnormalities and associated insulin-like growth factor overexpression are important in phyllodes tumours and fibroadenomas of the breast. Journal of Pathology 2003; 200: 627–632.

18. Nardelli GB, Lamaina V & Siliotti F. Steroid receptors in benign breast disease, gross cystic disease and fibroadenoma. Clinical and Experimental Obstetrics and Gynecology 1987; 14: 10–15.

19. Martin PM, Kutten F & Serment H. Progesterone receptors in breast fibroadenomas. Journal of Steroid Biochemistry 1979; 11: 1295–1298.

20. Ansahboatene Y & Tavassoli FA. Fibroadenoma and cystosarcoma phyllodes of the male breast. Modern Pathology 1992; 5: 114–116.

21. Ferrieres C, Cuny M & Simony-Fontaine J. Variation of bcl-2 expression in breast ducts and lobules in relation to plasma progesterone levels: overexpression and absence of variation in fibroadenomas. Journal of Pathology 1997; 183: 204–211.

22. Cericatto R, Pozzobon A, Morsch DM et al. Estrogen receptor-alpha, bcl-2 and c-myc gene expression in fibroadenomas and adjacent normal breast: association with nodule size, hormonal and reproductive features. Steroids 2005; 70: 153–160.

23. Canny PF, Berkowitz GS, Kelsey JL et al. Fibroadenoma and the use of exogenous hormones. American Journal of Epidemiology 1988; 127: 454–461.

24. Rohan TE & Miller AB. A cohort study of cigarette smoking and risk of fibroadenoma. Journal of Epidemiology and Biostatistics 1999; 4: 297–302.

25. Baildam AD, Higgins RM, Hurley E et al. Cyclosporin A and multiple fibroadenomas of the breast. British Journal of Surgery 1996; 83: 1755–1757.

26. Son EJ, Oh KK, Kim EK et al. Characteristic imaging features of breast fibroadenomas in women given cyclosporin A after renal transplantation. Journal of Clinical Ultrasound 2004; 32: 69–77.

27. Alkhunaizi AM, Ismail A, Yousif BM. Breast fibroadenomas in renal transplant recipients. Transplant Proceedings 2004; 36: 1839–1840.

28. Koerner FC & O'Connell JX. Fibroadenoma: morphological observations and theory of pathogenesis. Pathology Annual 1994; 29(Part 1): 1–19.

29. Cheatle GL. Hyperplasia of epithelial and connective tissues in the breast: its relation to fibroadenoma. British Journal of Surgery 1923; 10: 436–455.

30. Foster ME, Garrahan N & Williams S. Fibroadenoma of the breast – a clinical and pathological study. Journal of the Royal College of Surgeons (Edinburgh) 1988; 36: 16–19.

31. Devitt JE. Benign disorders of the breast in older women. Surgery, Gynecology and Obstetrics 1986; 162: 340–342.

32. Sandison AT. An autopsy study of the Human Breast National Cancer Institute monograph No. 8. US Department of Health, Education and Welfare; 1962.

33. Cyrlak D & Wong CH. Mammographic changes in post-menopausal women undergoing hormone replacement therapy. American Journal of Roentgenology 1993; 161: 1177–1183.

34. Meyer JE, Frenna TH, Polger M et al. Enlarging occult fibroadenomas. Radiology 1992; 183: 639–641.

35. Holcombe C, Pugh N, Lyons K et al. Blood flow in breast cancer and fibroadenoma estimated by colour Doppler ultrasonography. British Journal of Surgery 1995; 82: 782–788.

36. Wright IA, Pugh ND, Lyons K et al. Power Doppler in breast tumours: a comparison with conventional colour Doppler imaging. European Journal of Ultrasound 1998; 7: 174–181.

37. Wilkinson S & Forrest APM. Fibroadenoma of the breast. British Journal of Surgery 1985; 72: 838–840.

38. Dixon JM, Dobie V, Lamb L et al. Assessment of the acceptability of conservative management of fibroadenoma of the breast. British Journal of Surgery 1996; 83: 264–265.

39. Cant PJ, Madden MV, Close PM et al. Case for conservative management of selected fibroadenomas of the breast. British Journal of Surgery 1987; 74: 857–859.

40. Iwuagwu O & Drew P. Vacuum-assisted biopsy device – diagnostic and therapeutic applications in breast surgery. The Breast 2004; 13; 483–487.

41. Basu S, Ravi B, Kant R. Interstitial laser hyperthermia, a new method in the management of fibroadenoma of the breast: A pilot study. Lasers in Surgery & Medicine 1999; 25: 148–152.

42. Whitwoth PW & Rewcastle JC. Cryoablation and cryolocalization in the management of breast disease. Journal of Surgical Oncology 2005; 90: 1–9.

43. Viviani RS, Gebrim LH, Baracat EC et al. Evaluation of the ultrasonographic volume of breast fibroadenomas in women treated with tamoxifen. Minerva Ginecology 2002; 54: 531–535.

44. Tan-Chiu E, Wang J, Costantino JP et al. Effects of tamoxifen on benign breast disease in women at high risk for breast cancer. Journal of the National Cancer Institute 2003; 19: 302–307.

45. Moran CS. Fibroadenoma of the breast during pregnancy and lactation. Archives of Surgery 1935; 31: 688.

46. Dupont WD, Page DL, Parl FF et al. Long term risk of breast cancer in women with fibroadenoma. New England Journal of Medicine 1994; 331: 10–15.

47. Carney JA & Toorkey BC. Myxoid fibroadenoma and allied conditions (myxomatosis) of the breast. A heritable disorder with special associations including cardiac and cutaneous myxoma. American Journal of Surgical Pathology 1991; 15: 713–721.

48. Ashikari R, Farrow JH & O'Hara J. Fibroadenomas in the breast of juveniles. Surgery, Gynecology and Obstetrics 1971; 132: 259–262.

49. Hertel BF, Zaloudek C & Kempson RL. Breast adenomas. *Cancer* 1976; **37**: 2891–2905.

50. Powell CM, Cranor ML & Rosen PP. Multinucleated stromal giant cells in mammary fibroepithelial neoplasms – a study of 11 patients. *Archives of Pathology and Laboratory Medicine* 1994; **118**: 912–916.

51. Diaz NM, Palmer JO & McDivitt RW. Carcinoma arising within fibroadenomas of the breast – a clinicopathological study of 105 patients. *American Journal of Clinical Pathology* 1991; **95**: 614–622.

52. El-Wakeel H, Umpleby HC. Systematic review of fibroadenoma as a risk factor for breast cancer. *Breast* 2003; **12**: 302–307.

53. Sucic M, Boban D, Markovic-Glamocak M *et al.* Expression of cyclooxygenase-2 in fine-needle aspirates from breast carcinoma and benign breast diseases. *Breast* 2003; **12**: 51–57.

54. Zeladahedman N, Werer G, Collins P *et al.* High expression of the EGFR in fibroadenomas compared to breast carcinomas. *Anticancer Research* 1944; **14**: 1679–1688.

55. Goodal LRJ, Dawkins HJS, Robbins PD *et al.* Evaluation of the expression levels of NM23-H1 messenger RNA in primary breast cancer, benign breast disease, axillary lymph nodes and normal breast. *Pathology* 1994; **26**: 423–428.

56. Chan YJ, Chen BF, Chang CL *et al.* Expression of p53 protein and Ki-67 antigen in phyllodes tumor of the breast. *Journal of the Chinese Medical Association* 2004; **67**: 3–8.

57. Amiel A, Kaufman Z, Goldstein E *et al.* Application of comparative genomic hybridization in search for genetic aberrations in fibroadenomas of the breast. *Cancer Genetics Cytogenetics* 2003; **142**: 145–148.

58. Franco N, Picard SF, Mege F *et al.* Absence of genetic abnormalities in fibroadenomas of the breast determined at p53 gene mutations and microsatellite alterations. *Cancer Research* 2001; **61**: 7955–7958.

59. Franco N, Arnould L, Mege F *et al.* Comparative analysis of molecular alterations in fibroadenomas associated or not with breast cancer. *Archives of Surgery* 2003; **138**: 291–295.

60. Tibiletti MG, Sessa F, Bernasconi B *et al.* A large 6q deletion is a common cytogenetic alteration in fibroadenomas, pre-malignant lesions, and carcinomas of the breast. *Clinical Cancer Research* 2000; **6**: 1422–1431.

61. Tse GM, Tsang AK, Putti TC *et al.* Stromal CD10 expression in mammary fibroadenomas and phyllodes tumours. *Journal of Clinical Pathology* 2005; **58**: 185–189.

62. Otu AA. Benign breast tumours in an African population. *Journal of the Royal College of Surgeons of Edinburgh* 1990; **35**: 373–375.

63. Naraynsingh V & Raju GC. Familial bilateral multiple fibroadenomas of the breast. *Postgraduate Medical Journal* 1985; **61**: 439–440.

64. Williamson MER, Lyons K & Hughes LE. Multiple fibroadenomas of the breast – a problem of uncertain incidence and management. *Annals of the Royal College of Surgeons of England* 1993; **75**: 161–163.

65. Musio F, Mozingo D & Otchy DP. Multiple giant fibroadenoma. *The American Surgeon* 1991; **57**: 438–441.

66. Kuusk U. Multiple giant fibroadenomas in an adolescent breast. *Canadian Journal of Surgery* 1988; **31**: 133–134.

67. Stavrides S, Hacking A, Tiltman A *et al.* Gigantomastia in pregnancy. *British Journal of Surgery* 1987; **74**: 585–586.

68. Schneider B, Laubenberger J, Kommoss F *et al.* Multiple giant fibroadenomas. Clinical presentation and radiological findings. *Gynecologic and Obstetrics Investigation* 1997; **43**: 278–280.

69. Raganoonan C, Fairbairn JK, Williams S *et al.* Giant breast tumours of adolescence. *Australian and New Zealand Journal of Surgery* 1987; **57**: 243–247.

70. Nambiar R & Kannan-Kutty M. Giant fibroadenoma (cystosarcoma phyllodes) in adolescent females. A clinico-pathological study. *British Journal of Surgery* 1974; **61**: 113–117.

71. Naidu AG, Thomson SR & Nirmul D. Giant fibroadenomas in black and Indian adolescents. *South African Journal of Surgery* 1989; **27**: 171–172.

72. Mies C & Rosen PP. Juvenile fibroadenoma with atypical epithelial hyperplasia. *American Journal of Surgical Pathology* 1987; **11**: 184–190.

73. Holbrook WA & Ramsay JH. Giant fibroadenoma of the breast. *Bulletin of the School of Medicine of the University of Maryland* 1956; **41**: 58–63.

74. Hoffman SH. Giant fibroadenoma of the breast: immediate reconstruction following excision. *British Journal of Plastic Surgery* 1978; **31**: 170–172.

75. Daya M, Mahomva O, Madaree A *et al.* Reduction mammoplasty in cases of giant fibroadenoma among adolescent females. Case reports and literature review. *South African Journal of Surgery* 2003; **41**: 39–43

76. Kamei Y & Torii S. Natural skin reduction and breast recovery using a tissue expander after enucleation of a giant breast tumour. *Scandinavian Journal of Plastic Reconstructive and Hand Surgery* 2000; **34**: 383–385.

77. Hanson CA, Snover DC & Dehner LP. Fibroadenomatosis (fibroadenomatoid hyperplasia): a benign breast lesion with composite pathologic features. *Pathology* 1987; **9**: 393–396.

78. Neilsen BB. Fibroadenomatoid hyperplasia of the male breast. *American Journal of Surgical Pathology* 1990; **14**: 774–777.

79. Yamashita J, Ogawa M & Egami H. Abundant expression of immunoreactive endothelin-1 in mammary phyllodes tumour – possible paracrine role of endothelin-1 in the growth of stromal cells in phyllodes tumour. *Cancer Research* 1992; **52**: 4046–4049.

80. Auger M, Hanna W & Kahn HJ. Cystosarcoma phylloides of the breast and its mimics. An immunohistochemical

and ultrastructural study. *Archives of Pathology and Laboratory Medicine* 1989; **113**: 1231–1235.

81. Saleh HA & Klein LH. Cystosarcoma phyllodes arising synchronously in right breast and bilateral axillary ectopic breast tissue. *Archives of Pathology and Laboratory Medicine* 1990; **114**: 624–626.

82. Moffat CJC, Pinder SE, Dixon AR *et al.* Phyllodes tumour of the breast. A clinico-pathological review of 32 cases. *Histopathology* 1995; **27**: 205–218.

83. Sotheran W, Domjan J, Jeffrey M *et al.* Phyllodes tumours of the breast – a retrospective study from 1982–2000 of 50 cases in Portsmouth. *Annals of the Royal College of Surgeons of England* 2005; **87**: 339–344.

84. Treves N & Sunderland D. Cystosarcoma of the breast – a malignant and a benign tumour. A clinico-pathological study of 77 cases. *Cancer* 1951; **4**: 1286–1332.

85. Erhan Y, Zekioglu O, Ersoy O *et al.* p53 and Ki-67 expression as prognostic factors in cystosarcoma phyllodes. *Breast Journal* 2002; **8**: 38–44.

86. Keelan PA, Myers JL, Wold LE *et al.* Phyllodes tumour: Clinicopathologic review of 60 patients and flow cytometric analysis of 30 patients. *Human Pathology* 1992; **23**: 1048–1054.

87. Zurrida S, Bartoli C & Galimberti V. Which therapy for unexpected phyllodes tumour of the breast? *European Journal of Cancer* 1992; **28**: 654–657.

88. Rosen PP, Jozefczyk MA & Boram LH. Vascular tumors of the breast. IV. The venous haemangioma. *American Journal of Surgical Pathology* 1985; **9**: 659–665.

89. Ibrahim RE, Sciotto RC & Weidner N. Pseudoangiomatous hyperplasia of mammary stroma. *Cancer* 1989; **63**: 1154–1160.

90. Powell CM, Cranor ML & Rosen PP. Pseudoangiomatous stromal hyperplasia (PASH). A mammary stromal tumor with myofibroblastic differentiation. *American Journal of Surgical Pathology* 1995; **19**: 270–277.

91. Moore T & Lee AH. Expression of CD34 and bcl-2 in phyllodes tumours, fibroadenomas and spindle cell lesions of the breast. *Histopathology* 2001; **38**: 62–67.

92. Anderson C, Ricci A Jr, Pedersen CA *et al.* Immunocytochemical analysis of estrogen and progesterone receptors in benign stromal lesions of the breast. Evidence for hormonal etiology in pseudoangiomatous hyperplasia of mammary stroma. *American Journal of Surgical Pathology* 1991; **15**: 145–149.

93. Zanella M, Falconieri G, Lamovec J, Bittesini L. Pseudoangiomatous hyperplasia of the mammary stroma: true entity or phenotype. *Pathology Research and Practice* 1998; **194**(8): 535–540.

94. Salvador R, Lirola JL, Dominguez R *et al.* Pseudoangiomatous stromal hyperplasia presenting as a breast mass: imaging findings in three patients. *Breast* 2004; **13**: 431–435.

CHAPTER 8

Breast pain and nodularity

Key points and new developments

1. Mastalgia is now accepted as a common cause of morbidity, occasionally severe enough to interfere with quality of life, and then sufficient to justify careful investigation and treatment.

2. The basic cause of cyclical mastalgia is clearly endocrine in nature, but the precise mechanism(s) continues to elude investigators.

3. Cancer, sclerosing adenosis and postsurgery scars are rare but important causes, while referred pain often presents as mastalgia.

4. Most mild to moderate cases are seeking reassurance, and this is usually all that is required.

5. Management of more severe cases follows classification into cyclical and noncyclical cases, with the latter further divided into true noncyclical and musculoskeletal pain. Pain charts are an important aid to assessment.

6. Evening primrose oil for the mild to moderate case and danazol/tamoxifen for the moderate to severe case are the mainstays of treatment. Goserelin (an LHRH analogue) may be used for resistant and recurrent cases.

7. Lower than usual dosage has improved the therapeutic ratio with danazol and tamoxifen. Short courses, repeated if necessary, are preferred to longer, continuous therapy.

8. Cases refractory to standard treatment need careful individual assessment; some patients may benefit from psychological assessment and therapy.

9. Results of surgery, including mastectomy, are unpredictable, and surgery should be used only exceptionally.

10. Mastalgia in the postmenopausal period is being seen more frequently in women on hormone replacement therapy (HRT); it is usually self-limiting and not of great severity.

11. There is considerable overlap between cyclical mastalgia and premenstrual syndrome (PMS) but there are also significant differences, requiring differing approaches.

12. For further reading, refer to: Santen RJ & Mansel RE. Review of the aetiology and management. Current concepts: benign breast disorders. *New England Journal of Medicine* 2005; 353: 275–285.

Introduction

Mastalgia is one of the commonest symptoms in patients attending a breast clinic and is also the most frequent reason for breast-related consultation in general practice.[1,2] Many terms have been used to describe mastalgia in the past, including the term 'mastodynia' introduced by Heineke in 1821 and 'mazodynia' used by Birkett in 1850. The mixing of pathological with clinical terms noted in Chapter 4 has caused confusion in the past and it is better to use 'mastalgia' to denote the symptom of pain in the breast without any specific pathological connotation being implied.

Historical note

The literature amply demonstrates that breast pain is the commonest presenting symptom of breast conditions and it would be natural to assume that it was a well-documented subject with clear definitions and guidelines for management. Until recently this was not the case; the literature devoted to mastalgia has been poor both in quality and in clarity. Most of the problem has been due to attempts to relate poorly defined clinical presentations with pathological terms as previously discussed in Chapter 4.

Birkett, in 1850, in his textbook of breast diseases[3] described breast pain as 'mazodynia' and noted two subtypes: with induration (nodularity) or without induration. He noted premenstrual exacerbation of tenderness in the nodular group and suggested aperients and tonics as treatment. Cheatle and Cutler[4] in 1931 used the term 'mazoplasia' to describe bilateral painful nodular breasts, and suggested it was present to some degree in all women's breasts. Later authors used the all-embracing term 'chronic mastitis' to denote painful nodular breasts,[5,6] with some attempting to define degrees of severity.[7] Carl Semb described various degrees of painful nodularity in his exhaustive study of 1928,[8] but also mixed symptomatic terms with pathological descriptions. Geschickter devoted a whole chapter in his 1945 book to the subject of mastodynia (painful breasts) and described many of the clinical features of mastalgia,[7] but concluded, as had others before him, that mastodynia progressed into the various forms of chronic cystic mastitis.

Thus, despite a small number of exhaustive studies by these eminent clinicians and pathologists, there was no clear account of mastalgia as a symptom. In 1971, a special research clinic was set up within the Cardiff Breast Clinic, UK, in order to answer some of the questions regarding mastalgia and benign breast disease. The findings of this mastalgia clinic, which has continued to study this problem to the present, form the substance of this chapter.

Frequency of breast pain

Ader et al.[9] in 2001 attempted to establish the prevalence in the community. In this study 874 women between 18 and 44 were recruited for interview by random number dialling in Virginia. Sixty-eight per cent reported some cyclical mastalgia and in 22% this was described as mod-

erate or severe. Interestingly, patients on the oral contraceptive pill had less trouble, while there was a positive association with smoking, caffeine intake and perceived stress. Further, women with breast pain were twice as likely to have had a mammogram. The overall prevalence reflected these authors' previous experience from a gynaecology clinic.

The frequency of breast pain as a presenting symptom of breast disorders in various clinics is shown in Table 8.1.

The exact frequency is difficult to ascertain as many studies do not state the population from which the study group is drawn. An example is Geschickter's detailed account, which described 375 cases of mastodynia seen in Baltimore over a period of 50 years, but the incidence of other breast conditions is not stated.[7]

A study from the USA[12] shows a significant impact among a population of 1171 women attending a general obstetrics and gynaecology clinic. Sixty-nine per cent suffered regular discomfort and 36% had consulted about their breast pain. Current moderate-to-severe pain was found in 11% of women. Mastalgia interfered with usual sexual activity in 48% and with physical (37%), social (12%) and work (8%) activity.

In general, it can be concluded that breast pain is present in about 50% of patients presenting to surgical clinics with breast problems, but higher levels of around 65–70% were volunteered by women interviewed at a screening clinic and at screening carried out on site in a

Table 8.1 Frequency of breast pain as a presenting symptom in benign and malignant breast disease

Study	Percentage of patients complaining of mastalgia
Semb[8]	85
Southampton Breast Clinic[10]	50
Cardiff Breast Clinic	45
General practice[13]	47–52
Working population (Cardiff Marks & Spencer Study)	66
UK screening clinic[11]	70
US obstetric and gynaecology clinic[12]	69
USA questionnaire study[9] (Population study)	68

group of working women at a large retail chain store (the Cardiff Marks and Spencer Study).

Mastalgia in breast cancer

Although this text does not deal with cancer, the role of breast pain in the diagnosis of early breast cancer is of considerable importance. Classic teaching was that early cancers were not painful, so that patients presenting with pain were unlikely to have cancer. While this is generally true for bilateral cyclical mastalgia, more detailed work has shown that pain does not exclude cancer, and may occasionally be the only presenting symptom of a subclinical cancer. Several papers make the point that although breast pain is an uncommon symptom in breast cancer, it does not exclude the diagnosis.

Preece et al.[13] noted that mastalgia indicating an underlying cancer differed from cyclical premenstrual mastalgia in that it was unilateral, persistent and constant in position. Of 17 patients who presented with mastalgia alone out of a population of 240 operable breast cancers, they found five were T0 tumours and five T1 tumours, suggesting that mastalgia as a sole presenting symptom is associated with smaller tumours. Preece's work has been confirmed by an Italian study[14] of 200 patients presenting with local breast pain and negative physical examination. Mammography detected subclinical cancer at the site of the pain in five patients.

The literature on this topic is generally consistent, as is shown by Table 8.2.

The converse side of this question is whether cyclical mastalgia reflects a hormonal environment which predisposes to breast cancer. Studies attempting to answer this question raise many difficulties, but the bulk of evidence suggests that any such predisposition is minimal. However, one matched, case-control study of 420 women showed a relative risk of cancer of 2.12 (95% CI = 1.31–3.43) in those who gave a history of cyclical mastalgia, after allowing for confounding risks such as oral contraceptive use and pregnancies.[19] In a subsequent cohort study these authors reported an association between the duration of mastalgia and breast cancer risk, although the numbers are too small to allow generalization.[20]

Classification

Previous attempts at classification based on pathological terms did not give any practical help in the understanding

Table 8.2 Frequency of breast pain as a presenting symptom of operable breast cancer

Study	Percentage of cancers presenting with pain
Preece et al.[13]	7
River et al.[15]	24
Haagensen[16]	5
Smallwood et al.[10]	18
Yorkshire Group[17]	5
Chiedozie and Guirguis[18]	8

Table 8.3 Contents of the Cardiff Mastalgia Protocol

Feature	Examples
Descriptive terms	Tenderness/heaviness/burning
Periodicity	Continuous, intermittent
Duration	
Distribution in breast	
Radiation	
Aggravating factors	Physical contact
Relieving factors	Analgesics/drugs/well-fitted brassiere
Diurnal pattern	
Disturbance of lifestyle	Sleep loss/marital problem/can't hug children
Dominant hand	

or management of mastalgia. A pressing need was to classify accurately the symptom of mastalgia and this was initially done by drawing up a protocol in the Cardiff Mastalgia Clinic describing significant features of the symptom (Table 8.3).

In addition, a comprehensive gynaecological history was taken and careful physical examination performed. All the patients studied in the Mastalgia Clinic had already been examined clinically by an experienced breast surgeon and by mammography (when indicated) to exclude carcinoma of the breast and extramammary causes ranging from cervical spondylosis to biliary pain. These patients thus presented with painful breasts with or without nodularity. Cases with a discrete lump were managed as detailed in Chapter 5.

Analysis of the initial 232 patients studied with this protocol defined certain patterns of mastalgia.[21] The frequency of each type is shown in Table 8.4.

The general validity and utility of this classification has been confirmed, with some modifications, in 25 years' experience in the Cardiff Mastalgia Clinic.

Cyclical pronounced pattern

The commonest type of pain is related to the menstrual cycle, and particularly to ovulation (Fig. 8.1). Clearly, many women experience 2 or 3 days of premenstrual breast tenderness or heaviness every month and this should be regarded as normal (Fig. 8.2).

Fine nodularity which begins a short time before menstruation and regresses postmenstrually is equally normal; the difficult problem is deciding where normality ends and disease begins. When the normal discomfort is exceeded, we have used the term 'cyclical pronounced mastalgia'.

The cyclical group has been given the adjective 'pronounced' to denote the increased intensity of the symptom

defined either by duration (>1 week per cycle), or by severity documented using a pain chart (Fig. 8.3).

Severity is necessarily a subjective assessment, as is all assessment of pain in clinical practice, but obtrusive features in the lifestyle, such as sleep loss, work disturbance or interrupted sexual activity, can give some guide. This

Table 8.4 Frequency of patterns in 232 prospectively documented mastalgia patients

Pattern/diagnosis	Number (%)
Cyclical pronounced	93 (40)
Noncyclical	62 (27)
Tietze's syndrome	25 (11)
Trauma (post-biopsy)	19 (8)
Sclerosing adenosis	11 (4.5)
Cancer	1 (0.5)
Miscellaneous/non-breast	21 (9)

From Preece et al.[21]

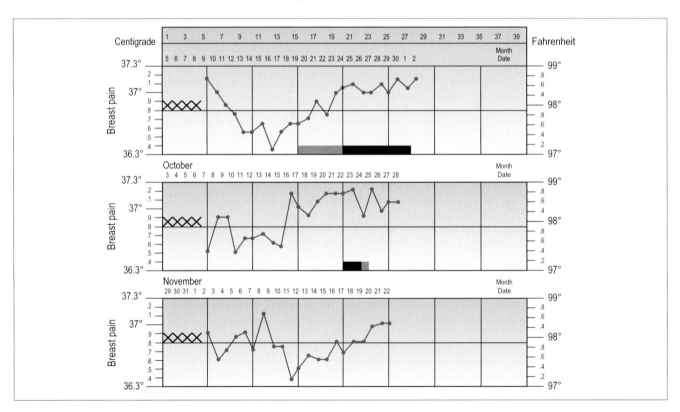

Fig. 8.1 Basal body temperature chart recorded by a patient with mastalgia. The first two cycles show a biphasic ovulatory pattern and breast pain (shown as black/grey shading) occurred for about 2 weeks premenstrually in the first cycle (*top level*) and for about 4 days in the second cycle. No pain occurred in the third cycle (*lower panel*) which appears to have a nonovulatory temperature pattern. This chart demonstrates the association of mastalgia with ovulation and the variation in one woman from cycle to cycle. XXXX = menstrual period.

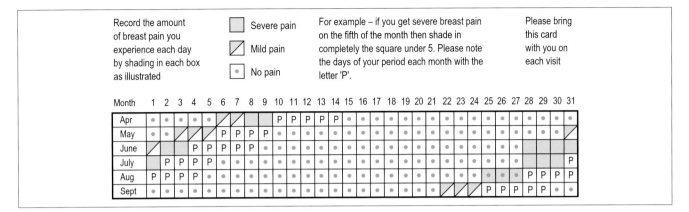

Fig. 8.2 Breast pain chart showing daily recording of breast pain. The chart shows 3–4 days of mild premenstrual pain per cycle, which would be regarded as normal. P, period.

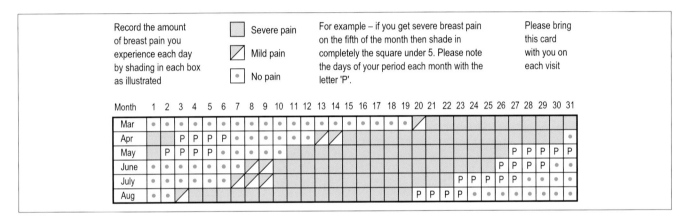

Fig. 8.3 Pain chart of a patient with cyclical pronounced mastalgia showing 2–3 weeks of severe premenstrual mastalgia per cycle over 6 months.

group probably represents the 'mastodynia' group of previous reports, although some authors state that associated nodularity excludes mastodynia. The cyclical pronounced patient almost invariably has nodularity of a varying degree which is maximal in the upper outer quadrant, and shows cyclicity similar to the pain.

Other characteristics of the cyclical pronounced group are shown in Figure 8.4 and it is worth noting that the terms 'heaviness' and 'tenderness to touch' are used frequently to describe symptoms of the pattern.

Bilateral pain and nodularity are also common. The pain often radiates to the axilla and down the medial aspect of the upper arm, presumably as a referred pain via the intercostobrachial nerve. A well-taken history will often reveal the temporal association with the menstrual cycle, but we have found a simple pain chart to be extremely useful in displaying this pattern (see Fig. 8.3). This is essential in patients who have had a hysterectomy.

A pain chart is readily completed by most patients and has the added advantage of giving a simple quantitation to the symptom (days of pain) which is useful for assessing effectiveness of therapy.

Mammography has proved unhelpful in the cyclical pronounced pattern, as the non-specific changes of radiological density ascribed to 'fibroadenosis' have been the main feature, and no specific radiological appearance correlates with the site or side of pain.

Noncyclical pattern

The second largest group (27%), the noncyclical pattern, is distinguished principally by its lack of relationship with events in the menstrual cycle and again is well shown by the pain chart (Fig. 8.5).

Detailed analysis of 72 noncyclic patients has shown that they fall into two main groups: true noncyclical mastalgia and musculoskeletal pain (Fig. 8.6).[22]

The two groups are roughly equal in frequency of presentation, although this varies with the efficiency of screening before reaching the mastalgia clinic. The mean age of the musculoskeletal group is greater (39 years vs 34 years) and the duration of pain shorter (15 months vs 35 months).

True noncyclical breast pain

This pattern occurs in both pre- and postmenopausal women in contradistinction to the cyclical pattern but the mean age of these patients is similar at 34 years. The noncyclical pattern differs in several respects from the cyclical. The pain tends to be well localized in the breast and is more frequently subareolar or upper outer quadrant. Simultaneous bilateral pain is not uncommon and the descriptive terms of 'burning, drawing or abscess-like'

are different. Other terms indicative of a transient sharp quality, such as pricking or stabbing, have also been commonly used, and such pain may last for minutes or days at a time. When the pattern was assessed quantitatively using a linear analogue scale (see later), it was scored by the patients at a lower intensity than the cyclical pattern. Nodularity is less prominent than in the cyclical group, but is still seen in 54% of patients. When differentiated from musculoskeletal pain, noncyclical breast pain has a better response to hormonal therapy than previously thought. About half will have a useful response to danazol, with a similar response rate reported for tamoxifen.[23] Half will have a spontaneous remission, but after a mean period of 27 months.

Mammography has been of some interest in the noncyclical group, as the radiological changes of coarse calcification and ductal dilatation attributed to duct ectasia or periductal mastitis have been commonly seen in this group. Of the 62 patients documented, no less than 42 showed radiological evidence of duct ectasia somewhere

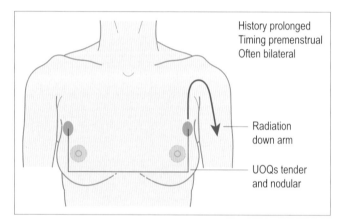

Fig. 8.4 The clinical features of cyclical mastalgia. It is premenopausal; mean age = 34 years. Descriptive terms are 'heaviness' and 'tenderness to touch', relieved by menstruation and menopause. UOQ, upper outer quadrant.

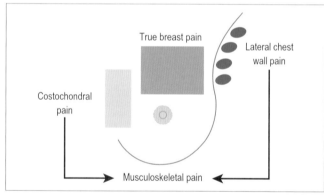

Fig. 8.6 The types of noncyclical mastalgia. (From Maddox et al.[22])

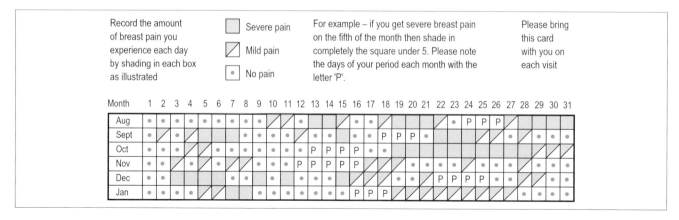

Fig. 8.5 Pain chart showing a noncyclical pattern of mastalgia. There is no demonstrable relationship to any phase of the menstrual cycle.

in the painful breast, and of these 20 showed the typical coarse calcification at the site of complaint. These findings led us initially to describe the noncyclical pattern as the 'periductal mastitis' pattern, but we prefer to use the 'noncyclical' term, firstly because it conforms to our principle of not mixing symptomatic with pathological terms, and secondly because we have no histological evidence that noncyclical pain is due to the pathological changes of duct ectasia.

A further term, 'the trigger spot', has been introduced for this pattern, or at least a subgroup of it,[24] based on the special feature that pressure by palpation at the indicated site of pain will reproduce the patient's pain. However, in our experience, while this picture is seen in some patients, it does not describe the overall group and there is no correlation with any histological finding at the site of complaint.[25] We feel it is best reserved as a small subtype of noncyclical mastalgia.

Chest wall (musculoskeletal) pain

Musculoskeletal pain is almost always unilateral (92%) and falls into two groups: Tietze's syndrome and lateral chest wall pain.[22] A good response is often obtained with an injection of steroid and local anaesthetic.

Tietze's syndrome[26] or painful costochondral junction syndrome is not a true breast pain but the pain is often felt in the region of the breast overlying the costal cartilages, which are the source of the pain (Fig. 8.7).

It has a characteristically chronic time course and, on examination, one or several costal cartilages are tender and feel enlarged. Typically, the pain is felt within the medial quadrants of the breast and increased pain occurs

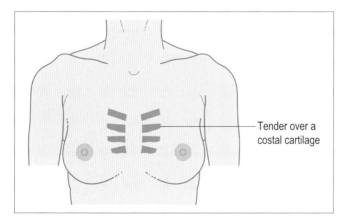

Fig. 8.7 The clinical features of Tietze's syndrome. It is often unilateral; any age; no time pattern; no palpable abnormality; chronic course.

on pressure over the affected cartilage. Radiological examination of these patients reveals no abnormality in the costal cartilages or specific features in the breast.

Lateral chest wall pain most commonly occurs in the anterior axillary line and is related to the slips of origin of the serratus anterior muscle. Less commonly the tender area is just lateral to the midclavicular line. These syndromes are treated by explanation and reassurance. In our experience local injections of steroid and local anaesthetic are not usually necessary, although they have been reported to be effective.[27] These noncyclical-type pains can be managed effectively with topical nonsteroidal application as was demonstrated in a trial of diclofenac gel in 48 women which showed that 50% of the women were pain free after 6 months of topical therapy.[28]

Trauma

The trauma group, 8% of the total, complained of a persistent noncyclical-type pain localized to a previous benign biopsy scar. There were no specific findings apart from the presence of the scar, but on enquiry it was revealed that several of the biopsies had been complicated by infection or haematoma, and some of the painful scars had been made across Langer's lines of tension. However, prolonged breast discomfort of annoying degree can follow even simple, uncomplicated biopsy. Indeed, the considerable incidence of long-term pain after all forms of breast surgery is not always appreciated. In a study of 282 patients undergoing major breast surgery, one-third to one-half still had pain after a year. It was particularly troublesome after mastectomy with reconstruction, and after subpectoral implant insertion.[29] Kudel et al. reported in 2007 a study of 278 women some years after mastectomy.[30] They identified three types of pain: phantom symptoms, scar pain and other pain, and found that such pains may cause considerable distress.

Other causes

Cancer was an uncommon cause of pain in the Cardiff series as these cases were filtered out in the general breast clinic. Thus, only one case of a cancer developing during observation in the Mastalgia Clinic was seen in Preece's original study. This patient had a well-localized pain with no lump at presentation and negative mammography, but the pain persisted for 1 year and a repeat mammogram showed an impalpable cancer. Cancer usually shows a noncyclical pain chart, as illustrated in Figure 8.8.

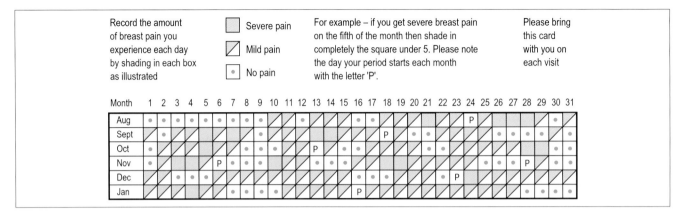

Fig. 8.8 Pain chart of a patient who subsequently developed a small palpable cancer at the site of pain. The chart shows a typical noncyclical but persistent pattern.

The miscellaneous group (see Table 8.4) consisted of patients who were unclassifiable into the preceding groups or were shown to have pain due to a non-breast cause, such as gallstones or angina. About 10–13% of patients presenting with breast pain will be found to have a cause outside the breast, particularly of musculoskeletal origin, such as cervical spondylosis.[31]

Other general findings for the whole group of patients were that mastalgia is commoner in the left breast and half of the patients had experienced pain for over 1 year prior to consultation. Thus, mastalgia is often prolonged and seems to have a predilection for the left breast, as does cancer and most breast pathology.

In summary, there are three major pain patterns: the cyclical pronounced, noncyclical and chest wall pain, and only these three will be considered further in the discussion of therapy.

Aetiology of mastalgia and nodularity

History

Many of the surgeons who wrote about the clinical description of mastalgia also speculated on the cause of the condition, but modern hormone estimations were unavailable and most of the conclusions remained pure speculation. Several workers suggested that some ovarian influence was responsible for the cyclical pattern of mastalgia as they had noted the association with the menstrual cycle and also the absence of the problem after the menopause.[4,7] Perhaps we should not be too critical of these scientists because aetiological terms coined by them have a very familiar ring today and endocrinology was far

less advanced. Cutler proposed a luteal abnormality and Geschickter described a relative hyperoestrogenism.

Other theories were those of excessive water retention and, more importantly, neuroticism. As early as 1829, Astley Cooper began the trend of describing mastalgia patients as 'being of a nervous disposition' but also added that this was a personal impression.[32] Unfortunately, this trend continued, without any rational scientific basis, and was brought up to date almost a century and a half later by a leading gynaecologist with the comment in an influential gynaecology textbook that mastalgia patients were 'frustrated, unhappy nulliparae'.[33] Even such an authority as Haagensen wrote that women with severe breast pain were 'in general, unstable and hypochondriacal although they are not frankly psychotic'.

These impressions and hypotheses have now been examined scientifically.

Studies of aetiology

Water retention

Oedema due to water retention has been suggested as a cause of both mastalgia and the premenstrual syndrome because women had reported weight gain and breast and ankle swelling in late cycle. As a result, treatment with diuretics was proposed.[34] There was, however, no study in the literature showing that general oedema was associated with mastalgia. At the Cardiff Mastalgia Clinic, we therefore carried out estimations of total body water using tritiated water in mastalgia patients and asymptomatic normal women.[35] The results clearly showed that there were no significant differences in water gain between the fifth and twenty-fifth days of the cycle when mastalgia patients were compared with normal controls, and this was true even for the cyclical group who displayed the typical premenstrual increase in breast pain. This suggests that simple retention of body water does not seem to be correlated with mastalgia, although it might be argued that intramammary oedema is more important. Breast swelling is common in the luteal phase when assessed volumetrically.[36,37] This work has been confirmed since it has been possible to study the water component of breast volume changes using magnetic resonance imaging (MRI).[38]

Psychoneurosis

We next turned our attention to the hypothesis that mastalgia patients were more neurotic than other patients, as suggested by Astley Cooper. Using the well-validated Middlesex Hospital Questionnaire (MHQ), specifically designed as a rapid screening test for differentiating between 'normals' and psychiatric cases,[39] the psychoneurotic profiles of 300 patients presenting to hospital with mastalgia (cyclical and noncyclical) and 156 patients presenting with varicose veins were tested.[40] The scores of the varicose vein and mastalgia patients were significantly lower than those of psychiatric out-patients, which had been published by the MHQ designers (Table 8.5).

Moreover, the only differences between mastalgia cases and varicose vein patients were in favour of the former (although a different pattern has been shown in treatment-resistant cases – discussed later in this chapter). This study showed conclusively that there is no scientific foundation for the impressions of those who believed mastalgia patients to be psychoneurotic. Psychological aspects of mastalgia are discussed more fully in Chapter 19.

Table 8.5 Neuroticism scores of mastalgia patients compared with patients with varicose veins, and psychiatric outpatients – mean (SD)

	Mastalgia (n = 300)	Varicose veins (n = 156)	Psychiatric outpatients (n = 173)
Anxiety	7.6 (0.23)	7.8 (0.30)	11.0 (0.26[a])
Depression	4.2 (0.16)	5.1 (0.21)	7.6 (0.29[a])
Phobia	5.0 (0.16)	5.7 (0.22)	6.8 (0.29[a])

a Significantly greater than mastalgia or varicose vein groups. High scores imply abnormality (MHQ questionnaire).

Endocrine abnormalities

The advent of accurate radioimmunoassays for estimation of blood hormones and the discovery of human prolactin as a separate entity from growth hormone caused a rapid upsurge in interest in the 'hormonal imbalance' hypotheses previously discussed. From previous work, three main theories emerged regarding the aetiology of painful nodular breasts:

- increased oestrogen secretion from the ovary
- deficient progesterone production ('relative hyperoestrogenism'[41])
- hyperprolactinaemia.

Early studies failed to support the first two theories, as steroid levels were found to be no different in patients and controls,[42–44] but a French group in 1979 showed a significantly depressed level of luteal progesterone,[41] thus supporting the second theory. Furthermore, the same group obtained symptomatic relief by correcting the depressed progesterone level with an exogenous progestogen. Unfortunately, no other group has been able to find a definite defect in luteal-phase progesterone and in all British and American studies there was no significant difference between mastalgia patients and controls.[43,45]

Our experience is similar, and in a study of 50 mastalgia patients and 18 controls we failed to show any difference in luteal-phase progesterone between the two groups.[46] Further studies of the free fraction of progesterone measured daily in the saliva failed to reveal any differences between controls and mastalgia patients in Wales or Scotland.[47,48] In contrast, a study of 671 patients on parenteral medroxyprogesterone acetate for contraception and 1433 controls showed a halving of clinically significant mastalgia in the contraception group.[49] The case for a luteal defect therefore remains unproven and the therapeutic value of progestogens is also debatable (see later). One review concludes that there are no significant differences in basal levels of ovarian steroids and gonadotrophins in women with benign breast conditions compared with controls.[50]

Prolactin was only accepted as a separate hormone from 1970 onwards, and a specific radioimmunoassay became available a year later, but has since received a great deal of attention. As the major lactogenic hormone, there are prima facie reasons for believing that it may play a role in a condition which is thought to be due to overstimulation of a normal physiological process. However, although several studies of random basal prolactin levels showed no significant differences between normals and patients with benign breast disorder (review by Wang and Fentiman[50]), analysis of prolactin secretion in normal women has shown that the hormone is secreted in a pulsatile manner and has a diurnal variation.[51] These factors suggest that random sampling of basal prolactin is inappropriate. In order to avoid these problems, Malarkey et al. measured 24-hour profiles, but again failed to find any differences between controls or biopsied benign disease cases at any time of the day or night.[44] One further study of daily sampling at a fixed time throughout the menstrual cycle revealed a small but statistically significant difference between women with cystic disease and controls.[52]

The above studies were performed on random or 24-hour basal prolactin levels, but a more recent approach is the examination of the dynamics of the pituitary release of prolactin.

Prolactin is almost unique in that its secretion is tonically inhibited by dopamine (Fig. 8.9), but neural control of prolactin is extremely complex.[53]

However, prolactin secretion by the pituitary can be stimulated by the use of thyrotrophin-releasing hormone (TRH) and domperidone. Both agents produce an immediate rise in serum prolactin in normals and test different sections of the control system, as TRH is directly stimulatory to the lactotrophs while domperidone antagonizes the inhibitory action of dopamine on prolactin secretion. Peters and colleagues examined the stimulated prolactin response to TRH in a mixed group of benign disease patients and found that the patients with mastalgia had a significantly greater rise in prolactin compared with controls.[54]

We also examined the pituitary control of prolactin secretion in 17 patients with cyclical mastalgia compared with 11 controls and confirmed Peters's findings that the TRH-induced rise of prolactin is significantly greater at 20 minutes (Fig. 8.10) and is maintained for up to 60 minutes postinjection.[55]

The basal prolactin levels were not significantly different between the groups. The enhanced prolactin response is also seen after domperidone administration (Fig. 8.11), whereas the thyroid-stimulating hormone (TSH) response to TRH is not different between mastalgia patients and controls.

These studies strongly suggest that there is a disturbance of hypothalamic control in women with cyclical mastalgia and this 'fine tuning' defect may be the primary problem in painful nodular breast disease. It is of interest that a similar defect has been demonstrated in the cyclical oedema syndrome, which has many similarities to cyclical mastalgia although they are distinct conditions.[56]

Many believe that stress may impact on the hypothalamus and thus produce elevated hormone levels, although there is no literature on breast pain to support this view (Fig. 8.9).

Caffeine and methylxanthines

Other theories that have been put forward include the overstimulation of breast cells due to interference with adenosine triphosphate (ATP) degradation by methylxanthines consequent on high caffeine intake.[57] There is some biochemical evidence to support this contention, but caffeine intake appears to be much lower in British women than is common in the USA and may not be relevant in the UK. Even in American women, the serum caffeine and theobromine levels were found to be identical, although the catecholamines were significantly raised in women with mastalgia.[58] The epidemiological evidence for the potential role of caffeine has been conflicting as case-control studies have both supported[59,60] and opposed[61-63] any association.

The methylxanthine intake varies between different cultures and a proper trial of withdrawal of a dietary substance is difficult to control, so these results need

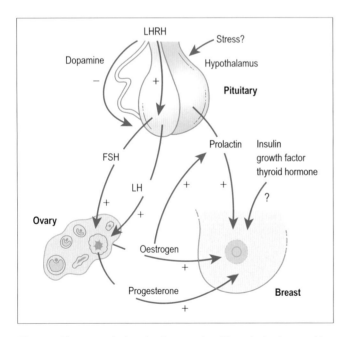

Fig. 8.9 The control of prolactin secretion. The principal control is the tonic inhibitory effect of dopamine, but note that oestrogen acts to elevate prolactin levels. In practice, the relationships are more complicated than depicted in this simple diagram.

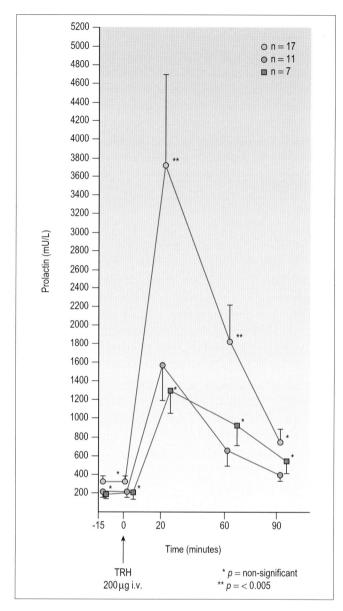

Fig. 8.10 TRH test in women with cyclical and noncyclical pain and controls. The cyclical mastalgia patients (n = 17) show a significantly increased peak release of prolactin at 20 minutes. The noncyclical patients (n = 7) have a similar response to controls (n = 11). Values given are the mean (1 SEM. Mann-Whitney U test). (From Kumar et al.,[55] with permission of *Cancer*.)

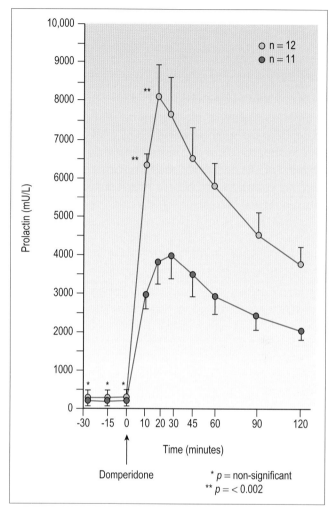

Fig. 8.11 Domperidone test in women with cyclical mastalgia (n = 12) compared with controls (n = 11). Domperidone 10 mg i.v. (bolus) gives a typical high peak of prolactin secretion but the cyclical mastalgia patients show a significantly higher peak prolactin release at 20 minutes. Values given are the mean (1 SEM. Mann-Whitney U test). (From Kumar et al.,[55] with permission of *Cancer*.)

further study. However, if a patient with mastalgia was found to have an intake in excess of 10 cups of coffee a day, it would seem worth suggesting a change to decaffeinated coffee.

The caffeine methylxanthine hypothesis has been challenged by several investigators. Two case-control studies, one of histologically diagnosed benign breast disease and one of 'fibrocystic' disease, both failed to show an association with coffee consumption.[63,64] A randomized trial of

caffeine reduction with non-blind assessment showed some reduction in breast nodularity in the coffee-abstaining group, but the changes were minor and there was no correlation of palpable nodularity at entry to the study with coffee consumption at that time.[65]

Several studies of caffeine restriction in the treatment of mastalgia have been performed, although some of these have been directed at reduction of benign proliferative disease. Minton and co-workers originally reported that caffeine restriction produced improvement in symptoms, but these studies were uncontrolled.[66] Subsequent randomized trials have failed to demonstrate a clear advantage for caffeine restriction.[65,67] Despite this, recommendations on caffeine restriction still appear in official publications on fibrocystic disease (California Pacific Medical Center leaflet, 2008).

Prostaglandins and essential fatty acids

Horrobin and Manku proposed an hypothesis that there is an abnormality of prostaglandin synthesis secondary to deficient essential fatty acid (EFA) intake in the diet.[68] This is supported by circumstantial evidence that other stigmata of EFA deficiency, such as increased sebum secretion, are commoner in benign breast disorder patients.[69] Measurements of plasma fatty acids[70] have confirmed abnormal profiles in patients with mastalgia, with proportions of saturated fatty acids increased, and EFA reduced. Treatment with evening primrose oil improved the profiles towards normal, but this was not necessarily associated with a clinical response. The end result of EFA deficiency is postulated to be amplification of prolactin effects on breast cells because of deficient production of prostaglandin E1.

Other workers have reported lipid abnormalities unrelated to EFAs, with elevation of HDL-C in cyclical mastalgia patients, but not in noncyclical patients.[71] They also report an improvement in symptoms consequent on a low-fat dietary regimen.

Miscellaneous factors

Mastalgia is reported in a wide and diverse range of conditions, mainly associated with events during reproductive life. Examples range from a 17% incidence of new or more severe mastalgia following tubal ligation[72] to the expected association with macromastia (see Ch. 15). An excess in patients who have not breastfed and in women not undertaking active exercise has been reported.[73]

An interesting observation was made by Peters[74] that breast pain correlated positively with degree of ductal dilatation, as demonstrated by ultrasound. Mastalgia is sometimes precipitated by prescription of drugs, especially psychotropic drugs, such as phenothiazines, herbal remedies such as ginseng, or recent commencement of hormone replacement therapy (HRT). These examples illustrate the importance of taking a comprehensive history, even though the majority of patients will have no specific underlying cause.

Pain in the nipple and areola, including that due to vasospasm, is discussed in Chapter 12.

In summary, it is clear that the cherished and widely accepted hypotheses of neuroticism and general water retention have found little support in experimental results, and modern work suggests that control mechanisms of pulsatile secretion of gonadotrophins and/or prolactin are abnormal in patients with painful nodular breasts. This, of course, just moves the basic questions back one stage, leaving the aetiology of such hormonal abnormalities as the next question to be answered. The possibility of an end-organ abnormality remains to be investigated in detail.

Management of patients with mastalgia

The first consideration in management is the taking of a careful history and examination of the breast. If a dominant or discrete lump is present, management is as detailed in Chapter 5. The group of patients remaining comprises those with mastalgia and nodularity and those with diffusely nodular breasts that are painless. The latter group requires nothing other than exclusion of significant pathology and can be discharged if there are no other indications for follow-up. The next section on therapy deals with patients with mastalgia irrespective of the presence of nodularity, and the term 'mastalgia' is used to denote pain with or without nodularity.

Each patient must have her symptomatology assessed carefully so that the pain can be designated as cyclical or noncyclical, and if the latter, true noncyclical breast pain or musculoskeletal pain.

Reassurance and other supportive measures

For patients with mastalgia of whatever pattern, the first and most successful treatment is reassurance that their symptoms are not due to cancer. Geschickter stated that 'cancer should be excluded; rule out infection, reassure and give support' and Billroth emphasized that 'friendly advice, reassurance and the banishment of suspicion and fear of dread disease is of great importance'. These quotations have been emphasized because the manner of delivery and conviction of the reassurance are very important, as it is certainly true that many women consult surgeons about their mastalgia because they fear there is cancer in their breasts. Reassurance of these patients does not cure their breast pain but it does alter their attitude to the pain, so that it is no longer a serious problem.

One of the difficulties with active reassurance is that many surgeons in the past disliked using the term 'cancer' in the patient's presence (even when discussing the absence of the condition), and so resorted to various euphemisms, which are open to misinterpretation. For example, the following statement of reassurance was actually made to a patient with painful nodularity: 'You have something in your breast; don't worry about it and as there is nothing I can do about it, there's no point in me seeing you again.' Most clinicians would translate this sentence as: 'You have fibroadenosis (ANDI); it is harmless and the cause is unknown, but as I don't know of any useful treatment for the pain, I don't think you need to come to out-patient's for a repeat visit.' However, the patient's translation was: 'I have cancer; it is incurable and the surgeon is abandoning me!' More recently, there is a readiness to discuss the issues around cancer in patient management.

These points are made to underline that sympathetic, detailed reassurance is required and in our Mastalgia Clinic we have successfully treated 85% of 1000 mastalgia patients by simple reassurance. In a recent review of the Edinburgh Breast Clinic, McFayden et al. found that of 797 patients referred to the breast clinic only 213 were deemed to have sufficiently severe pain to be referred to the Mastalgia Clinic.[75]

Some clinicians agree with Geschickter's recommendation of support for the painful breast. We generally find that our patients with persistent mastalgia have already fitted themselves with the most comfortable brassiere they could find. However, there is a report of the therapeutic value of a well-fitting brassiere,[76] although the placebo effect of fitting a specially designed brassiere in the hospital must have played a considerable part in the good results obtained. A more recent report suggested that a sports bra may be helpful,[77] but there are no randomized data examining support from a bra versus no support.

It is inevitable that patients attending a breast clinic with breast pain will be anxious, and the effectiveness of relaxation therapy has been investigated in Aberdeen.[78] Patients were randomized to receive relaxation therapy (via an audio tape) during the middle month of a 3-month observation period, against no therapy for the controls. Sixty-one per cent of the intervention group had a response at a Cardiff Breast Score grade I or II, compared with 25% in the control group.

The next step in management is concerned with those patients who have been reassured, but still find that mastalgia causes considerable interference to their lives. This group, in our experience, is about 5% of the new patient referrals to a breast clinic and the mastalgia in this group may be so severe as to cause relationship problems within the family because a husband is unable to touch his wife's breasts for 3 weeks every month or children are unable to hug their mother.

Since there is no clear-cut diagnostic pathophysiology in mastalgia, hormonal investigations have little place in management apart from a routine prolactin level in cases with galactorrhoea or amenorrhoea, to exclude a prolactinoma. It should also be remembered that a common presentation of both mastalgia and amenorrhoea is pregnancy, but this should have been excluded by an accurate history, and if necessary by a pregnancy test.

In cases where the onset of pain corresponds to institution of drug therapy, consideration should be given to stopping or substituting the drug, depending on the indications for the drug, and taking into account the fact that mild mastalgia of this type will frequently decrease spontaneously with time.

The contraceptive pill

The role of oral contraceptives in the epidemiology of breast cancer is hotly debated and, due to the long lag between hormonal events and breast cancer occurrence, the matter remains unresolved. However, in terms of benign breast disorders, most reports have indicated a protective effect.[79,80] We have recorded the type of oral contraceptive taken by our mastalgia patients but on analysis there are no correlations between pain patterns and brands. Some women may experience mastalgia for the first time on starting a new oral contraceptive but most mastalgia then tends to disappear or is minimal.

In a study of 44 patients suffering from mastalgia/nodularity at the time of starting oral contraception, 53% found an improvement in their mastalgia, but nodularity improved in only 8%.[81]

If a patient has severe mastalgia that starts for the first time on commencing oral contraception, it is worth advising either a change to a lower dose or, if already on a 30 μg pill, a change to a different brand. Little is known of the exact effects of exogenous 'balanced' mixtures of oestrogens and progestogens, as the controversy regarding the 'potency factors' of different progestogens has shown.[82,83] If mastalgia remains a major problem, then occasionally a change to mechanical methods of contraception may be helpful, but there is no guarantee of response and the risks of an unwanted pregnancy are increased. In our experience, the severity of the mastalgia dictates whether the patient will readily agree to stop taking the oral contraceptive.

Drugs available for treating mastalgia

The many different hypotheses of aetiology of benign breast disorders discussed in the previous section have given rise to a number of specific therapies which are perhaps more logical than the previous empirical treatments (Table 8.6).

However, it is important to distinguish clearly between controlled and uncontrolled studies because there is a powerful placebo effect in subjective symptoms such as pain. Our benchmark for studies is the double-blind, placebo-controlled trial and we have used this technique in nearly all of our therapeutic studies.

We have devised a number of objective methods of assessment which can be analysed and submitted to statistical analysis, including pain charts indicating number of days of symptoms per month, visual linear analogue (VLA) scales for patient assessment of severity, and clinician assessment of tenderness and nodularity. The results can be expressed in absolute and comparative terms, pre- and post-treatment, for each individual (Fig. 8.12).

We have also found it helpful to have an overall response grade – the Cardiff Breast Score (CBS) – to assess the benefit of treatment (Table 8.7).[84]

Doppler measurement of breast vascularity has been used to monitor response to drug therapy in mastalgia,

with a good correlation reported.[85] This may prove a useful approach, but requires wider confirmation in view of the operator dependency of this technique.

Diuretics

One of the popular treatments, certainly among primary healthcare physicians, is the administration of diuretics. These have no rational basis, as was demonstrated by the lack of correlation between retention of body water and symptoms.[35] As no placebo-controlled trial has shown any beneficial effect, it is likely that their apparent 'efficacy' in general practice is due to the placebo effect. Pain is the subjective symptom par excellence, and for this reason all studies in mastalgia should be at least placebo controlled and preferably randomized between the active and placebo therapies.

Progestogens

The luteal deficiency hypothesis, championed by Sitruk-Ware and his colleagues,[41] had also been considered by earlier workers and attempts were made to correct the progesterone deficiency by administration of luteal

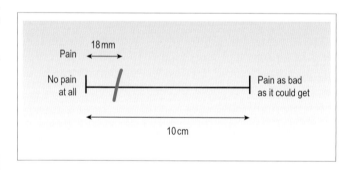

Fig. 8.12 A typical VLA scale. The patient has made a mark 18 mm from the 'no pain' end and so a reading of 18 is obtained. This scale is sometimes known as an LAS scale (linear analogue scale).

Table 8.6 Mastalgia: aetiological hypotheses and treatments

Hypothesis	Treatment
Hyperoestrogenism	Androgens/antioestrogens (tamoxifen)/LHRH agonists
Luteal insufficiency	Progesterone/progestogens
Hyperprolactinaemia	Bromocriptine (dopamine agonist)
Increased gonadotrophin	Danazol (antigonadotrophin)
Dietary methylxanthines	Caffeine restriction
Dietary essential fatty acids (EFA) deficiency	Evening primrose oil (EFA supplement)
Local inflammation or fibrosis	Local steroid injection
Miscellaneous	Pyridoxine/thyroid hormones/vitamin A/HRT

Table 8.7 The Cardiff Breast Score

CBS I	An excellent response leaving no residual pain
CBS II	A substantial response leaving some residual pain but considered by the patient to be easily bearable
CBS III	A poor response leaving substantial residual pain
CBS IV	No response

Thus, CBS I and II are considered useful responses; III and IV as nonresponders.

extracts with varying success. The apparent demonstration by the Paris group of a definite progesterone deficiency in benign breast disorders gave rise to hopes that simple correction by progestogens would be useful. Other groups had failed to find a progesterone deficiency.

Progestogens have been compared with placebo in premenstrual stress (PMS) and failed to show any benefit greater than the placebo effect.[86] A randomized, controlled trial of medroxyprogesterone acetate in patients with cyclical mastalgia showed no significant improvement in pain, tenderness or nodularity.[87] A double-blind, randomized study of 80 mastalgia patients using vaginal micronized progesterone showed a greater than 50% reduction in pain in 65% of the active group compared with 22% in the placebo group.[88] Breast nodularity was not affected. In a double-blind, placebo-controlled study of the application of progesterone gel to the breast, von Fournier et al. were unable to find an active effect despite the known absorption of progesterone through the skin,[89] and a similar study in Edinburgh gave similar results. Thus, the precise role of progesterone and progestogens remains unclear.

Bromocriptine

The discovery of a small elevation of basal prolactin in patients with benign breast disorders[52] and the availability of a specific prolactin-lowering agent, bromocriptine, suggested that the first truly specific treatment for mast-

algia was attainable. In fact, a report of the effectiveness of bromocriptine had already appeared, describing a good response in 10 or 15 patients in an open study.[90] Soon afterwards, a controlled study showed that the drug was effective in relieving breast swelling in patients with the premenstrual syndrome.

These encouraging results were tested in the Cardiff Mastalgia Clinic in a double-blind, placebo-controlled trial carried out on 53 patients using a bromocriptine dosage of 2.5 mg twice daily.[91] Assessment of response, which had been sketchy with the previous two bromocriptine trials, was improved by using a simple scale for the clinician's assessment, and a subjective, self-rating VLA scale for the patient's response (see Fig. 8.12).

The VLA scales were completed independently of the clinician's assessment. Unlike the previous studies, the patients were randomized into their respective pain patterns to see if any pattern responded preferentially. The results of this trial showed that the cyclical pattern of pain was significantly reduced by bromocriptine compared with placebo, but that the noncyclical pattern failed to respond (Fig. 8.13).

This trial demonstrated for the first time that patients classified according to a simple symptomatic classification responded differentially to a precise manipulation of the pituitary output of prolactin. Blood sampling during the trial confirmed the depression of prolactin levels on bromocriptine to subnormal levels as these patients were initially normoprolactinaemic as expected.

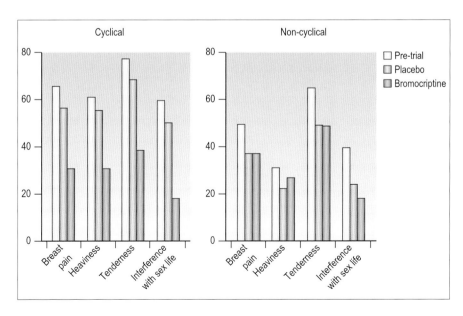

Fig. 8.13 VLA results of the Cardiff controlled trial of bromocriptine in mastalgia. Note the placebo response in both cyclical and noncyclical patients, but the significantly lower scores, i.e. improvement, on bromocriptine in the cyclical patients. (From Mansel et al.,[91] with permission of the *British Journal of Surgery*.)

It is currently not understood how lowering of prolactin levels produces amelioration of mastalgia, but the mechanism is presumed to be due to a reduction in the overall stimulation of breast cells by prolactin, because it is known that bromocriptine does not lower sex steroid levels. When the data on serum prolactin levels were analysed to see if there was a correlation between amount of depression and symptom improvement, no correlation could be found. This suggests that the effects may be more complicated than was first thought. As bromocriptine is a dopamine agonist, it is possible that there is a direct effect on breast tissue, independent of prolactin effects, if breast cells have dopamine receptors similar to those found on pituitary cells. However, recent studies in our laboratories have failed to detect dopamine receptors on human breast cells grown in monolayer culture.

Confirmation of the Cardiff results has come from other controlled trials,[92–94] and it is clear from review of the literature that this drug is consistently effective in reducing the symptoms of mastalgia.[95] The problem with bromocriptine is that some women experience severe side effects, the commonest being nausea, vomiting and dizziness, which have caused a 20% dropout rate in many trials. The severity of side effects can be reduced by introducing the drug slowly in an incremental scheme and avoiding doses higher than 2.5 mg twice daily.

The incidence of side effects is variable and some women have no problems even at high dosage. In our experience, of 216 patients treated with bromocriptine, 75 (35%) had significant adverse effects and 46 had to stop treatment (although 13 of these had already had a clinically useful response). This high level of side effects has led to the discontinuance of bromocriptine in the treatment of mastalgia.

Danazol

Danazol was introduced in 1971 by Greenblatt and co-workers, who suggested it may have a role in mastalgia.[96] This agent, like bromocriptine, is unique in its action on the pituitary–ovarian axis. It was originally described as an impeded androgen and in monkeys it was shown to act as an antigonadotrophin, as it depressed serum follicle-stimulating hormone (FSH) and luteinizing hormone (LH) and prevented ovulation. Its action in humans is not so clearly defined because it only interferes with FSH and LH levels at high dosage. It may have a local tissue effect as it has been shown to bind to both progesterone and androgen receptors but not to oestrogen receptors.

Greenblatt's group initially used the drug for treating endometriosis but a number of papers soon followed from the same group showing the usefulness of danazol in painful nodular breast disease.[97,98] All these reports were of uncontrolled studies and appeared to be cumulative, and were thus open to the criticisms of lack of placebo control. We therefore carried out a double-blind, placebo study in the Cardiff Mastalgia Clinic on 28 patients with cyclical mastalgia, using a detailed protocol similar to that described earlier.[99] This study showed that danazol was clearly beneficial in cyclical mastalgia, producing both relief of symptoms and reduction in nodularity, and these effects could be obtained with doses as low as 200 mg. The lower dose gave much lower side effects, and only a 10% dropout rate was recorded in the trial.

The hormonal effects of danazol treatment were a low luteal progesterone (suggesting anovulation) and an unchanged prolactin, so it appears the drug is working on the ovary or pituitary although only 30% of these patients were amenorrhoeic on the drug. The side effects are mainly amenorrhoea, the incidence of which increases with dose up to 100% at 600–800 mg, and various mild androgenic effects such as weight gain, acne and hirsutism. All of these effects are dose related and can be minimized by low-dose therapy.[100] Our current practice is to start at 200 mg daily and then use a maintenance dose of 100 mg daily on alternate days.

In our experience, of 295 patients treated with danazol, 88 (30%) complained of significant adverse events and 43 had to stop treatment. However, many of these were before we had developed the low-dose regimen. A recently reported side effect has been a lowering of the voice pitch which has been permanent in a small number of cases, but our experience is that only 5% of patients notice this symptom and it is generally reversible on stopping the drug. Danazol currently appears to be the best agent for severe breast pain and nodularity with an overall improvement rate of 70% in our total group of 295 treated patients.

Another double-blind, controlled study from Nottingham reported that danazol was superior to bromocriptine for cyclical breast pain.[101] A paper reporting the experience of a Brisbane mastalgia clinic also confirmed the efficacy of danazol in practice, with an overall success rate of 67% compared with the rates of 30–40% for other agents.[73]

Both Peters[102] and Stein et al.[103] showed a significant benefit from the somewhat similar agent gestrinone, which has androgenic, antioestrogenic and antiprogestogenic properties, and some androgenic side effects. Both double-blind, randomized, placebo-controlled studies used 2.5 mg twice weekly for 3 months, with benefits and side effects similar to danazol. The lower dosage necessary has potential advantages regarding side effects, but the drug does not yet have the benefit of the extensive and prolonged experience with danazol.

Evening primrose oil

The fatty acid deficiency hypothesis has led to the testing of treatment by supplementing the diet with an EFA. One preparation which has proved valuable is evening primrose oil (EPO) which is unique in containing 7% linolenic acid and 72% linoleic acid and represents the richest natural source of EFAs known (Fig. 8.14).

Early trials showed EPO to be useful for treating mild cases of cyclical mastalgia.[104] This agent is potentially useful in mild to moderate cases as it has virtually no side effects. Patient acceptance is high as it is viewed as a 'natural substance' rather than a hormone or drug. Interestingly, the trials of EPO also suggested that noncyclical pain is unresponsive to this therapy, as had been found in the bromocriptine trial, although this conclusion has been modified with further analysis of the noncyclical group, as discussed later. The positive balance of moderate effectiveness and minimal side effects leads us to use it as the first-line treatment in patients with mastalgia of moderate severity. In our own clinic experience, of 85 patients treated with EPO as first-line therapy, 58% had a clinically useful response (CBS I or II). In our overall experience of 241 patients treated only 9 (4%) complained of a significant adverse effect.

However, more recent studies have suggested that the efficacy of EPO may be limited. Blommers et al. carried out a study of evening primrose oil and fish oil in chronic severe mastalgia, and were not able to demonstrate a significant improvement on EPO.[105] Furthermore, a recent large multicentre UK study of EPO with and without antioxidants and multivitamins in the primary and secondary care settings showed a high placebo response, and EPO was not shown to be better than placebo.[106] As a result of these data and other equivocal results, EPO has been removed from prescription lists in the UK, but it remains available over the counter in a variety of chemists and health food stores. We still suggest that patients with mild/moderate mastalgia try this medication as the first-line therapy, as most women do have some response and side effects are minimal.

Tamoxifen

The antioestrogen drug tamoxifen was reported to be helpful in mastalgia in an Italian study,[107] but this drug is currently only licensed for the treatment of breast cancer. A double-blind study of tamoxifen in Guy's Hospital, London, showed that tamoxifen 10 mg daily significantly improved mastalgia, with response rates of 98% for cyclical and 56% for noncyclical pain. Side effects were reported to be 'minimal', but in this study about 15% of the patients dropped out on therapy.[108]

A further study from the Guy's group showed that 20 mg of tamoxifen was equally effective, but gave the same relapse rate and caused much higher side effects.[23] This study also compared 3- versus 6-month treatments; the longer period did not increase response rate, nor did it reduce the relapse rate (seen in up to half the patients by 2–3 months). The same group have investigated various metabolic side effects of tamoxifen in their patients, and found no significant alteration with short-term treatment.[109,110]

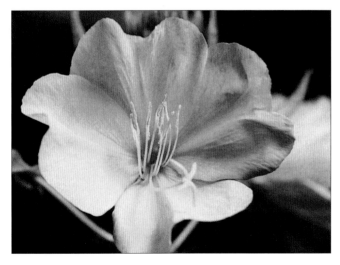

Fig. 8.14 The evening primrose flower (*Oenothera biennis*).

In the largest trial to date,[111] the dose has been reduced further to 11 days per cycle. Three hundred and one women were randomized to receive 10 mg or 20 mg daily from day 15 to day 25 in the cycle over a period of 3 months. There were no placebo controls. The response rate was no different in the two groups: three-quarters obtained a useful response. One-quarter had recurrence by 1 year, again with no difference between the groups. However, side effects were significantly greater in the 20 mg group, 66% versus 50%, although only 8% and 2% stopped treatment because of side effects.

A potential problem of tamoxifen therapy in premenopausal women is an elevation of serum oestradiol on tamoxifen, although this was not found by Ricciardi and Ianniruberto.[107] A further problem has been raised by a toxicology study which showed that a small number of rats developed liver tumours on high-dose tamoxifen. In contrast, there is a huge experience of the use of tamoxifen in prevention trials in premenopausal women in the IBIS-1 and P1 trials, and no problems relating to liver tumours have been reported. Indeed, in these placebo-controlled trials a reduction in benign breast conditions has been observed in the tamoxifen-treated women[112,113] Although the drug is currently mainly indicated for malignant disease, it is being used increasingly as a second-line drug for mastalgia, while recognizing that relapse is a significant problem at the end of the course. The appropriate dose on present experience is 10 mg daily for 3 months, repeated for relapse if necessary, with further courses given only after full consideration of the possible long-term effects. An alternative selective oestrogen (estrogen) receptor modulator (SERM), toremefine was studied in a recent trial in Guy's Hospital in London, and a high response rate was noted, but also a high incidence of associated side effects including flushes, nausea and vaginal discharge.[114] The authors concluded that the drug was effective, but not a drug of choice in mastalgia due to the increased side effects.

A newer SERM, Ormeloxifine, has been studied in India where it was developed. A nonrandomized pilot study was carried out in patients with mastalgia (70%) or fibroadenoma (30%) at a dose of 30 mg daily in 60 patients, and assessment was by a VAS scale. Unusually in this study, noncyclical pain was much more common than cyclical, but there was a good response with large declines in the VAS scores, with most patients free of pain after 1 month. There was a mixed response in the fibroadenoma group.[115]

Alternative routes of delivery of tamoxifen or SERMS may be possible by the transcutaneous route, in order to reduce side effects by avoiding transhepatic passage. This approach has shown some promise, using a gel containing 4 hydroxy tamoxifen applied to the breast morning and night. A placebo-controlled trial of this gel afimoxifine (Tamogel®) applied daily for four cycles, showed efficacy for pain and nodularity, with minimal side effects, in cyclical mastalgia, particularly in the late luteal phase of the cycle.[116] The progressive improvement in luteal peak pain can be seen in Figure 8.15, especially in the fourth cycle on treatment where the 4-mg preparation of afimoxifine shows a definite blunting of the normal peak of cyclical pain. This preparation is not yet available commercially, but has potential as a low-morbidity treatment in the future. It is clear that these series of studies of SERMS and the prevention studies confirm the active therapeutic role of these agents in benign conditions of the breast.

Luteinizing hormone-releasing hormone analogues

These are dealt with below in the section on refractory mastalgia.

Other therapeutic approaches

A number of groups report varying degrees of success with different dietary measures, particularly a low-fat diet.[71,117] Boyd and colleagues[117] have reported marked improvement in breast symptoms after a diet which limits fats to 15% of caloric intake. However, the practical difficulties in maintaining and monitoring such a diet probably explain the less enthusiastic interest among all but the most dedicated patients and centres.

The evidence for many other varied therapeutic approaches is generally poor and it is likely that the results reported are due to the placebo effect.

Leis has reported excellent results in a series of 721 mastalgia patients outside a formal study.[118] The low-fat, high-fibre diet, supplemented with vitamins A, C and selenium, gave an 81% response for pain and tenderness and 39% response for nodularity.

The caffeine/methylxanthine theory suggests that withdrawal of dietary coffee, cola and chocolate would help the symptoms of benign breast disorder, and this has been found in an open study by Minton et al.[66] While this may be relevant to cultures with a very high coffee intake, other experience is less convincing. This question is dis-

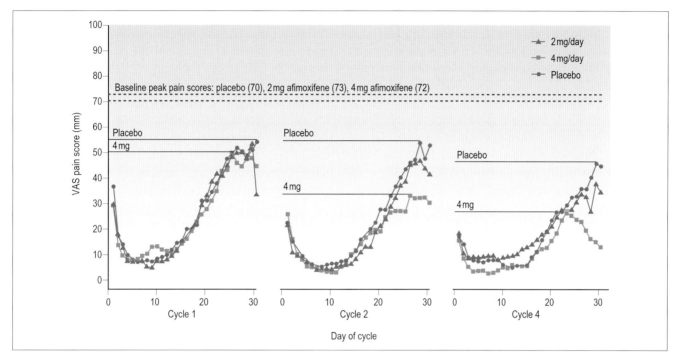

Fig. 8.15 The afimoxifine gel trial. Visual linear analogue scores for placebo gel, 2 mg afimoxifine, and 4 mg afimoxifine. In cycle 4, the blunting of the normal cyclical pain peak is achieved by the 4 mg afimoxifine gel, while the 2 mg preparation shows an intermediate blunting compared with placebo gel.[116]

cussed earlier in this chapter with consideration of aetiology.

Other dietary studies have looked at phytoestrogens or soy extracts, and a small randomized, placebo-controlled trial of isoflavones in only 12 patients suggested a reduction in breast pain of around 40%.[119] A trial of soy protein also suggested some efficacy.[120]

A randomized trial of *Vitus agnus castus* extract (castor oil), showed a modest fall in VAS scores on the plant extract (54% compared with 40% on placebo), with few side effects.[121] A small number of studies have suggested that pyridoxine (vitamin B₆) may be useful in treating mastalgia on the basis that pyridoxine will enhance the decarboxylation of dopa to dopamine and so inhibit prolactin levels. Most studies have been uncontrolled and furthermore it has been shown that pyridoxine treatment does not lower serum prolactin in patients with the amenorrhoea–galactorrhoea syndrome.[122] In contradistinction, a study has shown that pyridoxine lowers exercise-induced prolactin secretion.[123] A double-blind study using pyridoxine at a dose of 200 mg daily in cyclical mastalgia found that the vitamin did not significantly improve breast pain compared with placebo.[124]

Other studies of vitamin A administration and treatment with thyroid hormone[125] have been reported to show improvement of mastalgia, but the studies were open and involved a small number of heterogeneous patients and are thus difficult to interpret. There is still some interest in the role of the thyroid and iodine in the aetiology and management of mastalgia. It was reported many years ago that thyroid hormone abnormalities may be linked to benign breast change[54] and that correction of iodine deficiency may relieve symptoms. Additional iodine may be supplied as elemental dietary iodine or in combination with other metabolites. A recent randomized, controlled trial (RCT) reported that 3–6 mg of iodine daily was effective in treating breast pain with nearly 40% of patients reporting a >50% reduction in pain on iodine compared with only 8% on placebo.[126]

Vitamin E has been studied in a controlled trial using mammographic change as the outcome measure in 105 women, but no changes were found compared to the placebo group.[127]

Treatments for noncyclical mastalgia

All the above treatments have been directed at the cyclical group of patients whether the authors have realized this or not, but our studies suggest that the cyclical group appears to have an endocrine basis and, in turn, appears to respond to endocrine-directed therapy. It also seemed at first that the noncyclical group appeared to be unresponsive to manipulation of the endocrine system but results have been more encouraging when true noncyclical mastalgia has been differentiated from musculoskeletal pain of chest wall origin.

Our results show that it is worthwhile treating true noncyclical mastalgia in the same way as for cyclical mastalgia. This then leaves musculoskeletal pain, localized 'trigger-spot' pain, and refractory mastalgia. A report of five cases of breast pain relieved by surgical decompression of the thoracic outlet[128] emphasizes the need to exclude referred pain in general, and musculoskeletal pain in particular, in all cases. These patients all had typical arm pain as well as breast pain, so differentiation from mastalgia should not be difficult.

Attempts have been made to treat the generalized noncyclical group with nonsteroidal antiinflammatory agents but there is no published evidence of their efficacy. Our experience of nonsteroidal antiinflammatory drugs (NSAIDs) is similarly disappointing. As an extension of this approach, Crile suggested that a local injection of lidocaine and prednisolone may be effective in relieving the localized noncyclical pain.[129] His description corresponds to the trigger-spot subgroup mentioned previously and he found the steroid/local anaesthetic injection gave initial relief in two-thirds of the patients with continued relief in about one-half of the patients followed. Our experience has been similar; we have obtained a 70% response rate.

Surgical excision

More extensive surgical excision for mastalgia as a symptom is uncommon but prophylactic excision for premalignant disease has been performed more commonly and is considered in Chapter 18. For most types of mastalgia, except the trigger spot mentioned above, the symptom extends so widely in the breast that segmental resection is insufficient. Thus, most surgeons have used subcutaneous mastectomy, or total mastectomy in earlier times. Most of these operations are carried out for 'prophylaxis' of breast cancer by plastic surgeons and documentation of the numbers and results of operations performed solely for mastalgia is very poor, although nearly all authors list mastalgia as an indication for the operation. The Nottingham Breast Clinic reported that only four patients underwent subcutaneous mastectomies for mastalgia in 12 years, with only two patients obtaining relief and one patient developing a fibrous capsule.

Our experience is of only 15 cases over 33 years, all with severe mastalgia resistant to medication. Our first 12 cases were drawn from a pool including many tertiary referrals as well as our own cases.[130] They represent less than 1% of cases of mastalgia severe enough to require detailed investigation and treatment. The median age at time of surgery was 35 years (29–53) and duration of pain prior to surgery 6.5 (2–16) years. The procedures were two quadrantectomies, one bilateral subcutaneous mastectomy without reconstruction, and subcutaneous mastectomy with implant in eight patients, three bilateral. The results were not encouraging; only five patients (50%) were free of pain after mastectomy, and pain recurred in both patients with quadrantectomy. Five patients having mastectomy developed complications, wound dehiscence in two (eventually requiring musculocutaneous flap reconstruction), and capsular contraction in five. However, on review, those patients who were pain free were happy in the long term with the outcome, and considered the cosmetic deficiencies well justified by the relief of pain.

Surgery should only be undertaken after all drug therapies have been exhausted and have failed. The patient should be reviewed by a psychologist prior to surgery, and the complications of the procedure, which are common both early and in the long term, outlined by the surgeon. Particularly troublesome is fibrous contracture around implants, especially if they are placed subcutaneously. The patient should be warned that even mastectomy may not relieve her pain.

Additionally, nipple or areolar necrosis and infection of the prosthesis are not uncommon. Our view is that this operation is rarely indicated for breast pain because it has a modest chance of therapeutic success and a high incidence of complications. A review of the detailed results of this operation performed for mastalgia is urgently needed but perhaps the paucity of published figures reflects other surgeons' disquiet about surgery for this indication.

Natural history of mastalgia

One of the problems of therapeutic trials in mastalgia is that the natural history of the condition is poorly documented. Because spontaneous remissions can occur, these may give a false impression of treatment benefit. Geschickter[7] briefly described some features of the natural history of his mastodynia cases and noted that the majority found relief of pain at the menopause.

In an effort to correct this lack of knowledge, we undertook a review of all our mastalgia cases documented between 1973 and 1976 in the Cardiff Mastalgia Clinic.[131] There was a total of 258 patients and a follow-up of 66% was obtained by direct interview or postal questionnaire. Details regarding the duration of pain and spontaneous remission were obtained. The results showed that cyclical pain was most commonly relieved by hormonal events such as pregnancy and the menopause but this was not the case with noncyclical pain. It also appeared that patients with cyclical pain who started having symptoms at an early age (<20 years) tended to have persistent pain, often throughout reproductive life, whereas a late age of onset was associated with a shorter overall duration of pain. This implies that younger patients may require treatment for prolonged periods, as we had previously found that post-treatment recurrence of pain is common. In view of these findings, we aim to treat young patients with severe mastalgia in short intermittent bursts rather than continuous periods. However, patients near the menopause may be treated for longer periods in the expectation that their pain will be naturally resolved in the near future by their menopause.

It should be noted that patients investigated in the Mastalgia Clinic were by definition severe cases of long duration, so these findings do not apply to the many women who develop mild to moderate mastalgia in the fourth and fifth decades. In many of these patients, natural remission occurs within a few months.

Plan of management for patients with mastalgia

Our detailed management protocol and experience of treatment in nearly 300 mastalgia patients has been published[132] and later updated for 500 patients.[83] The improved response rate (92% with cyclical and 64% with noncyclical) in the second report compared with the earlier one reflects improved understanding of the diagnosis and classification of mastalgia, along with more accurate assessment of each of the drug therapies for particular patients (Figs 8.16 and 8.17).

The corresponding response rates to placebo have been CBS I 4%, CBS II 15%, CBS III 6% and CBS IV 75%.

The important points in management are shown in Table 8.8.

The first priority is exclusion of cancer by appropriate tests and firm reassurance of the patient. This will be

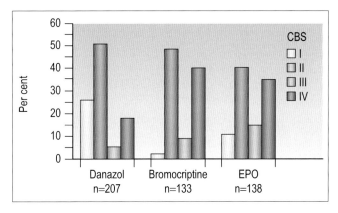

Fig. 8.16 Overall response of patients with cyclical mastalgia to drug treatment. EPO, evening primrose oil; CBS, Cardiff Breast Score. (From Gateley et al.[84] by permission of The Royal Society of Medicine Press, London.)

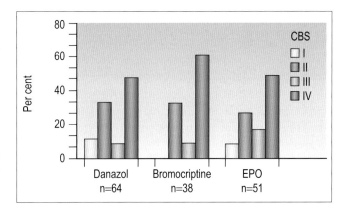

Fig. 8.17 Overall response of patients with noncyclical mastalgia to drug treatment. EPO, evening primrose oil; CBS, Cardiff Breast Score. (From Gateley et al.[84] by permission of The Royal Society of Medicine Press, London.)

Table 8.8 Principles of mastalgia treatment

1	Exclude cancer
2	Reassurance
3	Define pattern (pain chart or history)
4	Cyclical mastalgia (overall response 92%)
	(a) EPO: six capsules daily
	(b) Danazol: 100–300 mg daily then reduce
	(c) Bromocriptine: 1.25 mg, increasing to 3.75–5 mg daily
5	True noncyclical mastalgia (overall response 64%)
	(a) Danazol
	(b) EPO
	(c) Bromocriptine
6	Musculoskeletal chest wall pain Lidocaine/steroid injection to trigger spots and Tietze's syndrome
7	Consider surgery only as a last resort

adequate treatment for around 85% of patients with mastalgia presenting to hospital and probably higher in family practice.

The 15% of mastalgia patients with severe mastalgia who are not helped by reassurance should then be assessed initially by a pain chart to define the pain pattern to give a baseline measurement of the number of days of pain per cycle. Patients who are still troubled by their mastalgia after 2–3 months of charting (to allow for spontaneous remission) should be treated by one of the three main agents.

Cyclical mastalgia

Our current first choice for treatment of cyclical mastalgia is evening primrose oil (EPO), which we recommend the patient purchases from a pharmacy or health food store, as it has a reasonable response and is almost free of side effects. In addition it does not interfere with the menstrual cycle, but cost can be a problem in some countries. Our next option is danazol which has the best response rate overall (around 80%) but has significant side effects (Table 8.9), especially on the menstrual cycle. An alternative would be to use tamoxifen as a second-line treatment at a dose of 10 mg per day, as this drug is equally effective as danazol but has lower side effects. This prescription would, of course, be off label, as tamoxifen is not licensed for use in benign breast conditions in most countries.

Alternatively, low-dose maintenance regimens of danazol using 25 or 50 mg per day have many fewer side effects. The third agent we use is bromocriptine, which has an efficacy midway between danazol and EPO (see Fig. 8.16), but also gives side effects in some 20% of patients (see Table 8.9), principally nausea and dizziness. The drug does not disturb the menstrual cycle and this is a positive advantage to some patients. Our review of treatment has shown that failure of response to one drug does not predict subsequent failure on another drug, so it is worth trying all three drugs in turn in an individual before concluding that the mastalgia is unresponsive.

Patients are assessed after 2 months of treatment (4 months for EPO) and given a CBS grade. If a clinically useful grade (CBS I and II) has been achieved, treatment is continued for a full 6-month course (if danazol, on a reduced maintenance dose). With a CBS III score, treatment is continued for a further 2 months then reassessed. CBS IV patients are considered for an alternative therapy at 2 months.

Noncyclical mastalgia

The overall response with true noncyclical mastalgia to the three principal drug therapies is lower at around 50% overall, but rises to 64% if patients are carefully divided into true noncyclical and musculoskeletal. The order of efficacy of the agents is still danazol, bromocriptine and EPO (see Fig. 8.17); because the response rates are lower, we recommend using danazol first as this offers the best chance of response.

Again, it is worth trying the other agents in turn, but the evidence from the controlled studies shows that bromocriptine and EPO effects are only slightly better than placebo in noncyclical patients.

The use of local anaesthetic and steroid injection in noncyclical mastalgia is well worthwhile if a persistent localized painful area can be demonstrated on repeat visits to the clinic, and the same is true for musculoskeletal chest wall pain. We use Depo-Medrone with lidocaine injection (Upjohn) which contains methylprednisolone 40 mg and lidocaine hydrochloride 10 mg/mL. Medially located injections are conveniently performed with the patient supine, and laterally located injections are best made in the lateral position, affected side uppermost, in each case so that the breast falls into a dependent position, minimizing the thickness of traversed breast tissue. The localized tender area is marked and 1 mL of the injection is carefully infiltrated at the level of the pectoral fascia. (The injection should not be subcutaneous as this will cause skin atrophy.) The only side effect is mild local discomfort but this is quickly

Table 8.9 Side effects of the principal therapies

Therapy	Common side effects	Incidence (%)
Danazol (100–400 mg)	Weight gain Acne Amenorrhoea Hirsutism Reduction in breast size Voice change	25
Bromocriptine (2.5 mg twice daily)[†]	Nausea Dizziness Headache	20
Evening primrose oil (6 capsules daily)	Mild nausea	<2

†Not in routine use.

relieved by the local anaesthetic. Care should be exercised to make sure the injection is not too deep, as we have seen one small pneumothorax following an injection into the axillary tail.

More diffuse areas of tenderness can be treated with topical anti-inflammatory gel.[28]

Choice of drug with regard to side effects

The choice of drug should be generally as recommended in Table 8.8 but the attitude of the patient may indicate the final choice. Patients who are fertile must take mechanical precautions against pregnancy if taking bromocriptine or danazol as both of these agents is potentially teratogenic and may interfere with concomitant oral contraception pills. Thus, a patient who is unable or refuses to use barrier contraception should be treated with EPO, which can be taken with the oral contraceptive. If patients dislike the idea of drug-induced amenorrhoea, the choice of agents will be between EPO and bromocriptine, neither of which alters the menstrual cycle. These choices are illustrated in the flow diagram in Figure 8.18.

Length of drug treatment

It appears from our studies that the good response obtained with most of the endocrine treatments was short lived, as might be expected if the postulated endocrine defect is long term. In the danazol trial, recurrence of symptoms was appearing 3 months after finishing active treatment (Fig. 8.19).

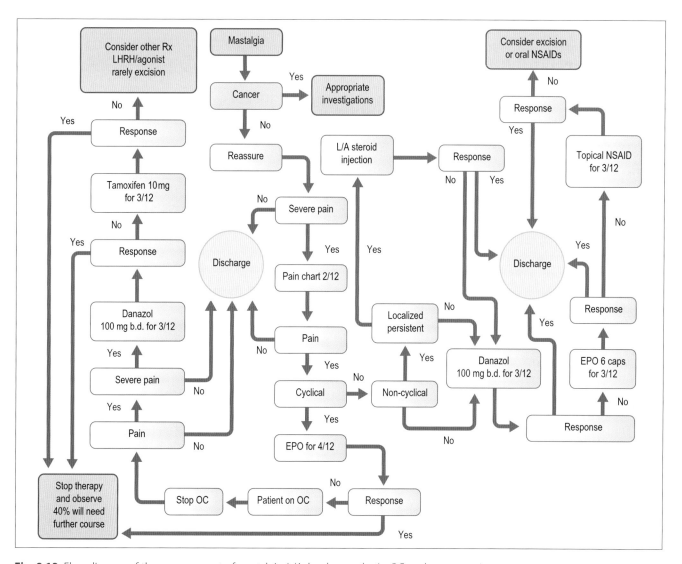

Fig. 8.18 Flow diagram of the management of mastalgia. L/A, local anaesthetic; OC, oral contraceptive.

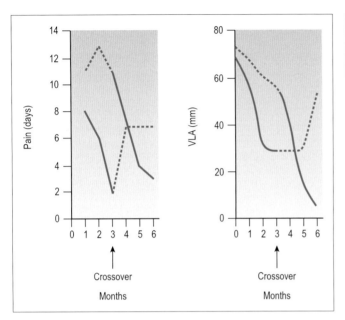

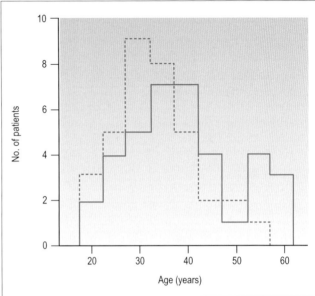

Fig. 8.19 The results of the Cardiff danazol trial for days of pain and VLA scores for tenderness. Note that symptoms return after 1–3 months when the patients took placebo (----) after a course of danazol (—).

Fig. 8.20 The age incidence of true non-cyclical mastalgia compared with musculoskeletal pain. ----, noncyclical mastalgia; —, musculoskeletal pain. (From Maddox et al.[22] by permission of the *British Journal of Surgery*.)

We have found that about one-half of the patients have recurrent mastalgia at 6 months but some of these had milder pain than before. Other authors have similar experience.[133]

Our current policy is to treat for 2–3 months (danazol or tamoxifen) or 4 months with EPO initially. If a clinically useful response (CBS I or II) is obtained, treatment is continued for a full 6 months (with reduced dose for danazol). If there is a CBS III response, treatment is continued for a further 2 months (provided side effects are not troublesome) with review after a further 2 months.

Of the 50% that recur, some will not require further therapy as the pain is milder but the patients with severe recurrences can be put back onto the original therapy if there had been a previous good response, or on to an alternative if the initial response had been poor.[83,134] (This change of therapy often had occurred already if the response had been poor.) These short treatment bursts limit drug costs and may be less suppressive to the pituitary–ovarian axis than continuous treatment, although studies of long-term usage and high dosage in both bromocriptine and danazol have not indicated any permanent suppression.

What happens to patients who defect during treatment? Of 99 such patients contacted from the Longmore Breast Clinic in Edinburgh, 36 said they were better, 19 felt no more could be done, 18 had learnt to live with

their pain, 14 did not want more treatment even if the pain recurred, 5 were still taking the medication prescribed, 2 were pregnant and 5 postmenopausal.

Mastalgia in the postmenopausal patient

Although mastalgia is seen much less frequently after the menopause, in recent years the widespread use of hormone replacement therapy (HRT) is leading to an increased incidence. The basic principles of assessment and management are similar to those in premenopausal patients, with some provisos.

Non-breast causes such as biliary pain, cervical spondylosis and shoulder lesions are more common and need careful exclusion. Likewise, the higher incidence of breast cancer requires careful assessment of persisting focal pain. Fortunately, diagnostic imaging techniques are more accurate in this age group, although HRT may cause obscuring parenchymal densities more typical of premenopausal women. Because true breast pain is uncommon in postmenopausal women (except on HRT), most are due to musculoskeletal pain (Fig. 8.20).

Management is the same as for premenopausal women.

Patients on hormone replacement therapy

In postmenopausal women, continuous oestrogen administration may stimulate ductal cell proliferation resulting in mild discomfort with fullness and nipple paraesthesia, but these symptoms do not persist.[135] In contrast, combined oestrogen and progesterone stimulates both ductal and alveolar cells to give fullness and tenderness. While this is usually modest and temporary, it may be severe and persist. Paradoxically, women who have breast tenderness at the start of HRT tend to have relief, whereas those without it before tend to develop tenderness after HRT, although this usually resolves by 6 months.[136] Where this requires active management, the following options can be tried:

- Stop the HRT, if this is appropriate.
- Try progesterone alone. As the level of oestrogen/progesterone receptors decreases, breast symptoms rapidly resolve as the cells undergo apoptosis. This option may not be acceptable to some women because progesterone may cause bloating, weight gain and depression.
- Try a medium dose of unopposed progestogens. This needs to continue for 3 months, as the initial effect is to cause a surge of mitosis, making symptoms worse, but then going on to secretory effects. Bromocriptine has proved ineffective in mastalgia due to HRT, and there are inadequate data on the efficacy of danazol in this situation.

Patients with refractory mastalgia

Every breast clinic has a small group of patients who appear refractory to normal therapeutic approaches and recognition as a centre with an interest in mastalgia leads to increasing numbers of such referrals from an increasingly wide geographical area. There is no single or simple answer to the management of these patients, but each needs to be assessed in greater than usual depth, and in an individual manner.

First, the classification and severity of the pain should be reassessed with the benefit of a new period of pain chart recording. Many such patients have had inadequate standard treatment, as a result of inadequate assessment, inappropriate prescription or failure to comply. Such patients merit a further episode of conventional treatment with full explanation. Our study of 126 patients

who failed to respond to first-line therapy with bromocriptine, danazol or EPO showed a 57% response to a second drug and a 25% response to a third drug.[137] The corresponding figures for noncyclical pain were 24% and 21% (little better than placebo). However, most of these secondary responses were to danazol; in patients who had previously had one of the other drugs, response rates were very low in patients who had failed to respond to danazol. Analysis of responders and nonresponders to first-line therapy failed to identify any factors which might help predict a secondary response.

When a patient fails to respond to danazol, it is probably best to move to tamoxifen or possibly a luteinizing hormone-releasing hormone (LHRH) analogue if the patient wishes to try further therapy, recognizing the possible side effects, especially with prolonged therapy. Tamoxifen can be given as 10 mg daily for 2–3 months, and possibly only on days 15–25 of the cycle. As it induces ovulation, contraception is particularly important if appropriate. Zoladex, a depot LHRH analogue, is given as a rod containing 3.6 mg Zoladex delivered into the subcutaneous space of the abdominal wall each 28 days for six doses, and has been shown to be effective in an early trial.[138] A recent larger, placebo-controlled trial of 147 women with cyclical mastalgia treated with Zoladex for 6 months showed significant reduction in breast pain.[139] The patients were then followed off treatment for 6 months and the breast pain gradually returned as did menstruation. The unpleasant menopause-like side effects and the risks to bone metabolism limit its prolonged use.

Can psychological testing help? Preece et al.,[40] using the MHQ to assess psychoneurotic tendency, identified an abnormal subgroup of patients (4%) who had failed to respond to reassurance and three treatment options. Their scores were close to those of psychiatric patients, in contrast to the normal scores of the average mastalgia patient. This test might be useful as a predictor of failure of response, but has not been prospectively tested in this way.

Jenkins et al.[140] carried out a similar study of patients with severe, refractory mastalgia using a structured, diagnostic psychiatric interview. In this group, they found a significant incidence of psychiatric abnormality, including anxiety, panic disorder, somatization disorder and depression, patterns common in other groups suffering from various types of chronic pain. They suggest that this subgroup might benefit from psychiatric assessment and trial of tricyclic antidepressants, particularly before any surgical approach for refractory mastalgia.

Can endocrine evaluation help? Kumar et al.[141] showed that the results of dynamic pituitary function testing correlated with the response to hormonal therapy in cyclical mastalgia patients, but this invasive test would not be suitable for routine use. Its efficacy raises the possibility that a simpler, noninvasive endocrine assessment may become available.

The example given below illustrates the diverse factors that can underlie refractory mastalgia. Such 'one-off' factors become more likely with increasing refractoriness, and require patient 'listening' to elucidate them.

A 35-year-old woman attending the breast clinic of a major institution was asked to undergo an open breast biopsy as part of an ongoing research project at that time. She reluctantly agreed, and the biopsy was complicated by a major haematoma requiring drainage under general anaesthesia and delayed healing. She did not see the original surgeon again, and staff were unwilling to discuss her complication, the details of the research project or her constant pain at the site of the scar. She consulted three breast surgeons of repute in different institutions, by whom she was treated unsuccessfully with a variety of hormonal and nonhormonal measures. Each lost interest when she failed to respond to their prescriptions, and her pain escalated.

It was clear that the patient suffered from modest pain in the scar (a common occurrence) but the severity and persistence of her pain were related to her anger at the unwillingness of the original team to accept responsibility for the complications of an unnecessary and unwanted procedure. After discussion of the background, the patient was able to tolerate the annoying discomfort.

A summary view of the extent of the clinical problem of mastalgia as seen in the Cardiff Breast Clinic 1973–1998 is given in Figure 8.21.[142]

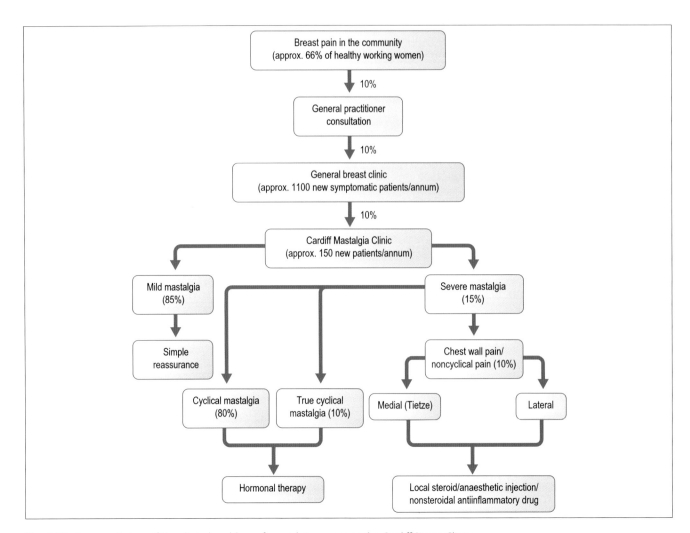

Fig. 8.21 An overall view of the clinical problem of mastalgia as seen in the Cardiff Breast Clinic.

The relationship of cyclical mastalgia to premenstrual stress

Premenstrual stress (PMS) has been defined as physical or psychological symptoms appearing during the luteal phase of the menstrual cycle, which improve during menstruation, but interfere with the person's well-being. On this definition, cyclical mastalgia is part of PMS, but in practice it is often seen in isolation from other aspects of PMS. Horrobin and Manku regard both as disorders of EFA metabolism.[68]

In general, PMS is a multisymptomatic complex which is dealt with by gynaecologists, and cyclical mastalgia by surgeons, although this varies from country to country. What is surprising is how little interaction there has been between the two specialities dealing with apparently closely related conditions, and how little interest has been shown in the relationship between PMS and cyclical mastalgia.

Some degree of PMS is extremely common,[143] and it probably affects all women. For example, 96% of 400 nurses surveyed in a Nairobi teaching hospital were affected, with 80% complaining of breast tenderness and 75% of abdominal bloating.[144] However, most did not consider it an illness, but rather part of their femininity. Only 6% changed their activities, and only 3% took medication.

It is clear from general clinical experience that PMS and cyclical mastalgia overlap, but equally that the two may occur independently, especially in the impact of the various elements on the patient's life.

Yet, while progestogens have generally been the mainstay of treatment for PMS, most trials of progestogens for mastalgia have shown no benefit over placebo. Danazol, on balance the most efficacious treatment for cyclical mastalgia, has also been advocated for PMS.[145] It has been found to work best in those with a marked cyclical mastalgia element but not effective in those with some of the other elements of PMS, particularly the psychological symptoms. This would suggest fundamental differences between the two.

Only recently have workers looked specifically at this problem. Goodwin et al. looked at the similarities, and not surprisingly found that PMS symptoms, and concern about breast problems, were more common in women with cyclical mastalgia.[146] Ader et al.[147] studied this relationship in 30 women with a recent history of cyclical mastalgia. As would be expected, PMS was significantly more likely when cyclical mastalgia is present than when it is not. But other PMS symptoms were not present in most cycles with mastalgia. They concluded that cyclical mastalgia is a chronic pain disorder where presentation, aetiology and effective therapy differ from those of PMS, and the two need to be investigated independently.

This is in keeping with our own experience; in most women presenting with cyclical mastalgia this is the dominant concern, rather than other aspects of PMS. It is important that those with cyclical mastalgia (and also noncyclical mastalgia) are assessed by a physician with experience of the full range of breast disease, and in particular by one who can confidently exclude the patient's fear of malignancy. It seems likely that a considerable degree of selection has already been undertaken by the referring physician, and this may be why the two conditions have been considered in isolation for so long. It is likely that the uncertainties relating to these two important conditions will continue.

Conclusion

A recent meta-analysis of therapies for mastalgia has confirmed that the active agents in mastalgia are bromocriptine, danazol and tamoxifen and suggests that tamoxifen may be the best drug due to the lower side effect profile.[148] The authors do note that many studies are either too small or suffer poor study design, and it is important in the future that only well-designed and sufficiently powered studies should be performed in mastalgia patients if we are to develop better treatment plans for these patients.

REFERENCES

1. Nichols S, Waters WE & Wheeler MJ. Management of female breast disease by Southampton General Practitioners. *British Medical Journal* 1980; **281**: 1450–1453.

2. Roberts MM, Elton RA, Robinson SE *et al.* Consultations for breast disease in general practice and hospital referral patterns. *British Journal of Surgery* 1987; **74**: 1020–1022.

3. Birkett J. *The Diseases of the Breast and their Treatment.* London: Longman, Brown, Green and Longmans; 1850:164.

4. Cheatle GL & Cutler M. *Tumours of the Breast.* London: Edward Arnold; 1931.

5. Atkins HJB. Chronic mastitis. *Lancet* 1938; **i:** 707–712.

6. Patey DH. Two common non-malignant conditions of the breast. *British Medical Journal* 1949; **i:** 96–99.

7. Geschickter CF. Mastodynia (painful breasts). In: *Diseases of the Breast,* 2nd edn. Philadelphia: JB Lippincott; 1945:183.

8. Semb C. Pathologico-anatomical and clinical investigations of fibro-adenomatosis cystica mammae and its relation to other pathological conditions in mamma, especially cancer. *Acta Chirurgica Scandinavica* 1928; **64** (suppl. 10): 1–484.

9. Ader DN, South-Paul J, Adera T *et al.* Cyclical mastalgia: prevalence and associated health behavioural factors. *Journal of Psychosomatics, Obstetrics and Gynaecology* 2001; **22:** 71–76.

10. Smallwood JA, Kye DA & Taylor I. Mastalgia: is this commonly associated with operable breast cancer? *Annals of the Royal College of Surgeons* 1986; **68:** 262.

11. Leinster SJ, Whitehouse GH & Walsh PV. Cyclical mastalgia: clinical and mammographic observations in a screened population. *British Journal of Surgery* 1987; **74:** 220–222.

12. Ader DN & Browne MW. Prevalence and impact of cyclical mastalgia in a United States clinic-based sample. *American Journal of Obstetrics and Gynecology* 1997; **177:** 126–132.

13. Preece PE, Baum M, Mansel RE *et al.* The importance of mastalgia in operable breast cancer. *British Medical Journal* 1982; **284:** 1299–1300.

14. Fariselli S, Lepera G, Viganotti P *et al.* Localised mastalgia as presenting symptom in breast cancer. *European Journal of Surgical Oncology* 1988; **14:** 213–215.

15. River L, Silverstein J, Grout J *et al.* Carcinoma of the breast: the diagnostic significance of pain. *American Journal of Surgery* 1951; **82:** 733–735.

16. Haagensen CD. *Diseases of the Breast,* 3rd edn. London: WB Saunders; 1986:502.

17. The Yorkshire Breast Cancer Group. Symptoms and signs of operable breast cancer. *British Journal of Surgery* 1983; **70:** 350.

18. Chiedozie IC & Guirguis MN. Mastalgia and breast tumour in Nigerian women. *West African Journal of Medicine* 1990; **9:** 54–58.

19. Plu-Bureau G, Thalabad JC, Sitruk-Ware R *et al.* Cyclical mastalgia as a marker of breast cancer susceptibility. *British Journal of Cancer* 1992; **65:** 945–949.

20. Plu-Bureau G, Le MG, Sitruk Ware R *et al.* Cyclical mastalgia and breast cancer risk: results of a French cohort study. *Cancer Epidemiology Biomarkers Preview* 2006; **15:** 1229–1231.

21. Preece PE, Hughes LE, Mansel RE *et al.* Clinical syndromes of mastalgia. *Lancet* 1976; **ii:** 670–673.

22. Maddox PR, Harrison BJ, Mansel RE *et al.* Non-cyclical mastalgia – an improved classification and treatment. *British Journal of Surgery* 1989; **76:** 901–904.

23. Fentiman IS, Caleffi M, Hamed H *et al.* Dosage and duration of tamoxifen for mastalgia. A controlled trial. *British Journal of Surgery* 1988; **75:** 845–846.

24. Bishop HM & Blamey RW. A suggested classification of breast pain. *Postgraduate Medical Journal* 1979; **55:** 59–60.

25. Dowle CS. Breast pain: classification, aetiology and management. *Australian and New Zealand Journal of Surgery* 1987; **57:** 43–48.

26. Tietze A. A peculiar accumulation of cases with dystrophy of the cartilages of the ribs. *Berliner Klinische Wochenschrift* 1921; **30:** 829–831.

27. Khan HN, Rampaul R & Blamey RW. Local anaesthetic and steroid combined injection therapy in the management of non-cyclical mastalgia. *Breast* 2004; **13:** 129–132.

28. Colak T, Ipek T, Kanik A *et al.* Efficacy of topical non-steroidal antinflammatory drugs in mastalgia treatment. *Journal of the American College of Surgeons* 2003; **196:** 525–530.

29. Wallace MS, Wallace AM, Lee J *et al.* Pain after breast surgery: a survey of 282 women. *Pain* 1996; **66:** 195–205.

30. Kudel I, Edwards RR, Kozachik S *et al.* Predictors and consequences of multiple persistent postmastectomy pains. *Journal of Pain Symptom Management* 2007; **34:** 619–627.

31. La Ban MM, Meerschaert R & Taylor S. Breast pain: a symptom of cervical radiculopathy. *Archives of Physical and Medical Rehabilitation* 1979; **60:** 315.

32. Cooper A. *Illustrations of the Diseases of the Breast,* Part I. London: Longman, Rees, Orme, Brown and Green; 1829:76.

33. Jeffcoate N. *Principles of Gynaecology,* 4th edn. London: Butterworths; 1975:550.

34. Israel SL. *Menstrual Disorders and Sterility,* 5th edn. New York: Harper & Row; 1967:160.

35. Preece PE, Richards AR, Owen GM *et al.* Mastalgia and total body water. *British Medical Journal* 1975; **iv:** 498–500.

36. Ingelby H & Gershon-Cohen J (eds). *Comparative Anatomy, Pathology and Roentgenology of the Breast.* Philadelphia: University of Pennsylvania Press; 1960.

37. Milligan D, Drife JO & Short RV. Changes in breast volume during normal menstrual cycle and after oral contraceptives. *British Medical Journal* 1976; **iv:** 494–496.

38. Fowler PA, Casey CE, Cameron GG *et al.* Cyclic changes in composition and volume of the breast during the menstrual cycle, measured by magnetic resonance

imaging. *British Journal of Obstetrics and Gynaecology* 1990; **97**: 595–602.

39. Crown S & Crisp AH. A short clinical diagnostic self-rating scale for psychoneurotic patients: the Middlesex Hospital questionnaire (MHQ). *Journal of Psychology* 1966; **112**: 917–923.

40. Preece PE, Mansel RE & Hughes LE. Mastalgia: psychoneurosis or organic disease? *British Medical Journal* 1978; **i**: 9–30.

41. Sitruk-Ware R, Sterkers N & Mauvais-Jarvis P. Benign breast disease. 1: Hormonal investigation. *Obstetrics and Gynecology* 1979; **53**: 457–460.

42. Swain MC, Hayward JL & Bulbrook RD. Plasma oestradiol and progesterone in benign breast disease. *European Journal of Cancer* 1973; **9**: 553–556.

43. England PC, Skinner LG, Cottrell KM et al. Serum oestradiol-17[b] in women with benign and malignant breast disease. *British Journal of Cancer* 1974; **30**: 571–576.

44. Malarkey WB, Schroeder LL, Stevens VC et al. Twenty four hour preoperative endocrine profiles in women with benign and malignant breast disease. *Cancer Research* 1977; **37**: 4655–4659.

45. Walsh PV, Bulbrook RD, Stell PM et al. Serum progesterone concentration during the luteal phase in women with benign breast disease. *European Journal of Cancer and Clinical Oncology* 1984; **20**: 1339–1343.

46. Preece PE. *A study of the aetiology, clinical patterns and treatment of mastalgia.* MD thesis, University of Wales, 1982:94–124.

47. Kumar S, Mansel RE, Wilson DW et al. Daily salivary progesterone levels in cyclical mastalgia patients and their controls. *British Journal of Surgery* 1986; **73**: 260–263.

48. Read GF, Bradley JA, Wilson DW et al. Evaluation of luteal-phase salivary progesterone levels in women with benign breast disease or primary breast cancer. *European Journal of Clinical Oncology* 1985; **21**: 9–17.

49. Euhus DM & Vyehara C. Influence of parenteral progesterones on the prevalence and severity of mastalgia in premenopausal women. *Journal of the American College of Surgeons* 1997; **184**: 596–604.

50. Wang DY & Fentiman IS. Epidemiology and endocrinology of benign breast disease. *Breast Cancer Research and Treatment* 1985; **6**: 5–36.

51. Nokin J, Vekemans M & L'Hermite M. Circadian periodicity of serum prolactin concentration in man. *British Medical Journal* 1972; **3**: 561–562.

52. Cole EN, Sellwood RA, England PC et al. Serum prolactin concentrations in benign breast disease throughout the menstrual cycle. *European Journal of Cancer* 1977; **13**: 597–603.

53. Lancranjan I & Friesen HG. The neural regulation of prolactin secretion. In: Veale WL & Lederis K (eds).

Current Studies of Hypothalamic Function, vol I. Basel: S Karger; 1978:131.

54. Peters F, Pickardt CR, Zimmerman G et al. PRL, TSH and thyroid hormones in benign breast disease. *Klinische Wochenschrift* 1981; **59**: 403–407.

55. Kumar S, Mansel RE, Hughes LE et al. Prolactin response to thyrotropin-releasing hormone stimulation and dopaminergic inhibition in benign breast disease. *Cancer* 1984; **53**: 1311–1315.

56. Young JB, Krownjohn AM, Chapman C et al. Evidence for a hypothalamic disturbance in cyclical oedema. *British Medical Journal* 1983; **286**: 1691–1693.

57. Minton JP, Abou-Issa H, Reiches N et al. Clinical and biochemical studies in methylxanthine-related fibrocystic breast disease. *Surgery* 1981; **90**: 299–304.

58. Farrar WB, Walker MJ & Minton JP. Common benign conditions of the breast. In: Donegan WL & Spratt JS (eds). *Cancer of the Breast*, 4th edn. Philadelphia: WB Saunders; 1995:48.

59. Odenheimer DJ, Zunzunegui MV, King MC et al. Risk factors for benign breast disease. A case control study of discordant twins. *American Journal of Epidemiology* 1984; **120**: 565–571.

60. Boyle CA, Berkowitz GS, LiVolsi VA et al. Caffeine consumption and fibrocystic breast disease: a case control epidemiologic study. *Journal of the National Cancer Institute* 1984; **72**: 1015–1019.

61. Marshall J, Graham S & Swanson M. Caffeine consumption and benign breast disease. A case control comparison. *American Journal of Public Health* 1982; **72**: 610–612.

62. Lawson DH, Jick H & Rothman KJ. Coffee and tea consumption and breast disease. *Surgery* 1981; **90**: 801–803.

63. Lubin F, Ron E, Wax Y et al. A case control study of caffeine and methylxanthines in benign breast disease. *Journal of the American Medical Association* 1985; **253**: 2388–2392.

64. Heyden S & Fodor JG. Coffee consumption and fibrocystic breasts: an unlikely association. *Canadian Journal of Surgery* 1986; **29**: 208–211.

65. Ernster VL, Mason L, Goodson WH et al. Effects of caffeine free diet on benign breast disease: a randomised trial. *Surgery* 1982; **91**: 263–267.

66. Minton JP, Foeking MK, Webster DJT et al. Response of fibrocystic disease to caffeine withdrawal and correlation with cyclic nucleotides with breast disease. *American Journal of Obstetrics and Gynecology* 1979; **135**: 157.

67. Russell LC. Caffeine restriction as medical treatment for breast pain. *American Journal of Primary Health Care* 1989; **14**: 36–37.

68. Horrobin DF & Manku MS. Premenstrual syndrome and premenstrual breast pain: disorders of essential fatty acid metabolism. *Prostaglandins, Leukotrienes and Essential Fatty Acids* 1989; **37**: 255–261.

69. Goolmali SK & Shuster S. A sebotrophic stimulus in benign and malignant breast disease. *Lancet* 1975; **i**: 428.

70. Gateley CA, Maddox PR, Pritchard GA *et al*. Plasma fatty acid profiles in benign breast disorders. *British Journal of Surgery* 1992; **79**: 407–409.

71. Sharma AK, Mishra SK, Salila M *et al*. Cyclical mastalgia – is it a manifestation of aberration in lipid metabolism? *Indian Journal of Physiology and Pharmacology* 1994; **38**: 267–271.

72. Saraiva J, Carvalho V, Almeida C *et al*. The quality of life after tubal ligation. *Acta Medica Portuguesa* 1995; **8**: 347–353.

73. Wetzig NR. Mastalgia: A 3 year Australian study. *Australian and New Zealand Journal of Surgery* 1994; **64**: 329–331.

74. Peters F, Diemer P, Mecks O *et al*. Severity of mastalgia in relation to milk duct dilatation. *Obstetrics and Gynecology* 2003; **101**(1): 54–60.

75. McFayden IJ, Forrest APM, Chetty U *et al*. Cyclical breast pain: some observations and the difficulties in treatment. *British Journal of Clinical Practice* 1992; **46**: 161–164.

76. Wilson MC & Sellwood RA. Therapeutic value of a supporting brassière in mastodynia. *British Medical Journal* 1976; **ii**: 90.

77. Hadi MSSA. Sports brassiere: is it a solution for mastalgia? *Breast J* 2000; **6**: 407–409.

78. Fox H, Walker LG, Heys SD *et al*. Are patients with mastalgia anxious, and does relaxation therapy help? *The Breast* 1997; **6**: 138–142.

79. Ory H, Cole P & MacMahon B. Oral contraceptives and reduced risk of benign breast diseases. *New England Journal of Medicine* 1976; **294**: 419–422.

80. Royal College of General Practitioners Study. *British Medical Journal* 1981; **282**: 2089–2093.

81. DiLieto A, De Rosa G, Albano G *et al*. Desogestrel versus gestodine in oral contraceptives. *European Journal of Obstetrics, Gynaecology and Reproductive Biology* 1994; **55**: 71–83.

82. Pike MC, Henderson BE, Krilo MD *et al*. Breast cancer in young women and use of oral contraceptives: Possible modifying effect of formulation and age at use. *Lancet* 1983; **ii**: 926–929.

83. Anderson TJ. Mitotic and apoptotic response of breast tissue to oral contraceptives. *Lancet* 1984; **i**: 99–100.

84. Gateley C, Miers M, Mansel RE *et al*. Drug treatments for mastalgia: 17 year experience in the Cardiff Mastalgia Clinic. *Journal of the Royal Society of Medicine* 1992; **85**: 12–15.

85. Madjar H, Vetter M, Prompeler H *et al*. Doppler measurement of breast vascularity in women under pharmacologic treatment of benign breast disease. *Journal of Reproductive Medicine* 1993; **38**: 935–940.

86. Day JB. Clinical trials in the premenstrual syndrome. *Current Medical Research and Opinion* 1979; **6** (Suppl 5): 40–45.

87. Maddox PR, Harrison BJ, Horobin JM *et al*. A randomised controlled trial of medroxyprogesterone acetate in mastalgia. *Annals of the Royal College of Surgeons of England* 1990; **72**: 71–76.

88. Nappi C, Affinito P, DiCarlo *et al*. Double blind controlled trial of progesterone vaginal cream treatment for cyclical mastodynia in women with benign breast disease. *Journal of Endocrinological Investigation* 1992; **15**: 801–806.

89. von Fournier D, Junkermann H, Warendorf U *et al*. In: Kubli F et al. (eds). *Breast Diseases*. Berlin: Springer-Verlag; 1989:499–506.

90. Schulz KD, Del Pozo E, Lose KH *et al*. Successful treatment of mastodynia with the prolactin inhibitor bromocriptine (CB 154). *Archiv für Gynaekologie* 1975; **220**: 83–87.

91. Mansel RE, Preece PE & Hughes LE. A double blind trial of the prolactin inhibitor bromocriptine in painful benign breast disease. *British Journal of Surgery* 1978; **65**: 724–727.

92. Blichert-Toft M, Anderson AN, Henriksen OB *et al*. Treatment of mastalgia with bromocriptine. A double blind crossover study. *British Medical Journal* 1979; **I**: 237.

93. Durning P & Sellwood RA. Bromocriptine in severe cyclical breast pain. *British Journal of Surgery* 1982; **69**: 248–249.

94. Mansel RE & Dogliotti L. European multicentre trial of bromocriptine in cyclical mastalgia. *Lancet* 1990; **335**: 190–193.

95. Mansel RE. A review of the role of bromocriptine in symptomatic benign breast disease. *Research Clinical Forum* 1981; **3**: 61–65.

96. Greenblatt RB, Dmowski WP, Mahesh VB *et al*. Clinical studies with an antigonadotrophin-Danazol. *Fertility and Sterility* 1971; **22**: 102–112.

97. Asch RH & Greenblatt RB. The use of an impeded androgen-Danazol in the management of benign breast disorders. *American Journal of Obstetrics and Gynecology* 1977; **127**: 130–134.

98. Greenblatt RB, Nezhat C & Ben-Nun I. The treatment of benign breast disease with danazol. *Fertility and Sterility* 1980; **34**: 242–245.

99. Mansel RE, Wisbey JR & Hughes LE. Controlled trial of the antigonadotrophin danazol in painful nodular benign breast disease. *Lancet* 1982; **i**: 928–931.

100. Harrison BJ, Maddox PR & Mansel RE. Maintenance therapy of cyclical mastalgia using low dose Danazol. *Journal of the Royal College of Surgeons of Edinburgh* 1989; **34**: 79–81.

101. Hinton CP, Bishop HM, Holliday HW *et al*. A double blind controlled trial of danazol and bromocriptine in

the management of severe cyclical breast pain. *British Journal of Clinical Practice* 1986; **40**: 326–330.

102. Peters F. Multicentre study of gestrinone in cyclical breast pain. *Lancet* 1992; **339**: 205–208.

103. Stein RC, Rawson NSB, Gazet J-C *et al.* Gestrinone in mastalgia. *The Breast* 1994; **3**: 90–94.

104. Pashby NL, Mansel RE, Hughes LE *et al.* A clinical trial of evening primrose oil in mastalgia. *British Journal of Surgery* 1981; **68**: 801.

105. Blommers J, DeLange-deKlerk ESM, Kulk DJ *et al.* Evening primrose oil and fish oil for severe chronic mastalgia: a randomised double-blind controlled trial. *American Journal of Obstetrics and Gynecology* 2002; **187**: 1389–1394.

106. Goyal A & Mansel RE. A randomized multicentre study of gamolenic acid (Efamast) with and without antioxidant vitamins and minerals in the management of mastalgia. *Breast Journal* 2005; **11**: 41–47.

107. Ricciardi I & Ianniruberto A. Tamoxifen induced regression of benign breast lesions. *Obstetrics and Gynecology* 1979; **54**: 80–84.

108. Fentiman IS, Caleffi M, Brame K *et al.* Double blind controlled trial of tamoxifen therapy for mastalgia. *Lancet* 1986; **i**: 287–288.

109. Fentiman I, Caleffi M, Rodin A *et al.* Bone mineral content of women receiving tamoxifen for mastalgia. *British Journal of Cancer* 1989; **60**: 262–264.

110. Caleffi M, Fentiman IS, Clark GM *et al.* Effect of tamoxifen on oestrogen binding, lipid and lipoprotein concentrations and blood-clotting parameters among premenopausal women with breast pain. *Journal of Endocrinology* 1988; **119**: 335–339.

111. GEMB Group. Tamoxifen therapy for cyclical mastalgia. Dose randomised trial. *The Breast* 1997; **5**: 212–213.

112. Cuzick J, Forbes JF, Sestak I *et al.* Long term results of tamoxifen prophylaxis for breast cancer – 96 month follow up of the randomised IBIS-1 trial. *Journal of the National Cancer Institute* 2007; **99**: 272–282.

113. Fisher B, Costantino JP, Wickerham DL *et al.* Tamoxifen for prevention of breast cancer: report of the National Surgical Adjuvant Breast and Bowel Project P-1 study. *Journal of the National Cancer Institute* 1998; **90**: 1371–1388.

114. Hamed H, Kothari A, Beechey-Newman N *et al.* Toremefine, a new agent for treatment of mastalgia: an open study. *International Journal of Fertility and Women's Medicine* 2004; **49**: 278–280.

115. Dhar A & Srivavastava A. Role of Centchroman in regression of mastalgia and fibroadenoma. *World Journal of Surgery* 2007; **31**: 1178–1184.

116. Mansel RE, Goyal A, Le Nestour E *et al.* and Afimoxifene (4-OHT) Breast Pain Research Group. A phase II trial of Afimoxifene (4-hydroxytamoxifen gel) for cyclical mastalgia in premenopausal women. *Breast Cancer Research and Treatment* 2007; **106**: 389–397.

117. Boyd NF, Maguire V, Shannon P *et al.* A clinical trial of low fat high carbohydrate diet in patients with cyclical mastalgia. *Breast Cancer Research and Treatment* 1987; **10**: 117.

118. Leis HP. Recommended current management of mastalgia. *British Journal of Clinical Practice (Symposium Suppl)* 1989; **68**: 50.

119. Ingram DM, Hickling West L, Mahe LJ *et al.* A double-blind randomised controlled trial of isoflavones in the treatment of cyclical mastalgia. *Breast* 2002; **11**: 170–174.

120. McFadyen IJ, Chetty U, Setchell KD *et al.* A randomised double-blind crossover trial of soya protein for the treatment of cyclical breast pain. *Breast* 2000; **9**: 271.

121. Halaska M, Gorkow C & Sieder C. Treatment of cyclical mastalgia with a solution containing a *Vitex agnus castus* extract: results of placebo controlled double-blind study. *Breast* 1999; **8**: 175–181.

122. Lehtovirta P, Ranta T & Seppala M. Pyridoxine treatment of galactorrhoea-amenorrhoea syndromes. *Acta Endocrinology* 1978; **87**: 682–686.

123. Moretti C, Fahri A, Gressi L *et al.* Pyridoxine (B_6) suppresses the rise in prolactin and increases the rise in growth hormone induced by exercise. *New England Journal of Medicine* 1982; **307**: 444.

124. Smallwood J, A-Kye D & Taylor I. Vitamin B_6 in the treatment of premenstrual mastalgia. *British Journal of Clinical Practice* 1986; **40**: 532–533.

125. Estes NC. Mastodynia due to fibrocystic disease of the breast controlled with thyroid hormone. *American Journal of Surgery* 1981; **142**: 764–766.

126. Kessler KH. The effect of supraphysiological levels of iodine on patients with cyclic mastalgia. *Breast Journal* 2004; **10**: 328–336.

127. Meyer EC, Sommers DK, Reitz CJ *et al.* Vitamin E and benign breast disease. *Surgery* 1990; **107**: 549–551.

128. Sutton GCJ, Palmer JD & Royce GT. Breast pain and the thoracic outlet compression syndrome. *The Breast* 1993; **2**: 250–252.

129. Crile G. Injection of steroids in painful breasts. *American Journal of Surgery* 1977; **133**: 705.

130. Davies EL, Cochrane RA, Sweetland HM *et al.* Is there a role for surgery in mastalgia? *The Breast* 1999; **8**: 285–288.

131. Wisbey JR, Kumar S, Mansel RE *et al.* Natural history of breast pain. *Lancet* 1983; **ii**: 672–674.

132. Pye JK, Mansel RE & Hughes LE. Clinical experience of drug treatments for mastalgia. *Lancet* 1985; **ii**: 373–377.

133. Rasmussen T, Doberl A, Rannevik G *et al.* The Hjorring project on fibrocystic breast disease. In: Baum M, George WD & Hughes LE (eds). *Benign Breast Disease*. London: Royal Society of Medicine Symposium Series; 1984:135.

134. Holland PA & Gately CA. Drug therapy of mastalgia. What are the options? *Drugs* 1994; **48**: 709–716.

135. Blankenstein MA, Szymczak J & Daroszewski J. Estrogens in plasma and fatty tissue from breast cancer patients and women undergoing surgery for non-oncological reasons. *Gynecology and Endocrinology* 1992; **6**: 13–17.

136. Marsh MS, Whitcroft S & Whitehead MI. Paradoxical effects of HRT on breast tenderness in post-menopausal women. *Maturitas* 1994; **19**: 97–102.

137. Gateley CA, Maddox PR, Mansel RE *et al.* Mastalgia refractory to drug treatment. *British Journal of Surgery* 1990; **77**: 1110–1112.

138. Hamed H, Chaudary MA, Caleffi M *et al.* LHRH analogue for treatment of recurrent and refractory mastalgia. *Annals of the Royal College of Surgeons of England* 1990; **72**: 221–224.

139. Mansel RE, Goyal A, Preece P *et al.* European randomised, multicenter study of goserelin (Zoladex) in the management of mastalgia. *American Journal of Obstetrics and Gynecology* 2004; **191**: 1942–1949.

140. Jenkins PL, Jamil N, Gateley C *et al.* Psychiatric illness in patients with treatment resistant mastalgia. *General Hospital Psychiatry* 1993; **15**: 55–57.

141. Kumar S, Mansel RE, Hughes LE *et al.* Prediction of response to endocrine therapy in pronounced cyclical mastalgia using dynamic tests of prolactin release. *Clinical Endocrinology* 1985; **23**: 699–704.

142. Davies EL, Gately CA, Miers M *et al.* The long term course of mastalgia. *Journal of the Royal Society of Medicine* 1998; **91**: 462–464.

143. Lurie S & Borenstein R. The premenstrual syndrome. *Obstetrical and Gynecological Survey* 1990; **45**: 220–228.

144. Rupani NP & Lema VM. Premenstrual tension among nurses in Nairobi, Kenya. *East African Medical Journal* 1993; **70**: 310–313.

145. Derzko CM. The role of danazol in relieving the premenstrual syndrome. *Journal of Reproductive Medicine* 1990; **35**(1 Suppl): 97–102.

146. Goodwin PJ, Miller A, DelGuidice ME *et al.* Breast health and associated premenstrual symptoms in women with severe cyclical mastalgia. *American Journal of Obstetrics and Gynecology* 1997; **176**: 998–1005.

147. Ader DN, Shriver CD & Browne MW. Relation of cyclical mastalgia to premenstrual syndrome. *Psychosomatic Medicine* 1997; **59**: 104.

148. Srivavastava A, Mansel RE, Arvind N *et al.* Evidence based management of mastalgia: a meta-analysis of randomised trials. *Breast* 2007; **16**: 503–512.

CHAPTER 9

Sclerosing adenosis, radial scar and complex sclerosing lesions

Key points and new developments

1. These lesions are important because they may be confused radiologically, macroscopically and histologically with cancer.

2. Sclerosing adenosis may present with mastalgia or as a mass, as well as an incidental radiological or histological finding.

3. Sclerosing adenosis is regarded as a component of ANDI.

4. Radial scar (RS) and complex sclerosing lesion (CSL) are the same process, and are arbitrarily differentiated on size, CSL being 1 cm or more in diameter.

5. With all three, the pathologist finds diagnosis easier on a low-power view than assessing high-power cytology.

6. Because cancer and RS/CSL cannot be differentiated reliably on radiological appearances, all such lesions should be biopsied.

7. The cancer risk associated with an individual lesion is that of associated pathology, such as atypical hyperplasia. The likelihood of such coexisting pathology is related to the size of the lesion and the age of the patient.

8. Whether stereotactic core needle or open surgical biopsy is utilized depends to some extent on the facilities and experience available. Even confirmed cases are better removed.

9. Oxytocin receptors are prominent in the myoepithelial cells seen in these conditions, possibly playing an aetiological role.

Introduction

These three lesions have long been recognized by pathologists under a variety of names. They have more recently attracted clinical attention (and some degree of uniformity of terminology) because they are diagnosed more frequently on mammography as screening abnormalities which simulate cancer. Simultaneously, pathologists have subjected them to greater scrutiny because of the intensified interest in differentiating histological patterns into those which may, or may not, be precancerous.

Sclerosing adenosis

This lesion was first described by Masson in 1923[1] and a number of excellent pathological descriptions have since

been published, one such being that by Dawson.[2] We regard sclerosing adenosis as one of the manifestations of aberrations of normal development and involution (ANDI) (an aberration of lobular involution; see Chapter 4), in which a well-ordered lobular involution is distorted by excessive myoepithelial proliferation, and accompanied by pronounced fibrous alteration of the specialized lobular stroma.

This is in keeping with the fact that sclerosing adenosis is present (unrecognized) in the breast much more frequently than it presents clinically. Among surgeons it has received little attention, being known mainly through notoriety as a cause of difficulty for pathologists in the diagnosis of cancer. Its surgical implications extend over a wider field for it may simulate cancer clinically, macroscopically and radiologically, as well as histologically. In addition, the condition shows an association with breast pain. Sclerosing adenosis may become particularly florid during pregnancy.[3]

Clinical presentation

The condition has four distinct modes of clinical presentation:

- presentation as a mass
- presentation with pain
- presentation on mammography
- chance histological finding.

Presentation as a mass

This may occur at any age from the mid-20s to the postmenopausal age group. The mass tends to be small, 2 cm or less, firm, poorly delineated and attached to surrounding breast tissue. There are no gross signs of cancer, such as skin retraction or lymphadenopathy, but these would not necessarily be expected with a small mass.

Presentation with pain

This is discussed in more detail in Chapter 8. In brief, sclerosing adenosis produces the same type of localized persisting pain that is seen in cancer, but sometimes having premenstrual exacerbation. Pressure also often causes exacerbation and, in some patients, it is severe enough to interfere with sleep.[4,5] The perineural invasion demonstrated histologically in some cases may be an explanation of the association with pain (Fig. 9.1).

In a series of 316 consecutive and unselected cases of benign mammary disorders, Davies found that sclerosing

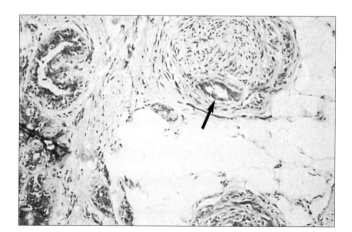

Fig. 9.1 Sclerosing adenosis with neural invasion (*arrow*).

adenosis was the condition most frequently found to show neural invasion by mammary epithelial cells.[6]

Presentation on mammography

With increasing use of mammography as a screening or semiscreening procedure, the radiological features typical of sclerosing adenosis are being detected more frequently, either in association with a mass or in asymptomatic patients. Where the radiological pattern is indistinguishable from cancer, biopsy is mandatory. Where unequivocal radiological signs of sclerosing adenosis are seen on mammography, 90% will have the condition on histology. Thus, in our experience, there is a 10% false-negative rate for the mammographic diagnosis.

Chance histological finding

Small patches of sclerosing adenosis are frequently found on histological sections of breast tissue. It has been estimated that these occur 20–30 times more commonly than palpable lesions. These small areas found on histology can be ignored.

Frequency of presentation

In our clinic, 43 patients were encountered over a 5-year period. The age range extended from 24 to 64 years. Eleven presented primarily with pain, although 25 of the patients experienced some pain at the site of the lesion. Nine presented with a mass and four were chance histological findings. The rest were detected on mammography. Undoubtedly, there would have been other cases detected on histological examination during this period which the pathologist did not bother to report.

Sclerosing adenosis appears to be particularly common in some developing countries, where it is also frequently associated with mastalgia. Ihekwaba found it in 52 of 657 women with benign breast disorders in Nigeria, and associated with mastalgia in 68% of them.[7]

Radiological criteria

Three patterns of radiographical change are seen[8] (see also Ch. 6):

- Increased density with irregular margins, very similar to cancer but without fine microcalcification.
- Fine, smooth calcification scattered widely throughout the breast, usually bilateral.

- Smooth microcalcifications, up to 10 in number, arranged in a small group (Fig. 9.2). This may or may not be associated with widespread calcification. This pattern cannot be differentiated from that of cancer, and biopsy is mandatory.

The ultrasound characteristics of sclerosing adenosis are variable and may show features suggestive of both benign and malignant breast disease.[9] Mass effects may have either clearly demarcated or irregular outlines and occasionally focal acoustic shadowing without a visible mass.

Pathology

Careful macroscopic examination will suggest the diagnosis. Sclerosing adenosis occurs as a firm, ill-defined fibrotic mass, but is not as hard, cartilaginous or gritty as cancer and it has a nodular, circumscribed appearance rather than the stellate pattern of cancer. Azzopardi[3] points out that examination with a fine hand lens will often demonstrate clearly the nodular and whorled appearance. The nodules have a brownish tinge and the greyish or creamy streaks of necrotic debris in ductules typical of cancer are not seen.

The microscopic criteria outlined by McDivitt et al.[10] have been summarized by Davies[6] as nodular epithelial lesions in which lobular units are enlarged by an increased number of acini, but the normal two cell population and basement membrane are maintained. The normal lobular structure is distorted by the fibrosis, particularly in the centre of the lesion, where epithelial cells may appear to

be isolated and simulate the appearance of invasive malignancy, especially on frozen section. The problem is compounded by mitoses sometimes seen in the early cellular phase, and neural and vascular invasion may occur. Microcalcification, similar to that seen in malignancy, is common. The problem is now well recognized by experienced pathologists, but was the cause of much overdiagnosis of malignancy in the past.

The histological similarities between sclerosing adenosis and cancer are illustrated in Figure 9.3, in which the two are shown side by side.

The maintenance of a lobular architecture on low-power evaluation is an essential feature used to differentiate the two lesions. Figure 9.4 shows the extensive microcalcification which is the basis of one of the radiological patterns.

The development of techniques for localizing oxytocin receptors has shown these to be prominent in the myoepithelial cells, which themselves are prominent in sclerosing adenosis.[11] This raises the possibility that oxytocin and its receptors may play a role in the aetiology and evolution of sclerosing adenosis.

Management

Because sclerosing adenosis and cancer cannot be differentiated with certainty on imaging, histological confirmation is essential. This may be done with a core biopsy using either ultrasound or a stereotactic technique. An alternative, particularly for mass lesions, is to use the mammotome. We agree with Gill et al.[12] that provided adequate tissue sampling has been performed there is no indication for excision. If open biopsy is required for a nonpalpable, mammographic lesion a standard prearranged procedure involving surgeon, radiologist and pathologist must be followed to ensure that the correct tissue is removed. The steps are described in Chapter 18.

Radial scar and complex sclerosing lesions

Radial scar (RS) and complex sclerosing lesions (CSL) are similar to sclerosing adenosis in that they present most commonly as mammographic or incidental histological findings simulating malignancy, and may also present as a mass. Histologically, sclerosing adenosis lacks the elastosis and epithelial proliferation notable in these two

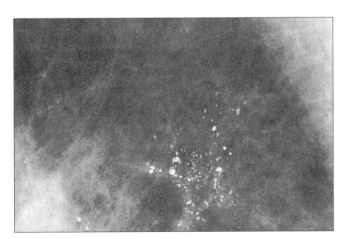

Fig. 9.2 Mammogram showing microcalcifications typical of a focus of sclerosing adenosis – variable in size, shape and density in a segmental distribution.

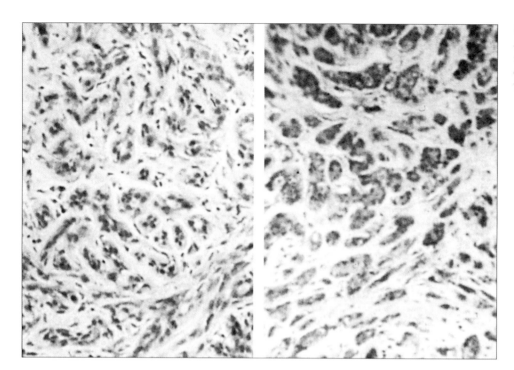

Fig. 9.3 Sclerosing adenosis (*left*) and invasive cancer (*right*) shown side by side, illustrating difficulties encountered in differentiation on frozen section.

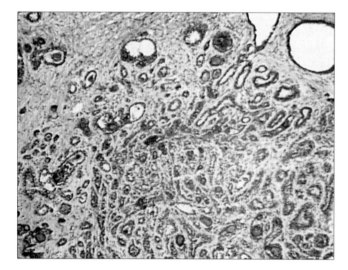

Fig. 9.4 Sclerosing adenosis showing numerous areas of microcalcification, providing the pathological basis for the typical X-ray appearance.

lesions, while the maintained lobular orientation typical of sclerosing adenosis is lost in the greater complexity and distortion of RS and CSL.

These terms were defined much more recently than sclerosing adenosis, the term radial scar being used first by Linell et al. as recently as 1980,[13] although the lesions had been described previously under various names by a number of workers.

For practical purposes, RS and CSL are interchangeable terms[14] differentiated arbitrarily on the basis of size, lesions smaller than 1 cm being designated as RS, and those larger as CSL. They may be multiple.

The reported incidence in screening programmes is from 0.1 to 0.5 per 1000 women attending. The incidence is much higher in autopsy studies; Nielsen et al.[15] found RS in 28% of unselected autopsies, two-thirds multiple and one-half bilateral.[12] It is well recognized that typical pathological lesions may show no mammographic abnormality, even though in practice the majority are found in this way.

Pathology

Macroscopically, small RS may be unremarkable, but larger lesions show the induration, retraction and greyish-white colour typical of cancer. There has been a tendency to regard RS/CSL as impalpable, the presence of a mass being considered to indicate cancer. However, Wallis et al.[16] found a quarter of benign lesions detected on screening to be palpable.

Microscopically, the lesion has a stellate appearance around a central core. The core is of fibrous and elastic tissue with entrapped distorted glandular elements. Radiating from this central core are ducts that may show cystic dilatation. This arrangement suggests that the lesion may develop by sclerosis around a small duct where it branches into terminal ducts. Page and Anderson[17] describe the typical appearance as 'the arrangement of parenchyma around a fibrosing spindle, rather in the manner of a central purse string having been pulled'. The distortion of the epithelial cells caught in the central sclerosis is the reason for the confusion with malignancy. The surrounding ducts frequently show benign hyperplasias, adenosis or sclerosing adenosis.

As the lesion becomes larger, the complexity of the surrounding tissues drawn in makes the term complex sclerosing lesion appropriate. The histological appearances of RS are reproduced in the larger lesions, but the greater complexity arises from other changes being drawn in, such as papilloma, sclerosing adenosis and apocrine change.

As with sclerosing adenosis, pathologists report that they make the diagnosis by viewing at low power, rather than by studying high-power cytological detail. In a multicentre study where pathologists reviewed slides of breast screening abnormalities 'blind', RS and CSL were lesions that were diagnosed by different pathologists with a high degree of consistency.[18] Davies and Kulka[19] have drawn attention to small false arterial aneurysms associated with these lesions. They believe them to be traumatic, resulting from diagnostic needle puncture.

Diagnosis

The lesion is seen in a wide pre- and postmenopausal age group, typically 35–65 with a mean of 55 years.[20] They rarely present as a lump, but after identification on a mammogram, a quarter can be palpated. The typical radiological features are a lucent centre with radiating spicules, with or without microcalcification, and varying appearances on different mammographic views (Figs 9.5 and 9.6). These typical features may also occur with early cancers. Ultrasound[21] and contrast enhanced magnetic resonance imaging[22] may help to differentiate these lesions from cancers but are not sufficiently accurate to preclude histological confirmation.

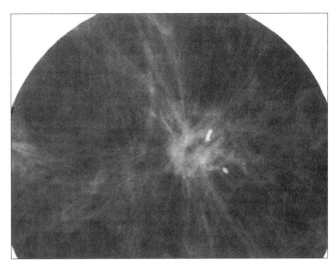

Fig. 9.5 Mammogram of a radial scar, showing the typical features of central lucent area and long, radiating strands described in the text.

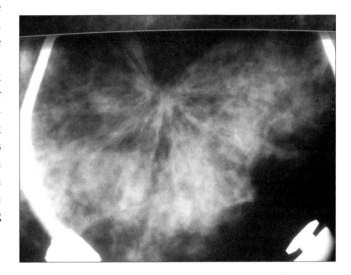

Fig. 9.6 Radial scar shown on compression mammography.

Management

The diagnostic work-up is similar to that for sclerosing adenosis. Histological examination of core biopsy material obtained with either ultrasound or stereotactic guidance is essential. For example, Frouge et al.[23] reported the pathological findings in 40 RS lesions diagnosed on mammography. Pathology showed 20 pure RS, 12 pure cancers and 8 cancers (7 tubular) associated with an RS. On review of the mammograms, it was not possible to differentiate the three groups on the size and shape of the spicule, the size of the central core or the calcifications. Patterson et al.[14] reviewed the Northern Ireland experience of imaging diagnosed RS/CSL and found that 7% of screening cases had either ductal carcinoma in situ (DCIS) or invasive cancer; the figure for symptomatic patients was 32%.

The experience from our own screening unit is similar: 32 lesions showing radiological features of RS were excised after detailed mammography, ultrasound and fine needle aspiration (FNA); four were well-differentiated cancers and three had small areas of in situ cancer in the breast tissue adjacent to an RS. Brenner et al.[24] have performed a useful analysis of 157 radial scars diagnosed by core biopsy. Nine per cent (5/58) of those diagnosed by spring-loaded biopsy device were found to have cancer on following excision biopsy (this reduced to zero if 12 cores were performed). None of 70 mammotome biopsies had cancer. On this evidence, we and most others believe that all RS/CSL lesions should be excised. Some advocate a stereotactic biopsy and watch policy (e.g. Cawson et al.[25]) Mammotome excision is an attractive alternative to core biopsy and subsequent excision biopsy although only the study of Brenner et al.[24] has systematically evaluated this. A further indication for excision of radial scars may be derived from the studies of Jacobs et al.[26] These authors showed similarities in mRNA expression, encoding for vascular stroma, in patients with radial scars and breast cancer.

Significance

The implications for malignancy of these lesions have been the subject of some controversy, but the balance of opinion at present is that they are not precancerous, although the findings of Jacobs et al.[26] suggests that it may be. Local excision to ensure accurate diagnosis and eliminate the lesion is appropriate management. It is generally agreed that the cancer risk is that of the individual elements; thus, if an area of atypical hyperplasia or cancer in situ is included, the prognosis would be that of the individual processes.[27] Sloane and Mayers have drawn attention to the importance of the size of the lesion and the age of the patient in the likelihood of such associated pathology being present.[28] In a study of 126 radial scars in 91 women, atypical hyperplasia and intralesional cancer were rare in lesions less than 6–7 mm in diameter and in women younger than 50 years old, but was much higher with larger lesions in older women.

The suggestion that the central epithelial cells represent the earliest stage of a tubular or other breast cancer cannot be excluded; autopsy studies have shown that RS is significantly commoner in cancerous than noncancerous breasts.[15] On the other hand, follow-up studies have shown no increase in cancers after excision of radial scars[29] and there is insufficient evidence to support a precancerous potential.

REFERENCES

1. Masson P. *Traite de Pathologie-Medicale*. Paris: A. Malione; 1923.

2. Dawson EK. Fibrosing adenosis: a little recognised mammary picture. *Edinburgh Medical Journal* 1954; **61**: 391–401.

3. Azzopardi JG. *Problems in breast pathology*. London: WB Saunders; 1979: 168.

4. Preece PE, Fortt RW, Gravelle IH et al. Some clinical aspects of sclerosing adenosis. *Clinical Oncology* 1979; **2**: 192.

5. Preece PE. Sclerosing adenosis. *World Journal of Surgery* 1989; **13**: 721–725.

6. Davies JD. Neural invasion in benign mammary dysplasia. *Journal of Pathology* 1973; **109**: 225–231.

7. Ihekwaba FN. Benign breast disease in Nigerian women: a study of 657 patients. *Journal of the Royal College of Surgeons of Edinburgh* 1994; **39**: 280–283.

8. Evans KT & Gravelle IH. *Mammography, Thermography and Ultrasonography in Breast Disease*. London: Butterworths; 1973.

9. Gunhan-Bilgen I, Memis A, Ustun EE et al. Sclerosing adenosis: mammographic and ultrasonographic findings with clinical and histopathological correlation. *European Journal of Radiology*. 2002; **44**: 232–238.

10. McDivitt RW, Stewart FW & Berg JW. Tumours of the breast. *Atlas of Tumour Pathology*, vol 2. Washington DC: 2nd Series Fascicle; 1968:133–137.

11. Bussolati G, Cassoni P, Ghisolfi G et al. Immunolocalisation and gene expression of oxytocin receptors in carcinomas and non-neoplastic tissues of the breast. *American Journal of Pathology* 1996; **148**: 1895–1903.

12. Gill HK, Ioffe OB & Berg WA. When is a diagnosis of sclerosing adenosis acceptable at core biopsy? *Radiology* 2003; **228**: 50–57.

13. Linell F, Ljungberg O & Andersson I. Breast carcinoma: aspects of early stages, progression and related problems. *Acta Pathol Microbiol Immuno Scand* 1980; **272**: 199–217.

14. Patterson JA, Scott M, Anderson N et al. Radial scar, complex sclerosing lesion and risk of breast cancer.

Analysis of 175 cases in Northern Ireland. *European Journal of Surgical Oncology* 2004; **30**: 1065–1068.

15. Nielsen M, Jensen J & Andersen JA. An autopsy study of radial scars in the female breast. *Histopathology* 1985; **9**: 287–295.

16. Wallis MG, Devakumar R, Hosie KB *et al.* Complex sclerosing lesions (radial scars) of the breast can be palpable. *Clinical Radiology* 1993; **48**: 319–320.

17. Page DL & Anderson TJ. *Diagnostic Histopathology of the Breast.* Edinburgh: Churchill Livingstone; 1987:91.

18. Sloane JP, Ellman R, Anderson TJ *et al.* Consistency of histopathological reporting of breast lesions detected by screening. *European Journal of Cancer* 1994; **30A**: 1414–1419.

19. Davies JD & Kulka J. Traumatic arterial biopsy after fine needle aspirational cytology in mammary complex sclerosing lesions. *Histopathology* 1996; **28**: 65–70.

20. Patel A, Steel Y, McKenzie J *et al.* Radial scars: a review of 30 cases. *European Journal of Surgicical Oncology* 1997; **23**: 202–205.

21. Cawson JN. Can sonography be used to help differentiate between radial scars and breast cancers? *Breast* 2005; **14**: 352–359.

22. Pediconi F, Occhiato R, Venditti F *et al.* Radial scars of the breast: contrast-enhanced magnetic resonance mammography appearance. *Breast Journal* 2005; **11**: 23–28.

23. Frouge C, Tristant H, Guinebretiere JM *et al.* Mammographic lesions suggestive of radial scars: microscopic findings in 40 cases. *Radiology* 1995; **195**: 623–625.

24. Brenner RJ, Jackman RJ, Parker SH *et al.* Percutaneous core needle biopsy of radial scars of the breast: when is excision necessary. *American Journal of Roentgenology* 2002; **179**: 1179–1184.

25. Cawson JN, Malara F, Kavanagh A *et al.* Fourteen-gauge needle core biopsy of mammographically evident radial scars: is excision necessary? *Cancer* 2003; **97**: 345–351.

26. Jacobs TW, Schnitt SJ, Tan X *et al.* Radial scars of the breast and breast carcinomas have similar alterations in expression of factors involved in vascular stroma formation. *Human Pathology* 2002; **33**: 29–38.

27. Nielsen M, Christensen L & Andersen J. Radial scars in women with breast cancer. *Cancer* 1987; **59**: 1019–1025.

28. Sloane JP & Mayers MM. Carcinoma and atypical hyperplasia in radial scars and complex sclerosing lesions: importance of lesion size and patient age. *Histopathology* 1993; **23**: 225–231.

29. Andersen JA & Gram B. Radial scar in the female breast: a long term follow-up of 32 cases. *Cancer* 1984; **53**: 2557–2560.

CHAPTER 10

Cysts of the breast

Key points and new developments

1. Macrocysts constitute the commonest discrete benign breast mass, estimated to occur in 7–10% of all women.

2. Microcysts develop from apocrine metaplasia of a single lobule throughout most of reproductive life; a few go on to form macrocysts, mainly in the last decade of reproductive life.

3. Macrocysts fall into two broad groups: those with a persisting apocrine cell lining and active secretion/concentration of many substances; and those lined by flattened cells and metabolically much less active.

4. Gross cysts are associated with a small but definite increase in subsequent breast cancer, but opinions about, and evidence for, the details of the associated cancer risk are not uniform.

5. Simple cysts are adequately treated by aspiration; ultrasound is helpful with poorly defined cysts and to ensure complete emptying of recurrent cysts.

6. Cysts yielding bloodstained fluid are investigated by cytology and sonography, and warrant exploration even if triple assessment is negative. Most are due to intracystic papillary tumours of benign histology or low-grade malignancy.

7. Recurrent cysts may be aspirated as often as necessary, without further therapy or investigation.

8. Leakage from a cyst gives surrounding inflammation with altered sonographic appearances (complex cyst) and may give a residual mass after aspiration. Where painful cysts are a problem, a trial of danazol is worthwhile.

9. Since the increased risk of cancer is small, and most patients are in their fifth decade, standard breast screening is appropriate follow-up for most cases.

10. Cysts per se are not premalignant, so do not need excision, and screening should be directed at both breasts.

11. Galactoceles cause few clinical problems, being readily managed by aspiration. They may cause greater problems with imaging, because of the variety of appearances seen on sonography and mammography.

Introduction

Cysts are the commonest abnormality found in patients presenting to a breast clinic, a fact of little surprise since it has been estimated that 7–10% of all women will develop a symptomatic breast cyst during their reproductive life.

Like many other breast lesions, cysts were described by Sir Astley Cooper in 1831.[1] The French surgeon Reclus provided a comprehensive description in 1883[2] in an account so accurate that the disease is still known by his name among French surgeons. Bloodgood[3] has achieved surgical immortality more easily than most with his attention-catching description of the 'blue-domed cysts' that bear his name.

A large majority of breast cysts are a manifestation of aberrations of normal development and involution (ANDI) – aberrations of normal lobular involution as described in Chapters 1 and 4. Unless otherwise specified, this chapter refers to these lesions. Some of the less common forms of cysts and pseudocysts shown in Table 10.1 are dealt with in Chapter 17.

The reasons for regarding cyst formation as an aberration of normal involution, and therefore part of the spectrum of ANDI, have been set out in Chapter 4. Haagensen[4] and many others use the term 'cystic disease' to include other elements of ANDI such as mastalgia and cyclical nodularity, but this can further confuse the issue, and it is preferable to consider each aspect separately. The management of macroscopic cysts is specific to that clinical presentation and unrelated to the other elements of ANDI.

Pathology

The pathology of breast cysts was only too familiar to surgeons when biopsy excision was the standard management of all cysts. Now the surgical trainee brought up on needle aspiration will see only the small cysts encountered by chance during breast surgery. These vary in size from those just visible to the naked eye to others up to 4–5 mm in diameter. They often occur in a cluster over an area 2–3 cm in diameter. These are the 'blue-domed' cysts (Fig. 10.1), which have classically been considered to denote benign disease.

These small cysts have no intrinsic significance except the potential to form larger cysts in due course.

Larger cysts are thin walled and more brown than blue in colour, from the brownish opalescent fluid within them. They usually present as an individual cyst but the single palpable cyst is likely to be the overt presentation of multiple, bilateral cysts, the majority of which are impalpable (Fig. 10.2).

The cysts may be uni- or multilocular but, even in unilocular cysts, constricting fibrous bands provide evidence of their origin from a single lobule or group of lobules (see Ch. 4). Cysts are lined by a single layer of epithelium that may be of two types: tall columnar secretory epithelium or attenuated, flattened cells. Sometimes they have no epithelial lining at all.

The fluid content of the cysts shows a wide range of appearances from clear to heavily turbid, and from light brown, through grey, to almost black (Fig. 10.3).

These fluids consist of a variety of chemical substances, including pigmented products of apocrine secretion, lipofuscin products of peroxidated lipoprotein, breakdown

Table 10.1 Breast cysts

TRUE BREAST CYSTS	
1	ANDI
	Microcysts
	Apocrine macrocysts
	Nonapocrine macrocysts
2	Juvenile cysts
3	Secondary cysts
	Galactocele
	Oil cysts of fat necrosis
	Liquefied haematoma
	Implant-related loculated fluid collections
4	Papillary cystadenoma
CONDITIONS THAT REQUIRE DIFFERENTIATION FROM BREAST CYSTS	
1	Dilated ducts/chronic abscess associated with duct ectasia/periductal mastitis
2	Cysts of the dermis and areola
3	Cysts associated with tumour necrosis
	Phyllodes tumour – benign and malignant
	Necrotic carcinoma
4	Hydatid cysts

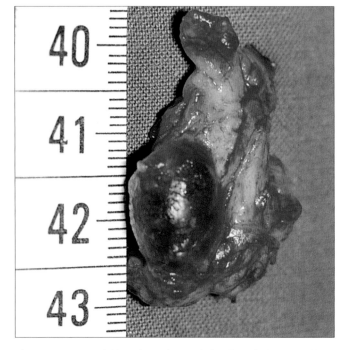

Fig. 10.1 A typical 'blue-domed cyst of Bloodgood' discovered by chance at biopsy for dominant nodularity. It has already reached the size when its colour is closer to brown than blue. It should have been found by a needle point!

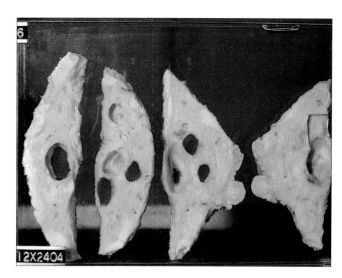

Fig. 10.2 A breast autopsy. The breast was asymptomatic during life. This illustrates the multiplicity of macroscopic cysts and the diffuse nature of the involutional stromal changes of ANDI.

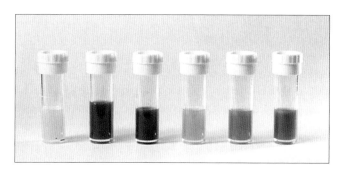

Fig. 10.3 The range of colours of cyst fluid. The first specimen of opalescent fluid is common; the blood-stained fluid is uncommon and requires further investigation.

products of haemoglobin and possibly secretory products related to diet.[5] They do not contain blood unless there is an associated neoplasm. Crystal clear watery fluid is not seen in the common cysts of ANDI.

Multiple cysts are frequently impalpable due to the laxity of the cyst, allowing it to merge into surrounding breast tissue of similar consistency. But a very small increase in volume has a disproportionate effect on the intracystic pressure, explaining how a small increase in fluid can cause a large cyst to become tense and clinically apparent in a few days. This also explains the surprising fact that most cysts do not recur after aspiration. In fact, many do not disappear after aspiration but merely revert to their lax, impalpable state, as is readily shown by repeat imaging. Both increase and decrease in size may be seen

on serial imaging over a short period, suggesting that the balance between secretion and reabsorption or duct obstruction must be variable, so obstruction of the ductule draining the cyst is not a complete or irreversible process. Little is known of the dynamics of secretion and reabsorption of fluid by the cyst epithelium or through the cyst wall, the other process that might lead to rapid volume change.

There is an extensive literature on the biochemistry of cyst fluid. It contains many steroid hormones, beta human chorionic gonadotrophin (βHCG) and relaxin, tumour markers such as fetoprotein and carcinoembryonic antigen (CEA) and 'gross cystic disease proteins', many of which are found in much higher concentrations than in blood, suggesting an active secretory process. Manello et al.[6] have provided a useful review of the topic.

There is growing evidence that, firstly, breast cyst fluid is not merely the result of filtration from plasma, its composition being strikingly different from that of plasma or extracellular fluid, and secondly, active (though not yet clarified) secretory and/or concentrating mechanisms are involved.[7] Epidermal growth factor (EGF) can also be measured and its level appears to act as a marker for epithelial proliferation elsewhere in the breasts.[7]

Incidence

There are surprisingly few satisfactory data on incidence of cysts in the general population. One autopsy study[8] of 225 women without overt clinical breast disease showed a 19% incidence of macroscopic cysts 1–2 mm or more in diameter; in half of these cases the cysts were bilateral. Sandison[9] put the figure rather higher but put together both ectasia and cysts. Ultrasound examination will show further impalpable cysts, particularly in pre- and postmenopausal women taking hormone replacement therapy (HRT). Foote and Stewart[10] reported 27% incidental cysts in 300 breasts removed for cancer. Haagensen[4] estimates that 7% of white women in Western countries will develop a palpable cyst, because this is the incidence of cancer, and in his practice cyst and cancer are seen with equal frequency. This must be a very rough approximation, although the figure of 7% is quoted almost universally. Others believe 10% to be a better estimate. Even complex cysts seem to occur in about 5% of ultrasound examinations.[11] Whatever the true incidence, cysts are so common that they should be considered as part of the normal involution of the breast.

Pathogenesis and cyst types

There is such a large body of research data relevant to the aetiology of breast cysts that it is easier if a summary of the conclusions is given first, with the data to follow.

The current view is that all macrocysts start with an area of apocrine epithelium in a terminal ductal lobular unit (TDLU). Excessive secretion of the apocrine epithelium, probably compounded by osmotic effects of the secretion products, leads to progressive dilatation of the TDLU to give a microcyst. The dilatation is at first confined to the acini containing apocrine epithelium. (These contrast with involutional microcysts, without apocrine epithelium and common in postmenopausal patients.)

If the apocrine microcyst enlarges, it does so in one of two directions: type 1 macrocyst containing actively secreting apocrine epithelium and with contents similar to intracellular fluid, and type 2 macrocysts, with flattened epithelium and contents more akin to extracellular fluid. Type 1 cysts are more prone to occur in patients with multiple or recurrent cysts, and carry a small increase in subsequent cancer risk.

Many early workers and some recent writers have regarded cysts as dilated ducts. However, the clinical course and complications of duct ectasia and involutional cysts are very different, as is the underlying pathology of the two conditions. They should not be linked in any way, although they frequently coexist as different aberrations of involution.

Sir Alan Parks was one of the first workers to shed light on the problem when he described the process of cystic lobular involution.[12] In this process lobules develop microcysts during their involution, while maintaining some of the specialized lobular stroma around the epithelial acini. As long as this remains, the lobule may go on to complete involution, but if the specialized stroma is replaced by fibrous tissue before the small cysts have regressed, the cystic change is likely to persist. With time, the many small cysts representing the acini of the lobule will coalesce to form a smaller number of larger cysts (see Ch. 4). This is the simplest form of microcystic change, and is common in postmenopausal women. The lobular origin of macroscopic cysts is described by Azzopardi,[13] who shows the value of elastic stains in demonstrating that each cyst derives from a lobule, enormously distended in the case of large macrocysts. Most macrocysts are seen in premenopausal women and disappear at the menopause.

Many workers have noticed a second type of microcyst lined by apocrine metaplastic epithelium, and concluded that obstruction of the outflow from the lobule leads to distension and conversion of the columnar apocrine cells to a flat cuboidal epithelium, or little epithelium at all. It was assumed that all macrocysts arose by this single mechanism.

Further work has cast doubt on this simplistic approach from a number of directions, but there is still much uncertainty about detailed mechanisms. Studies from Bradlow's unit[14] have shown that cysts fall into two main groups, dependent on the ratio of Na^+ and K^+ in the cyst fluid. One group of cysts has a low Na^+ and high K^+, resembling intracellular fluid, and is designated type 1; the other (type 2) has a high ratio, resembling extracellular fluid. Different cut-off points for classifying type 1 and 2 cysts have been used, using $Na:K$ ratios varying from 1.5 to 3. In a large study,[15] 52% had type 1, 41% had type 2, and 7% had both. Type 1 cysts occurred more in younger women who had fewer births. Estimation of the $Na^+:K^+$ ratio in our own series of 725 patients shows a similar bimodal distribution (Fig. 10.4). These findings, now confirmed by other workers, suggest that there may be at least two populations of cysts, possibly corresponding to those lined with apocrine epithelium (Fig. 10.5) which is actively secreting in the high K^+ group, while in the others the flat epithelium (or no epithelium lining at all) acts more as a passive membrane (Fig. 10.6). The type

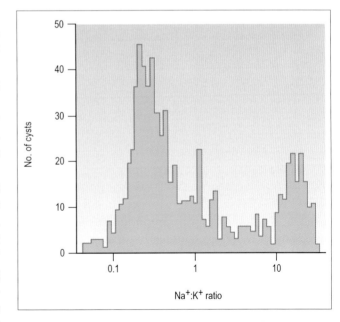

Fig. 10.4 The bimodal distribution of breast cysts when characterized by $Na^+:K^+$ ratio of cyst fluid – Cardiff series.

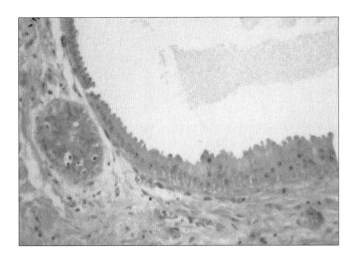

Fig. 10.5 Wall of apocrine cyst, lined by tall, pink columnar epithelium.

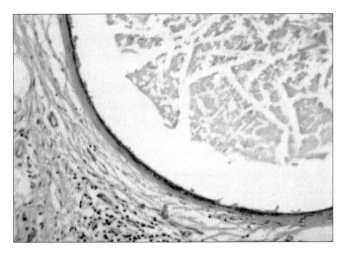

Fig. 10.6 Cyst lined by flattened epithelium (sometimes the epithelial lining of the cyst wall is lost completely).

1 apocrine cysts are characterized by tight junctions, so all transport is by cellular pore, while type 2 cysts have loose junctions and secretions can move directly, to some extent, from plasma into cyst fluid. A further extension of the different cyst types is the demonstration by Parish et al.[16] that the cytokine profiles differ and that type 1 cysts have higher levels of EGF.

This would suggest that the progression from micro- to macrocyst is dependent on the balance between secretion and outflow or reabsorption, and this balance might be upset in two ways. In one, obstruction of the ductule draining the original lobule would lead to back pressure and dilatation. A number of possible obstructing mechanisms have been suggested, including benign epithelial hyperplasia and fibrous obliteration of the lumen. But in

many cases, the normal involutional fibrosis around the ductule, perhaps augmented by kinking, may alone be sufficient. It seems likely that some obstructive element is important, particularly with large, tension cysts. In the second group, apocrine secretion in excess of the reabsorptive capacity of the cyst may be important. Patients with apocrine-lined cysts are more likely to have multiple cysts and to develop further cysts.[17]

It is these cysts with apocrine lining, particularly where the lining is papillary, which Haagensen[4] has suggested have a small but definite increase in malignancy associated with macroscopic cyst disease. This view has long been disputed, but many studies of this question have now been performed, and there is increasing acceptance that gross cystic disease is associated with a small, but definite, increase in cancer risk.[18]

In this context, it is interesting to note that type 1 cysts have higher concentrations of hormones, androgen and oestrogen conjugates, as well as EGF. Conjugated bile acids can also be detected in breast cyst fluid, with significantly higher concentrations in the apocrine-type cyst (with the higher cancer risk) than the flattened walled cyst.[19] Torrisi et al. found that EGF levels in breast fluid were a better indicator of proliferative epithelial hyperplasia elsewhere in either breast than $Na^+:K^+$ ratio.[7] Mannello et al. have shown that breast cyst epithelium secretes and accumulates large amounts of prostate-specific antigen.[20] Dixon et al.[21] have shown that intravenously administered tritiated hormone (dihydroepiandrosterone sulphate) appears in the fluid of apocrine cysts within 2 hours, and persists within the cysts for up to 2 years. Furthermore, danazol, spironolactone and evening primrose oil (EPO) can inhibit this process,[22] opening possible therapeutic approaches. A majority, but not all, of type 1 cysts are metabolically active in this way; type 2 cysts are inactive. In contrast, type 2 cysts have been found to concentrate transforming growth factor beta 2,[23] which is reported to have an inhibitory effect on epithelial tumour cell growth. Thus breast cysts, with their active transluminal transport mechanisms, may well act as a 'window' on what is going on within the rest of the breast.

However, the diversion of cysts along the two paths of high or low $Na^+:K^+$ ratio occurs during macrocyst development, and not from the beginning. Dixon and co-workers[24] have studied 40 microcysts, and found that all had high concentrations of androgen conjugates and a high $K^+:Na^+$ ratio. They have shown that microcysts form a single population lined by apocrine secretory epithelium. The two types of macrocysts thus appear to develop from a single, apocrine type of microcyst. Even the type 2 cysts with flattened epithelium may show gradients with protein concentrations higher than serum, showing that they do not act as pure passive membranes.

Wellings and Alpers[25] have contributed further to our understanding of this process with their elegant technique of subgross whole-organ sampling. The definitive lesion is the apocrine cyst, in which apocrine metaplasia occurs in hyperplastic/hypertrophic cystically dilated lobules. At first, only part of a TDLU may contain tufts of apocrine epithelium, and only this portion of the lobule will show dilatation. They postulate that pressure of apocrine secretion, compounded by the osmotic effects of breakdown products, leads to progressive 'unfolding' of the acini, until the whole lobule may be affected. As patients grow older, the cyst tends to enlarge, and the lining epithelium flattens or atrophies. This confirms the general view of the pathogenesis of cysts, but does not elucidate the mechanism for progression to macrocyst, or the differentiation into types 1 and 2.

Surprisingly, they have shown that the extralobular terminal duct (ETD) is dilated, so that any obstructive element must be beyond the TDLU/ETD junction. Alternatively, the dilatation may be due only to secretory pressure, and Molina et al.[26] add evidence that secretion from hyperplastic apocrine epithelium initiates microcysts, and osmotic mechanisms lead to progression to macrocysts.

Bundred et al.[27] showed that zinc alpha-2 glycoprotein, a marker of apocrine epithelium, is raised in breast fluids, highest in microcysts, intermediate in type 1 cysts, and lowest in type 2 cysts. Nevertheless, levels are still 10 times higher than in serum, confirming the view that all cysts are derived from apocrine epithelium. Levels were also higher in cyst fluid of patients who subsequently developed recurrent cysts.

Aetiology

Cyst formation can be regarded as a minor aberration of normal lobular involution, but the specific aetiological factors responsible for this aberration are unknown. There is some indirect evidence to implicate hyperoestrogenism, either absolute or relative. There is also evidence that acini dilate towards the end of the menstrual cycle, and that this is an oestrogen effect. It has been suggested that excess unopposed oestrogen in premenopausal patients maintains the acini in a dilated state, which is accentuated by the pressure of apocrine secretion. A number of cases seem to be related to oestrogen therapy, particularly in postmenopausal patients. Haagensen[4] regards the administration of oestrogen for menopausal symptoms as a potent cause of cysts in women over the age of 50. There is also some direct evidence in that England et al.[28] demonstrated raised mean levels of serum oestradiol-17β in 13 women with cysts, although among these patients seven had high levels, four were normal and two were reduced. Both basal and stimulated levels of biologically active prolactin are raised in patients with breast cysts, and this may prove important.[29] This view is not supported by more systematic assessment of breast changes in patients receiving HRT. For example, neither Yenen et al.[30] nor Ozdemir et al.[31] found any difference in cystic change from a range of hormone replacement therapies. At present, a hormonal basis for involutional cysts remains unproven. The cause of this condition is undetermined, and there is no conclusive evidence to support hormonal therapy for cysts, although it is reasonable to withdraw oestrogen supplements in such patients if it otherwise seems appropriate.

Simpson and Page[32] have demonstrated the absence of fodrin in the wall of all cysts. Since fodrin is a cytoskeletal structural protein which binds actin and plays a role in the establishment of cellular orientation and polarity, it is attractive to suggest that this loss may be a significant factor in cyst formation, although the loss could be a secondary rather than primary phenomenon.

Clinical features

Macroscopic cysts are frequently asymptomatic, the patient often noting the mass accidentally when touching the breast. In other cases, sudden pain draws the attention of the patient to a large cyst, probably due to sudden distension or to leakage of fluid into the surrounding tissue, giving chemical irritation. Pain may also be associated with disappearance of the cyst, which has presumably ruptured or discharged its contents into a duct. Pain is not usually related to the menstrual cycle, nor is variation in the size of the cyst. Nipple discharge is uncommon but does occur and duct injection has sometimes demonstrated communication with a cyst in such a case. The discharge will then be typical of cyst fluid.

Fifty-five per cent of cysts are found in the left breast and 45% in the right, a ratio identical to that for fibroadenoma. Two-thirds occur in the upper outer quadrant, with the upper inner quadrant being next most common. Cysts are uncommon in the lower half of the breast.

On examination, the physical characteristics vary widely according to a number of factors: size, intracystic pressure, depth and situation in the breast, and the characteristics of surrounding breast tissue.

Large cysts are frequently visible when the patient lies down (Fig. 10.7).

Generally, the cyst is felt as a smooth, tense structure, readily palpable against the chest wall, and to some extent attached to breast tissue (see Ch. 5). Large cysts may be palpably multilocular. Lax cysts are palpated only with difficulty or not at all. Very tense cysts are so hard that carcinoma may be simulated closely. A large cyst may displace surrounding Cooper's ligaments, producing apparent skin attachment or even retraction (false retraction of Haagensen[4]). The diagnostic problem is fortunately solved readily by routine use of needle aspiration and ultrasonography for all lumps.

A deep cyst may feel much more superficial in a youngish patient with pliable breast tissue and be missed entirely by timorous needling. Likewise, only the fore-most loculus of a lobulated cyst may be felt from the surface, so that needling produces surprisingly more fluid than expected. Conversely, needling of one of a cluster of cysts will produce less fluid than expected.

There is a strong clinical impression that multiple cysts are seen most commonly in larger breasts, but no habitus is exempt and simple cysts are common in patients with small, dense breasts. There seems to be no relationship between age and multiplicity or recurrence.

It is difficult to obtain a representative study group to assess the true incidence of subclinical cysts, since all populations are biased to some extent. Of women presenting with painful nodularity to a breast clinic, ultrasound examination will show about 20% to have cysts, of which 20% will be small (<5 mm), and 40% medium (5–15 mm) or large (>15 mm).

Age

Cysts occur predominantly in the middle and late reproductive period, increasing in frequency from 35 years to a maximal incidence between 40 and 50 years. They are rarely seen before the age of 30, although we have seen a 5-cm cyst behind the areola in a 16-year-old girl, which did not recur after a single aspiration. Perhaps the pathogenesis differs in such juvenile cysts, although the clinical features were typical in this case. Cysts disappear rapidly after the menopause, unless the patient is taking hormone preparations. Of Haagensen's 2511 patients, 78% presented between 35 and 50 years and only 2.3% before the age of 30.[4]

The rare cysts seen in the elderly tend to be large, and associated with a papillary tumour, when the fluid will be bloodstained. It seems likely that the even rarer cysts in the elderly not associated with tumour have a different aetiology to the premenopausal cyst, although little has been written about large non-neoplastic cysts in the elderly. Devitt[33] found that only 6% of symptomatic women over the age of 60 had breast cysts, compared with 15% of those less than 55 years presenting to a breast clinic. Furthermore, a majority of the older patients with cysts were taking hormone supplements. It is interesting that this premenopausal concentration of clinical cysts is not seen with histological apocrine microcysts, which are much more uniformly distributed from 25–30 years until the ninth decade.[25]

Brenner et al. studied the development of new cysts in women undergoing mammographic screening, and found

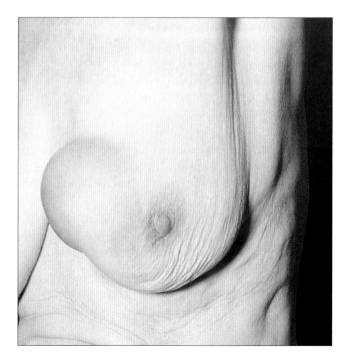

Fig. 10.7 A large, visible cyst. This is an extreme example, but smaller cysts may also produce an eccentric contour when the patient lies down.

that 1% of women developed new cysts between screens, with a clear relationship to hormone replacement therapy (HRT) in those over the age of 50.[34] Only one of 20 women with cysts under the age of 50 was on HRT, compared with 17 of 33 over 50.

Natural history

The natural history can be presented no better than through the results of Haagensen's unique study,[4] in which he has followed 2511 patients, 2235 for 5–30 years. Seventeen were multiple at first presentation on clinical examination (ultrasound or surgery would show much higher figures); 40% developed new cysts, the interval to a further cyst being progressively shorter with age from an average of 10 years in the third decade to 2 years in the sixth. As would be expected, the greater the number of cysts, the shorter the interval to recurrence. With a minimum 5-year follow-up, 30% had only one cyst, 30% had 2–5 cysts, and the remainder had 6 or more. A further excellent paper is that of Jones and Bradbeer, who followed 322 cases for a minimum of 5 years, and obtained similar results.[35] Sterns[36] reported on a series of 4207 patients observed over 14 years. Two hundred and eighty-six women had cysts on 561 occasions. Cysts did not recur in 60% of the patients. There were two to five recurrences in 36% and more than five recurrences in 4%. Patients with more than five recurrences were 5 years younger than the overall group when the first cyst appeared and the events developed over a period of time ranging from 51 to 161 months (mean of 96 months) and appeared at intervals averaging 17 months.

In our clinic, half the patients develop a further palpable cyst (new or recurrent) in the 12 months following aspiration, and 6% will develop a new cyst for the first time more than 5 years after the initial aspiration. The number of new cysts presenting clinically (i.e. not detected only by imaging) within a period of 5 years after aspiration is shown in Table 10.2.

There is considerable controversy about the homogeneity of cyst type for any given patient with multiple recurrent cysts. One group[37] found that concentrations of EGF and insulin growth factor-1 (IGF-1) were concordant when taken from multiple cysts, whether ipsi- or contralateral.

Brenner et al. showed that over 5 years only 12% of new cysts detected between mammographic screenings increased in size, while 60% of the cysts had resolved by

Table 10.2 Number of clinically detected cysts (after aspiration) per patient with a minimum follow-up of 5 years

No. of cysts	No. of patients (%)
1	164 (46.6)
2	66 (18.8)
3	31 (8.8)
4	25 (7.1)
5	22 (6.2)
6 or more	44 (12.5)
Total	352 (100)

1 year, and 80% by 4 years without treatment.[34] All those that increased in size did so within 2 years, and this was twice as likely to occur in patients on HRT.

Investigation

In practice, cysts are adequately managed by mammography, ultrasound, needle aspiration and inspection of the aspirated fluid. Radiological examination is not strictly necessary for cysts, but we utilize mammography for all cyst patients over the age of 35 years as a form of screening, to exclude an incidental cancer. We found five incidental cancers in 352 patients presenting for aspiration of a breast cyst (1.4%).

Ultrasound will usually show cysts to be multiple and bilateral with numbers in excess of those detected clinically or mammographically. Cysts are rounded, ovoid or lobulated with characteristics so similar to fibroadenoma as to make radiological differentiation impossible, emphasizing the superiority of ultrasound in managing cysts. Leakage of cyst fluid into the surrounding tissues gives altered sonographic appearances due to an inflammatory reaction (termed complex cyst by sonographers). Ultrasound of the abnormal rim can confirm inflammation rather than neoplasm.

Pneumocystography has been used when cyst aspiration reveals bloodstained fluid, but has been replaced by ultrasound. Ultrasound provides similar information more easily, with the added bonus of allowing accurate sampling of any associated solid component.

Differential diagnosis

Cysts are readily differentiated from solid lesions by ultrasound and needling. Three other cystic conditions need to be considered: the cystic form of fat necrosis (page 274), galactocele (page 157) and cystic papillary tumours, adenoma and carcinoma (page 158). It cannot be stressed too often that a tense cyst can closely simulate cancer on palpation. The question of cancer should never be raised with a patient before a cyst has been excluded by ultrasound and/or needling.

Management

The last 40 years has seen the management of cysts pass from mandatory excision, through selective aspiration with cytological examination, via routine (and if necessary repeated) aspiration alone and now, if there are classic features of a cyst without any other risk factors, leaving the cyst alone. Patey and Nurick[38] had an early influence in the UK in managing cysts conservatively, and this development of a conservative regimen for managing breast cysts has been one of the truly major advances in breast surgery. Nevertheless, no aspect of breast disease management is without pitfalls and strict rules must be followed to avoid an occasional disaster. The exact sequence of management will be determined by the arrangements of individual clinics. In our unit all patients over 35 have a mammogram prior to their consultation. Patients with discrete lumps have an ultrasound. If a cyst is identified it is either aspirated under ultrasound guidance or left alone if the patient wishes and there are no atypical features.

Aspiration

The majority of cysts are now aspirated with ultrasound guidance. If immediate ultrasound is not available, the first investigation of an easily palpable lump in the breast should be the insertion of a needle, and if this is practised cysts will be diagnosed at first consultation. A 21-gauge needle with a syringe of appropriate size to the estimated cyst volume is plunged directly into the cyst, fixed by two fingers of the opposite hand (Fig. 10.8).

No anaesthetic is necessary. The average cyst volume is 5–10 mL, but this varies from less than a millilitre to 75 mL or more. A 10-mL or 20-mL syringe is usually

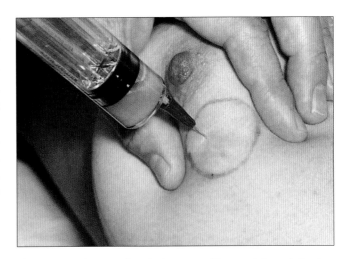

Fig. 10.8 Technique of aspirating a cyst. The cyst is immobilized by fingers of the left hand.

convenient. If the mass proves to be solid, a cytological specimen is obtained, and this is facilitated if a syringe holder designed for obtaining cytology specimens is used. If the fluid is not bloodstained, the cyst is aspirated to dryness, the needle removed and the fluid discarded. Cytological examination of cyst fluid is not useful or cost effective unless the fluid is bloodstained. Many early workers advocated cytological examination of all cyst fluid,[38] but it is now recognized to be unnecessary and most large units have abandoned it except when bloodstained.[39,40] The breast is carefully palpated to exclude a residual mass. If one exists, an ultrasound guided biopsy of any residual abnormality should be performed.

If the fluid is bloodstained, 1–2 mL only of fluid is taken for cytology in Cytospin fluid. The mass is then imaged with ultrasound and a core biopsy taken from any solid area in the cyst. The presence of blood is usually obvious, but in cysts with black fluid (usually not due to blood), any doubt should be eliminated by examining the fluid for blood by microscopy or a chemical occult blood test. Blood must be regarded as synonymous with tumour (usually benign, but sometimes malignant). Malignancy is more likely to occur in the elderly but even then the prognosis is favourable.

If mammography has not already been performed it is advisable to do so to evaluate pathology elsewhere in the breast. The radiologist should be informed that an aspiration has taken place so that allowance can be made for any artefacts produced by the aspiration.

Recurrent cysts

Early recurrence is not rare but is less common than might be expected. Because aspiration might not be expected to influence the natural history, one might anticipate universal recurrence. In fact, only about 10% of cysts refill to become palpable, although almost one-half of patients will develop another cyst elsewhere in the breast, and about one-third will develop more than one. We treat a recurrent cyst by repeated aspiration, and are not particularly concerned at the number of aspirations required. Fortunately, cysts rarely refill after two or three aspirations. Recurrence is an indication for mammography but not for excision. Because recurrence usually occurs in patients with multiple cysts, excision is not appropriate treatment. A persistent mass, or bloodstained fluid, remains the only indication for excision.

If recurrence becomes tedious for the patient, injection of air after aspiration may reduce the chances of further recurrence.[41] Gomes et al.[42] advocated the injection of a sclerosant to prevent recurrence and, like Dixon and co-workers,[17] have found that apocrine-lined cysts, characterized by a high $K^+:Na^+$ ratio, are more prone to be multiple and to recur than nonapocrine cysts. In practice in our clinic we have found little need for such interventions.

Hormone therapy

The hormonal background to cysts is not defined sufficiently precisely to justify any form of hormone therapy on a routine basis. One study of patients with recurrent cysts has reported a remarkable reduction (75%) in the number of cysts requiring aspiration after a course of danazol, 100 mg three times per day for 3 months.[43] Benefit was even greater at 6 months, i.e. 3 months after cessation of therapy, and persisted at 3-year follow-up, but had disappeared at 5 years. This indicates that this treatment might prove worthwhile in severe cases with recurrent painful cysts. A controlled trial of EPO in our unit had no effect on the incidence of recurrent cysts.[44]

Mastectomy

In the past, some surgeons recommend subcutaneous mastectomy with silicone implant for extensive or recurrent cystic disease, either on the basis of reduction of cancer risk or for the physical and psychological benefit of the patient. We believe this practice should be con-

demned except in the most exceptional circumstances. Although cysts are a nuisance, they cause the patient relatively little morbidity when they are managed conservatively by repeated aspiration. This is entirely different to the complications, short and long term, which may trouble patients after bilateral subcutaneous mastectomy with silicone implants or autogenous tissue reconstruction. The presence of cysts alone would not justify mastectomy on grounds of cancer risk, and should be considered as one aspect only of cancer risk, in weighing up the very difficult decisions in this area.

Follow-up and breast cancer risk

This is another area of clinical practice undergoing reevaluation as the result of increased knowledge over the past decade. Although Haagensen[4] gave evidence many years ago that macroscopic cysts are associated with a definite, but quite small, increase in cancer risk, other workers did not confirm this. Several studies have demonstrated a definite, though relatively small, increase in risk. Bundred et al.[18] showed an increase in subsequent cancer of 4.4 times in women having a cyst aspirated over the expected risk. The risk was even greater in women with multiple or bilateral cysts. This finding has recently been confirmed by a prospective study[16] in which the cyst type was determined by fluid examination at entry. These workers found a similar degree of overall risk, but this was confined to type 1 apocrine cysts, and there was no increase with multiple cysts. However, not all studies reflect this increased risk of breast cancer, e.g. the study of 1312 high risk women with and without gross cystic disease failed to show an increased risk for those with cysts.[45]

Thus, while the small increase in overall cancer risk seems definite, the further effect of individual factors remains controversial. A further, larger study by Dixon and colleagues[46] showed a similar increase in overall risk, but no relation to cyst type. The main factor affecting cancer risk in this study was age, with the greatest risk in women presenting with a cyst before the age of 45. The differences in these studies – age versus multiplicity versus cyst type – will probably prove to be due to methodological problems. For example, Dixon relied on cancer registry data for his follow-up.

These data provide some basis for devising a follow-up policy. The overall risk is not great: only 14 cancers occurred in 352 patients followed an average of 7 years in the Bundred series. It would be reasonable to enter such women in a screening programme at the age of 40, rather than the age of 50 generally recommended in the UK. This would be an appropriate age since cysts are uncommon before 40. It should be emphasized that this is a pragmatic approach that requires validation. Follow-up of all patients with cysts below the age of 40 is not cost effective, so at present patients are discharged after assessment provided that no other risk factors have been demonstrated.

Haagensen et al. reported the prognostic influence of the presence of high blood levels of the cyst fluid protein GCDFP-15.[47] Over a 10-year follow-up period, the relative risk of cancer for women who developed 10 or less cysts increased from 1.8 to 4.2 if they showed elevated plasma levels of the protein. The corresponding figures for those developing more than 10 cysts were 2.0 and 7.1. Since this protein is secreted by apocrine epithelium, it is further evidence for the influence of apocrine metaplasia on cancer risk.

There is considerable scope for defining a high-risk population even more closely by adding data on family history, age and cyst type, and with further study of hazards associated with various constituents of cyst fluid. It is important to appreciate that a cyst is an indicator of increased risk, and is not itself a premalignant condition; hence there is no need to excise cysts, and screening must encompass both breasts.

Galactocele

A galactocele is an uncommon lesion in which a cyst filled with milky material develops after a period of lactation. There is a surprising paucity of information about this condition, compared with other aspects of breast pathology. Such literature as exists is often obscured by a tendency to confuse galactocele with duct ectasia and recurrent subareolar abscess. The confusion extends down to some of the most recent papers, particularly those which state that galactoceles are prone to lead to chronic sinuses. The first use of the term 'galactocele' has been attributed by Fitzwilliams to de Lambell, who defined it in 1845 as a 'form of tumour which springs from one of the milk ducts, forming a cyst'.[48]

The term is best confined to a specific clinical syndrome in which a woman develops a painless swelling of the breast from a few weeks to some months after ceasing lactation. The swelling is smooth and mobile and in fact has the exact physical characteristics of the usual breast cyst. Aspiration produces what is clearly milk, instead of one of the variety of fluids commonly found in breast cysts. The lesion disappears completely and is usually cured by a single aspiration but, like ordinary cysts, will occasionally require two or three aspirations. It may be found anywhere in the breast, but commonly towards the areola.

In one series of 10 cases[49] the age range was from 27 to 36, the duration 1 week to 6 months; six cases were postpartum and five still feeding.

The mammographic appearances have been described[50] and are complex, with three distinctive radiological patterns. Ultrasound is more appropriate as the first examination in this group, and again the appearances are complex, with 50% cystic or multicystic, 37% mixed cystic/solid and 13% solid.[49]

The aetiology and pathology are obscure. Lactation is an essential antecedent in the typical case (although the condition has been described in male infants!). It is usually stated to follow abrupt artificial cessation of lactation.

A simple explanation of the pathogenesis is that a pre-existing cyst that connects with the duct system fills with milk, either by secretion or retrograde filling, but the ductule draining the cyst becomes blocked, trapping the milk. This may become slightly thicker by absorption of water, but retains the obvious characteristics of milk. Since some cysts can be demonstrated to connect with the duct system, it is surprising that galactocele is not more common, given the frequency of cysts in the breasts. Presumably the reason is that cysts are an aberration of involution and less common during the usual childbearing period. It also has been reported that macroscopic cysts resolve during pregnancy along with the well-recognized improvement in mastalgia and nodularity. An interesting insight into the pathogenesis comes from the controlled trial reported by Auvichayapat et al.[51] who passed a nylon probe into the duct obstructed by a protein plug. Although the probing took longer than simple aspiration there were no recurrences as opposed to two of five in the aspiration group.

A neglected galactocele may present at a later stage when they are filled with inspissated material. If there is not a clear history of the lump persisting since lactation, cysts containing inspissated pus or infected material are better regarded as a separate group, most of which fall into the categories of duct ectasia, periductal mastitis or chronic cystic disease.

Papillary tumours associated with macrocysts

Pathology

Papillary tumours within the wall of a cyst are rare, yet by no means excessively so. We see approximately one such tumour a year, yet there is remarkably little written on this subject. Hart first drew attention to the subject in 1927.[52] He described 124 cases and emphasized that the majority were benign. However, the report does not differentiate between duct papillomas and intracystic tumours, but since 69 of 95 benign cases had nipple discharge and 75 a lump, it must have included both. That confusion, or at least lack of differentiating the two groups, persists today.

Haagensen[4] regards them all as duct papillomas within grossly dilated ducts, yet this is not consistent with our experience. Cystic dilatation of ducts due to intraductal papilloma (sometimes also called papillary cystadenoma) is commoner than the true isolated cyst containing a tumour, but in our experience the two conditions are clinically distinct, and this is important in management. Cyst puncture and pneumocystography (a technique now replaced by ultrasound) shows no connection with the duct system with the isolated lesion, nor is there any nipple discharge. Azzopardi[13] mentions that papilloma can be seen within cysts, i.e. of lobular derivation, but gives no details apart from mentioning a single case he had encountered. Devitt[53] discusses the problem of carcinoma in association with a cyst.

Perhaps the most important point is whether they are single or multiple. Intracystic tumours in the elderly are usually solitary and of low-grade malignancy. Intraductal tumours are usually multiple, and more likely to be associated with multifocal intraduct cancer. Calvert et al.[54] described a solitary huge intracystic papillary lesion (18 cm in diameter) which they regarded as intraductal, in spite of the lack of nipple discharge, because fragments of elastic tissue could be identified in its wall. Whether this finding is definitive in such a large lesion is probably less important than the fact that it was solitary, and hence likely to behave as an intracystic tumour and more likely to be suitable for local excision.

A second problem causing confusion is the use of the term intracystic cancer, since this by definition excludes benign lesions. A series of 48 cases of intracystic cancer was reported from the Mayo Clinic[55] where it constituted 0.5% of all breast cancers. However, 31 cases were excluded because they were benign, suggesting that intracystic papilloma has approximately the same incidence as the malignant version. The report gives evidence of the excellent prognosis of the lesions regarded as malignant; only 1:3 showed invasion of the cyst wall, and only 6% had axillary metastases. A series of 16 cases reported in 1969[56] were all reported as malignant, although 12 showed 'orderly papillary epithelium with little mitotic activity', reflecting the tendency to err on the side of diagnosing cancer at that time.

Carter et al.[57] describe 41 cases of intracystic cancer without mention of benign cases. They divide them into three groups: (1) noninvasive intracystic cancer and with no surrounding ductal carcinoma in situ (DCIS), (2) intracystic cancer with cyst wall invasion but no DCIS, and (3) intracystic cancer with associated DCIS. They point out the differing prognosis for the first group; none had recurrence, including eight who had biopsy only. It is clear that these form a biologically favourable group.

In summary, intracystic papillary tumours need to be differentiated from multiple ductal papillomas, to be assessed very carefully in terms of malignancy, and assessed in terms of tumour invasion into the surrounding breast.

Clinical features

Papilliferous cysts usually arise in patients a decade or more after the menopause. The patient presents with a soft mass that is usually large and often apparently of recent onset. Aspiration yields old, bloodstained fluid and cytology will usually show epithelial cells of benign or degenerate appearance. Ultrasound will demonstrate the cyst, and a small papilloma within its wall. Estabrook et al. reported mammographic features in 10 such cases.[58]

Ultrasound with guided biopsy can give considerable information regarding differential diagnosis and malignancy of the cyst and its contained tumour, and has replaced pneumocystography (Figs 10.9 and 10.10) as the main diagnostic technique. Invasion of the wall can be assessed, although caution is needed in relying entirely on ultrasound for assessment. It can help target any suspicious area for FNA cytology. The series of 56 tumours with a cystic appearance on ultrasound studied by Omori et al. contained a wide variety of pathology. Ten of the 56 were intracystic cancers; other lesions included necrotic cancers and phyllodes tumours, simple cysts and abscesses.[59] Yamamoto et al.[60] have described a technique of endoscopy in which a fibreoptic ductoscope is intro-

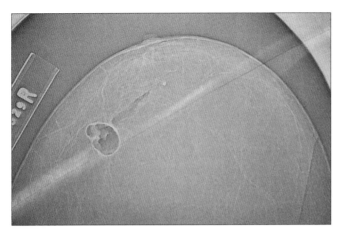

Fig. 10.9 This historical pneumocystogram nicely demonstrates an intracystic papilloma, and also air in a major duct.

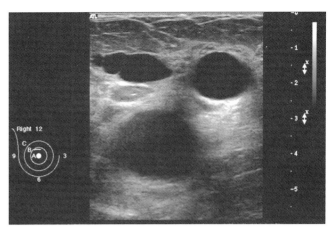

Fig. 10.11 Ultrasound image of multiple cysts.

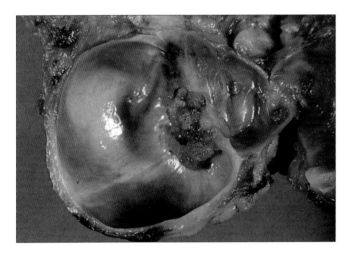

Fig. 10.10 Typical papillary tumour in the wall of a cyst in an elderly woman.

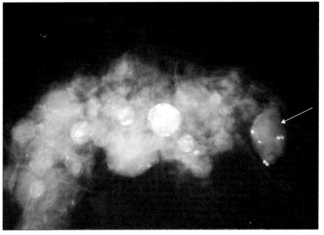

Fig. 10.12 Mammogram showing florid breast cysts, some are partly calcified; a fibroadenoma is seen (*arrow*).

duced via a cannula into the cyst. Although we doubt that this approach is justifiable in a routine clinic, the authors were able to separate the benign papilloma from the malignant ones on the basis of their surface appearance.

Management

Fortunately, the majority of papillary tumours associated with macrocysts are benign, even (or especially) in the elderly. The local nature of the lesion, as a confined cyst,

will usually be apparent on clinical examination, and imaging (Figs 10.11 and 10.12). Mammography will give some indication of the presence of invasive cancer or DCIS.

Where the lesion appears to be a confined cyst, in this age group it is best treated by total cyst excision, with a 1-cm resection margin as for phyllodes tumour. This will provide material for adequate histological assessment in all cases, and definitive treatment in the majority proved benign or with minimal invasion on histology.

REFERENCES

1. Cooper A. On diseases of the breast. *Cooper Lectures* 1831; **2**: 125.

2. Reclus P. La maladie kystique des mammelles. *Revue de Chirurgie* 1883; **3**: 761.

3. Bloodgood JC. The bluedomed cyst in chronic cystic mastitis. *Journal of the American Medical Association* 1929; **93**: 1056.

4. Haagensen CD. *Diseases of the Breast.* Philadelphia: WB Saunders; 1986.

5. Petrakis NL, Miike R, King EB *et al.* Association of breast fluid coloration with age, ethnicity, and cigarette smoking. *Breast Cancer Research and Treatment* 1988; **11**: 255–262.

6. Mannello F, Tonti GA, Papa S. Human gross cyst breast disease and cystic fluid: bio-molecular, morphological, and clinical studies. *Breast Cancer Research and Treatment* 2006; **97**:115–129.

7. Torrisi R, Zanardi S, Pensa F *et al.* Epidermal growth factor content of breast cyst fluids from women with breast cancer or proliferative disease of the breast. *Breast Cancer Research and Treatment* 1995; **33**: 219–224.

8. Frantz VK, Pickren JW, Melcher GW *et al.* Incidence of chronic cystic disease in so-called normal breasts. *Cancer* 1951; **4**: 762–783.

9. Sandison AT. An autopsy study of the adult human breast. *National Cancer Institute*: Monograph No 8 Bethesda; 1962.

10. Foote FW & Stewart FW. Comparative studies of cancerous versus non-cancerous breasts. *Annals of Surgery* 1945; **121**: 6–53.

11. Houssami N, Irwig L, Ung O. Review of complex breast cysts: implications for cancer detection and clinical practice. *Australian and New Zealand Journal of Surgery* 2005; **75**: 1080–1085.

12. Hayward JL & Parks AG. Alterations in the microanatomy of the breast as a result of changes in the hormonal environment. In: Currie AR (ed.). *Endocrine Aspects of Breast Cancer.* Edinburgh: Livingstone; 1958: 133–134.

13. Azzopardi JG. *Problems in Breast Pathology.* London: WB Saunders; 1979.

14. Bradlow HL, Fleisher M, Schwartz D *et al.* Biochemical classification of patients with gross cystic breast disease. *Annals of the New York Academy of Sciences* 1990; **586**: 12–16.

15. Bruzzi P, Dogliotti L, Naldoni C *et al.* Cohort study of risk of breast cancer with cyst type in women with gross cystic disease of the breast. *British Medical Journal* 1997; **314**: 925–928.

16. Parish DC, Ghilchik MW, Day JM *et al.* Cytokines in human breast cyst fluid. *Journal of Steroid Biochemistry and Molecular Biology* 2007; **104**: 241–245.

17. Dixon JM, Miller WR, Scott WN. Natural history of cystic disease: the importance of cyst type. *British Journal of Surgery* 1985; **72**: 190–192.

18. Bundred NJ, West RR, Dowd JO *et al.* Is there an increased risk of breast cancer in women who have had a breast cyst aspirated? *British Journal of Cancer* 1991; **64**: 953–955.

19. Mannello F, Sebastiani M, Amati S *et al.* Conjugated bile acids in breast cyst fluid. Relationship to cation-related cyst sub-populations. *Cancer Letters* 1997; **119**: 21–26.

20. Mannello F, Bocchiotti G, Bianchi G *et al.* Quantification of prostate-specific antigen immunoreactivity in human breast cyst fluids. *Breast Cancer Research and Treatment* 1996; **38**: 247–252.

21. Dixon JM, Telford J, Elton RA *et al.* Uptake of dihydroepiandrosterone sulphate into human breast cyst fluid. *The Breast* 1997; **6**: 12–16.

22. Dixon JM, Telford J & Miller WR. Effects of spironolactone, danazol and efamast on the uptake of tritiated dihydroepiandrosterone sulphate into human breast cyst fluid. In: Mansel RE (ed.). *Recent Developments in the Study of Benign Breast Disease.* Carnforth: Parthenon; 1993: 265–270.

23. Lail C, Siraj AK, Erbas H *et al.* Relationship between basic fibroblast growth factor and transforming growth factor beta-2 in breast cyst fluid. *Journal of Clinical Endocrinology and Metabolism* 1995; **80**: 711–715.

24. Dixon JM, Scott WN & Miller WR. An analysis of the content and morphology of human breast microcysts. *European Journal of Surgical Oncology* 1985; **11**: 151–154.

25. Wellings SR & Alpers CE. Apocrine cyst metaplasia: subgross pathology and prevalence in cancer-associated versus random autopsy breasts. *Human Pathology* 1987; **18**: 381–386.

26. Molina R, Fillella X & Herranz M. Biochemistry of cyst fluid in fibrocystic disease of the breast. *Annals of the New York Academy of Sciences* 1990; **586**: 29–42.

27. Bundred NJ, Scott WN, Davies SJ *et al.* Zinc alpha-2 glycoprotein levels in serum and breast fluids: a potential marker of apocrine activity. *European Journal of Cancer* 1991; **27**: 349–352.

28. England PC, Skinner LG, Cottrell KM *et al.* Sex hormones in breast disease. *British Journal of Surgery* 1975; **62**: 806–809.

29. Gately CA, Maddox PR, Jones DL *et al.* Biologically active prolactin in patients with macroscopic breast cysts. *British Journal of Surgery* 1992; **79**: 1238.

30. Yenen MC, Dede M, Goktolga U *et al.* Hormone replacement therapy in postmenopausal women with benign fibrocystic mastopathy. *Climacteric* 2003; **6**: 146–150.

31. Ozdemir A, Konus O, Nas T *et al.* Mammographic and ultrasonographic study of changes in the breast related to HRT. *International Journal of Gynaecology and Obstetrics* 1999; **67**: 23–32.

32. Simpson JF & Page DL. Loss of expression of fodrin (a structural protein) in cystic changes in the human breast. *Laboratory Investigation* 1993; **68**: 537–540.

33. Devitt JE. Benign disorders of the breast in older women. *Surgery, Gynecology and Obstetrics* 1986; **162**: 340–342.

34. Brenner RJ, Bein ME, Sarti DA *et al.* Spontaneous regression of interval benign cysts of the breast. *Radiology* 1994; **193**: 365–368.

35. Jones BM & Bradbeer JW. The presentation and progress of macroscopic breast cysts. *British Journal of Surgery* 1980; **67**: 669–671.

36. Sterns EE. The natural history of macroscopic cysts in the breast. *Surgical Gynecology and Obstetrics* 1992; **174**: 36–40.

37. Wang DY, Hamed H & Fentiman I. Epidermal growth factor and insulin growth factor 1 in human breast cyst fluid. *Annals of the New York Academy of Sciences* 1990; **586**: 158–160.

38. Patey DH & Nurick AW. Natural history of cystic disease of the breast treated conservatively. *British Medical Journal* 1953; **I**: 15–17.

39. Forrest APM, Kirkpatrick JR & Roberts MM. Needle aspiration of breast cysts. *British Medical Journal* 1975; **3**: 30–31.

40. Cowen PN & Benson EA. Cytological study of fluid from benign breast cysts. *British Journal of Surgery* 1979; **66**: 209–211.

41. Gizienski TA, Harvey JA, Sobel AH. Breast cyst recurrence after postaspiration injection of air. *Breast Journal* 2002; **8**: 34–37.

42. Gomes C, Amaral N, Marques C *et al.* Sclerosis of gross cysts of the breast: a three-year study. *European Journal of Gynaecology and Oncology* 2002; **23**: 191–194.

43. Locker AP, Hinton CP, Roebuck EJ *et al.* A long term follow up of patients treated with a single course of Danazol for recurrent breast cysts. *British Journal of Clinical Practice* 1989; **43**: 100–101.

44. Mansel RE, Harrison BJ, Melhuish J *et al.* A randomized trial of dietary intervention with fatty acids in patients with categorized cysts. *Annals of the New York Academy of Sciences* 1990; **586**: 288–294.

45. Chun J, Joseph KA, El-Tamer M *et al.* Cohort study of women at risk for breast cancer and gross cystic disease. *American Journal of Surgery* 2005; **190**: 583–587.

46. Dixon JM, McDonald C, Elton RA *et al.* Breast cancer risk with cyst type in cystic disease of the breast. Larger study found no association between cyst type and breast cancer [letter]. *British Medical Journal* 1997; **315**: 545–546.

47. Haagensen DE, Kelly D & Bodian CA. GCDFP-15 blood levels for stratification of risk of breast cancer development in women with active gross cystic disease. *Breast* 1997; **6**: 113–119.

48. Fitzwilliams DCL. *On the Breast*. London: William Heinemann; 1924:173.

49. Stevens K, Burrell HC, Evans AJ *et al.* The ultrasound appearance of galactoceles. *British Journal of Radiology* 1997; **70**: 239–241.

50. Gomez A, Mata JM, Donozo C *et al.* Galactocele: 3 distinctive radiological patterns. *Radiology* 1986; **158**: 43–44.

51. Auvichayapat P, Auvichayapat N, Tong-un T *et al.* A controlled trial of a new treatment for galactocele. *Journal of the Medical Association of Thailand* 2003; **86**: 257–261.

52. Hart D. Intracystic papillomas of the breast – benign and malignant. *Archives of Surgery* 1927; **14**: 793–835.

53. Devitt JE. The clinical recognition of cystic carcinoma of the breast. *Surgery, Gynecology and Obstetrics* 1984; **159**: 130–132.

54. Calvert RJ, Kashi SH & Quinn CM. Giant intra-duct papilloma of the breast. *The Breast* 1994; **3**: 193–194.

55. Gatcher FG, Dockerty MB & Clagett OT. Intracystic carcinoma of the breast. *Surgery, Gynecology and Obstetrics* 1958; **106**: 347–352.

56. McKittrick JE, Doane WA & Failing KM. Intracystic papillary carcinoma of the breast. *American Surgeon* 1969; **35**: 195–202.

57. Carter D, Orr SL & Merino MJ. Intracystic papillary carcinoma of the breast. *Cancer* 1983; **52**: 14–24.

58. Estabrook A, Asch T, Gump F *et al.* Mammographic features of intracystic papillary lesions. *Surgery, Gynecology and Obstetrics* 1990; **170**: 113–116.

59. Omori LM, Hisa N, Ohkuma K *et al.* Breast masses with mixed cystic-solid sonographic appearances. *Journal of Clinical Ultrasound* 1993; **21**: 489–495.

60. Yamamoto D, Ueda S, Senzaki H *et al.* New diagnostic approach to intracystic lesions of the breast by fiberoptic ductoscopy. *Anticancer Research* 2001; **21**: 4113–4116.

CHAPTER 11

The duct ectasia/periductal mastitis complex

Key points and new developments

1. The duct ectasia/periductal mastitis (DE/PDM) complex covers a number of processes which may exist alone or in combination. Some are subclinical and minor variants of normality (ANDI) while the spectrum extends to disease with severe morbidity.

2. Much confusion has arisen through failure to differentiate between histological findings (not clinically overt) and the very overt syndromes of the clinical disease entities.

3. The processes include duct dilatation (ectasia), histological PDM, bacterial mastitis and periductal fibrosis. Associated conditions are nipple inversion and squamous metaplasia of the ducts.

4. Clinical manifestations include nipple discharge (bloody and non-bloody), inflammation, abscess, fistula, mastalgia and nipple retraction. Bilateral involvement is not uncommon.

5. Secondary bacterial invasion shows mixed flora (aerobes and anaerobes) typical of (and probably coming from) those in the mouth and vagina.

6. Cigarette smoking is a powerful facilitator of severe inflammatory complications.

7. Established infections are rarely cured without surgery to the underlying duct abnormality, directed towards a single duct or to multiple ducts, depending on the individual findings.

8. Recurrence is not uncommon, often due to inappropriate or inadequate surgery. Management of recurrence requires a planned sequential approach to find and deal with the persisting pathology.

9. Granulomatous mastitis shows a close resemblance to peripheral perilobular mastitis, and at least some cases are best managed by surgery directed to proximal ectatic ducts.

Introduction

The terms 'duct ectasia' and 'periductal mastitis' cover the second major group of benign breast disorders. Mild duct ectasia is part of the normal involution of the breast and as such forms part of ANDI (aberrations of normal development and involution). The term 'mammary duct ectasia' introduced by Haagensen in 1951[1] is useful in that it has a single simple connotation – the presence of dilated mammary ducts – using terminology consistent with that of bronchiectasis and sialectasis. To this has been added periductal mastitis to describe the frequent occurrence of periductal inflammation in association with duct ectasia. This term has advantages over others used such as plasma cell mastitis or comedo mastitis because these specific elements are not present in all cases. Hence, the condition is best known as the duct ectasia/periductal mastitis complex even though this by no means covers all the pathological or clinical aspects of the disease. Understanding of disease has been held back by attempts to confine the clinical manifestations within the straight-jacket of a single all-embracing disease process or, alternatively, attempts to remove the straight-jacket completely and regard the condition as one aspect of 'fibrocystic disease'. Both approaches are incompatible with the breadth of clinical manifestations or the observed pathology.

While the exact aetiology is still uncertain, recent work has demonstrated that a number of pathological processes contribute to the clinical manifestations, including duct dilatation, stagnant secretions, duct obstruction by nipple inversion or epithelial squames, epithelial metaplasia, nonbacterial inflammation, bacterial inflammation and periductal sclerosis. These diverse processes, individual but interrelated, explain the protean clinical presentations. Evolution of thought and practice continues, and quite recent demonstration of anaerobic bacteria in many cases is having a major impact on understanding and management, as is the recognition that infective complications are much more common and severe in cigarette smokers. This disease complex presents clinically in many ways, at times giving rise to all three common breast symptoms: lump, nipple discharge and pain. The main manifestations are set out in Table 11.1 and any concept of the disease complex must be able to encompass this wide range of clinical presentations.

There are a number of other chronic inflammatory conditions, such as lymphocytic mastopathy and granulomatous mastitis, which may be unrelated, but which also may overlap with periductal mastitis. These are further discussed in Chapter 17. In view of the confusion in nomenclature and understanding, it is useful and salutary to look at it from a historical point of view.

Historical survey

This condition has been recognized and well described in the surgical literature over many decades, yet remained unrecognized in clinical practice to a surprising degree. It was recorded by many early writers but they were unable, on the whole, to conceive it as a distinct process, confusing it with tuberculosis, galactocele, cystic disease and fat necrosis. Even today, many endocrinology texts confuse the nipple discharge of duct ectasia with galactorrhoea.

John Birkett, surgeon to Guy's Hospital and President of the Royal College of Surgeons of England in 1877, gave a description of the condition in his book on breast disease:[2] 'In the breast of a middle-aged woman it is not uncommon to find the ducts dilated and filled with mucous greenish fluid.' Bloodgood described several cases in 1921[3] in a paper dealing primarily with chronic cystic disease. He returned to the subject in 1923, presenting 31 cases. His description of an advanced case could hardly be bettered:[4] 'The characteristic picture when the dilated ducts are situated in the nipple zone is the palpation of a doughy, worm-like mass beneath the nipple. When explored, one can recognize large and small dilated ducts with distinct wall, containing brown, green, milky or cream-like material, of various degrees of viscosity and consistency.' He went on to describe nipple discharge, palpable tumours, some with skin and nipple fixity resembling malignancy, others resembling subareolar abscesses and peripheral breast masses. He even described a case of eczema of the areola apparently due to nipple discharge.

Bloodgood made no contribution to aetiology and stated that the condition could be classed as part of chronic cystic mastitis, an area of confusion which persists in some present-day literature. He noted that patients with dilated ducts were often postmenopausal and that the condition seemed to have no relation to parity or breastfeeding. He recognized that the condition could present as nipple discharge or a mass which could be evanescent, but that it could also simulate cancer exactly, that it often settled spontaneously and that it had a tendency to be bilateral.

According to Cutler,[5] it was James Ewing, of the Memorial Hospital in New York, who drew attention to 'plasma cell mastitis' in the 1920s. It is not surprising that a

Table 11.1 The clinical spectrum of duct ectasia/periductal mastitis

Underlying pathology	Clinical manifestations
Duct ectasia	Nipple discharge – thick, creamy, bloody
Periductal mastitis	
Single duct	Recurrent subareolar abscess Mammary duct fistula
Multiple ducts	Inflammation and/or abscess formation – evanescent – recurrent – chronic Duct fistula Mastalgia
Periductal fibrosis	
Inflammatory	Nipple retraction
Involutional	Nipple retraction
Secondary to nipple discharge	Eczema of the nipple/areola

All the above manifestations may rarely occur in the male.

pathologist should so do, for radical mastectomy was not infrequently carried out mistakenly for a chronic inflammatory mass simulating cancer. He used this term because he was impressed with the number of plasma cells infiltrating these lesions. Cheatle and Cutler[6] recorded it in the literature survey in their book on breast tumours. Adair[7] reported 10 cases from the records of the Memorial Hospital, highlighting the clinical problem of inappropriate mastectomy. Further reports added the names comedo mastitis and mastitis obliterans. Each name stressed one particular aspect of the condition, but the different terminology did little to develop a unifying concept of the condition.

The subject was reviewed from the Mayo Clinic in 1948.[8] This paper gave a good review of the literature and reflected the usual attitude at that time: of 172 cases, the great majority had been identified from a retrospective study of pathology specimens usually found as a chance finding in mastectomy specimens for cancer. Only 19 of this series had undergone treatment for clinical manifestations of the condition. The consequences of failure to appreciate the pathology in the past is vividly illustrated in Sandison and Walker's paper from Glasgow.[9] Of 38 juxta-areolar inflammatory lesions studied, eight were incorrectly considered to be neoplastic and seven to be tuberculous, with nine inappropriate mastectomies. In this series, 12 had shown periductal mastitis (PDM) without duct ectasia (DE), 12 had shown DE with PDM, and 14 cases had shown ectopic squamous epithelium. These figures may reflect the relative frequency of the different pathologies underlying periareolar infection.

The increasing recognition of the clinical manifestations was not matched by understanding of pathogenesis, or even of pathology. Rodman and Ingleby[10] tried to produce it experimentally, claiming that a similar condition was produced by injection of pancreatized milk into the mammary duct of rabbits.

Three important papers appeared in 1951, which was a vintage year for this condition. Frantz and colleagues[11] reported an autopsy study of apparently normal breasts, and found an incidence of substantial DE of 25% and almost 50% in women over the age of 60. It was clear that the condition of DE was common, a disease of ageing, and often subclinical.

Zuska et al.[12] described the condition now known as recurrent subareolar abscess or mammary duct fistula, recognizing its pathological basis for the first time, and reporting successful management by simple excision or laying open of the fistula. Earlier, Deaver and McFarland[13] had noted that persistent sinuses were sometimes seen after drainage of nonlactational abscesses, but they could only advise wide drainage, antiseptics and simple mastectomy for resistant cases. Even earlier cases of fistula have been reported in France and England in 1835 and 1892.[14,15] Zuska and co-workers considered the condition to be a complication of DE ('comedo mastitis') because they saw dilated ducts containing the typical material seen in DE, which in its thicker form resembles a comedo. They also noted that it occurred in younger women, could be bilateral and was associated with squamous cell lining of the affected duct.

Haagensen[1] completed the 1951 trio by publishing his first paper on the subject, and suggested the term 'mammary duct ectasia'. His views are expanded in his textbook.[16] It is surprising that the youngest patient he had seen with the disease was 34 years old, and the mean age of the group was 55. He saw only 67 patients with clinical disease in 30 years' practice, reflecting either the specialized nature of his practice with a bias towards cancer, or suggesting that the disease is becoming more common, because we operated on some 200 cases in 15 years.

Haagensen supported the classic view that duct dilatation was the primary abnormality, leading to stagnation of secretion and nipple discharge, with leakage of material outside the duct leading to a chemical PDM. He regarded it as a rather benign condition and did not discuss severe abscesses, or recurrent inflammation or fistula after surgical excision. He also regarded recurrent subareolar abscess as a separate condition of trivial importance and criticized Zuska et al. for 'confusing it with duct ectasia'.

Atkins[17] drew the attention of British surgeons to recurrent subareolar abscess with a report of 28 cases. He introduced the unfortunate term 'mammillary fistula', suggesting a fistula into the nipple, which soon became corrupted to mammillary duct fistula. The term seems inappropriate because the external opening of the fistula is along the edge of the areola (or more peripheral) and the internal opening is into a duct under the areola rather than within the nipple. It is a term better dropped in favour of the simpler and more accurate term 'mammary duct fistula'. Atkins saw the condition in simple mechanistic terms as an obstruction to the exit of the duct, with build-up of secretions leading to infection which burst out through the skin. Again, he reported it in younger patients, often with inverted nipples, and sometimes beginning during pregnancy and lactation. He recommended a simple laying open technique, allowing the wound to heal by granulation. He noted no recurrence but gave no details of follow-up.

Three years later, Patey and Thackray[18] reported a detailed histological study of the ducts excised from seven specimens. They found the terminal portion of the involved duct lined by squamous epithelium instead of the normal columnar epithelium and believed this replacement to be congenital rather than acquired, partly because one case also showed multiple sebaceous glands opening into the track.

Hadfield[19] introduced the operation of major duct excision for a number of benign breast conditions, including DE. He paid tribute to having learned the operation from Adair and Urban at the Memorial Hospital of New York, and 3 years later Urban[20] reported his own technique and results, again giving precedence to Adair. The operation slowly became the standard management for all the syndromes of DE/PDM except localized mammary duct fistula.

Two papers from Sandison and Walker in Glasgow in 1962 and 1964[9,21] did much to increase the knowledge of chronic inflammatory conditions of the breast. They helped to fit PDM into an overall picture of breast disease and also suggested that recurrent subareolar abscess might have more than one aetiology. It is well worthwhile studying their papers in detail for their description of the disease complex. However, they do not appear to have used duct excision, preferring wide en bloc excision of diseased tissue. They infer that the results were satisfactory but give no details of follow-up.

Ewing[22] reviewed the syndrome and the relevant literature to move full circle away from Haagensen, suggesting that mammary duct fistula is not a separate entity, but just a manifestation of DE. Habif and his colleagues[23] came down strongly in favour of the other view, reporting 146 cases of mammary duct fistula without seeing a single case with dilated ducts. They were all associated with squamous metaplasia of the terminal duct, and it is clear that these authors fell into the classic error of expecting all manifestations to be based on a single pathological process.

Davies[24] carried out elegant studies of the role of inflammatory cells in the genesis of periductal disease and provided new insights into the frequency of subclinical periductal inflammation, and the possible role this might play in normal duct involution, as well as the clinical manifestations of this condition.

The last 25 years have seen two new developments with an impact on management: the recognition of the importance of cigarette smoking in inflammatory complications, and recognition of the importance of anaerobic bacteria (particularly those normally found in the mouth and vagina). Both of these are leading to the possibility of control by more conservative measures than have been necessary in the past.

Most of the advances in past years have come from detailed correlations of clinicopathological findings with outcome in individual cases, in studies that have emphasized the diversity of the clinical and pathological spectra of these conditions. More recent studies utilize computer analysis of large databases of retrospective case material, with a resulting simplification of concept and management that does not sit comfortably with clinical experience. It remains important to respect the diversity seen in clinical practice, so that individual patients are assessed and managed on an individual basis.

Pathology and pathogenesis of duct ectasia/periductal mastitis

This condition exhibits a paradox. The pathology of the disease at a point in time – surgical biopsy or autopsy – is well established and well described, yet there is almost total ignorance of the sequence of events leading to or from that point in time. It is useful to summarize the position as understood at present and important to recognize that no single pathological process can explain, or should be asked to explain, the whole clinical spectrum. As with other benign breast disorders, it must be considered in relation to interaction of a number of aberrations of normal processes with added complications, sometimes pushing it from the area of disorder to disease (see Ch. 4). There are a number of pathological processes that require consideration, all closely interrelated: DE with stagnation of secretion, and periductal inflammation which may be histological or clinically overt and in the latter case may be sterile or bacterial. Squamous metaplasia of the terminal duct epithelium may be an aetiological factor in some cases, and periductal fibrosis a common outcome.

Stagnation of duct contents, obstructive or passive, is the common factor in all cases, while the tough structure of the nipple/areolar complex obstructs the direct drainage which allows abscesses elsewhere in the body to cure themselves.

Ectatic ducts: pathology

The dilatation seen in ectatic ducts may be considerable, varying from just above normal diameter (about 0.5–1 mm) up to 5 mm or more. Typically three or four of the ducts are ectatic. It is unusual for more than a few of the ducts to be involved and it is not clear why only some are dilated. Similarly, dilatation is often confined to the 2–3 cm closest to the nipple, although it may extend further into the breast; occasionally the dilated ducts extend right to the periphery. Not surprisingly, the older the patient the greater the number of ducts affected, and the further ectatic ducts are likely to extend into the breast. Sometimes the wall of the dilated duct is thin and uninflamed; much more commonly the wall is thickened with fibrosis and disruption of the elastic lamina.

Although ectatic ducts may look like cysts on section, the ducts are more uniformly dilated than cystic. It is now realized that the two conditions are quite separate, though they frequently coexist. Cystic disease is a condition of lobules, DE of the ductal system.[25] The secretion in the ducts may be amorphous, representing cellular debris and fatty acid crystals, or cellular, packed with colostrum cells and inflammatory cells. These colostrum cells are thought by many to be macrophages and by others to be myoepithelial cells. Changes in the epithelial cells lining the ducts tend to be non-specific; sometimes they are hyperplastic in the early stages, later flattened and atrophic or shed completely. Our studies of the duct epithelial cell surface by scanning electron microscopy showed a normal microvillous surface in most cases.

Ectatic ducts: pathogenesis

A number of possible mechanisms for the development of ectatic ducts have been suggested.

Hormonal effect

Endocrine-induced relaxation of contractile, myoepithelial elements of the duct wall, similar to relaxation of the ureter in pregnancy, has been suggested to be implicated in the development of ectatic ducts and, in the past, pregnancy and breastfeeding have frequently been considered as important in the aetiology of DE. However, the evidence of this is poor and Dixon et al.[26] found no relation between parity or breastfeeding and DE.

Obstruction

A second theory incriminates duct obstruction by epithelial squames. Patey and Thackray[18] investigated seven cases of duct fistula and found the terminal portion of the duct to be blocked by squamous epithelium. They concluded that obstruction of the terminal duct due to desquamation of squamous cells was the cause and that the squamous lining was probably a congenital abnormality.

Other authors have not confirmed this finding, and cases are commonly seen where secretion can readily be expressed through the terminal duct with no obstruction to the passage of a probe, although this does not exclude stagnation due to desquamated cells. The common association of subareolar abscess with congenital inversion of the nipple in young girls suggests that the inversion contributes to stagnation. It is not clear whether this is due to mechanical blockage or a greater frequency of squamous metaplasia.

Tedeschi et al.[27] produced experimental evidence which combines obstruction and hormonal effects but suggested that hormonal effects were more important than obstruction in the pathogenesis. They found that ligation of the mammary ducts in rabbits produced no DE, whereas administration of hormones (oestrogen, progesterone or gonadotrophin) produced DE equally alone, or combined with duct ligation. No rabbits developed PDM.

Secondary to inflammation

A third theory is that dilatation results from destruction of the duct wall elastica and myoepithelial cells by inflammation. Two suggested causes of the inflammation are autoimmunity and bacterial infection. Davies induced an autoimmune model in mice[28] and he has also described widespread periductal inflammation with muscle disruption in the normal breast, although often associated with duct obliteration.[29] An interesting insight into a possible mechanism for involutional duct ectasia is provided by the studies of Hanayama and Nagata.[30] Mice deficient in lactadherin (in humans encoded for at 15q 25) failed to undergo normal postpartum involution. Such mice failed to remove aptototic cells, retained large quantities of milk fat globulin in the breast ducts accompanied by a sterile periductal mastitis. Although their studies were in mice it is not difficult to see how this might be relevant to the development of duct ectasia in postmenopausal involution. Studies of the role of lactadherin in patents with duct ectasia and periductal mastitis are awaited. Whatever the exact pathogenesis at the cellular level, this would appear to be part of the normal ageing or involutional process. More overt inflammation is discussed below.

Lymphatic blockage

Yet another theory incriminates failure of absorption of duct secretions due to inadequate lymphatic flow.

The bulk of evidence supports squamous metaplasia/nipple inversion as the cause of mammary duct fistula in the young, while DE in older life seems to be an aberration of the processes of normal duct involution.

Squamous metaplasia and nipple inversion

Squamous metaplasia requires more detailed consideration, especially in relation to mammary duct fistula. Normal squamous epithelium extends into a nipple duct no further than 2 mm from the surface with a sharp linear junction between squamous and columnar epithelium.[31] Patey and Thackray[18] describe this squamous epithelium extending down the duct in surgical specimens for a variable distance into the dilated portion of the duct; they found no significant squamous down-growth in the fistula itself. Finding fully developed sebaceous glands in the area in two cases led them to come down on the side of congenital aetiology and their arguments are convincing for at least some cases. They found the affected duct lined by squamous epithelium throughout the whole length of the duct from the nipple to the point of junction with the fistula in five of seven cases, and the other two were lined by granulation tissue. The squamous epithelium even extended into some secondary branches of the affected duct. It is of interest that only one duct was involved. This might seem to argue against a congenital aetiology, but would explain the usual success of an operation directed towards a single duct.

Another paper which discusses the problem of squamous metaplasia is that of Habif et al.[23] and this paper is worth studying in detail for its pathological material. In contrast to Patey and Thackray, they show cases where more than one duct is lined by squamous epithelium.

Toker[31] argued that the metaplasia was an acquired condition (although from study of only one case) and likened it to the squamous replacement of columnar epithelium seen in the uterine cervix and other body areas.

Nipple inversion

A number of workers have noted that nipple inversion is commonly associated with both DE/PDM and mammary duct fistula. Likewise, PDM is often associated with, or followed by, the development of retracted nipple. Our experience leaves no doubt that both relationships exist. There is a high incidence of congenital nipple inversion in young girls with recurrent subareolar abscess and we have frequently documented the progressive retraction of a previously normal nipple during the evolution of severe PDM.

This association is confirmed from the observations of Schaffer et al.[32] who noted nipple retraction in 8% with a first abscess, 22% with recurrent abscesses, and 47% with a fistula. Some of this may be due to more severe cases occurring in patients with nipple inversion, but it also supports the progressive nature of nipple retraction in many cases.

Mammary duct fistula

This condition, described by Zuska et al.,[12] is seen in typical form when a young woman develops an abscess under the edge of the areola of one breast. Simple drainage of the abscess results in persisting discharge, or recurrent abscesses presenting at the same point. The condition has been likened to a perianal fistula with a sinus lined by granulation tissue leading down to a dilated sumplike duct (Fig. 11.1).

It seems likely that the discrepancies are best explained by at least two separate pathologies: a congenital lining of squamous epithelium in the terminal duct and stagna-

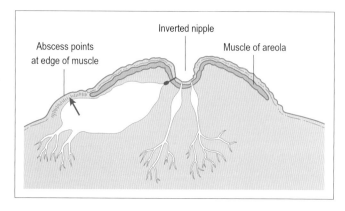

Fig. 11.1 Basic concept of mammary duct fistula. Squamous debris blocks the duct leading to dilatation of the subareolar portion. Because of the tough muscle of the areola skin, an abscess will tend to burst through the skin at the edge of the areola.

tion of duct contents due to DE. The first is commonest in young women, and is frequently accompanied by congenital nipple inversion. The pathology was well described by Patey and Thackray.[18] The second is seen in older patients, without nipple inversion. While some patients have a fistula always discharging from the same duct, others will have external openings communicating with different ducts. In this group, nipple retraction usually follows the inflammatory process. It is important that this dual pathology is recognized, because treatment of multiple duct disease by operation directed towards one duct will lead to recurrence, while failure to recognize the solitary congenital duct abnormality will lead to unnecessarily radical surgery.

Periductal inflammation: pathology

Histological periductal mastitis

Histological changes of periductal inflammation with periductal histiocytes and inflammatory cells are usually present with dilated ducts but may be seen whether the ducts are dilated or not. There is sometimes a granulomatous reaction, and often a lipophagic reaction with a picture similar to fat necrosis. Plasma cells may or may not be prominent among the infiltrate.

Davies[29] has stressed the relationship of cellular infiltration with focal ulceration, disruption of elastic tissue and subsequent fibrosis. In the presence of clinical PDM, these changes spread into the surrounding breast tissue to form an inflammatory mass.

Davies[24] has made a detailed study of periductal inflammation in both ectatic and nonectatic ducts. In the latter group, the paradoxical aspect of this condition can be seen in the presence of narrow sclerosing ducts, which led to the old term 'mastitis obliterans' or 'mazoplasia obliterans'. He has demonstrated a striking periductal infiltration by four cell types, apparently of macrophage origin, which can lead to total obliteration of the duct. Their presence is associated with marked damage to the duct wall and epithelial lining. The lumen may be filled with the colostrum cells typical of DE, but the eventual outcome is fibrosis and obliteration of the ducts. The study shows a predominance of fibrous obliteration occurring in young women, although the study was biased towards this group because it derived from biopsy material for benign breast disorders. It was present in a wide variety of benign breast conditions, including those with no clinical evidence of PDM.

It is not clear what relation this intense periductal inflammation and duct wall damage has to the ectatic form of duct disease, but both duct obliteration and duct dilatation could be seen to result in different areas of the same breast. This process probably explains the shortening of ducts leading to nipple retraction; it may be part of normal ductal involution or an aberration of that process. Hence, histological PDM can be seen as a normal process, which may contribute to DE, to duct obliteration or to duct shortening, and also as a possible precursor of clinical PDM.

The histological picture of PDM shows a further spectrum of changes from the 'normal' juxtaductal infiltration of macrophage-derived cells, through a more extensive spread of inflammation characterized by plasma cells or lymphocytes. The final stage is frank abscess formation when more acute inflammatory cells are obvious, often along with lipid-laden foreign body giant cells and granulomas. These latter changes were responsible for confusion with tuberculosis in earlier literature.

A histological grading system (grades 1–3) for severity of each of the two main pathological processes – dilated ducts and periductal inflammation – has been put forward,[26] although, confusingly, grade 1 is most severe for periductal inflammation but least severe for DE.

Clinical periductal mastitis

Abscesses from PDM are usually subareolar or juxtaareolar. They are typically single, small (1–2 cm), well localized and unilocular. (In contrast, puerperal abscesses are commonly large, poorly localized and multilocular.) In the rare case of peripheral abscess (usually multiple) associated with PDM, the ducts are macroscopically dilated to the site of the abscess. Abscesses may be sterile, or associated with a wide range of bacteria; the latter is more likely as the process increases in severity or recurrence.

In younger women, PDM is often associated with congenital inverted nipple without evidence of gross DE; in the latter half of reproductive life, it is more likely to be associated with multiple ectatic ducts. These should be differentiated from the peripheral staphylococcal abscesses sometimes seen in postmenopausal women, without anaerobes. It is not clear whether these are associated with PDM or represent a random infection. The ducts are not grossly dilated, and the abscess can be expected to resolve with drainage and antibiotics, without duct surgery. This is discussed in Chapter 14.

Bacteriology

Until recently there has been remarkably little work done on the bacteriology of PDM and it is still a matter of some controversy. For many years it was believed that most cases were sterile early in the disease and that the inflammation was due to chemically irritant fatty acids leaking into the periductal tissue. The histological picture, similar to fat necrosis, supported this.

In recurrent cases a variety of bacteria have been found. Anaerobes, *Staphylococcus aureus, Proteus* sp. and streptococci have been reported. Many are undoubtedly secondary invaders. With the advent of techniques for reliable demonstration of anaerobic organisms, it became clear that these bacteria were sometimes present in earlier cases. Beigelman and Rantz[33] reported growth of *Bacteroides* sp. and anaerobic streptococci from a breast abscess as early as 1949.

More recently, several detailed studies of the microbiology have been reported.

Walker et al.[34] have carried out a prospective study in 29 patients aged 20–85 and report the detailed culture results. A total of 108 strains were recovered, anaerobes outnumbered aerobes by 2 to 1. Only two abscesses were sterile; both had had antibiotics. The commonest anaerobes were peptostreptococci (47%). These and the other anaerobes found are normally inhabitants of the vagina or oropharynx; gut anaerobes are rarely present. Many of their patients reported oro-nipple contact. Anaerobic cocci usually occur together with other anaerobes and facultative microorganisms in a mixed flora. The synergistic pathogenicity of anaerobic cocci in mixed infections is well documented. The commonest aerobe (60%) was *Staph. epidermidis*; *Staph. aureus* was found in only 8%. *Staph. epidermidis* adheres to the squames of the skin and nipple, so it is not surprising that it finds its way into these abscesses.

Interesting work has been conducted on enzyme production by peptostreptococci.[35] *Peptostreptococcus magnus* is an opportunist organism often found in abdominal infections (where it does not seem to cause serious problems), non-puerperal breast abscesses and diabetic foot infections. *P. magnus* obtained from abdominal infections is relatively inactive enzymatically, whereas the strains grown from non-puerperal abscess and foot infections are much more active, particularly in producing collagenase and gelatinase. This may explain the burrowing activity seen in these infections.

Leach and co-workers have reported anaerobic subareolar abscesses after vaginal manipulation,[36] suggesting

bloodstream spread of bacteria to settle in the stagnant duct secretions. The same organisms found in an acute subareolar abscess have been cultured from a high vaginal swab, in this case bacteraemia from sexual activity and direct oral transfer of vaginal organisms to the nipple were possible modes of transmission.[37]

Bundred and colleagues[38] studied the bacteriology of spontaneous discharge from 51 patients and of pus from 17 patients with abscess or fistula. Bacteria were isolated from 62% of patients with discharge due to DE and only 5% from those with discharge due to other causes. (The separation of patients into 'duct ectasia' and 'other causes' was made rather arbitrarily on 'clinical and radiological' grounds.) All the patients with abscesses or fistulas grew bacteria. The bacteria included enterococci, anaerobic streptococci, *Bacteroides* sp. and *Staph. aureus*.

There is clearly room for further investigation into whether all clinical PDM is bacterial since there are still some discrepancies.

The clinical, painful masses of evanescent PDM resolve without treatment and with surprising rapidity for a bacterial infection. This sequence would be far more compatible with a chemical reaction to leaking duct contents as suggested by Haagensen, as is the histological picture, which is so similar to fat necrosis.

Dixon has argued strongly that bacterial infection is primary in all cases, and DE secondary or unrelated, even though evidence from that unit is conflicting.[39] He bases his view on histological studies,[26] on the fact that they were able to grow pathogens from nipple discharge in 62% of patients with DE,[38] and on an increased incidence of wound infection in patients with DE/PDM (10%) compared with 2% with other breast conditions.

There seems to be a discrepancy between 10% wound infections and 62% growing pathogens. Furthermore, another worker in the same unit using the same bacteriological methods grew a pathogen (*Staph. aureus*) from retroareolar biopsy material from only one of 11 patients with overt and histological DE/PDM, and no biopsy grew the typical mixed aerobic and anaerobic organisms.[40] This latter study is much more in keeping with our own experience, in which careful examination with immediate bacteriological culture for aerobic and anaerobic organisms has failed to demonstrate bacteria in a significant proportion of our cases with overt inflammatory masses on initial presentation, and many such cases fail to respond to appropriate antibiotics. In contrast, we find it usual to grow bacteria in recurrent inflammatory lesions.

It is also important to distinguish between PDM diagnosed on histology, and the gross inflammatory complications seen clinically. Dixon reported 108 patients with a histological diagnosis of DE/PDM.[26] He found histological PDM to occur at a younger mean age than DE (although the difference in mean ages was small). From this he has argued that PDM is the primary cause of DE.[39] This study confirms the earlier work of Davies[24,29] that periductal inflammation is common in unselected breast biopsies, and the many earlier studies that have shown that DE is a common involutional occurrence. It is misleading to suggest that either finding is relevant to the severe inflammatory complications encountered in clinical practice.

Operative findings have been recorded prospectively in all cases in the author's series of primary and recurrent PDM. The patterns are quite clear, and fall into two main groups, although with some overlap. In young women, typically 20–30 years old, the pathology is restricted to a single sumplike duct, associated with congenital nipple inversion or squamous metaplasia. In older women, typically 40–50 years, there are obviously dilated ducts, usually three or four, sometimes many more. The degree of DE, and the recent onset of the active inflammation, leaves little doubt that the ectatic duct precedes the onset of inflammation.

Not all cases conform to these patterns; we have seen multiple grossly ectatic ducts at 26 years, and multiple typical ectatic ducts as young as 20. Conversely, some older women have a single ectatic duct, and are cured by fistulectomy directed to that single duct.

It is possible that subclinical periductal inflammation leads to ectatic ducts, but there is no direct evidence. It is more likely that it leads to duct sclerosis, the outcome clearly demonstrated by Davies. So there is no reason based on evidence to abandon the classic view that stagnation of secretion, for differing reasons in the young and old, is the primary cause of clinical PDM.

Current evidence is that in some cases, particularly early inflammatory masses or the first abscess, the inflammation is nonbacterial whereas the incidence of bacterial involvement rises with repeated abscesses and drainage. It is likely that stagnation, from any of the causes above, favours leakage of duct contents into periductal tissue to give chemical inflammation, and also provides a focus for bacterial colonization. Equally, there is no doubt that bacteria play a major role in more overt cases, even from the outset of clinical presentation, as discussed in detail later in this chapter.

Periductal mastitis: pathogenesis

Is there a hormonal basis to periductal mastitis?

Unlike most breast conditions, hormonal abnormalities have not generally been associated with the DE complex, although DE itself is generally regarded as part of the perimenopausal involutional process. However, Peters and Schuth have been a strong advocate of hyperprolactinaemia as an important aetiological factor in PDM.[41] Their group measured serum prolactin levels in 108 patients before, during and after therapy for non-puerperal mastitis. One-quarter of the patients exhibited transient rises in serum prolactin during the period of inflammation, which returned to normal levels, 22 presented with higher levels of hyperprolactinaemia, and 15 were found to have pituitary microadenomas; in 11, the inflammatory episode was the first symptom. In a second study from this unit, 83 patients known to be hyperprolactinaemic were questioned about symptoms of PDM; one in five reported such symptoms, compared with none of the controls.

Thus, established hyperprolactinaemia appears to be a cause of PDM, while this can be a cause of transient hyperprolactinaemia. However, the situation is clouded by the very wide symptom complex that these workers include within the scope of PDM. Shousa et al.[42] also reported three postmenopausal patients with prolactinomas who had an unusually florid degree of DE.

It is surprising that so little interest has been shown in these findings; it would seem to be an area requiring further investigation.

Cigarette smoking

A recent development of considerable interest is the recognition that cigarette smoking is related to the more serious inflammatory complications of DE. The association was first noted in Switzerland[32] when a case-control study showed that 85% of patients with recurrent subareolar abscess were smokers compared to 37% of the controls, with relative risks of 9 for light smokers and 26 for heavy smokers. Only 10% had never smoked; most had smoked for many years, even a 15-year-old girl had smoked heavily for 3 years.

Bundred and co-workers have studied the clinical and pathological implications in greater detail.[43–45] Cigarette smoking is associated with the presence of histological evidence of PDM, development of non-puerperal breast abscess, recurrent abscess after treatment and development of mammary duct fistula. Heavy smokers are more likely to have anaerobic bacteria and severe inflammatory complications. Smokers also seem to have a greater chance of squamous metaplasia in the ducts.

Smoking was not associated with the degree of ductal dilatation or with recurrence after lactational abscess. About 30% of patients with histological PDM are not current smokers, so smoking is more related to clinical complications than the underlying process.

Although histological changes of PDM were associated with smoking in patients with this diagnosis, the same changes were not associated with smoking in patients presenting with a duct papilloma,[46] so smoking is only one element of a multifactorial pathogenesis.

The mechanism by which smoking causes these changes is not clear at present. A number of possibilities may be relevant. Toxic products have been demonstrated in ductal secretions of smokers. These may damage the duct epithelium, facilitating extravasation of secretions. Smoking also has an antioestrogenic effect, producing an early menopause, and inhibits Gram-positive bacteria in vivo and in vitro, which may facilitate overgrowth of anaerobic bacteria. The altered bacterial spectrum in the mouth of smokers may be relevant to the oro-nipple route of infection.

Of relevance to these theories is the fact that the relationship of smoking to severe inflammatory complications of PDM also holds for males. All five male patients with periareolar abscess or fistula seen in our clinic were heavy smokers.[47]

The development of the duct ectasia/periductal mastitis complex

The classic view (Fig. 11.2)

Each of the ducts opening on to the nipple normally has a diameter only of 1 mm or less and the subsegmental and terminal ducts become progressively narrower.

In the sequence proposed by Haagensen[1] and developed by Ewing (Table 11.2),[22] the first change to occur is DE, commonly restricted to the portion of the duct deep to the areola.

In a few cases dilatation extends peripherally to involve segmental and even subsegmental ducts. The dilated ducts fill with stagnant secretion, leading to nipple discharge. Persisting stagnation may lead to ulceration,

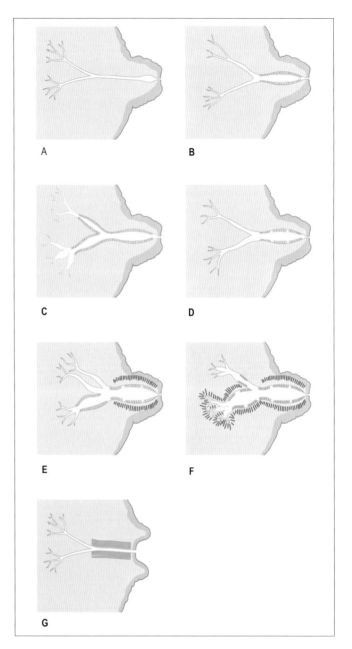

Fig. 11.2 Classic view of the pathogenesis of the clinical spectrum of duct ectasia. (See text for more recent alternative theories.) (**A**) A normal segmental duct, uniformly narrow except for the terminal sinus, and breaking up into subsegmental and finally terminal ducts. (**B**) The proximal subareolar part of the duct dilates with stagnation of secretion. Intact mucosal epithelium is seen lining the dilated ducts. (**C**) The dilatation may extend into the subsegmental ducts. (**D**) The stagnant secretions lead to patchy mucosal ulceration which may give bloody discharge. (**E**) The contents of the duct leak through the ulcerated areas, giving a chemical inflammatory response. (**F**) This may affect subsegmental ducts or even occur peripherally beyond the major duct system. (**G**) Inflammation leads to fibrosis of the duct wall, and as the fibrous tissue contracts, nipple retraction is produced.

Table 11.2 The classic view of the pathology of duct ectasia/periductal mastitis

Process	Clinical manifestations
Duct ectasia (?A hormonal effect)	Stagnation of secretions Nipple discharge
Epithelial ulceration	Bloody nipple discharge
Leakage of secretion into periductal tissue	Evanescent painful mass
Granulomatous reaction + secondary bacterial infection	Abscess/fistula
Periductal fibrosis	Nipple retraction

resulting in bloodstained nipple discharge and in leakage of stagnant secretions into the periductal tissue; the irritant fatty acids then induce an inflammatory response, which is chemical rather than bacterial. This is usually seen beneath the edge of the areola, but where dilatation extends into the subsegmental ducts, PDM may occur more peripherally, or even form a granulomatous mass more peripheral to the obviously dilated ducts. In severe cases the inflammation progresses to abscess formation. Simple drainage is unlikely to be curative and gives an increasing likelihood of secondary bacterial infection.

Some cases may develop a chronic indurated mass stopping short of abscess formation, and the clinical signs in this situation may simulate cancer exactly. The periductal inflammation leads to fibrosis, and subsequent contracture leads to nipple retraction.

The current view

Any mechanisms of pathogenesis must be compatible with the findings (1) that within one breast some ducts are normal and some dilated; (2) that most workers have been able to demonstrate bacterial infection in only a proportion of cases; and (3) that obstruction must be due mainly to stagnation rather than mechanical obstruction, since most patients show no obvious duct obstruction on radiology or at surgery. In addition, the primary symptom according to the classic view, nipple discharge, is seen mainly in older women, while the supposedly secondary symptom, mastitis and abscess formation, is seen at all ages, often in quite young women.

The frequent occurrence of bilateral involvement must be taken into consideration in any discussion of pathogenesis, and the frequency with which the disease starts in the second breast shortly after control of that in the first breast is a striking observation.

No single mechanism which meets these requirements has yet been put forward. A clinicopathological picture consistent with evidence and experience is best based on a number of processes, which may occur individually or in combination with others, and with differing emphases in the young, the mature and the elderly. These are:

- Stagnation of secretion due to squamous metaplasia, either congenital or acquired, seen particularly in young women, and often associated with congenital nipple inversion.
- Stagnation due to dilatation of the ducts, probably due to a hormone effect or damage by periductal inflammation, possibly autoimmune, possibly an exaggeration of the normal involutional process.
- Histological periductal inflammation as is found in 1 in 5 'normal' breasts, and which leads to fibrous obliteration of ducts as well as DE. Together with simple DE, this can be considered as part of normal involution, so that nipple discharge and nipple retraction can be regarded as manifestations of ANDI.
- Exacerbation of periductal inflammation from leakage of duct contents, and further exacerbation from bacterial colonization.
- Colonization by bacteria probably from sexual contact, oro-nipple or intercourse-related bacteraemia.
- Fibrosis related to bacterial inflammation, or normal duct involution, which leads to secondary nipple retraction.
- Cigarette smoking, which plays an important role in facilitating bacterial invasion.

The clinical spectrum of duct ectasia/periductal mastitis (See Table 11.1)

Nipple discharge

Considering the pathology of DE, it is not surprising that it is sometimes associated with nipple discharge. The commonest complaint is a small amount of purulent discharge, which is confirmed by the patient expressing material from the nipple. Rarely it is so profuse as to cause severe social embarrassment (Fig. 11.3).

The colour varies over the spectrum seen in the ducts at operation: off-white, creamy, brown, grey or green; sometimes it is as thick as toothpaste (Fig. 11.4).

Bloodstained discharge is less common than these coloured discharges, although Dixon et al.[26] found positive occult blood in about half of their cases with nipple discharge. Certainly, in our experience a bloodstained discharge, even from a single duct, in the older age group (35 and over) is more commonly due to DE than to duct papilloma. Typically, it comes from a number of ducts; it is then even more likely to be due to DE (Fig. 11.5).

Patients with nipple discharge and palpable ducts tend to be in the peri- or postmenopausal age group.

Breast masses associated with periductal mastitis (Table 11.3)

Palpable subareolar ducts were described by Bloodgood as very characteristic of this condition. He likened it to a varicocele. This degree of gross duct dilatation is rather uncommon in our experience.

Evanescent mass

This is a very common presentation of the disease. The patient notices a small, slightly tender mass in the subareolar region. By the time she is seen in a clinic 7–10 days later, the mass has often disappeared. Such rapid development and regression of a breast mass is uncommon in any other breast condition. These masses are typically 1–2 cm in diameter, firm, tender and not attached to surrounding tissues. The subareolar situation distinguishes

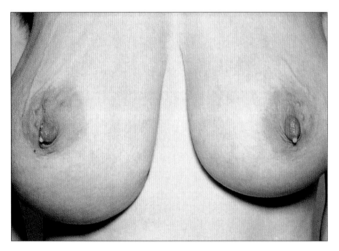

Fig. 11.3 The discharge of DE is often bilateral and sometimes so severe as to be socially embarrassing.

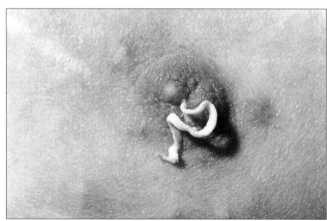

Fig. 11.4 Thick grumous nipple discharge of DE.

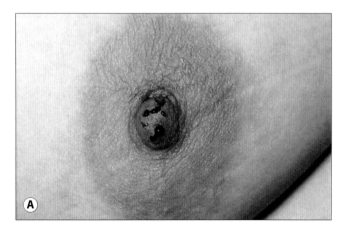

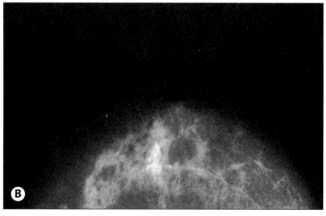

Fig. 11.5 (**A**) Blood-stained nipple discharge from multiple ducts is usually due to DE. (**B**) Mammogram of postmenopausal patient with bloodstained discharge and segmental-shaped opacity. Histology of the excised segment showed DE only.

Table 11.3 Breast masses associated with duct ectasia/periductal mastitis

Palpable ducts

Subareolar or periductal mass

    evanescent

    recurrent

    persistent → subareolar abscess

    chronic → simulating cancer

Peripheral mass

    peripheral abscess

evanescent PDM from the pain of leakage of fluid from a cyst which is usually a little more peripheral in the breast and is not associated with a small localized mass; in fact a palpable cyst may disappear with the onset of pain. Masses of PDM may progress to reddening of the overlying skin and still regress in a few days. As Haagensen[16] commented: 'The most remarkable thing about these episodes is the rapidity with which they develop, and, if left alone, the promptitude with which they subside.' This pattern of behaviour makes it very difficult to assess any form of medical treatment. The patients have often been given antibiotics and naturally attribute their improvement to the treatment.

Recurrent mass

While an evanescent mass may not recur, it has a tendency to do so at the same site at intervals of a few months to 10 years or more. The condition also has a tendency to become more severe with each recurrence. There is an appreciable incidence of bilateral involvement and it is not uncommon for the opposite breast to become involved shortly after successful control of one breast, although we have also seen an involvement of the contralateral breast as long as 10 years after the first one.

Persistent mass

If a mass persists for some weeks, it is usually firm and fairly well defined. Aspiration cytology is characteristic, showing foamy macrophages and inflammatory cells. Cancer cannot be excluded absolutely, but this cytological appearance (i.e. inflammatory cells without epithelial cells) is highly characteristic and justifies a short course of appropriate antibiotics. If the mass does not resolve

rapidly, biopsy excision is desirable in women of cancer age group. Provided there is no overt abscess formation, a periareolar biopsy wound will heal satisfactorily and there is no need to perform a formal duct excision. In fact, macroscopically dilated ducts are not particularly common in the presence of a simple PDM mass.

Some people have split off a condition which has been called granulomatous mastitis.[48] It is far from certain that this is not a variant of PDM, but it is discussed more fully in Chapter 17.

Chronic mass

This is the lesion that simulates cancer closely. It is a hard, oedematous mass fixed to the skin, with nipple retraction and sometimes with axillary node enlargement. In the past, many such cases were subjected to radical mastectomy because the lesion could show some resemblance to cancer even when cut across. It may also be impossible to distinguish the two on mammography, but aspiration cytology will allow a presumptive diagnosis to be made and a trial of antibiotics given before biopsy. In these cases, the typical large ducts with their pultaceous contents are more likely to be present. A formal duct excision procedure, together with excision of the mass, is usually indicated. This should be done under appropriate antibiotic cover. This lesion is seen less frequently than 30 years ago, probably because of the more widespread use of antibiotics effective against anaerobes.

Abscess

Any of these subareolar masses may proceed to abscess formation. The underlying mass becomes attached to the skin which first becomes reddened and then shows bluish discoloration. Nipple retraction will often develop if not already present, and nipple oedema may be marked. These abscesses are associated with discomfort which varies from mild to severe, but not usually as severe as with pyogenic abscess. Aspiration will yield creamy or dirty, watery pus and bacteriological culture may be sterile on the first occasion.

If not treated, the abscess will burst spontaneously with considerable relief, but a persistent sinus remains, or the abscess recurs sooner or later and usually at the same site. A typical disease sequence is shown in Figures 11.6–11.8.

Recurrent abscesses are more likely to grow bacteria – anaerobes or staphylococci.

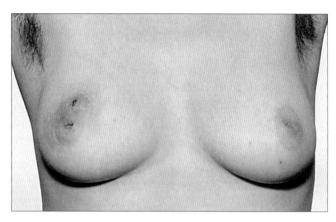

Fig. 11.6 A 28-year-old woman presenting with a diffuse periareolar abscess which has burst spontaneously while she was taking antibiotics. Note the bilateral congenital nipple inversion. The patient was successfully treated by major duct excision because of the diffuse nature of the sepsis.

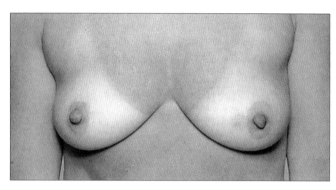

Fig. 11.8 The result (patient in Figs 11.6 and 11.7) 2 years later. The small scar of conservative drainage is visible medial to the left nipple. She has had no further problems.

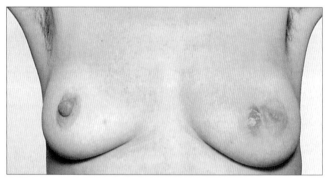

Fig. 11.7 The patient (as in Fig. 11.6) had no further problem with the right breast. Eight years later she presented with a similar condition of the left breast unresponsive to appropriate antibiotics. Treatment was by local drainage, followed by major duct excision 6 weeks later. (This was done in preference to fistulectomy at the patient's request, so that the inverted nipple could be corrected.)

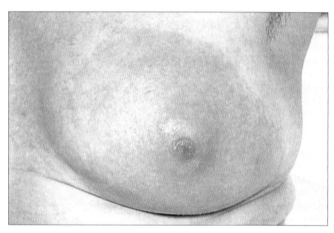

Fig. 11.9 A diffuse breast abscess associated with DE. The patient had relatively little pain, despite the gross inflammation.

While most sinuses are situated in the juxta-areolar region and are reasonably well localized, more severe abscesses may occur in association with DE, sometimes involving most of the breast (Fig. 11.9).

Peripheral mass

While most masses arise in relation to major ducts near the areola, similar masses are occasionally seen in the periphery of the breast. Figure 11.10 shows a large tender mass in the mid, upper, right breast, which slowly increased in size over 2 months.

Mammography and cytology were both consistent with benign diagnosis, but the patient requested excision because of constant aching. Figure 11.11 shows the pres-

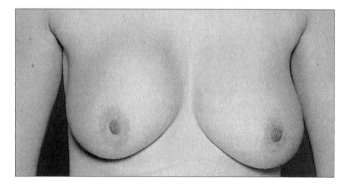

Fig. 11.10 A 28-year-old woman with a peripheral mass in the upper aspect of the right breast, due to perilobular mastitis.

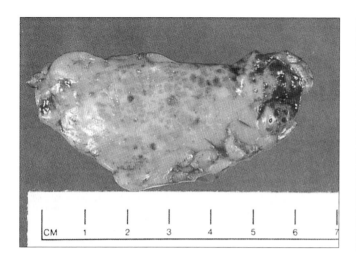

Fig. 11.11 The cut specimen from Figure 11.10 showing multiple small abscesses, sterile on culture.

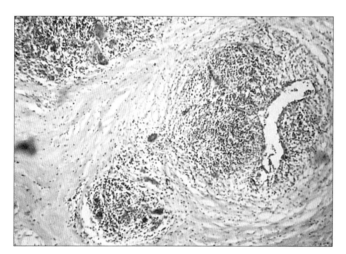

Fig. 11.12 The histological picture of Figure 11.11, which shows intense focal inflammation.

ence of multiple small abscesses and Figure 11.12 shows the typical histology of intense inflammatory infiltration around duct remnants.

The clinical pattern resembles that recorded with 'granulomatous mastitis'. It was cured by excision of the mass in continuity with duct excision, an approach we believe should be considered in cases of apparent granulomatous mastitis.

Figure 11.13 shows a 45-year-old woman who presented with recurrent abscesses involving a large area of the upper, outer quadrant of the right breast.

Each abscess was painful and discharged to leave a chronic sinus and to be followed by further abscesses. At operation the mammary ducts were grossly distended into the axillary tail and filled with thick, dark-green

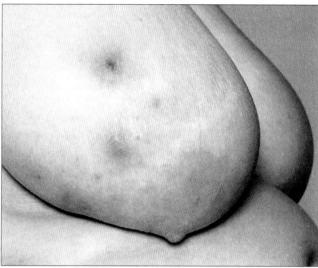

Fig. 11.13 Multiple peripheral sinuses following abscesses due to DE/PDM.

material. The abscesses were sufficiently incapacitating for the patient to request a large segmental excision. A few further small abscesses later developed adjacent to the excision margin, but were not sufficiently incapacitating to warrant further treatment. This clinical pattern may be confused with hidradenitis suppurativa.

Mammary duct fistula

The major papers describing this condition have been outlined in the historical survey. The typical features are classic. A young woman – of average age in the early thirties but sometimes as early as the teenage years – presents with a history of having several abscesses in one breast which have been treated by surgical drainage or have discharged spontaneously. The appearance is so typical that a spot diagnosis can usually be made (Fig. 11.14).

The features are partial inversion of the nipple and a sinus or scar at the edge of the areola. In cases recurrent on many occasions, the areola is distorted, scarring having reduced the distance between the nipple and the edge of the areola in the radius of the fistula.

Hanavadi et al.[49] have reported our own experience of 35 cases diagnosed between 1990 and 2001. This shows how difficult it is to obtain good results in this troublesome condition. The observation that seven of these cases followed duct excision for other conditions emphasizes the need for caution when advising patients about duct excision. A majority of patients developing the condition have nipple inversion, for example 19 of 28 in Atkins's series[17] and 23 of 40 in the series by Bundred et al.[50] However, neither states the number of these in which inversion was congenital. In our experience many of the patients have always had inverted nipples, but the history is sometimes vague in patients developing abscesses in their thirties, with inversion of long standing. About one in five of patients first develop an abscess in association with pregnancy or lactation.

Bundred et al.,[50] in a retrospective case note study, reported 13 of 40 patients developing a fistula after breast biopsy, by implication in the absence of a prior abscess. This is an unusual finding and, in our experience, biopsy of nonsuppurative PDM usually heals uneventfully.

Almasad[51] provided a useful classification of fistula into deep (associated with disease of the breast ducts) and superficial (associated with infection of the areolar glands). The first group require total duct excision; the latter will heal with more conservative surgery.

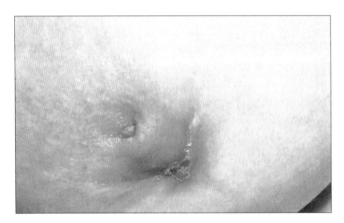

Fig. 11.14   The classical picture of late-diagnosed mammary duct fistula.

Nipple retraction

There is a complex relationship between nipple inversion or retraction and the syndrome of DE/PDM. It occurs in about one-third of patients requiring surgery for DE/PDM but it is difficult to estimate its incidence in patients with asymptomatic DE. There are at least three aspects of this complex relationship:

- There can be little doubt that congenital inversion of the nipple predisposes to the development of subareolar abscess and fistula (see Fig. 11.6 and Table 11.3), and that this is a very significant factor in the pathogenesis of the condition in teenagers and young women.
- There is frequently a close temporal relationship between overt PDM and the development of nipple retraction. The nipple inversion is characteristically transverse and of minor extent in the early stages (Fig. 11.15), but subsequently progresses to more complete retraction over a period of 1 or 2 years. It not infrequently commences following a pregnancy. The initial changes may precede, coincide with, or follow the development of overt PDM.
- Nipple retraction is frequently seen as an isolated event, without other evidence of DE. These cases are usually around or beyond the menopause. The retraction is circular (Fig. 11.16) and progresses over 1 or 2 years, often followed by the same process in the other breast. It seems likely that this type of retraction is due to the obliterative changes described by Davies[29] where microscopic periductal inflammation leads to disruption and periductal fibrosis without clinical ectasia or inflammation,

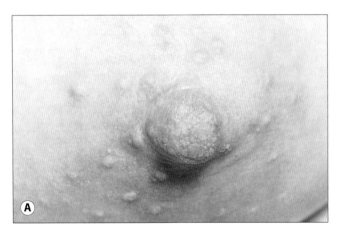

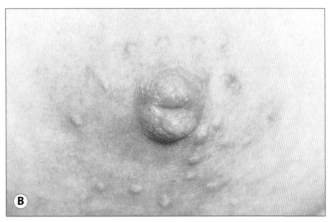

Fig. 11.15   The classical transverse central retraction of early nipple involvement in DE (**B**). The right nipple (**A**) developed retraction 2 years later.

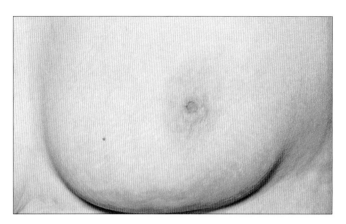

Fig. 11.16 Well-advanced nipple retraction due to periductal fibrosis in a postmenopausal woman.

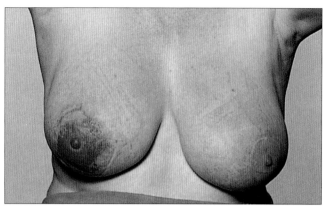

Fig. 11.17 Severe, recurrent eczema of the areola and surrounding breast which the patient claimed always followed nipple discharge. Note the scar of a major duct excision on the left breast.

probably more a normal involutional process than a disease.

We have previously described the clinical features of nipple retraction in this condition.[52] Thirty patients were seen in a 3.5-year period and an incidence of one case of nipple retraction due to DE per 100 new patients seen in the breast clinic was noted. The age range of the patients was 25–75 years with a mean of 52 years. The duration of retraction ranged from 3 months to 16 years. The incidence of parity and breastfeeding did not differ from that of other conditions presenting to the breast clinic. Retraction was partial in 12 cases, complete in 18. The left nipple was affected in 14, the right in 11 and was bilateral in 5. Early transverse retraction is easily withdrawn but the eversion becomes more difficult as retraction becomes more complete with the passage of time. However, eversion is still sometimes possible in advanced cases of long duration. The second nipple may show similar changes which may lag months or years behind the first in the development of retraction.

Some clinical features help in the differentiation from carcinoma. Retraction is more likely to be complete in carcinoma and to be accompanied by distortion of the areola when the breast is examined in different positions, while central and symmetrical retraction favour a diagnosis of DE. Eversion of the nipple by pressure behind the areola is more likely to be possible in DE. Pain is of little help in differential diagnosis because two-thirds of patients with nipple retraction due to DE have no pain. The presence of nipple discharge of the type typical of DE favours this diagnosis, as does a long history of a year or

more, particularly when no mass is palpable. Bilateral retraction favours DE. However, it must be stressed that no feature is absolutely diagnostic and cancer must always be excluded with care.

Mammography will usually exclude cancer in the fatty radiolucent postmenopausal breast, but this may not be so easily achieved in the dense breast of the young patient. Typical radiological features of DE (see below) may be present.

Mastalgia

We believe that a considerable proportion of cases of noncyclical mastalgia are associated with DE and PDM, although it is difficult to prove this except in acute episodes. It would not be surprising if the intense periductal inflammation and subsequent fibrotic process, described by Davies,[24] was a cause of chronic pain.

The evidence associated with the two conditions is derived largely from an association of radiological signs of DE with pain.[53] Sometimes, serial mammograms have shown the subsequent development of typical calcification of this disease at the site of pain.

Eczema

Bloodgood[3] described a case of eczema of the areola which was ascribed to nipple discharge. Azzopardi[25] mentioned similar cases. We have also seen this phenomenon (Fig. 11.17) in a 35-year-old woman who was adamant that the eczema always followed nipple discharge.

After some hesitation, duct excision was performed and the typical changes of DE were demonstrated. The condition promptly developed on the other side, but again responded to duct excision. Several years later the patient complained of recurrent discharge and recurrent eczema in the right breast. The operation was repeated with a further period of relief. (The question of the reconnection of divided ducts is discussed later.)

While there seems to be good evidence from these cases for an association between eczema and nipple discharge, it is very difficult to exclude a factitial element. However, on balance, we accept the likelihood that some areolar eczema may be due to sensitization of the skin to some element in nipple discharge.

Neonatal duct ectasia

The hypertrophy of breast tissue seen in neonates results from the transplacental passage of maternal hormone and both males and females respond in the same way. The degree of secretory change may be sufficient to induce considerable DE. The changes regress spontaneously in most cases but have been described as a cause of bloody nipple discharge.[54]

Duct ectasia in the male

The male breast may occasionally show much of the clinical spectrum of DE/PDM, including nipple discharge, nipple retraction, recurrent subareolar abscess and bilateral involvement.[55] As in women, inflammatory complications are usually associated with heavy cigarette smoking.[47] Tedeschi and McCarthy[56] reported a patient presenting with a tender lump which showed a typical histological picture of PDM. Habif et al.[23] also reported

two cases. The condition is further discussed in the section on the male breast (see Ch. 16).

Frequency of duct ectasia/periductal mastitis

Simple duct ectasia is very common. Sandison[57] found 'gross DE with much dilated and thickened ducts containing grumous, yellowish green material, ramifying through the fibro-fatty parenchyma of the organ' in 11% of women at autopsy, with the greatest incidence in the elderly. Clearly, the great majority of these had never experienced clinical disease in relation to these ducts. One group[58] encountered 40 cases requiring surgery over a 10-year period, during which time 732 breast operations of all types were performed. The frequency of presenting features in their series and three other series are given in Table 11.4.

Dixon et al.[26] found the mean age of presentation for pain, lump and nipple discharge to be similar at about 40 years, while nipple retraction was seen at a mean age of 53 years. However, in all these series, it is difficult to assess the figures given because it is not possible to differentiate between congenital and acquired nipple retraction, and mammary duct fistula is not considered.

Non-puerperal breast abscess associated with DE is becoming more common, and now exceeds the incidence of puerperal abscess,[59] perhaps associated with the increase in cigarette smoking among young women.

The disease probably occurs in all races, although literature from developing countries is scant. It occurs with approximately equal frequency in whites, blacks and Hispanics.[60]

Table 11.4 Presenting features of mammary duct ectasia/periductal mastitis

	Cromar & Dockerty[61]	Haagensen[16]	Walker & Sandison[21]	Thomas et al.[58]
No. of patients	24	110	34	78
Mean age (years)	40	54		45
Nipple discharge (%)	21	20	47	44
Nipple inversion(%)	42	25	8	32
Mass(%)	100	90	8	32
Sepsis(%)		18	9	9

The large discrepancy in the incidence of a mass between the older and more recent series reflects increasing awareness of this condition.

Radiology

The changes on mammography have been described by a number of authors.[62,63] Nipple retraction will be obvious and prominent ducts will be shown as a conical opacity with the apex of the cone towards the nipple. The individual ducts may be seen leading into this opacity but it is not possible to distinguish radiologically between DE, intraductal hyperplasia and periductal collagenosis.[64] In a few cases of gross dilatation, the fatty contents may be sufficiently radiolucent to outline the ducts and confirm their ectatic nature.

DE is frequently associated with characteristic coarse calcification. This may be ringlike – the calcification lying on the duct wall – or circular or needle shaped, when the duct contents are calcified (Figs 11.18 and 11.19).

The ultrasound appearances have also been described.[65]

Plasma cell mastitis gives moderately dense opacities, usually in the subareolar region and often flame shaped. Overlying skin and nipple oedema or retraction are sometimes seen (Fig. 11.20).

Management

Although there is a very large literature on this subject, many record results of retrospective case-note studies, provide no details of operative technique or long-term follow-up, and hence tend to confuse or to be misleading rather than helpful.

Medical management

There can be little hope for efficacious medical management until more is known about the causes of DE and PDM, in both sterile and suppurative forms. Because simple DE with nipple discharge causes trivial symptoms, and other cases are asymptomatic, no active treatment is necessary in many cases. In the more troublesome cases with gross infective lesions, medical management is unlikely to give long-term control, while dilated ducts act as a sump with stagnant secretions forming a nidus for persisting bacterial colonization. It is difficult to assess reports of medical therapy because of the evanescent nature of early PDM and also because diagnosis is imprecise

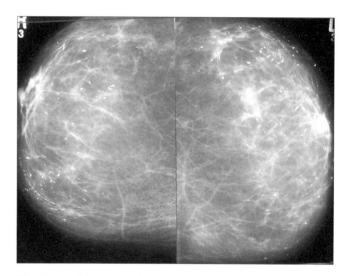

Fig. 11.19 Mammographic images of typical periductal calcifications.

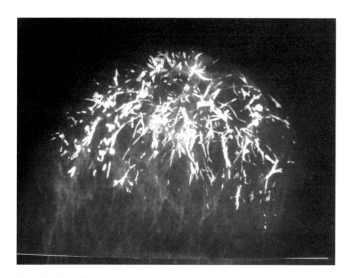

Fig. 11.18 Mammogram showing florid periductal calcification.

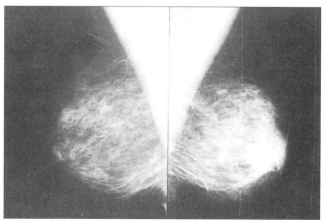

Fig. 11.20 Mammogram showing the typical features of plasma cell mastitis with an associated flame-shaped subareolar opacity and oedema of skin and Cooper's ligaments (left breast).

in the absence of biopsy material. These factors militate against meaningful controlled trials.

Nipple discharge

Galactorrhoea is usually readily distinguished from the nipple discharge in DE by the volume and consistency of the fluid, but, where any doubts exists, serum prolactin measurement should be performed to exclude a prolactinoma. We have not seen benefit from bromocriptine therapy in patients with profuse discharge due to DE and this drug is often poorly tolerated by patients with a normal serum prolactin.

The late Dr JP Minton of Columbus, Ohio, reported that nipple discharge may be associated with excess caffeine ingestion. He reported that exclusion of caffeine and other xanthines from the diet may result in resolution of the nipple discharge due to DE, although it took 6–9 months for an effect to be seen (personal communication). We have no experience of this approach to management.

Painful periductal mastitis

Peters and his co-workers[66] reported rapid resolution of non-puerperal mastitis after prescribing bromocriptine at a dose of 7.5 mg per day for 3 days, reducing to 5 mg per day for 11 days. The group was a mixed one but included some patients with typical PDM. Symptoms relapsed on stopping treatment but responded again to a 6-month maintenance course of bromocriptine 2.5 mg daily. There is no obvious rationale for this treatment and the results take no account of spontaneous remission, related to the evanescent nature of many early attacks of PDM. We have not had such satisfactory results but further results of this approach will be watched with interest.

Antibiotics

Many patients with painful breast lumps have already been started on antibiotics before attending a breast clinic and will report that symptoms have improved. By the time the patient is seen, it is impossible to determine whether this was spontaneous resolution or the result of antibiotic therapy. However, if the work quoted earlier[35] reflects the bacteriology of mild PDM, the antibiotics generally used in general practice, such as ampicillin and erythromycin, would not be effective. This suggests that any benefit of such antibiotic therapy may be due to

spontaneous resolution. Because anaerobic bacteria and staphylococci are the commonest organisms, metronidazole and flucloxacillin would be the appropriate combination with the addition of a broad-spectrum antibiotic such as erythromycin if these two are not effective. Augmentin is another option. The result of this therapy has been variable in our experience and we are not aware of any reported controlled trial.

A controlled trial would be difficult to organize because of the diagnostic uncertainty in presuppurative cases. It is likely from general principles that the efficacy of antibiotic therapy is dependent on the underlying pathology. Early bacterial PDM could be expected to respond while nonbacterial mastitis would not benefit. Advanced cases with grossly dilated ducts might be expected to be resistant because bacteria in the thick duct secretions would not be reached by the antibiotics. This variable response due to diverse pathology would be consistent with our results. In practice, we would recommend the following approach.

Mildly painful and tender masses behind the areola should be observed initially with the likelihood that they would resolve spontaneously. More painful masses should be explored with a 21-gauge needle and any fluid aspirate submitted to cytology and culture with meticulous use of transport medium appropriate to the detection of anaerobic organisms. In the absence of pus, patients are started on a combination of metronidazole and flucloxacillin while awaiting the results of culture. Antibiotics are continued on the basis of sensitivity tests and many of these mild cases respond satisfactorily, especially in the short term. Where there is more than a minimum amount of pus, it is best to proceed to conservative surgical drainage with continuing antibiotic cover. Once a large amount of pus has formed, repeated aspiration is unlikely to lead to resolution (although some recommend it) but results in destruction of breast tissue and skin with a less satisfactory cosmetic result in the long term. Antibiotic therapy is particularly useful in recurrent inflammation after formal duct excision and a prolonged course – at least 2 weeks and repeated once if necessary – should always be tried before resorting to further surgery.

Surgery

A striking feature of reports of surgical treatment of the DE/PDM complex is the variation in the frequency with which operations are performed and the varying indications given for surgery and for individual operations. Thus, Cox et al.[67] reviewed 753 consecutive new outpatient referrals to a breast clinic. No operation was performed specifically for this condition, and only one case of mammary duct fistula and one case of DE were diagnosed, although no fewer than 332 patients in this group had some form of surgical operation. In contrast, another recent series[58] reports 78 major duct excisions in a series of 732 breast operations, 40 being for DE. Urban[20] was able to report 160 major duct excisions in 150 patients, while Hadfield[19] reported 139 similar operations.

We operated on 200 cases over 15 years, giving an average operation rate of 15 cases per 1000 new referrals to the breast clinic. However, this figure is undoubtedly higher because of the tertiary referrals to our unit, but conversely we find it necessary to operate on only a proportion of clinically significant cases. Indications for surgery in 148 cases of major duct excision in our unit are shown in Table 11.5.

Recently, some workers have reported that surgery can be avoided in most cases by antibiotic therapy. Our own experience does not support this view in the longer term and suggests that the more enthusiastic reports of successful antibiotic therapy reflect cases of mild severity followed for a short time.

Surgeons reporting large series of total duct excision have tended to use this operation very freely, many being performed for simple non-bloody discharge or for an otherwise straightforward lump which lies behind the areola. Hadfield[19] and Thomas et al.[58] both used total duct excision as the procedure of choice for recurrent subareolar sepsis in preference to the operation of fistulotomy or fistulectomy favoured by other surgeons.

With such a diversity of thought and practice, it is not possible to give a consensus from the literature. Hence, we give our own views derived from an experience of some 200 operations for DE and its complications, performed over 15 years and from a considerable experience of tertiary referrals of problem cases following earlier surgery.

Indications for surgery

Surgery may be required in the following clinical situations:

- Nipple discharge – coloured, opalescent, bloody, serous
- Correction of nipple inversion
- Diagnosis of a retroareolar mass
- Subareolar abscess
- Fistula
- Eczema
- Recurrence after previous surgery.

Non-bloody nipple discharge

This condition, typically from several ducts and sometimes bilateral, is a benign condition with no increased cancer risk. It is not normally an indication for surgical treatment. We do not believe that investigation or treatment is necessary except in those rare cases where discharge is so profuse as to require constant wearing of a pad and to cause significant social embarrassment. In this situation, we would exclude a prolactinoma, and then offer the patient the operation of total duct excision, bilateral if necessary.

Table 11.5 Indications for operation in the 148 patients undergoing major duct excision

Indication	Total	Right	Left	Bilateral	
				Simultaneous	Sequential
Nipple discharge	83	29	41	11	2
Discharge plus inflammation	9	3	3	0	3
Discharge plus mass	2	1	1	0	0
Subareolar inflammation	32	10	16	4	2
Mass	15	6	9	0	0
Other	7	4	3	0	0
Total	148	53	73	15	7

Blood-related discharge

The management of this symptom is dealt with more fully in Chapter 13. Over the age of 40 years there is a significant risk of cancer or hyperplastic lesions and the operation of total duct excision has some advantages over more conservative procedures. It provides a good histological specimen and relieves the anxiety of the symptom. Where the cause proves to be one which is potentially multifocal, such as DE or a hyperplastic epithelial lesion, it pre-empts further discharge from other ducts.

Correction of nipple inversion

Patients are more likely to request correction of congenital nipple inversion than retraction due to DE occurring later in life, but some patients request correction of retraction for this condition. Although the results are usually satisfactory, patients seeking correction for cosmetic reasons should be aware of the possibility of nipple necrosis, of interference with sensation, of the inability to breastfeed and the possibility that postoperative fibrosis will lead to late reinversion.

Because the condition is due to shortening of the ducts, it can only be corrected permanently by a complete division of the subareolar ducts.

We usually do not encourage operative correction on cosmetic grounds alone, but when patients have had the procedure carried out for complications of PDM, the resulting correction of nipple inversion has been a much appreciated side effect. Such patients may then press for operative correction of a contralateral inverted nipple. Accumulation of debris in an inverted nipple can be malodorous; this provides another indication for correction.

Diagnosis of a retroareolar mass

The tender acute retroareolar mass of PDM frequently resolves spontaneously, so surgery should be delayed if aspiration biopsy is suggestive of this diagnosis. Where a mass persists for several weeks, we would treat it by simple excision biopsy, even if dilated ducts filled with pultaceous material are encountered. Primary healing is the rule; only in the presence of an overt abscess is postoperative sepsis likely. If such an abscess is encountered at operation, we would either undertake simple drainage with a view to formal surgery should the problem recur, or proceed immediately to formal total duct excision under appropriate antibiotic cover. We tend to the first course in young women and to the latter in women past the child-bearing period.

Subareolar abscess

The diagnosis is confirmed by needle aspiration, which also provides a specimen for cytology and bacterial culture. In our experience, aspiration under antibiotic cover rarely leads to a satisfactory long-term result with an established abscess, which is best treated by conservative open drainage. Drainage is conservative because, unlike puerperal abscess, the infection is usually unilocular and often associated with a single duct system, and it is desirable to confine the process to a single segment. More radical drainage may spread the infection or damage adjacent normal ducts.

A majority of patients with anaerobic bacteria will develop recurrent infection and/or a fistula, so in most cases it is advisable to proceed to a definitive procedure (fistulotomy or duct excision) when the infection has settled after 6–8 weeks. The resulting wound can be managed satisfactorily by open healing by secondary intention, or by primary closure under antibiotic cover,[68] depending on the acuteness and extent of inflammation.

If the patient prefers a more conservative approach, aspiration under antibiotic cover is a reasonable alternative, and has been advocated by Dixon.[69] Aspiration is facilitated by ultrasound guidance. Repeated aspirations are often necessary, and in his series, 40% of cases with anaerobic bacteria had recurred after a short follow-up period. Scholefield et al., reporting a 10-year follow-up, found that 90% of patients with anaerobes suffered recurrent infection.[59] It is not yet clear if cessation of cigarette smoking will lessen the risk of recurrence.

Recurrent abscess with fistula

This situation provides a difficult problem of surgical judgement, the decision whether a fistula with recurrent sepsis should be treated by fistulotomy or by major duct excision. Some of the factors bearing on this decision are set out in Table 11.6.

When a small localized periareolar abscess recurs at the same point, and a fistula is clearly present, the operation of choice is fistulotomy (or fistulectomy – see Ch. 18). It is a simple procedure with minimal complications and a

Table 11.6 Treatment of recurrent subareolar sepsis

Suitable for fistulectomy	Suitable for total duct excision
Abscess small and localized to one segment	Abscess large, affecting >50% of areolar circumference
Recurrence always at the same site	Recurrence involving a different segment
Probe passes easily from fistula through nipple at interval operation	Probe may be 'lost' in cavity
Mild congenital nipple inversion or no inversion	Gross nipple inversion
Patient unconcerned about nipple inversion	Patient requests correction of nipple inversion
Younger patient	Older patient
No discharge from other ducts	Purulent discharge from other ducts between episodes
	Recurrence after fistulectomy

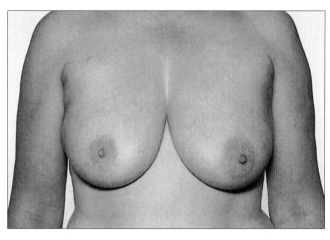

Fig. 11.21 A typical long-term postoperative result of (right-sided) major duct excision of nipple discharge. Operation for sepsis often leaves a less satisfactory result.

high degree of success. Should it fail (in spite of being carried out correctly), total duct excision can still be used. Some authors are still advocating formal duct excision in all cases,[70] rather than the selective approach which allows many patients a simple effective procedure with minimal disruption to the breast.

Where subareolar sepsis is diffuse rather than localized to one segment or where more than one fistula opening is present, total duct excision is the procedure of choice. The former situation is likely to be seen in young women with squamous metaplasia of a single duct, the latter in an older woman with multiple ectatic ducts. However, age is not a reliable guide and we would recommend fistula excision as the initial procedure for localized lesions irrespective of age. One exception is where there is marked nipple inversion and the patient wishes to have this corrected. This tips the balance towards total duct excision, particularly if the patient does not wish to breastfeed in the future. Figures 11.6, 11.7 and 11.8 show a case where duct excision was considered appropriate in a young patient.

Eczema

Where there is good evidence that eczema of the areola follows nipple discharge, total duct excision is the only procedure likely to give relief. However, other forms of eczema and factitial injury should be considered carefully

before resorting to surgery, since DE is a rare cause of areolar eczema.

The consequences and results of operations for duct ectasia

Patients should be aware of the consequences of these operations before undergoing surgery, particularly where this is recommended for conditions other than sepsis, because a patient is unlikely to be satisfied if a less than optimal result is obtained. With severe or recurrent sepsis, the morbidity of the disease is such that most patients happily accept the results of surgery which relieves them of their episodes.

Consequences

Cosmesis

In general, the cosmetic effect is excellent when performed for nipple discharge, but less satisfactory when done for sepsis, especially for longstanding sepsis. In the first group the nipple is not distorted, and a typical result is shown in Figure 11.21.

Satisfactory results may also be obtained when operating for sepsis, provided the operation is done before gross scarring has occurred and if the cosmetic result is considered when performing operations (see Fig. 11.8). Once skin destruction is allowed to occur and multiple abscesses have been drained, severe distortion of the nipple has occurred and cannot be readily corrected. The situation is

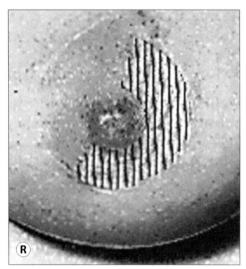
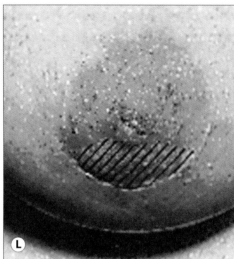

Fig. 11.22 Patient following bilateral major duct excision for severe recurrent sepsis, multiple on the patient's right side. The stippled area outlines the loss of sensation.

even worse when recurrent sepsis occurs more peripherally in the breast after duct excision and this is discussed below in relation to operations for recurrent disease.

Although failure to lactate after the operation suggests that glandular atrophy must occur with time, there is no change in size of the breast after the operation.

Sensation

Tactile sensation is usually lost in part over the half of the nipple raised as a flap (Fig. 11.22).

Multiple incisions around different segments are likely to increase the sensory loss, so should be avoided if possible. It is possible to perform the operation through small incisions, with less effect on sensation, but these carry a risk of leaving residual ducts unless performed meticulously.

Lactation

Patients cannot breastfeed after this operation and there are few reports of the consequences of pregnancy following duct excision. Urban[20] reported that four of his 150 patients became pregnant after the operation. Minimal engorgement occurred following delivery but this rapidly subsided when lactation was suppressed with hormones. Hadfield[71] recommended patients to defer pregnancy for a year after the operation. He reports an unspecified number of pregnancies after the operation. Lactation occurred normally on the unoperated side, but no discharge from the operated breast. When pregnancy

occurred within a year of operation, there were varying degrees of enlargement from activity in the operated breast which subsided quickly after delivery.

We also advise our patients to avoid pregnancy for 1 year after operation and have seen no problem under these circumstances. One of our patients had proximal duct excision for sepsis of the left breast, and the same procedure of the right breast 2 years later. She became pregnant 2 months after the second procedure. She had no problem with the left breast, but the right became engorged, and the infection flared up. This was controlled temporarily by antibiotics and drainage, but left two fistulas requiring reoperation after suppression of lactation. The typical chronic abscess was found under the nipple.

Restoration of duct continuity

Duct discharge sometimes recurs after the operation and it must be assumed that occasionally the ducts reconnect to an aperture in the nipple. Indeed, one of our patients claimed to breastfeed successfully for 9 months after this operation, but the breast at this time was involutional to palpation compared to the normal breast and we saw no milk from the operated nipple. Collection of debris in an inverted nipple can lead a patient to believe discharge has recurred.

Behaviour of residual ducts

There is a surprising lack of information about what happens to the remainder of the breast ducts after subareolar duct excision. Haagensen[16] makes no comment nor do the writers of any of the other series. In our experience, the small number of patients coming to further operation has shown that the ducts remain dilated and filled with the same material seen at the primary operation. Since most cases of reoperation have been for recurrent sepsis, this group may behave differently to the majority of patients without further trouble, but the same dilated ducts have also been encountered occasionally where reoperation has been performed for causes other than infection.

The fact that dilated ducts can remain in this state for years following major duct excision throws doubt on the suggestion that bacteria can be cultured from most cases of PDM. In contrast to the persistence of dilated collecting ducts, the minimal response of the breast to pregnancy after longstanding division of the ducts suggests that back-pressure may lead to atrophy of the secretory acinar elements of the duct system.

Cancer risk

The longstanding presence of secretions stagnant in ducts completely obstructed by major duct excision would seem to provide a background for carcinogenesis. However, Haagensen[16] and Urban[20] both state that there have been no excess cases of cancer in their patients having duct excision, many of whom were followed for a long time. Our experience would support this although it must be admitted that there are inadequate data based on documented long-term follow-up to provide a definitive answer to the question.

The results of operations for duct ectasia

Major duct excision

Early authors reported excellent results from operations for DE and PDM, which are somewhat surprising, especially because many such operations were performed before the importance of anaerobic organisms and appropriate antibiotic therapy was realized. Urban[20] concludes his study of 167 major duct excisions by stating that the operation 'results in satisfactory cosmetic appearance. There have been no recurrence of symptoms and no complications in our hands.' Hadfield[71] reported equally satisfactory results. All patients were left with a normal-looking breast and nipple, there was no instance of recurrent disease on the operation side, and no case of cancer developing during follow-up of 1–7 years.

More recent series have not been so encouraging. Thomas et al.[58] reported good results when the operation was performed for nipple retraction, nipple discharge and subareolar mass, although nine of their patients continued to have nipple discharge for up to 1 year after the operation. One patient required reoperation to correct nipple reinversion. However, they had 100% recurrent infection following major duct excision for abscess, and two of their patients eventually had a mastectomy.

Hartley et al.[72] also report a considerable postoperative complication rate after careful surgery (by a single operator) for all indications. This was despite operating only when sepsis was quiescent and using antibiotic cover routinely. Wound drainage was avoided in all cases.

Donegan[73] found that results deteriorate with time: 45% of 26 patients had recurrent sepsis at 1 year, 60% by 7 years. He believes that recurrence is due to downgrowth of epithelium of the nipple into the cavity, and advocates the radical approach of excision of the nipple with secondary reconstruction. In his hands, this is always associated with long-term cure. While agreeing with the thesis that residual ductal epithelium facilitates recurrence, we feel that the operation of core excision of the nipple (see Ch. 18) almost always achieves the same result without cosmetic deformity and avoids the need for reconstruction.

The sole dissenting recent authors are Dixon and Thomson,[74] who obtain excellent results with minimal recurrence. It is not clear why their results differ, or whether they will hold up in the longer term.

In our unit 122 patients have had formal examination and follow-up at 1–10 years after major duct excision. Thirty-four patients (28%) had suffered a problem affecting the breast subjected to major duct excision (Table 11.7).

Nineteen of the patients have required further surgery to the breast related to the original operation, eight drainage of an abscess, five required further duct excision, four laying open of the fistula, four biopsies and two mastectomies. Hence, it is also our experience that most recurrent problems are related to surgery for subareolar sepsis.

This high problem rate falls with increasing operator experience and is also now lower because of better use of appropriate antibiotic therapy. The interval between operation and development of further problems varies from a few weeks to several years. Recent papers also report improving results, probably reflecting the

Table 11.7 Breast problems following major duct excision

Mastalgia	9
Infection	9
Discharge	7
Lump	6
Haematoma	3
Recurrent eczema	1
? Raynaud's disease of the nipple	1

Table 11.8 Causes of recurrent disease following fistulectomy and major duct excision for duct ectasia/periductal mastitis

Persisting abscess cavity

Persistent proximal ducts

Persistent distal ducts

Persisting or recurrent nipple inversion

Early pregnancy

Contralateral disease

Factitial disease

recognition for the need to remove completely the affected duct(s). Passaro et al.[60] reported satisfactory results in 47 of 48 patients, although some had needed up to three operations, and some follow-up was short. They used a radial incision through areola and nipple to ensure complete removal of the terminal ducts, reinforcing the prime importance of this element of the operation.

Fistulotomy/fistulectomy

Atkins[17] had no recurrence following his operation of fistulotomy with saucerization, although length of follow-up was not detailed. Lambert et al.[75] reported 48 fistulas: 13 were laid open, 25 were excised and allowed to granulate, eight were excised with primary closure. One recurrence occurred 6 weeks after a primary closure. They made no attempt to correct inversion of the nipple. Like many series reporting good results, follow-up is relatively short at a mean of 25 months and the operations were performed in a specialist breast centre. Bundred et al.[68] reported results in 36 women with mammary duct fistula, 12 of whom had fistulectomy with two recurrences. Our experience of tertiary referral cases suggests that the results from less specialized centres are far from uniformly satisfactory, and surgical experience has a marked influence on the outcome.

Complications of operations

The complications of fistulectomy are slow healing and recurrent abscess and fistulas. Both are commonly due to inadequate technique.

The complications of major duct excision are haematoma, infection, flap necrosis, nipple inversion, cosmetic deformity, pain and recurrence of the original condition.

The commonest problem calling for further surgery is recurrent infection; less common is persisting nipple discharge or reinversion of the nipple.

Recurrent infection after surgery for periductal mastitis

Aetiology of recurrent sepsis after duct surgery

Recurrent sepsis tends to be more common after major duct excision than after simple fistulotomy, but this probably reflects the fact that the fistulotomy operation is more appropriate to less severe degrees of sepsis, and those which are confined to a single duct. Nevertheless, the underlying cause of recurrent sepsis is basically the same for both operations. The common denominator is a chronic abscess lined by granulation tissue, under the nipple, but a number of disparate factors may contribute to the persistence of this chronic abscess (Table 11.8).

The commonest cause of persisting problems following surgery is incorrect or inappropriate surgery. Intractable disease, in spite of adequate surgery, is less common. The first approach to a patient with recurrent problems is careful inspection for evidence of inadequate surgery. If this is found, revisional surgery is usually the best approach. Where surgery appears to have been satisfactory, a trial of prolonged antibiotic therapy for recurrent sepsis is preferable to early operation. The causes of recurrence of symptoms in patients referred to us are shown in Table 11.8.

Persistent abscess cavity

Any chronic abscess with a thick rigid wall must be eradicated either by opening the cavity so widely that it granulates from its base, or by excising any rigid cavity wall back to pliant tissues so that the cavity obliterates. It may be associated with persistent proximal duct.

Persistent proximal duct

When infection recurs after laying open of a fistula, it is not uncommon to find that the incision extends only half way on to the areola; a recurrent abscess will then discharge through the proximal end of the incisional scar. Operation in such a case is likely to show a persistent segment of terminal duct which may be only 7 or 8 mm in length (Fig. 11.23).

The essential feature of the fistulotomy operation is to pass a probe through the fistula and out of the opening of the duct on to the nipple, and then use a small racket-shaped incision to ensure that the whole of the terminal portion of the duct is removed. Attempts to perform this procedure by subareolar dissection of the tract invite recurrence (and make assessment more difficult), while the ultimate cosmetic appearance is more related to eradication of the infection than a transareolar incision.

The same mistake can occur with a major duct excision. It is easy to leave terminal elements of duct attached to the under surface of the nipple after transecting the duct cone and this has been the cause of several recurrent cases in our experience (Fig. 11.24). As well as

forming an entry site for bacteria, it provides a focus for epithelial downgrowth into the cavity. It can be prevented by inverting the nipple with a fingertip and removing the terminal portion of all the ducts with scissors (see Ch. 18), or more certainly by central core excision of the nipple.

Residual ducts

It is also common for inexperienced operators to miss some of the breast ducts, especially those furthest from the incision, when performing major duct excision (Fig. 11.25).

This must be assumed to be the case when nipple discharge persists immediately following surgery. Details of technique to avoid this are given in Chapter 18.

If the symptoms merit further treatment, operation to remove the residual ducts may be indicated. We have found this necessary occasionally both for eczema of the

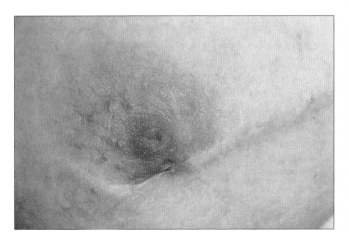

Fig. 11.23 A patient with recurrent sepsis following operation for mammary duct fistula. Note that the incision does not reach the centre of the nipple. The causative pathology has not been eliminated.

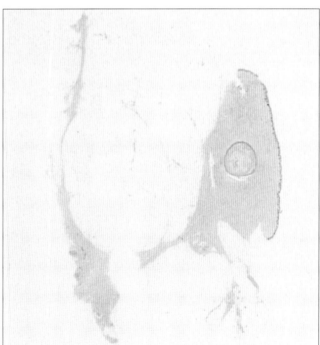

Fig. 11.24 Histological section after excision of a persisting fistula. The patient had previously undergone major duct excision but a terminal portion of duct had been left under the nipple.

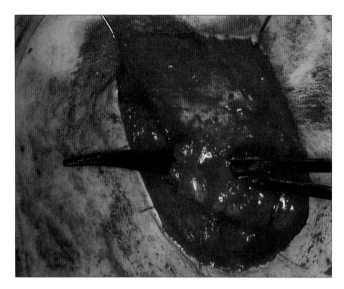

Fig. 11.25 At operation for persisting nipple discharge after major duct excision; some ducts have been left at the far end of the dissection.

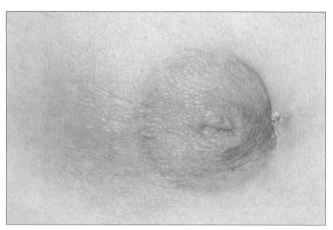

Fig. 11.26 A patient with recurrent sepsis following major duct excision. Note the nipple inversion has not been corrected.

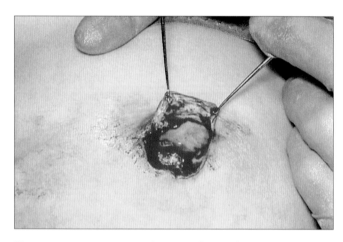

Fig. 11.27 At reoperation there is a chronic abscess under the nipple with sepsis extending out into the breast. Several ducts had been missed at the original operation.

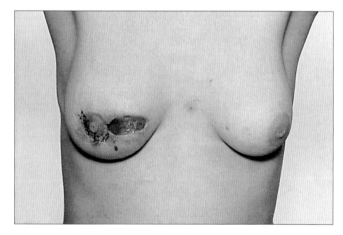

Fig. 11.28 This was treated by re-excision of the ducts and segmental excision in continuity.

nipple related to nipple discharge and for recurrent infection.

Residual peripheral ducts

The surprising aspect of operations on the major ducts for DE is that the residual distal ducts give so little trouble. Haagensen[1] noted this as early as 1951 and it has proved to be general experience. Even when dilated ducts are cut across and drain into the wound, late trouble from the residual breast is uncommon. Nevertheless, most authors report recurrent disease in a proportion of cases, some being sufficiently severe to lead to mastectomy. We have seen a number of similar cases. An example, and the way it was managed, is shown in Figures 11.26–11.29.

Intensive antibiotic therapy should be the first approach in such cases, but will not control all. It is of interest that some of these inflammatory attacks occurring after duct excision settle without treatment even when quite severe, resolving in 3 or 4 days in exactly the same manner as can be seen in the initial evanescent attacks of PDM. Once again, this seems to be incompatible with heavy bacterial colonization of the residual ducts and suggests a 'chemical' inflammatory response to irritant materials.

Where inflammation persists and pus can be aspirated, and antibiotics have not given control, a further wedge excision is the appropriate treatment because inflammatory changes in the residual breast tend to be segmental in outline. At the same time as this wedge excision is

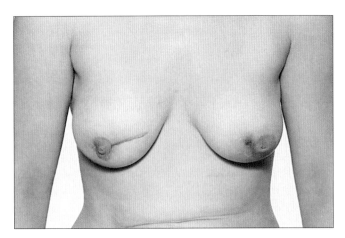

Fig. 11.29   The patient 1 year later. The right breast has healed satisfactorily but the patient has developed the same condition in the left breast, reflecting the frequent bilateral incidence of this condition.

carried out under antibiotic cover, the subareolar area should be explored to exclude persisting ducts or a hidden abscess cavity.

We have performed only two mastectomies for DE. With further experience, we now believe that local incisions under antibiotic cover will control most cases if the proximal duct excision has been correctly performed and core nipple resection may avoid mastectomy. However, there are some patients whose disease is sufficiently intractable and peripheral to warrant mastectomy. The complications are not inconsiderable because of scarring of previous operations, and any reconstructive procedure is better delayed to allow all sepsis to settle.

Persisting nipple inversion

The inverted nipple, so often associated with periareolar sepsis, becomes normally everted after total duct excision, and this is a bonus of the operation which is greatly appreciated by the patient. However, in longstanding cases with much sepsis the nipple remains fixed in the inverted position even after the terminal ducts have been excised.

Persisting nipple inversion leads to collection of grumous material in the inverted cavity which discharges periodically and leads the patient to believe that she has recurrent duct discharge. The material is sometimes offensive. Collection of material in an inverted nipple undoubtedly predisposes in some cases to further subareolar sepsis, particularly staphylococcal. Presumably, organisms ingress through the old duct openings in the nipple.

For this reason, and for reasons of cosmesis, we believe that complete nipple eversion should always be ensured as part of the operation of major duct excision. If inversion, or a tendency to inversion, persists after excision of all the terminal ducts on the undersurface of the nipple, a purse-string suture is inadequate to give correction. It is necessary to excise the central dense fibrotic core of the nipple, only 5–6 mm in diameter, leaving normal supple nipple (external skin) which everts easily and shows no tendency to reinvert. The defect in the apex of the nipple is closed loosely with a couple of fine absorbable sutures.

One of the disadvantages of the simple fistulotomy operation of Atkins is that marked nipple inversion is not corrected. This fact may tip the balance of choosing major duct excision in favour of simple fistulotomy, especially in the older woman who is not concerned with future breastfeeding.

Once nipple inversion is corrected by total duct division, it usually remains everted but a few cases will reinvert after some time, presumably due to formation of scar tissue and subsequent fibrous contraction. It does not occur after core excision of the nipple.

Contralateral disease

It is an unfortunate feature of PDM that it is frequently bilateral. It is not easy to determine the true frequency, since few series give long-term follow-up, and the incidence of bilateral disease increases with time, sometimes occurring as long as 10 years after operation on the first side. Our best estimate is that about 20% of patients will eventually develop bilateral disease. It will be interesting to see if patients can be persuaded to give up cigarette smoking with a beneficial effect.

Results of treatment are often better on the second side because the patient recognizes what is happening, and presents earlier to a surgeon who is familiar with the condition. It is our practice to treat the abscess on the second side by early drainage under antibiotic cover, proceeding to definitive operation after about 6 weeks when infection is quiescent, again under antibiotic cover. This allows primary wound closure with a good cosmetic result.

Factitial disease

The problem of self-inflicted disease is discussed in Chapter 17. This question must always be considered when recurrent sepsis becomes a problem after operation for DE. The presence of bowel organisms, such as *Escherichia coli*, *Streptococcus faecalis* and colonic *Bacteroides* sp. (as opposed to the oral or vaginal organisms commonly found) should raise the possibility of a factitial basis. Persistent bleeding from the nipple after major duct excision, particularly if no epithelial lesion was demonstrated, is also suggestive of this condition. Ill-advised mastectomy is likely to be followed shortly by bleeding or other problems with the other nipple so the whole process is repeated.

The patients often seem rather odd, but as is the case with other chronic painful conditions, their psyche may take a turn for the better if the condition is corrected. Most of the cases we have seen where factitial disease has been suspected have been shown to have had inadequate surgery and have healed uneventfully after reoperation. In one case it has been necessary to resort to excision of

nipple and areola with secondary reconstruction, with a satisfactory result.

Management of recurrent sepsis

Because of the role of mixed bacterial infection in persistent cases, the first approach to recurrent sepsis following surgery should be to give a 2-week course of antibiotics. A combination of flucloxacillin or erythromycin and metronidazole usually provides a satisfactory spectrum to cover these organisms.

Occasionally, long-term control will be obtained but more commonly one of the causes set out above will underlie the recurrence and require correction.

Mastectomy should be considered only as a last resort, and reconstruction delayed for some months if prosthetic material is to be used.

REFERENCES

1. Haagensen CD. Mammary duct ectasia – A disease that may simulate cancer. *Cancer* 1951; **4**: 749–761.

2. Birkett J. *The Diseases of the Breast and their Treatment.* London: Longman; 1850.

3. Bloodgood JC. The pathology of chronic cystic mastitis of the female breast with special consideration of the blue-domed cyst. *Archives of Surgery* 1921; **3**: 445–452.

4. Bloodgood JC. The clinical picture of dilated ducts beneath the nipple frequently to be palpated as a doughy, worm-like mass in the varicocele tumour of the breast. *Surgery, Gynecology and Obstetrics* 1923; **36**: 486–495.

5. Cutler M. Benign lesions of the female breast simulating cancer. *Journal of the American Medical Association* 1933; **101**: 1277–1282.

6. Cheatle GL & Cutler M. *Tumors of the Breast.* Philadelphia: Lippincott; 1931.

7. Adair FE. Plasma cell mastitis, a lesion simulating mammary carcinoma. *Archives of Surgery* 1933; **26**: 735–749.

8. Tice GI, Dockerty MB & Harrington SW. Comedomastitis. A clinical and pathological study of data in 17 cases. *Surgery, Gynecology and Obstetrics* 1948; **87**: 525–540.

9. Sandison AT & Walker JC. Inflammatory mastitis, mammary duct ectasia and mammillary fistula. *British Journal of Surgery* 1962; **50**: 57–64.

10. Rodman JG & Ingleby H. Plasma cell mastitis. *Annals of Surgery* 1939; **109**: 921–930.

11. Frantz VK, Pickren JW, Melcher GM *et al.* Incidence of chronic cystic disease in so-called normal breasts. *Cancer* 1951; **4**: 762–783.

12. Zuska JJ, Crile G Jr & Ayres WW. Fistulas of lactiferous ducts. *American Journal of Surgery* 1951; **81**: 312–317.

13. Deaver JB & McFarland J. *The Breast: Its Anomalies, its Diseases and their Treatment.* Philadelphia: Blakiston; 1917.

14. Bonnet. Memoire sur les fistules des conduits du lait. *Archives Gènèrales de Mèdècine Paris* 1835; **IX**: 451–464.

15. Waters JJ. Mammary sinus subsequent to abscess; treatment by a listerian method; cure. *British Medical Journal* 1892; **ii**: 209.

16. Haagensen CD. *Disease of the Breast*, 3rd edn. Philadelphia: WB Saunders; 1986.

17. Atkins HJB. Mammillary fistula. *British Medical Journal* 1955; **2**: 1473–1474.

18. Patey DH & Thackray AC. Pathology and treatment of mammary duct fistula. *Lancet* 1958; **ii**: 871–873.

19. Hadfield GJ. Excision of the major duct system for benign disease of the breast. *British Journal of Surgery* 1960; **47**: 472–477.

20. Urban JA. Excision of the major duct system of the breast. *Cancer* 1963; **16**: 516–520.

21. Walker JC & Sandison AT. Mammary duct ectasia. *British Journal of Surgery* 1964; **51**: 350–355.

22. Ewing M. Stagnation in the main ducts of the breast. *Journal of the Royal College of Surgeons of Edinburgh* 1963; **8**: 134–142.

23. Habif DV, Perzin KH, Lipton R *et al.* Subareolar abscess associated with squamous metaplasia of lactiferous ducts. *American Journal of Surgery* 1970; **119**: 523–526.

24. Davies JD. *Periductal mastitis*. MD thesis, University of London, 1971.

25. Azzopardi JC. *Problems in Breast Pathology*. London: WB Saunders; 1979.

26. Dixon JM, Anderson TJ, Lumbsdon AB *et al.* Mammary duct ectasia. *British Journal of Surgery* 1983; **70**: 601–603.

27. Tedeschi LG, Ouzouman G & Byrne JJ. The role of ductal obstruction and hormonal stimulation in main duct ectasia. *Surgery, Gynecology and Obstetrics* 1962; **114**: 741–744.

28. Davies JD. Histological study of mammae in oestrogenized rats after izoimmunization. *British Journal of Experimental Pathology* 1972; **53**: 406–414.

29. Davies JD. Inflammatory damage to ducts in mammary dysplasia: a cause of duct obliteration. *Journal of Pathology* 1975; **117**: 47–54.

30. Hanayama R, Nagata S. Impaired involution of mammary glands in the absence of milk fat globule EGF factor 8. *Proceedings of the National Academy of Science of the United States of America* 2005; **102**: 16886–16891.

31. Toker C. Lactiferous duct fistula. *Journal of Pathology and Bacteriology* 1962; **84**: 143–146.

32. Schaffer P, Furrer G & Mermillod B. An association of cigarette smoking with recurrent subareolar breast abscesses. *International Journal of Epidemiology* 1988; **17**: 810–813.

33. Beigelman PM & Rantz LA. Clinical significance of Bacteroides. *Archives of Internal Medicine* 1949; **84**: 605–631.

34. Walker AP, Edmiston CE Jr, Krepel CJ *et al.* A prospective study of the microflora of non-puerperal breast abscess. *Archives of Surgery* 1988; **123**: 908–911.

35. Krepel CJ, Gohr CM, Walker AP *et al.* Enzymatically active *Peptostreptococcus magnus*: association with site of infection. *Journal of Clinical Microbiology* 1992; **30**: 2330–2334.

36. Leach RD, Eykyn SJ & Phillips I. Vaginal manipulation and anaerobic breast abscesses. *British Medical Journal* 1981; **282**: 610–611.

37. Bennett KW, Wistanley TG, Taylor AKM *et al.* Anaerobic curved rods in breast abscess and vagina. *Lancet* 1989; 1: 564.

38. Bundred NJ, Dixon JM, Lumsden AB *et al.* Are the lesions of mammary duct ectasia sterile? *British Journal of Surgery* 1985; **72**: 844–845.

39. Dixon JM. Periductal mastitis/duct ectasia. *World Journal of Surgery* 1989; **13**: 715–720.

40. Aitken RJ, Hood J, Going JJ *et al.* Bacteriology of mammary duct ectasia. *British Journal of Surgery* 1988; **75**: 1040–1041.

41. Peters F & Schuth W. Hyperprolactinaemia and nonpuerperal mastitis (duct ectasia). *Journal of the American Medical Association* 1989; **261**: 1618–1620.

42. Shousa S, Backhouse CM, Dawson PM *et al.* Mammary duct ectasia and pituitary adenomas. *American Journal of Surgical Pathology* 1988; **12**: 130–133.

43. Bundred NJ, Dover MS, Coley S *et al.* Breast abscesses and cigarette smoking. *British Journal of Surgery* 1992; **79**: 58–59.

44. Bundred NJ, Dover MS, Aluwihari N *et al.* Smoking and periductal mastitis. *British Medical Journal* 1993; **307**: 772–773.

45. Bundred NJ. The aetiology of periductal mastitis. *The Breast* 1993; **2**: 1–2.

46. Furlong AJ, Al-Nakib L, Knox WF *et al.* Periductal inflammation and cigarette smoke. *Journal of the American College of Surgeons* 1994; **179**: 417–420.

47. Thomas JA, Williamson MR & Webster DJT. The relationship of cigarette smoking to breast disease in the Cardiff experience. In: Mansel RE (ed.) *Recent Developments in the Study of Benign Breast Disease.* Carnforth: Parthenon; 1994:221–226.

48. Kessler E & Wolloch Y. Granulomatous mastitis: a lesion clinically simulating cancer. *American Journal of Clinical Pathology* 1972; **58**: 642–646.

49. Hanavadi S, Pereira G, Mansel RE. How mammillary fistulas should be managed. *Breast Journal* 2005; **11**: 254–256.

50. Bundred NJ, Dixon JM, Chetty U *et al.* Mammillary fistula. *British Journal of Surgery* 1987; **74**: 466–468.

51. Almasad JK. Mammary duct fistulae: classification and management. *Australia and New Zealand Journal of Surgery* 2006; **76**: 149–152.

52. Rees BI, Gravelle IH & Hughes LE. Nipple retraction in duct ectasia. *British Journal of Surgery* 1977; **64**: 577–580.

53. Preece PE. *A study of the aetiology, clinical patterns and treatment of mastalgia*. MD thesis, University of Wales, 1982.

54. Stringel G. Infantile mammary duct ectasia – a cause of bloody nipple discharge. *Journal of Pediatric Surgery* 1986; **21**: 671–676.

55. Mansel RE & Morgan WP. Duct ectasia in the male. *British Journal of Surgery* 1979; **66**: 660–662.

56. Tedeschi LG & McCarthy PE. Involutional mammary duct ectasia and periductal mastitis in the male. *Human Pathology* 1974; **5**: 232–236.

57. Sandison AT. *A postmortem study of the adult breast*. MD thesis, University of St Andrews, 1957.

58. Thomas WEG, Williamson RCN, Davies JD *et al.* The clinical syndrome of mammary duct ectasia. *British Journal of Surgery* 1982; **69**: 423–425.

59. Scholefield JM, Duncan JL & Rogers K. Review of hospital experience of breast abscess. *British Journal of Surgery* 1987; **74**: 469–470.

60. Passaro ME, Broughan TA, Sebek BA *et al.* Lactiferous fistula. *Journal of the American College of Surgeons* 1994; **178**: 29–32.

61. Cromar CDL & Dockerty MB. Plasma cell mastitis. *Proceedings of the Staff Meeting of the Mayo Clinic* 1941; **16**: 775–782.

62. Evans KT & Gravelle IH. Mammography, Thermography and Ultrasonography in Breast Disease. London: Butterworths; 1973.

63. Sweeney DJ & Wylie EJ. Mammographic appearances of duct ectasia that mimic breast carcinoma in a screening programme. *Australasian Radiology* 1995; **39**: 18–23.

64. Mansel RE, Gravelle IH & Hughes LE. The interpretation of mammographic ductal enlargement in cancerous breasts. *British Journal of Surgery* 1979; **66**: 701–702.

65. Matricardi L & Lovati R. Ultrasonic appearance of a case of mammary duct ectasia. *Journal of Clinical Ultrasound* 1991; **19**: 568–570.

66. Peters F, Hilgarth M & Brecknoldt M. The use of bromocriptine in the management of non-puerperal mastitis. *Archives of Gynecology* 1982; **233**: 23–29.

67. Cox PJ, Li MKW & Ellis H. Spectrum of breast disease in outpatient surgical practice. *Journal of the Royal Society of Medicine* 1982; **75**: 857–859.

68. Bundred NJ, Webster DJT & Mansel RE. Management of mamillary fistula. *Journal of the Royal College of Surgeons of Edinburgh* 1991; **36**: 381–383.

69. Dixon JM. Outpatient treatment of non-lactational breast abscesses. *British Journal of Surgery* 1992; **79**: 56–57.

70. Khoda J, Lantsberg L, Yegev Y *et al*. Management of periareolar abscess and mamillary fistula. *Surgery, Gynecology and Obstetrics* 1992; **175**: 306–308.

71. Hadfield GJ. Further experience of the operation for excision in the major duct system of the breast. *British Journal of Surgery* 1968; **55**: 530–535.

72. Hartley MN, Stewart J & Benson EA. Subareolar dissection for duct ectasia and periareolar sepsis. *British Journal of Surgery* 1991; **78**: 1187–1188.

73. Donegan WL. In: Donegan WL & Spratt JS (eds). *Cancer of the Breast*, 4th edn. Philadelphia: WB Saunders; 1995:98.

74. Dixon JM & Thomson AM. Effective surgical excision for mammary duct fistula. *British Journal of Surgery* 1991; **39**: 1185–1186.

75. Lambert ME, Betts CD & Sellwood RA. Mammillary fistula. *British Journal of Surgery* 1986; **73**: 367–368.

CHAPTER 12

Disorders of the nipple and areola

Key points and new developments

1. Nipple inversion is common, but self-correcting changes often occur during pregnancy and lactation, allowing breastfeeding.

2. Nipple retraction is more commonly due to duct ectasia/periductal mastitis (DE/PDM) than cancer, although exclusion of the latter is the prime consideration.

3. PDM causes progressive retraction (initially a transverse slit) in young women; DE is associated with circular retraction in the perimenopausal period.

4. Erosive adenomatosis of the nipple has a distinct appearance, which usually allows clinical differentiation from prolapsing duct papilloma and Paget's disease. It is not premalignant, but is associated with an increase in cancer elsewhere in the breast.

5. Nipple pain associated with breastfeeding may be associated with candidal or staphylococcal infection.

6. Raynaud's phenomenon and CRPS (complex regional pain syndrome) are rare causes of nipple pain, sometimes occurring after surgery.

7. Secretions from Montgomery's glands, milklike, serous or bloodstained, are easily mistaken for nipple discharge, especially in younger patients.

Introduction

The nipple and the areola constitute an area of skin modified by the underlying breast tissue and ducts. In addition, the nipple has an extensive network of smooth muscle whose fibres are mainly arranged in circular fashion. The areola surrounds the nipple, both having more pigment than the surrounding skin, and contains the glands of Montgomery which provide a protective lubrication during lactation. The areola also has circular smooth muscle fibres and may contain auxiliary breast tissue which secretes milk during lactation. The blood supply to the nipple is mainly from the internal thoracic artery although the anterior intercostals and lateral thoracic arteries may make a significant contribution.[1] The nerve supply is also variable although the most constant supply is via the deep branch of the anterior division of the fourth lateral cutaneous nerve.[2] This, together with other nerves that pass subcutaneously, forms a subdermal plexus under the areola.

In the past there has been debate regarding the number of lactiferous ducts opening on to the nipple. Haagensen[3] stated that there were about 20, but others have put the number at seven. The difference of opinion arose from the fact that 20 ducts are seen in cross-section at the nipple, but experience with lobar excision shows that a single duct system occupies much more than one-twentieth of the breast parenchyma. The discrepancy is due to the fact that the lobular systems extending from individual ducts vary greatly in extent. Some of the ducts are rudimentary, only about seven developing to form fully functional lobes.

Koernecke[4] found that the functional ducts are arranged around the periphery of the nipple, the rudimentary ducts opening on to the centre of the nipple. More light has been thrown on the subject from another detailed study of a single breast, where the extent of individual ductolobular segments is very variable, confirming the view that some ducts lead to small glandular systems.[5] Love and Barsky[6] confirmed the arrangement of central and peripheral groups and found that 905 women had between 5 and 9 ducts, each opening communicating with a separate nonanastomosing peripheral duct system.

Some confusion arises from failure to appreciate the sebaceous glands and tiny milk-producing glands that also open directly on to the nipple.

Nipple inversion and retraction

The failure of full nipple eversion during breast development is common. It is termed 'inversion' and is discussed with other congenital conditions of the nipple in Chapter 15. Alexander and Campbell[7] have reviewed the prevalence of nipple inversion and non-protractility. They found that such changes occurred in almost 10% of 3006 women. The prevalence was lower in those who had previously breastfed and they attributed this to changes occurring during pregnancy and lactation. In a longitudinal study, 238 women were investigated and it was found that protractility increased during gestation. In most cases the changes were bilateral, but they were unilateral in a significant minority. Park et al.,[8] in Korea, found 53 inverted nipples in 1625 (3.5%) unmarried women between 18 and 26. Nine of 53 requested surgical correction.

It is clear that in most cases nipple inversion is a self-limiting condition that does not preclude breastfeeding. Attempts to increase the effectiveness of breastfeeding by using nipple shells or Hoffman's exercises does not seem to be helpful.[9] For those who find the changes unacceptable a plastic procedure is required. Han & Hong[10] have attempted to rationalize the indications by a grading classification depending on the degree that the inverted nipple can be everted and presume that the higher grades are due to fibrosis. They maintain that grade 2 lesions may be corrected by division of these fibrous bands without damaging the terminal ducts. The range of available options suggests that none is entirely effective.

Nipple retraction is an acquired condition and occurs after previous normal nipple development. The patients will give a clear history that a previously normal nipple has changed shape, and become retracted.

Bryant[11] made an appeal for careful assessment of nipple retraction over a hundred years ago, pointing out that many cases were not due to malignancy. Nevertheless, the erroneous view that most cases of recent nipple retraction are due to malignancy is still sometimes held. Recent changes in the appearance of the nipple do portend an underlying pathological process that requires evaluation. The principal diagnoses to be considered are malignancy and duct ectasia (DE). The presence of a clinical lump associated with nipple changes increases the likelihood of an underlying carcinoma, but is also seen with periductal mastitis (PDM). In the absence of clinical or mammographic malignancy, nipple retraction is likely to be due to some aspect of the DE/PDM syndrome.

The relation between nipple inversion and retraction and DE/PDM is complex. In younger women, congenital inversion predisposes to overt inflammatory complications of PDM, while the same process may cause progressive retraction of a previously normal nipple. We have observed this progression over a period of 2 years or so in many patients. In this situation, the retraction is typically transverse, especially in the early stages.

In older, peri- or postmenopausal women, recent nipple retraction (circular in outline) is frequently seen in the absence of inflammation. This appears to be due to the periductal fibrosis element of the DE syndrome, and as such is considered to be an aberration of normal mammary involution (ANDI).

Few women are sufficiently concerned to wish to undergo surgery for retraction alone. For those cases due to DE, a formal excision of the major ducts is necessary.

Assessment of nipple retraction

Although the early retraction of DE typically produces a transverse crease (see Fig. 11.15), in established cases the appearance is not sufficiently clear-cut to allow reliable distinction from cancer. If the changes are bilateral the diagnosis is more likely to be DE. Carcinoma is uncommon when the retraction has been present for more than 1 year, but even in DE the signs may be of recent onset. Associated masses may be difficult to assess clinically, but core biopsy is usually diagnostic. Cytology of any associated discharge may provide helpful information. Mammography is helpful because it will either show the typical features of cancer or a notable absence of these features in patients with DE.

The pathology, differential diagnosis and management of nipple retraction due to the DE complex are considered more fully in Chapter 11.

Cracked nipples

Cracked nipples are the bane of nursing mothers, for these are the source of entry of bacteria in lactational breast infection. Pain in the nipple on suckling is a common event in the first few days of breastfeeding and may occur in up to 17% of nursing mothers.[12] In most of these, careful examination, using a magnifying lens if necessary, will reveal a small erosive lesion.[13] The mechanism suggested is that during vigorous suckling the skin of the nipple exposed between tongue and hard palate is subjected to a high negative pressure – if the milk does not flow easily the infant will suck harder – which produces a small blood blister. This lesion usually regresses spontaneously but, if the trauma is repeated, especially if the nipple skin becomes macerated due to the moist environment that often occurs, the lesion may progress to the typical fissure often referred to as a cracked nipple, seen about 1 week postpartum. This is often infected with bacteria or with *Candida* sp. Livingstone & Stringer[14] carried out a randomized trial of four strategies to treat painful nipples during lactation; oral antibiotics provided significantly more symptomatic relief and reduced the incidence of subsequent mastitis. As in many such conditions, prevention is better than cure, and recognition of the predisposing factors is important. Good hygiene and a pattern of cleansing in the preconfinement period are helpful. The nipples should be washed gently in water and dried secretions removed. The breasts are then dried by dabbing rather than rubbing. Care needs to be taken in establishing suckling; the infant will find an overengorged breast difficult to empty and short or inverted nipples may also lead to overvigorous suckling. If one breast is painful, feeding should commence on the unaffected side, so that by the time the infant is applied to the affected breast, the draught reflex will allow easy flow of milk. After feeding, the breasts should be cleaned and dried carefully, and then kept as dry as possible until the next feed.

In the established case, correct feeding habits need reinforcing and in addition an antibiotic-based cream should be applied to the nipple. If candidal infection is suspected a nystatin-containing cream should be used. With care, the fissure will heal and breastfeeding can be maintained, although manual expression for a few days may be necessary. Neglect at this stage may lead to the development of an abscess as described in Chapter 14.

Nipple crusting

This symptom (Fig. 12.1) usually represents dried up secretions which may accumulate, particularly in association with inverted or retracted nipples.

Sometimes it hides an underlying nipple lesion such as Paget's disease, eczema or erosive adenomatosis. Beyond reassurance, having excluded the conditions mentioned above, no action is required other than advice about cleaning the nipple.

Verrucous nipple (naevoid hyperkeratosis)

The nipple and areola may be affected by verrucous change, a benign condition in which the nipple and areola show hyperkeratotic thickening with dark pigmentation. This rare condition is seen in women of child-bearing age, when it is thought to be related to oestrogens or their metabolites. (A similar condition may arise in males having oestrogen treatment for prostatic cancer.) It also takes a naevoid form, appearing in young women after puberty.[15]

A verrucous nipple may cause itching, malodour and interference with breastfeeding. A number of dermatological measures have been used, but treatment is difficult to assess because most reports only refer to single cases.

Erosive adenomatosis

This is a rare condition that is also described as papillary adenoma, florid papillomatosis of the nipple, subareolar

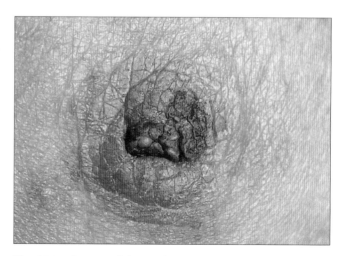

Fig. 12.1 Crusting of the nipple.

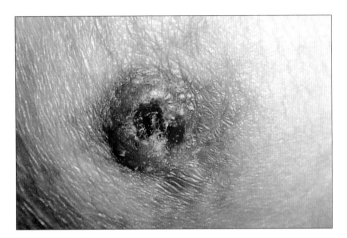

Fig. 12.2 Erosive adenomatosis of the nipple.

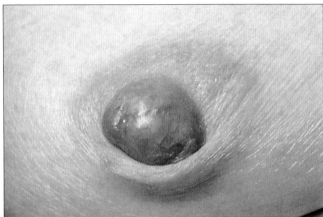

Fig. 12.3 A large benign papilloma of the terminal duct, distending the nipple of an elderly woman.

papillomatosis and erosive adenomatosis of the nipple.[16] While usually seen in the middle aged to elderly, it can occur at any age and has been reported as early as 9 years. It has been described in an accessory nipple.[17]

Erosive adenomatosis is termed 'adenoma' by Haagensen,[3] who points out the difficulties of diagnosis and records that many of the early cases were treated by radical mastectomy in the belief that the lesion was a carcinoma. It usually presents as a papilliferous lesion of the nipple, often with ulceration which may be concealed under a crust (Fig. 12.2).[18]

The condition is sometimes painful, the commonest descriptions being burning or itching,[19] although Perzin and Lattes[18] only recorded pain in one of their 51 cases. Our own experience with this condition would favour the view that it is relatively painless.

On examination, the whole nipple may be indurated, has an expanded appearance and may be ulcerated. The main differential diagnoses are prolapsing intraductal papilloma, Paget's disease of the nipple, artefactual disease and eczema. The differential diagnosis from Paget's disease can only be made with certainty by biopsy, although the characteristic clinical features are different. Pinto and Mandreker[20] have described a case in which the diagnosis was made on fine needle cytology. Erosive adenomatosis does not extend on to the areola like established Paget's disease, and it has the appearance of a deeper lesion eroding through the nipple; early Paget's disease is superficial in appearance. When a papilliferous lesion erodes through the nipple duct, it is more likely to represent this condition than an intraductal papilloma (Fig. 12.3).

An intraductal papilloma tends to expand the nipple rather than erode it, but if a papilloma prolapses through the opening of a duct, the nipple remains normal; it is not ulcerated.

Azzopardi[16] describes this lesion as being an extensive ramifying proliferation of two-layered tubules: an outer layer of myoepithelial cells and an inner layer of cuboidal cells. Although associated malignant breast disease has been described in about 8% of 200 collected cases, the lesion is not itself usually regarded as premalignant.[18] Associated benign duct papilloma has also been reported to occur more commonly than would be expected by chance. This incidence of associated breast cancer calls for careful assessment of both breasts. Erosive adenomatosis is adequately treated by local excision of the affected part of the nipple; there is no need to remove the whole nipple as advocated by some.[21]

Syringomatous adenoma

Rosen[22] has described a benign infiltrating lesion of adnexal skin origin, which he differentiates from erosive adenomatosis, in four women and one man. It is more likely to recur than erosive adenomatosis so adequate treatment may require nipple resection. We have no experience of this condition. Carter and Dyess[23] have reported a case and reviewed the literature to 2003.

Nodular mucinosis

This rare condition presents as a subareolar myxoid mass in young women. Sanati et al.[24] have reported a further case and reviewed the literature. It is most likely to be confused with a myxoid fibroadenoma.

Simple fibroepithelial polyp

This not uncommon condition was first described by Hutchinson,[25] who thought it arose from Montgomery's tubercles, although the polyps are found more frequently on the nipple than the areola. They are pedunculated dry lesions resembling the skin tags seen elsewhere in the body (Fig. 12.4).

Neurofibromas occurring at this site may also be pedunculated. They are readily treated by local excision and do not recur.

Eczema

There are many causes of red, oozing and crusted nipples recognized by dermatologists, including psoriasis, seborrhoeic dermatitis, contact dermatitis, neurodermatitis and atopic dermatitis. It is particularly common in atopic patients. Scabies and chronic friction require exclusion. Chronic infection, e.g. with *Staphylococcus aureus* or *Candida*, can persist in the moist, traumatized conditions of breastfeeding and can give rise to unusual clinical and histological appearances.[26]

Eczema may occur in a form localized mainly or completely to the nipple and areola (Figs 12.5 and 12.6) and requires to be distinguished from the non-eczema

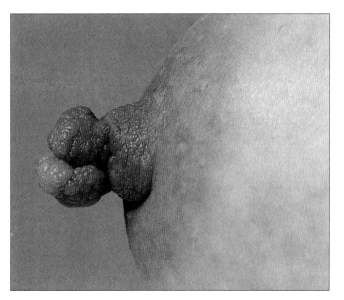

Fig. 12.4   Benign pedunculated fibroepithelial polyp.

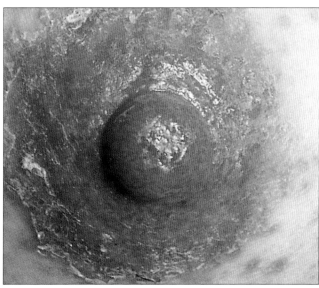

Fig. 12.5   Eczema of the nipple and areola; note the uniform involvement.

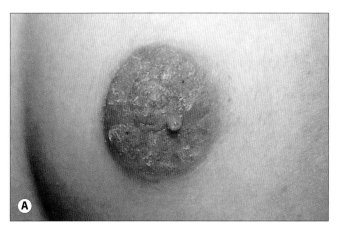

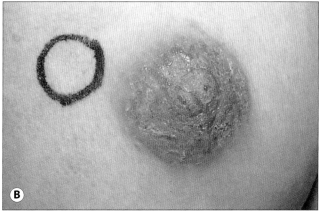

Fig. 12.6   Eczema of both areolae, with an unrelated benign cyst in the right breast.

conditions of Paget's disease and erosive adenomatosis which also have an eczematous appearance.

Paget's disease and eczema can usually be differentiated on clinical grounds (Table 12.1).

In spite of this, Paget's disease is still often neglected because of an erroneous diagnosis of eczema. It is important to think of Paget's disease in every inflammatory condition of the nipple and areola and to be aware of the range of appearances of Paget's disease (Figs 12.7 and 12.8).

Even so, biopsy in all cases is the safest course to follow. Eczema is confirmed by a punch biopsy although a core nipple biopsy as described by Aryal et al.[27] may be preferable. The typical Paget cells (Fig. 12.9) usually allow the pathologist to make the diagnosis without difficulty.

In patients with eczema of the nipple and areola, the condition is bilateral and in many patients there is evidence of eczema elsewhere. When this is not the case, eczema is usually symmetrical and does not extend beyond the areola (see Fig. 12.6). The possibility of an artefactual syndrome (see Ch. 17) should not be overlooked.

Treatment in cases of eczema follows the same guidelines as eczema elsewhere in the body.

Other general skin conditions may cause concern when the first, or only, manifestation of the condition occurs

Table 12.1 Clinical features of eczema of the nipple and Paget's disease

Eczema	Paget's disease
Usually bilateral	Unilateral
Intermittent history, with rapid evolution	Continuous history with slow steady progression
Moist	Moist or dry
Indefinite edge	Irregular but definite edge
Nipple may be spared	Nipple always involved and disappears in advanced cases
Itching common	Itching common

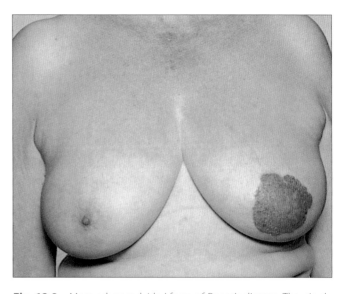

Fig. 12.8 More advanced, 'dry' form of Paget's disease. The nipple is disappearing.

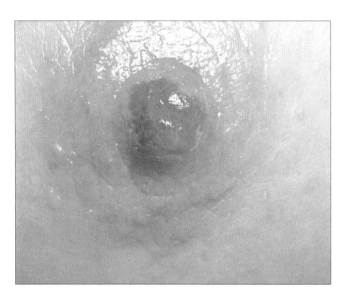

Fig. 12.7 The moist, erosive form of early Paget's disease.

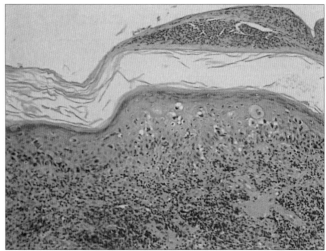

Fig. 12.9 Typical Paget cells, large pale vacuolated cells distributed along the squamous epithelium of the nipple.

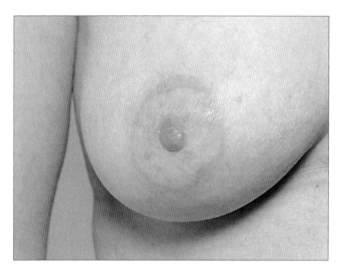

Fig. 12.10 *Vitiligo of the nipple as the first manifestation of the condition.*

on the nipple or areola. Figure 12.10 shows a patient with vitiligo confined to the areola that showed such concern.

Leiomyoma

Leiomyoma of the nipple is surprisingly uncommon in view of the large quantities of smooth muscle present. When it occurs it appears as a smooth round lump, obviously within the skin of the areola or nipple. It can occur at any age, is usually about 6–7 mm in diameter and may have been present for some years. Haagensen[3] distinguishes between this superficial leiomyoma, arising in the smooth muscle of the nipple and areola, and deep leiomyoma which arises from smooth muscle associated with blood vessels. Both are adequately treated by local excision.

Traumatic lesions

The nipple is occasionally the site of trauma and the condition of jogger's nipple is well recognized.[28] This lesion is presumably the result of constant friction of an unprotected warm and moist nipple on ill-fitting clothing. It is sometimes severe enough to produce bleeding. Related conditions are cyclist's nipple[29] which appears to be a cold injury with the subsequent pain lasting for several days, and tassel dancer's nipple.[30] Rings placed in the nipple (and the tracks thus created) may produce

unusual radiological artefacts;[31] this is not a problem with the ring in situ but may cause concern if it has been removed. We experienced one case in which a patient presented with intermittent periareolar inflammation. No track was apparent clinically but was demonstrated on ultrasound. Subsequent questioning revealed these attacks only followed her occasional use of the ring; the inflammation was due to a metal allergy. Artefactual trauma of the nipple is also seen occasionally.

Nipple pain

Around the time of the menopause, patients often describe various sensations of irritation, pricking and burning in the nipple region. They are usually irritating rather than of greater severity. No clear aetiological basis has been put forward; the most likely explanation relates to the histological periductal inflammatory changes regarded as part of the normal involutional process. In favour of this explanation is the fact that these sensations may accompany the circular nipple retraction also seen in the perimenopausal period. Another possible explanation is hormonal imbalance associated with declining ovarian function, since similar nipple sensations may be experienced with hormone administration. Paget's disease must also be carefully excluded, since itch, pricking and irritation are commonly experienced in the early phase of this condition.

Raynaud's phenomenon

Raynaud's phenomenon has also been described in the breast. It is probably more common than is usually recognized. In one series from New Zealand, it was thought that up to 1 in 20 pregnant women had symptoms suggestive of Raynaud's phenomenon during cold weather.[32] The changes typically occur in lactating women after or between feeding.[33]

Lawlor-Smith and Lawlor-Smith[34] have described five patients with Raynaud's phenomenon affecting the nipple presenting to an Australian general practice in a 2-year period. All patients experienced severe pain and nipple changes; in three the classic triphasic response of colour change was exhibited. In two patients, symptoms antedated their first pregnancy. Strangely, affection of the nipples does not seem to be associated with the typical changes in the extremities, questioning whether or not it is the same condition.

Reynaud's phenomenon of the nipple is now recognized as one of the causes of nipple pain during lactation and Anderson et al.[35] saw 11 cases in a single paediatric service in 1 year. They also raised the possibility that such events may be more common in those who have had previous breast surgery. In this series symptomatic relief was obtained with nifedipine.

The nipple necrosis described after vasopressin is also presumably due to vascular spasm.[36]

Postsurgical pain

It is now well recognized that complex regional pain syndrome may affect parts of the body other than the limbs, where it has long been recognized as a reflex sympathetic dystrophy of the causalgia type. Similar changes have been reported in the breast, especially the nipple area after surgery.

We have seen such a case after major duct excision, which was related to cold. Even though the patient was warmly clothed, the nipples were subjectively intensely cold and objectively so to examination. The attacks gradually abated over a period of 4–5 years. A case following breast reduction surgery has been reported.[37] The 27-year-old patient had pain, swelling, epidermal scaling and temperature changes persisting for a year. Liquid crystal thermography scanning confirmed a hypothermic region in the breast. Intravenous phentolamine gave temporary relief, with long-term relief provided by stellate ganglion blockade. Recent interest in this condition has led to consensus statements on classification and taxonomy.[38]

Pain during breastfeeding

Pain is common during breastfeeding, especially following the first pregnancy. The various causes are well recognized, but the importance of *Candida* infection as a cause is not always appreciated. The relationship of *Candida* infection to persistent nipple pain (burning in nature and radiating to the breast) has recently been investigated by Amir et al.[39] Microbiological assessment (culture of nipple and baby's mouth, and of expressed breast milk) was carried out in 61 lactating women with breast pain, 64 women without breast pain and 31 non-lactating women. Candida was grown from 19% of women with breast pain, but only 3% of those without. Nipples affected by *Candida* did not have the usual appearance of thrush elsewhere, but looked mildly inflamed and were tender to touch. *Candida* infection was associated with recent use of antibiotics (usually for mastitis), with *Candida* in the baby's mouth, and with use of a dummy. Treatment was with topical miconazole oral gel to nipple and baby's mouth and oral nystatin.

Staph. aureus was also associated with breast pain, and independently with cracked nipple.[10]

Nipple disease and HIV infection

Nipple disease is very common among African HIV-positive women suckling HIV-positive infants, and the status of the infant is the most important determinant of nipple disease in the mother.[40] Kambarami and Kowo reported that 31% of such mothers had nipple disease, 22% eczema, 11% cracked nipples and 11% painful nipples.[40]

Montgomery's glands

Montgomery, an Irish obstetrician, in 1837 gave a classic description of the changes in the areolar tubercles occurring during pregnancy. These structures, which now bear his name, had in fact been described by Morgagni in 1719. There are three types of gland in the areola: (1) apocrine sweat glands; (2) modified sebaceous glands; and (3) rudimentary mammary glands.

There is clear evidence that apocrine sweat glands are a normal finding in the areolar skin.[41] The modified sebaceous glands which lie under the tubercles of Montgomery are similar to sebaceous glands elsewhere, except that they are associated with a lactiferous duct extending from a more deeply placed mammary gland.[42] The rudimentary mammary glands and the sebaceous glands both undergo changes during pregnancy which lead to typical changes in the tubercle described by Montgomery. The position and relative sizes of these glands are depicted in Figure 12.11.

In addition to the areolar glands, there are dermal sebaceous glands of the nipple and occasional deep ectopic sebaceous glands which open into the main breast ducts. These are discussed below and in Chapter 11 in relation to the aetiology of mammary duct fistula.

When the detailed anatomy of the glandular components of Montgomery's tubercles is considered, the clinical problems of retention cysts (Fig. 12.12) and milk-like discharge are not surprising.

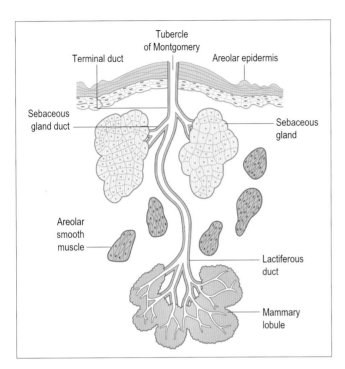

Fig. 12.11 The anatomy of the subareolar glands. (After Smith et al.[42] by permission of *Archives of Pathology and Laboratory Medicine*.)

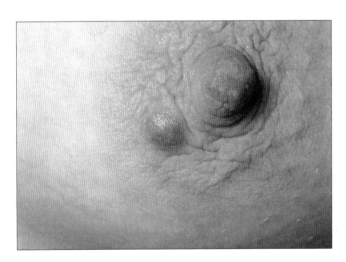

Fig. 12.12 A retention cyst of Montgomery's gland.

It is perhaps more surprising that discharge from the tubercles is as rare as it seems to be in the literature.[43] Infection of the tubercles may mimic subareolar abscess associated with DE and the persisting lesion suggests a mammary duct fistula, although it will present on the areola rather than at the periphery of the areola as occurs with mammary duct fistula.

Histological sectioning of the areola in mature females shows that the mammary elements of Montgomery's

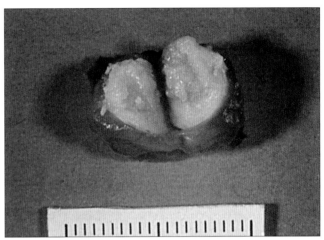

Fig. 12.13 A sebaceous cyst presenting as a lump within the nipple, treated by conservative enucleation.

glands are subject to many of the conditions affecting the mamma, including hyperplasia, cyst formation, periductal fibrosis and apocrine metaplasia.[42]

Bleeding from Montgomery's glands is occasionally seen in young girls and may be confused with bleeding from the nipple.

No obvious cause is usually found on biopsy and the bleeding may be due to trauma.

Sebaceous cyst of the nipple

This rare condition presents as a painless lump palpable immediately below and attached to the nipple (Fig. 12.13).

Because this lies deeper than the dermal sebaceous glands of the nipple, its origin can be explained by the findings of Patey and Thackray[44] that ectopic sebaceous glands may occasionally be found deep in the nipple, opening into the terminal portion of the duct. It is satisfactorily treated by excision. However, this is obviously a more extensive operation than that necessary for a retention cyst of the dermal sebaceous glands. Some authors have considered that all mammary duct fistulas arise on the basis of infection of these deep sebaceous glands. However, in our experience, the two conditions are quite separate. Sebaceous glands lie more centrally and when infected give a local juxtanipple mass, not a mass at the edge of the areola, as is seen with recurrent subareolar abscess secondary to mammary duct fistula.

The use of nipple rings is likely to be associated with occasional complications such as dermoid inclusion cysts and infection.[45]

Viral infections

Molluscum contagiosum occasionally occurs in the skin of the nipple. It produces a discrete lump which may ulcerate,[3] and is readily recognized on histopathology. It is uncommon,[46] which is perhaps surprising as this poxvirus is usually transmitted sexually. Herpesvirus lesions[47] and genital warts of the nipple (condyloma acuminatum)[48] are also seen occasionally.

Hidradenitis suppurativa of the areola

The areola is one of the classic sites for hidradenitis in most descriptions of the disease, presumably because apocrine-like sweat glands are found there. Despite a very large experience of hidradenitis, including many cases involving the breast, we have not seen a single case involving the areola. Li et al.[49] have described a case which required complex plastic surgery to obtain a satisfactory cosmetic result. It remains a very rare condition and it is likely that at least some of the confusion arises from misdiagnosis of a mammary duct fistula (see Ch. 11).

REFERENCES

1. van Deventer PV. The blood supply to the nipple-areola complex of the human mammary gland. *Aesthetic Plastic Surgery* 2004; **28**: 393–398.
2. Sarhadi NS, Shaw Dunn J, Lee FD et al. An anatomical study of the nerve supply of the breast, including the nipple and areola. *British Journal of Plastic Surgery* 1996; **49**: 156–164.
3. Haagensen CD. *Diseases of the Breast*, 3rd edn. Philadelphia: WB Saunders; 1986.
4. Koernecke IA. An anatomical study of the mammary gland twenty four hours post-partum. *American Journal of Obstetric Gynecology* 1934; **27**: 584–592.
5. Moffatt DF & Going JJ Three dimensional anatomy of complete duct systems in human breast – pathology and developmental implications. *Journal of Clinical Pathology* 1996; **49**: 48–52.
6. Love SM & Barsky SH. Anatomy of the nipple and breast ducts revisited. *Cancer* 2004 1; **101**: 1947–1957.
7. Alexander JM & Campbell MJ. Prevalence of inverted and non-protractile nipples in antenatal women who intend to breast feed. *Breast* 1997; **5**: 88–89.
8. Park HS, Yoon CH, & Kim HJ. The prevalence of congenital inverted nipple. *Aesthetic Plastic Surgery* 1999; **23**: 144–146.
9. Alexander JM, Grant AM & Campbell MJ. Randomised controlled trial of breast shells and Hoffman's exercises for inverted and non-protractile nipples. *British Medical Journal* 1992; **304**: 1030–1032.
10. Han S, Hong YG. The inverted nipple: its grading and surgical correction. *Plastic Reconstruction and Surgery* 1999; **104**: 389–395; discussion 396–397.
11. Bryant T. On the diagnostic value of the retracted nipple as a symptom of breast disease. *British Medical Journal* 1866; **2**: 635–637.
12. Gans B. Breast and nipple pain in early stages of lactation. *British Medical Journal* 1958; **2**: 830–832.
13. Gunther M. Sore nipples. Causes and prevention. *Lancet* 1945; **ii**: 590–593.
14. Livingstone V, Stringer LJ. The treatment of *Staphyloccocus aureus* infected sore nipples: a randomized comparative study. *Journal of Human Lactation* 2001; **17**: 115–117.
15. Alpsoy E, Yilmaz E & Aykol A. Hyperkeratosis of the nipple: report of two cases. *Journal of Dermatology* 1997; **24**: 43–45.
16. Azzopardi JG. *Problems in Breast Pathology*. London: WB Saunders; 1979.
17. Civatte J, Restout S & Delomenie D-C. Adenomatose erosive sur mamelon surnumeraire. *Annals Dermatologie et Venerologie* 1977; **104**: 777–779.
18. Perzin KH & Lattes R. Papillary adenoma of the nipple (florid papillomatosis, adenoma, adenomatosis). *Cancer* 1972; **29**: 996–1009.
19. Taylor HB & Robertson AG. Adenomas of the nipple. *Cancer* 1965; **18**: 995–1002.
20. Pinto RGW & Mandreker S. Fine needle aspiration cytology of adenoma of the nipple: a case report. *Acta Cytologica* 1996; **40**: 789–791.
21. Blamey RW (ed.) *Complications of Breast Surgery*. London: Baillière Tindall; 1986.
22. Rosen PP. Syringomatous adenoma of the nipple. *American Journal of Surgical Pathology* 1983; **7**: 739–745.
23. Carter E & Dyess DL. Infiltrating syringomatous adenoma of the nipple: a case report and 20-year retrospective review. *Breast Journal* 2004; **10**: 443–447.
24. Sanati S, Leonard M, Khamapirad T et al. Nodular mucinosis of the breast: a case report with pathologic,

ultrasonographic, and clinical findings and review of the literature. *Archives of Pathology and Laboratory Medicine* 2005; **129**: 58–61.

25. Hutchinson J. Polypoid outgrowths of the nipple areola. *Archives of Surgery*, London 1897; **8**: 37–39.

26. Paslin D. *Staphylococcus aureus* induction of inflammatory plaques of nipples and areolae. *American Academy of Dermatology* 1989; **20**: 932–934.

27. Aryal KR, Lengyel AJ, Purser N *et al.* Nipple core biopsy for the deformed or scaling nipple. *Breast* 2004; **13**: 350–352.

28. Levit F. Jogger's nipples. *New England Journal of Medicine* 1977; **297**: 1197.

29. Powell B. Bicyclist's nipples. *Journal of the American Medical Association* 1982; **249**: 2457.

30. Collins RE. Breast disease associated with tassel dancing. *British Medical Journal* 1981; **283**: 1660.

31. Healey T. Nipple piercings – unusual artefacts. *Radiography* 1979; **45**: 164–165.

32. Hood L. Raynaud's phenomenon of the nipple. *New Zealand Medical Journal* 1983; **84**: 294–295.

33. Gunther M. *Infant Feeding.* London: Methuen; 1972.

34. Lawlor-Smith L & Lawlor-Smith C. Vasospasm of the nipple – a manifestation of Raynaud's phenomenon: case reports. *British Medical Journal* 1997; **314**: 644–645.

35. Anderson JE, Held N & Wright K. Raynaud's phenomenon of the nipple: a treatable cause of painful breastfeeding. *Pediatrics* 2004; **113**: 360–364.

36. Reddy KR, Iskandarani M, Jeffers L *et al.* Bilateral nipple necrosis after vasopressin therapy. *Archives of Internal Medicine* 1984; **144**: 835–836.

37. Papay FA, Verghese A, Stanton-Hicks M *et al.* Complex regional pain syndrome of the breast in a patient after breast reduction. *Annals of Plastic Surgery* 1997; **39**: 347–352.

38. Stanton-Hicks M, Janig W, Hassenbusch S *et al.* Reflex sympathetic dystrophy: changing concepts and taxonomy. *Pain* 1995; **63**: 127–133.

39. Amir LH, Garland SM, Dennerstein L *et al. Candida albicans:* is it associated with nipple pain in lactating women? *Gynecologic and Obstetric Investigation* 1996; **41**: 30–34.

40. Kambarami RA & Kowo H. The prevalence of nipple disease among breast feeding mothers of HIV sero-positive infants. *Central African Journal of Medicine* 1997; **43**: 20–22.

41. Craigmyle MBL. *The Aprocrine Glands and the Breast.* Chichester: John Wiley & Sons; 1984.

42. Smith DM, Peters TG & Donegan WL. Montgomery's areolar tubercle. A light microscopic study. *Archives of Pathology and Laboratory Medicine* 1982; **106**: 60–63.

43. Heyman RB & Rauch JL. Areolar gland discharge in adolescent females. *Journal of Adolescent Health Care* 1983; **4**: 285–286.

44. Patey DH & Thackray AC. Pathology and the treatment of mammary duct fistula. *Lancet* 1958; **ii**: 871–873.

45. Fiumara NJ & Capek M. The brustwarze, or nipple ring. *Sexually Transmitted Disease* 1983; **9**: 138–139.

46. Carrahlo G. Molluscum contagiosum in a lesion adjacent to the nipple. Report of a case. *Acta Cytologica* (Baltimore) 1974; **18**: 532–534.

47. Quinn PT & Lofberg JV. Maternal herpetic breast infection: another hazard of neonatal herpes simplex. *Medical Journal of Australia* 1978; **2**: 411–412.

48. Wood C. Condyloma accuminatum of the nipple. *Journal of Cutaneous Pathology* 1978; **5**: 88–89.

49. Li EN, Mofid MM, Goldberg NH *et al.* Surgical management of hidradenitis suppurativa of the nipple–areolar complex. *Annals of Plastic Surgery* 2004; **52**: 220–223.

Nipple discharge

1. The visual assessment of the discharge is still of prime importance because it correlates with clinical significance.

2. Of the three groups, milk (galactorrhoea), coloured opalescent discharge and blood-related (serous, bloodstained and watery) discharge, only the third group carries a risk of serious breast disease.

3. Galactorrhoea is most commonly due to mechanical breast stimulation or drugs, and rarely to prolactinoma.

4. Blood-related discharge is usually due to papillary lesions (duct papilloma or carcinoma) or duct ectasia (DE).

5. Duct papillomas fall into three main categories: 'solitary' papilloma, in major ducts and with little malignant risk; multiple papillomas, in peripheral ducts with risk of recurrence and malignancy; and juvenile papillomatosis, a rare but distinctive condition.

6. Galactography is gaining popularity, in spite of few data on effectiveness – cost and therapeutic – with routine use.

7. Galactography is also combined with adjunctive techniques, such as hook-wire insertion, and ultrasound-guided fine needle aspiration (FNA) or percutaneous dye injection.

8. High-resolution ultrasound, fibreoptic ductography and intravenous enhanced MRI galactography appear to be promising developments.

9. Ductolobular segmental resection is sometimes an alternative to the standard operations of microdochectomy or major duct excision.

10. There is some evidence of increased risk of malignancy with benign papillomas, but not sufficient to warrant routine long-term follow-up.

Introduction

Nipple discharge is important when it occurs spontaneously and as the dominant symptom. Spontaneous presentation is important, because a high incidence will be recorded if milky discharge that occurs only following squeezing or expression of the breast is included in series of patients with nipple discharge. Such a discharge is common in parous women and will often be reported on direct questioning. This is not galactorrhoea and can be safely ignored.

Nipple discharge loses its significance when it is accompanied by a dominant lump. The lump then takes precedence in assessment and management.

A patient may present with discharge because she fears she may be developing malignancy, because the amount may be sufficient to cause social embarrassment, or as an incidental accompaniment of other breast symptoms. In general, the patient will delay no longer before presenting with discharge than with a lump.

Management will be directed at relieving the patient's concern regarding malignancy, and providing treatment for the minority of women who require treatment for the discharge itself. The ratio of patients falling into the two groups varies considerably in the literature because of different referral patterns and different views as to what constitutes discharge. For example, Gulay et al.[1] found that with an overall referral rate of 5%, the nipple discharge was spontaneous in only half; the other half had expressed the discharge themselves. In some African and Asian countries, nipple discharge accounts for a smaller proportion of referrals.[2]

Definition

Nipple discharge is defined as spontaneous efflux of fluid from the nipple apart from the physiological function of the puerperium and lactation. Discharge can be elicited by squeezing in about 20% of patients, and application of negative pressure with a pump can increase this to 50%.[3] Some patients report that nipple discharge follows mammography.

This chapter considers spontaneous nipple discharge in the absence of a dominant lump. In the latter case, the lump takes precedence in assessment and management. An associated discharge does not increase the likelihood of a mass being malignant at any age.[4]

Several conditions may simulate nipple discharge, especially skin exudate as from eczema of the nipple, and discharge from Montgomery's tubercles, seen particularly in adolescent girls.

Incidence

Nipple discharge is a relatively uncommon presenting complaint in a breast clinic. Devitt[5] has reviewed the literature of nipple discharge in breast clinics. About 5% of referrals are concerned with this symptom, and of these about 5% will prove to have cancer. Haagensen[6] reported that 3% of patients referred to him complained of nipple discharge. Our own experience is that 6.4% of referrals were for nipple discharge (Table 13.1). Since many of these cases fall outside the guidelines produced for general practitioner referrals to hospital in the UK[7] it seems likely that many are unnecessary. The guidelines recommend referral for cases in women over 50 years, for younger women with bloodstained discharge, and for persistent single duct discharge. The BRIDGE study group (1999)[8] in South Wales found that 5.5% of breast consultations,

in general practice, were for nipple discharge. Seltzer[9] reported an incidence of 9% in 10 000 self-referred patients.

Leis[10] reported that 7.4% of 8703 breast operations were performed for the indication of nipple discharge. In a study from Guy's Hospital over a 10-year period, 6.6% of referrals were for nipple discharge and of the 6000 operations performed 4.5% related to treatment of nipple discharge.[11]

Character and significance of discharge

The character of the discharge should be recorded accurately, as a good correlation exists between macroscopic appearance and underlying pathology (Table 13.2). Failure to be specific has led to confusion in much of the literature.

Table 13.1 Diagnosis and type of discharge

Referred cases	4012
Nipple discharge	259 (6.4%)
Cancer	14: 57% bloody
Duct papilloma	15: 60% bloody
Duct ectasia	87: 17% bloody

Table 13.2 Relationship of discharge type and pathological diagnosis

Type of discharge	Main cause	Less common cause
Blood-related Bloody	Hyperplastic lesions[a]	Duct ectasia, pregnancy
Serous	Hyperplastic lesions	Duct ectasia
Watery	Hyperplastic lesions	Duct ectasia
Coloured opalescent	Duct ectasia	Cyst
Milk	Physiological	Galactorrhoea of endocrine origin

[a]Hyperplastic lesions include hyperplasia, papilloma, carcinoma in situ and invasive ductal carcinoma.

Nipple discharge can be assigned to one of four groups:

- Physiological galactorrhoea
- Secondary galactorrhoea
- Coloured opalescent (or grumous)
- Serosanguineous and watery.

Only the last carries a risk of serious breast disease. The commoner causes of the different types of discharge are given in Table 13.3.

Galactorrhoea

The thin, off-white, modestly opalescent quality of human milk is characteristic. There is a 'grey' area between milk and the thicker creamy discharge of duct ectasia (DE), but it is not commonly difficult to distinguish the two.

Physiological galactorrhoea

Galactorrhoea is defined as milk secretion unrelated to breastfeeding. Many patients complaining of milky discharge are suffering from physiological rather than pathological conditions. Pathology within the breast is so rarely the cause of the discharge within this group that the cause should be sought elsewhere.

Milk production may continue long after lactation has ceased and a regular menstrual cycle has been re-established. This discharge is usually bilateral and may occasionally be copious. It is of no pathological significance and is usually due to stimulation of the breast by continued maternal attempts at expression. This is sometimes carried out in the belief that it will prevent further milk production, or that milk should not be allowed to lie in the breast. Milk discharge may result from mechanical stimulation of the breasts during sexual activity, especially in young girls. Milky discharge associated with other mechanical forms of stimulation is occasionally encountered, explaining the anecdotal reports of successful breastfeeding in the absence of prior pregnancy, and even reports of successful suckling by men!

Treatment is by reassurance and explanation of the sequence of events, that the condition is self-limiting and that cessation of expression or other mechanical stimulation will allow resolution. Occasionally, physiological milk discharge is seen at the extremes of reproductive life. At the menarche, during the period of rapid breast development, and at the menopause, squeezing of the breasts

Table 13.3 Causes of nipple discharge

| | Bloody | Blood related | | Opalescent | Milk |
		Serous	Watery		
PHYSIOLOGICAL					
Neonatal	–	–	–	–	+
Lactation	–	–	–	–	+
Pregnancy	±	–	–	–	+
Postlactational	–	–	–	–	+
Mechanical stimulation	–	–	–	–	+
Hyperprolactinaemia	–	–	–	–	+
DUCTAL PATHOLOGY					
Duct ectasia	±	±	±	+	–
Cysts	–	–	–	+	–
Papilloma	+	+	±	–	–
Cancer	+	+	±	–	–

+, common or likely cause; ±, rare but well defined; –, unusual or unknown.

may produce small quantities of fluid. Again, explanation and reassurance are all that is required.

The appearance of 'witch's milk' in the neonate has been dealt with in Chapter 3 and is due to the transplacental transport of maternal lactogenic hormones.

Secondary galactorrhoea

The appearance of a milky discharge is occasionally seen apart from the conditions mentioned above. A careful history and examination will usually reveal the cause (Table 13.4).

These causes are mostly related to those situations in which there is an increase in the levels of circulating prolactin. The important causes are prolactinoma and various drugs. Vorherr[12] reviewed the literature and gives a list of 17 causes of galactorrhoea. It is likely that some of these are in reality pituitary microadenomas secreting prolactin, a condition which was unrecognized at the time of the original descriptions. The diagnosis of prolactinoma is suggested by the history of galactorrhoea, amenorrhoea

Table 13.4 Causes of galactorrhoea

PHYSIOLOGICAL

   Mechanical stimulation
   Extremes of reproductive life (puberty, menopause)
   Postlactational
   Stress

DRUGS

Association with hyperprolactinaemia
   Dopamine receptor-blocking agents
      Phenothiazines, e.g. chlorpromazine
      Haloperidol
      Metoclopramide, domperidone
   Dopamine-depleting agents
      Reserpine
      Methyldopa
Others
   Oestrogen (including the contraceptive pill)
   Opiates

PATHOLOGICAL

   Hypothalamic and pituitary stalk lesions
   Pituitary tumours
      Adenoma
      Microadenoma

MISCELLANEOUS

   Ectopic prolactin secretion (e.g. bronchogenic carcinoma)
   Hypothyroidism
   Chronic renal failure

and relative infertility. If the tumour is large, expansion of the pituitary fossa, and possible erosion of the floor of the sella, may be seen on radiography and help to confirm the diagnosis. More often the lesions are microadenomas and skull radiology is normal. Diagnosis is then dependent on dynamic hormonal studies of prolactin, and on imaging of the pituitary fossa. The galactorrhoea disappears following appropriate treatment with a dopamine agonist such as bromocriptine or cabergolamine.[13] Surgical removal of the adenoma may be indicated in some patients.[14]

Drug-induced galactorrhoea is not uncommon and occurs with a number of tranquillizing agents, particularly of the phenothiazine group, oral contraceptives and antihypertensives as well as drugs which have a direct action on the hypothalamic–pituitary axis such as domperidone and metoclopramide.[15] The mechanism of action of some of these changes is obscure. Drugs which have been implicated in the production of galactorrhoea are listed in Table 13.4.

In clinical practice, quite gross galactorrhoea can occur for which no cause can be found on extensive investigation, or on long-term follow-up.

Coloured opalescent discharges

It is generally agreed that all coloured opalescent discharges, after sanguineous discharges and milk have been excluded, may be put into a single group in relation to significance. In particular, they are associated with no increased cancer risk. Such discharges are common in late reproductive life, often intermittent, sometimes persisting and occasionally very profuse. Multiple ducts of one or both breasts are often involved and with discharge of differing appearance from individual ducts. They show a wide range of colours and consistency from a creamy purulent appearance through yellow, brown, green and black. In general, the brown, green and black discharges tend to be of fluid consistency, the creamy discharge is more grumous, sometimes as thick as toothpaste (see Fig. 11.4). The coloured discharges resemble the range of appearances seen in cyst fluid (see Fig. 10.3).

When a pathological entity can be defined, this is most commonly due to duct ectasia (see Ch. 11). At operation for DE, it is noticeable that some ducts are of normal calibre and others dilated, while the material in adjacent dilated ducts of the same breast will be of widely differing appearance; creamy, brown and green material may be seen in the same patient.

Nipple discharge associated with DE is dealt with further in Chapter 11.

In some cases, nipple discharge is clearly due to cysts; occasionally, a ductogram for nipple discharge will show the dye entering a cyst from the duct (Fig. 13.1). Other circumstantial evidence in support of this view comes from patients who relate the appearance of nipple discharge to the disappearance of a previously palpable lump, sometimes during mammography.

Coloured discharges are usually readily distinguished from sanguineous ones, but where a brownish discharge causes difficulty a urine dipstick to test for blood is helpful.

Composition of coloured opalescent discharges

Ogan et al.[16] have studied the biochemical nature of these discharges. They found that nipple discharge fluid usually contained casein, suggesting that such discharges are derived from glandular epithelium secreting milk. Petrakis et al.[17] have measured nipple aspirates for the presence of GCDFP-15, a marker for apocrine metaplasia. GCDFP-15 was found in all but one of 115 women. This suggests that gross cystic disease fluid and nipple duct fluid have a similar composition and therefore a common origin. Petrakis et al.[18] extensively studied nipple aspirates from both asymptomatic women and those with benign breast disease. They found no difference in the constitution with respect to lactose, Na^+, K^+ and colour; they did, however, find changes that were age related. Lactose concentrations fell with age while the discharges became darker. In a previous study, Petrakis et al.[19] considered that the colour was likely to be due to pigmented products of apocrine gland secretion, lipofuscin complexes of peroxidated lipoprotein and breakdown products of haemoglobin. Interestingly, they also showed a positive correlation between smoking and dark colour of discharge.

Blood and serosanguineous discharge

Serous discharge is characterized by the yellow colour and sticky quality of serum (Fig. 13.2). Serous, serosanguineous (pink) (Fig. 13.3) and heavily blood-stained discharges (Fig. 13.4) carry the same significance.

Such discharge is due either to a hyperplastic epithelial lesion or to duct ectasia. The epithelial hyperplasia is usually benign, one or more duct papillomas, less commonly malignant. The risk of malignancy increases with age, being much greater after 55 years than before the menopause. In the original series of Selzer et al.[4] the overall incidence of cancer in patients presenting only with nipple discharge was 12%. The incidence of cancer was 3% in patients under the age of 40, 10% between 40 and 60 and 32% for patients over 60 years.

In patients with duct ectasia, it is assumed that the bleeding arises from areas of ulceration within the stagnant ducts, although we are not aware of any formal study of this question.

In many series, a percentage of cases with sanguineous discharge show no clear-cut pathology, even after operations such as major duct excision. Hence, it is not surprising that conditions of low specificity in pathological terms have been invoked to explain the bloody discharge. Older series often specify cystic disease as the cause. Some seem to refer to macroscopic cysts, others to the micropapillomatosis element that we now regard as part of aberrations of normal development and involution (ANDI). With these conditions that are part of the spectrum of normality, specificity as to the cause of bleeding is suspect, and the same must be true of a condition as common as DE, the diagnosis we believe to be most common. Hence, the cause of some serosanguineous discharges must remain uncertain, even after surgery. At least the satisfactory long-term follow-up of such cases shows that they are not associated with significant pathology that has been missed at surgery.

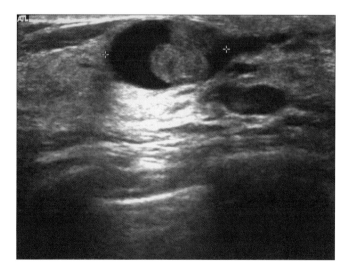

Fig. 13.1 Intraductal papillomata; ultrasound image of two small papillomata within a distended duct close to the nipple; patient presented with discharge.

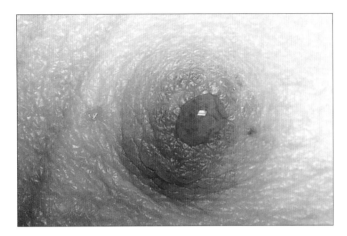

Fig. 13.2 Serous discharge, showing the characteristic straw colour.

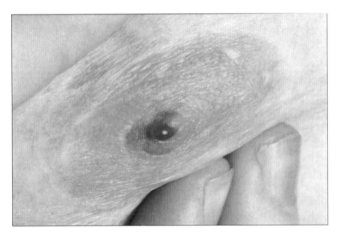

Fig. 13.3 Serosanguineous discharge, due to a duct papilloma, with characteristic pink colour.

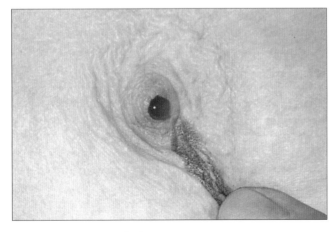

Fig. 13.4 Dark bloody discharge.

Haagensen's experience with serous and bloody discharge showed an identical significance for both types.[6] Duct papilloma was the cause in 70% and breast cancer in 10%, with both types of discharge. Likewise, 50% of benign papillomas presented with each type of discharge, and cancer cases with nipple discharge were divided evenly between the two. In the Philadelphia series the incidence of cancer was also the same for serous or bloody discharge.[4] Our experience is similar, although a higher proportion (29%) of our cases of serous or bloody discharge is associated with DE.

Chaudary et al.[11] have described the role of routine use of an occult blood test in patients admitted for operation for discharge from a solitary duct. In 292 microdochectomies, 215 were positive for blood. All 16 carcinomas were in this group but, in the benign conditions, the presence of blood did not usefully help to distinguish DE from benign papillomas.

Postsurgery nipple discharge

Lee et al.[20] draw attention to spontaneous nipple discharge that appears shortly after breast surgery. It can be due to communication with the operation site, or to a second undiagnosed pathology. Galactography was helpful in demonstrating a communication with the operation site, and the discharge subsequently ceased spontaneously.

Blood-stained nipple discharge of pregnancy

A little-recognized problem that occurs occasionally in pregnancy is bloodstained nipple discharge due to epithelial proliferation as the breasts respond to pregnancy. At term, the proliferation ceases, the cells swell and develop into secretory cells under hormonal control from prolactin, and milk is produced.

This bloodstained discharge is typically bilateral, as have been the cases in our experience, but can be unilateral, when it occurs in the larger of the two breasts.[21] It usually starts in the second or third trimester of the first or second pregnancy. When bilateral, the condition carries no serious significance and requires simple explanation and reassurance that it is self-limiting. It rarely persists for more than 2 months postpartum.[22] Further investigation and treatment should be avoided because cytology may be misleading in this situation. It often shows epithelial cell clusters similar to those of intraductal papilloma and the cells may appear to be cytologically active.[23] As it is self-limiting and disappears with breastfeeding, firm reassurance is all that is required.

It has been suggested recently that bloodstained discharge from a single breast during pregnancy should also be managed expectantly. Lafreniere[21] has reviewed the literature and found no example where this symptom has led to a subsequent diagnosis of cancer. This is reassuring, although clinical judgement should be exercised in a unilateral case. Breast examination and monitoring with ultrasound might be wise.

Watery discharge

This is a rare but very distinctive type of discharge (Fig. 13.5) which carries the same significance as serous or bloodstained discharge.

Why a blood-related discharge should be watery rather than serous is not obvious. It is crystal clear, copious and associated in our experience in four cases with multiple papillomas of the large ducts: with macroscopic papillomas in one case and with florid microscopic papillomatosis in the others. As yet, none has developed cancer (after 5 years of follow-up). Haagensen believes the large papilloma condition to be premalignant, although he could only record one such case, which was associated with papillary intraduct cancer. We have also had a case where the only pathology on duct excision was a gross degree of DE. Lewison and Chambers[24] present evidence that this type of discharge is associated with breast cancer and Leis[10] found cancer in a third of 15 cases with watery discharge.

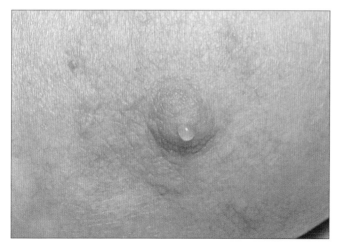

Fig. 13.5 Clear watery discharge, distinct from serous and sanguineous.

Pathology underlying nipple discharge

Duct papilloma

Benign duct papillomas occur in three main forms: solitary (discrete) duct papilloma, multiple duct papillomas and juvenile papilloma. These are three reasonably discrete clinicopathological complexes, but because of overlapping features, these terms are not ideal in terms of descriptiveness or specificity. For example, 'solitary' duct papilloma is often multiple. However, these are the terms proposed by Haagensen, who was primarily responsible for defining the three conditions. As these are now in general use and we cannot suggest better terms, we retain them. Being familiar with, and understanding, the three clinicopathological pictures and their implications is the priority, so that a patient can be put into the appropriate group.

It is also important to differentiate these macroscopic lesions from the microscopic papillary hyperplasia often referred to in the past as papillomatosis in the American literature, and as hyperplasia or epitheliosis (without atypia) in the British literature. This latter condition, part of ANDI, is not related to the duct papillomas described here.

In summary, discrete 'solitary' papillomas are the most common of the three; they occur in a large subareolar duct, frequently cause blood-related nipple discharge, and have little malignant potential. Multiple papillomas are rare, more peripheral, less likely to cause nipple discharge and have greater malignant potential. Juvenile papillomatosis is an exceedingly rare condition with yet another clinical picture.

Solitary (discrete) duct papilloma

The commonest hyperplastic lesion causing a serous or sanguineous discharge is discrete duct papilloma: single or multiple. The defining feature is its occurrence in a large duct. In about half the cases, the discharge is bloody; in the other half it is serous. A subareolar lump is palpable in less than half of the cases. The history is sometimes a long one; the discharge may have been present for several years.

The typical ductal papilloma is just 2–3 mm in diameter (Fig. 13.6), but as it grows it elongates and extends along the duct system so that it may be 1 cm or more in length.

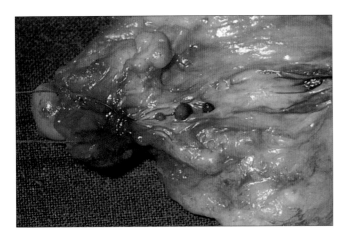

Fig. 13.6 Microdochectomy specimen opened to show three small duct papillomas.

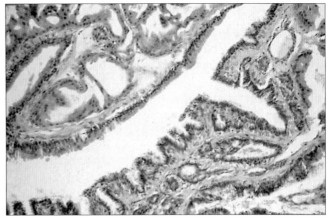

Fig. 13.8 Histology of benign large duct papilloma showing the typical core vascular stroma with covering epithelium.

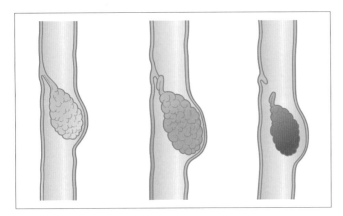

Fig. 13.7 Schematic representation of torsion and infarction of a duct papilloma.

Larger papillomas tend to cause, and lie within, a local pocketing of the duct, a diverticulum which alters the normal line of the duct. Fine probes passed into the duct tend to get side-tracked into these diverticula. The papilloma has a narrow, fragile stalk and delicate fronds. The narrow stalk predisposes to torsion, which may result in infarction and this is not uncommonly seen on histology. It is presumably the reason why bloody discharge frequently remits spontaneously, particularly in young women. The sequence of events is summarized in Figure 13.7.

The delicate fronds account for the marked tendency to haemorrhage. As the papilloma elongates and grows along the duct, torsion becomes less likely but partial ischaemia may lead to fibrosis and adhesion to the duct wall, making differentiation from papillary carcinoma

more difficult. Some authorities believe this to be the origin of ductal adenoma. Typical small lesions have many fronds with a fibrovascular core and a covering of regular epithelium, although mitoses may be quite frequent (Fig. 13.8).

Although a well-known lesion, solitary papilloma is relatively uncommon. There were only 15 'solitary' duct papilloma cases in the 259 nipple discharge patients in our Cardiff study and the figure of 29% of operations for nipple discharge is similar to the 37% of operations for nipple discharge described by Leis.[10] Most papillomas appear in the fourth to sixth decades with a peak age incidence in the fifth decade. However, it has a wide range of age incidence and we have seen it at the age of 16 and in an octogenarian. Sandison,[25] in his postmortem study of 800 women, found an incidence of duct papilloma of 1.6%. This suggests that many papillomas go undetected through life.

The usual location of a duct papilloma is in the subareolar major ducts, within 5 cm of the nipple. Macroscopic papillomas are usually solitary, but it is not uncommon to find two or three distinct papillomas in the one segment of duct (see Fig. 13.6). In fact this is commoner than most reports suggest, and depends on the assiduousness with which the duct is dissected (and the state of the specimen presented to the pathologist!). This is also the reason why the term 'solitary' papilloma is not entirely appropriate; perhaps 'discrete' is a better term since each is a small discrete lesion as seen in Figure 13.6.

In older patients there may be 10 or more such lesions distributed throughout the larger ducts of a single segment, with the whole segmental system distended to its periphery. But the papillomas remain small, discrete and with benign histology, and so represent the extreme of the spectrum of 'solitary' papilloma. They are still better included in the 'solitary' group than the 'multiple papilloma' group, which has a different clinicopathological picture, as discussed below.

Duct papillomas are sometimes bilateral. Seven of the 173 cases reported in Haagensen's series[6] were bilateral, and bilateral involvement was simultaneous in one case. In the remainder, the average time to presentation in the opposite breast was 8 years.

Solitary intraduct papilloma is not usually considered to be premalignant. Many recent studies have shown no increased incidence of cancer, but it must be admitted that there is a paucity of sound long-term follow-up data. The American College of Pathologists (ACP) consensus statement[26] puts papilloma with a fibrovascular core in the group with a slightly increased risk of cancer.

Occasionally, a papilloma develops in the terminal subareolar duct, when it may distend the nipple or prolapse through the duct orifice on to the nipple. When this occurs, usually in an elderly patient, it requires separation from a distinct entity, erosive papillomatosis (see Ch. 12). The characteristic feature of a prolapsed ductal papilloma is that the surface of the nipple is unaffected. With erosive papillomatosis, the nipple itself is eroded. Haagensen[6] gives clear guidelines for distinguishing the two.

Multiple duct papillomas

The term 'multiple duct papilloma' is better reserved for the uncommon condition of papillomas occurring in small peripheral ducts. They occur in a ratio of about one case to eight cases of solitary, large duct papilloma. They are more commonly palpable, more peripheral in the breast, more likely to be bilateral and less likely to give rise to nipple discharge than the 'solitary' or discrete type. The condition is of such rarity that few have a significant experience of it, and it is difficult to be certain that the small series reported are homogeneous with regard to the type of cases included.

A distinctive group described in detail by Haagensen differed from common experience in that almost all were large enough to be palpable and clustered together with obvious multiplicity. Haagensen[6] described 53 examples of this condition and found the mean age to be slightly younger than those with solitary papilloma though with a similar age range of 20 to 70+. A tumour was usually palpable with a diameter >2 cm, only a quarter were central compared with 90% of 'solitary' lesions, while local recurrence and subsequent carcinoma were respectively 15 and 3 times as common. For this reason, Haagensen considered this lesion to be premalignant, and 15 of his 39 patients developed carcinoma. In general, both benign local recurrence and subsequent malignancy occurred in the same segment of the breast as the original lesion, but this was not always the case. Nevertheless, Haagensen advises a conservative approach, reserving mastectomy (somewhat reluctantly) for multiple recurrences.

In more recent reports, cases have been diagnosed earlier, when tumours are smaller and less likely to be palpable than cases reported by Haagensen, but the implications are similar. Thus, a subclinical variant where tumours are less likely to be palpable may be a halfway house between intraduct cancer and Haagensen's palpable benign tumours. The smaller lesions have common features with the larger ones: multiplicity, peripheral location (often in continuity with the terminal ductal lobular unit, TDLU), and a distinct association with cancer. Because these lesions are uncommon, and reported series are retrospective or of few cases, it is difficult to put together a coherent picture. However, there is a general uniformity regarding a high recurrence rate after local excision, the presence of atypical hyperplasia in association with the lesions,[27–29] and a considerable subsequent incidence of cancer. Haagensen's series probably included cases of juvenile papillomatosis, which was a less well-defined entity before the publication by Rosen et al.[30]

In our small experience, this syndrome was associated with a watery discharge, and the tumours involved multiple breast segments. It seems likely that this is often a multisegmental system, in contrast to the unisegmental single duct system involved by 'solitary' papillomas, and this is at least part of the reason for the high local recurrence rate. For this reason it has seemed appropriate to us to advise local mastectomy, with immediate reconstruction where desired, but a more segmental resection seems reasonable where the pathology appears to be well localized.

Juvenile papillomatosis (Swiss cheese disease)

Although most patients with this condition present with a lump rather than nipple discharge it is convenient to consider it here because of its relationship to multiple papillomatosis and doubt about the distinction of these conditions. Nipple discharge has been described in 15% of cases of juvenile papillomatosis. The clinical diagnosis is often fibroadenoma, because of the age of the patient, and the first suggestion of the diagnosis may come when fine needle aspiration (FNA) produces watery fluid.

Haagensen first described eight patients with multiple intraductal papillomas which were unusual in that they were palpable, occurred in young women (age 14–24) and in which the epithelium was entirely apocrine in nature. He treated all cases by local excision without recurrence.[6]

Rosen and colleagues reported a collected series of 32 cases, and applied the term 'Swiss cheese disease' because of the multicystic nature of the masses.[30] They started a registry for these cases, and in 1985 gave a further report.[31] The patients were a little older than Haagensen's group (mean age 23 years) and typically presented with multiple small masses (1–3 cm) in the upper outer quadrant, sometimes bilateral, and because of the age group, were usually diagnosed as having fibroadenomas. The first suggestion that this might not be so was the finding of watery fluid on FNA. There was a family history of breast cancer in 25% of cases.

Macroscopically, the tumours are firm, cystic swellings with a circumscribed margin, but not enough to shell out at operation. Histology showed benign proliferative epithelium with half the cases showing a degree of histological atypia which would be regarded as precancerous in an older patient. The term papillomatosis is used in the American sense of 'epitheliosis'; it does not show a papillomatous structure with a central stromal core. A third paper reported follow-up of 41 patients after a mean period of 14 years.[32] In this group 58% had a family history (usually mother or maternal aunt) and six of 41 were bilateral. Ten per cent had developed breast cancer, and all of these had bilateral and recurrent papillomas and a family history of breast cancer. So those without these features seem to be at low risk. Complete excision with a small margin is recommended management at present, although recurrence does not seem to show a close relationship to clearance margins. Annual surveillance and breast self-examination are recommended for most cases, with more intensive follow-up for the high-risk cases (bilateral/recurrent/family history).

Papillary carcinoma

Papillary carcinoma is the usual type of malignancy associated with nipple discharge. However, most papillary carcinomas do not present in this way. Only 26% of Haagensen's cases presented with a nipple discharge; in 80% it was sanguineous or serosanguineous, and in the remaining 20% the discharge was serous. This diagnosis becomes much more likely over the age of 50 than in younger patients, and forms a continuum with the second type of multiple papilloma described above. This condition is outside the scope of this text but an excellent description can be found in Haagensen's textbook.[6]

Duct ectasia

Duct ectasia may give rise to blood-related discharges as well as the typical cream/brown/green/black colours. It is uncommon for more than a few of the ducts to be affected. The ducts are usually about 2–5 mm in diameter, often very thin walled but sometimes become thick walled. The discharge varies in consistency from thin to thick to grumous (toothpaste-like), which has to be squeezed out, and the colour is usually creamy coloured but is often brown or greenish. Analysis of the discharge shows fatty crystals and large foamy macrophages and much amorphous cell debris. Pigmented cells termed 'ochrocytes' by Davies[33] are also presumed to be macrophages which have ingested the ceroids produced by degeneration of the fatty material in the ducts which gives this type of discharge its wide variety of colour.

It is not always realized that duct ectasia is also a common cause of blood-related discharge, both serous and bloodstained. It is presumed that this arises from small ulcerated areas of duct mucosa. We have also had a case with profuse watery discharge which required major duct excision, and no pathology was found in the specimen except markedly dilated ducts.

The pathology is dealt with in detail in Chapter 11.

Cysts and 'fibrocystic disease'

It is uncertain how commonly cysts are the cause of nipple discharge. They are undoubtedly responsible in some cases, because injection for nipple discharge may show the duct communicating with the cyst (see Fig. 10.9). Sometimes aspiration of the cyst will be followed immediately by discharge of similar material through the nipple; presumably, release of intracystic tension allows the draining duct to open. Occasionally, the nipple discharge is elicited during mammography. The frequency of multiple duct involvement with coloured opalescent discharge suggests that DE is a more common cause than cyst, as does the frequency of ectatic ducts at operation where this type of discharge has been seen.

The situation is confused by the fact that cysts have often been regarded in the past as a variant of DE, with both being merely a part of the spectrum of 'fibrocystic disease', especially in the American literature. It is now well demonstrated that cysts arise from lobules, and have a different pathogenesis from DE.

Many series also describe 'fibrocystic disease' as the cause of up to 25% of blood-related discharge. There is no obvious explanation as to the underlying pathogenesis, and since this is no more than part of the spectrum of normality, the possibility that a conservative microdochectomy may have missed the true cause should be considered. With full preoperative evaluation of the patient, including fibreoptic ductoscopy in selected cases, negative histological findings at duct excision become less frequent.[34]

Nipple discharge in children and adolescents

Duct papilloma is occasionally seen in the later teenage years, but 'nipple' discharge in the earlier years is more likely to come from the surface of the nipple or from the areola. The commonest cause is probably related to Montgomery's tubercles.[35,36] The discharge may be clear to brown or bloody, with an associated lump. The discharge usually resolves spontaneously over a few weeks, but the lump may take several months to resolve. The cause is not obvious, but may be related to trauma to the duct orifice, since irritating clothing is another cause of nipple discharge in this age group.[37] We have also seen bloody discharge from Montgomery's tubercle in an adolescent with no underlying pathology. Again, the probable cause was trauma. Rogerson et al.[38] have reported on 16 cases of adolescent areolar discharge but found that in some surgical excision was necessary.

In children under the age of 5, duct ectasia is well recognized, and probably the most common cause of bloody discharge in this age group.[39] It is associated with a mass, the histology of which shows cystically dilated ducts with thickened walls and containing acellular material with cholesterol clefts, and blood. The duct lining shows focal ulceration and granulation tissue. Most settle spontaneously, although this may take months. It is particularly important to avoid surgery in young girls; otherwise breast development may be compromised.

Assessment

History

The history will cover duration, frequency, associated symptoms (pain, lump and nipple inversion) and precipitating causes. Careful questioning will usually reveal the nature of the discharge, its spontaneity and whether single or multiple duct openings are involved. Note should be made of menstrual irregularities and medication, particularly oral contraception in young women and hormone replacement therapy in older women. In women with a milky discharge, particular attention needs to be paid to previous lactation, breastfeeding and history of mechanical stimulation of the breast.

Physical examination

A useful sequence is as follows:

- Inspection should reveal whether discharge is from a solitary duct (and, if so, which duct) or from multiple ducts, and the colour and nature of the fluid. It is usually most convenient for the patient to express a little fluid herself while the physician watches. Where discharge is scant, a magnifying glass may be useful. Where no discharge is produced, inspection of the brassiere may reveal sufficient staining to determine whether or not it is sanguineous.
- Palpate slowly and systematically around the areola to determine where pressure will produce discharge and which duct is involved. If this is successful, a smear may be taken for cytology. When the segment has been localized, feel carefully for a palpable mass or dilated duct, especially under the areola. By pinching the areola between finger and thumb an assessment of the bulk of the ductal tissue can be made and the two sides compared.
- Careful standard examination of both breasts and axillae.

Investigations

Mammography

Mammography is advisable in all patients over 35 years with nipple discharge, and particularly so where the discharge is serous, bloody or watery. The most important finding is microcalcification along the line of ducts as it may draw attention to an otherwise unsuspected intraduct carcinoma. Prominent ducts may be noted together with the coarse, large calcifications which are typical of duct ectasia (see Fig. 11.19).

Galactography

Small papillomas may be demonstrated by cannulation of the duct and injection with contrast material (or by a percutaneous, ultrasound-guided technique if the duct cannot be cannulated[40]) but false positives and false negatives are not uncommon, in spite of some series reporting a strong correlation between radiological and pathological findings.

Debris or blood clot may masquerade as papillomas, while others may be missed in dilated ducts. Baker et al.[41] found that 20% of lesions seen on galactography could not be found in the pathology specimen. Duct injection is distinctly uncomfortable for the patient and, for this combination of reasons, we do not use the procedure as a routine investigation. It rarely alters management, but it does have a role in unusual or difficult cases. Ultrasound-guided FNA can be used to obtain cytology of a lesion demonstrated on galactography, and Sardanelli et al. found this twice as accurate as nipple discharge cytology.[42]

An extension of the technique is to insert a Kopan's spring-hookwire into the duct at galactography, to facilitate locating a lesion at surgery.[43] These authors found the technique satisfactory in 29 of 34 patients; in the other five the wire was dislodged.

Another option is to inject methylene blue into the duct at the time of galactography, to aid the identification of the affected duct system.[44] This requires galactography to be scheduled on the day of surgery to give maximum effectiveness. A bloody discharge will outline the duct without methylene blue, which can also cause problems if accidental damage to the duct leads to extravasation of the dye into the wound. For this reason, we advocate that no attempt should be made to elicit the discharge in the 24 hours prior to surgery.

In a comparative study of three-dimensional magnetic resonance imaging, ultrasound and galactography in 55 patients Nakahara et al.[45] found three patients with malignant lesions that were not identified by galactography. The optimum role for galactography remains uncertain.

Ultrasound

In our experience ultrasound has a limited role in assessment of nipple discharge. It may be used to amplify information about palpable or radiological abnormalities defined during initial assessment. Ultrasound can demonstrate dilated subareolar ducts. In the study of Nakahara et al.[45] ultrasound correlated less well with eventual pathological diagnosis than three-dimensional magnetic resonance imaging.

Fibreoptic ductography

A silica fibrescope of 0.48 mm diameter enables the breast ducts to be directly visualized.[46,47] Small intraduct carcinomas, intraduct papillomas and other benign lesions can be seen. Pereira and Mokbel[48] have reviewed the history and likely future developments of this technique, which can be performed as an office procedure under local anaesthetic. While it is an attractive concept it is not yet clear that it offers significant advantage over other diagnostic techniques such as helical computed tomography.[49] We have no experience of this technique but it would appear to offer an ability to refine the preoperative diagnosis in some cases of bloodstained nipple discharge.[50]

Exfoliative cytology

Cytological examination of nipple discharge has been used for a long time: the first report of diagnosing a carcinoma by this technique was in 1914.[51] This investigation will sometimes indicate intraduct carcinoma as the cause of the discharge. However, there are too many false negatives for it to be regarded as a completely reliable investigation. For example, Kjellogren[52] found a 16% false-negative and a 4% false-positive rate. Aspiration cytology of any associated mass is obviously appropriate (see Ch. 5) and is considered more reliable.[53]

Groves et al.[54] have carried out an audit of nipple discharge cytology and found that although the test has a low sensitivity for carcinoma (46.5%) it does have a high specificity (99.5%). They conclude that this approach is of limited value but in view of the ease with which it may be performed it should not be discarded completely. Dunn et al.[55] reviewed a 12-year experience in Bristol and found similar sensitivity (55%) and specificity (100%) rates. Two cancers in this series were diagnosed by cytology alone. This investigation is particularly appropriate for patients with blood-related discharge.

An expanded approach to exfoliative cytology is directed at samples obtained by suction rather than those of spontaneous discharge. Wrensch et al. have studied the factors affecting ability to obtain cytological specimens by suction.[56] Specimens are more likely to be obtained during ages 35–50 years, from women with an early menarche, non-Asian patients (versus Asian) and those with a history of lactation (parity alone has no effect). King et al.[3] have shown that it is possible to identify atypical cells as well as those which are unequivocally malignant. However, satisfactory specimens were obtained in less than half of the patients they studied so the value of this technique in routine practice is limited. Because of the very active epithelium in pregnancy, false positives are particularly likely at that time. In a study of 1948 nipple aspirates Gupta et al.[57] found that 624 had benign cells, 492 were inadequate, 96 were inflammatory, 229 showed papilloma, 22 were suspicious and 67 malignant. The authors concluded that the technique was reasonably specific for malignant disease but it is worth noting that there were two false positives in their 67 malignant cytology (a woman with a fibroadenoma and a man with florid gynaecomastia). It would seem prudent to obtain confirmatory evidence of the diagnosis before proceeding to definitive treatment. Another route to increased cellular material for examination is ductal lavage;[58] while this technique has been used in association with fibreoptic ductoscopy it remains to be seen if it is helpful in routine practice.[59] One problem with this approach is that atypical cells identified on one examination may not be elicited on subsequent tests. For example, when Johnson-Maddux et al.[60] repeated the ductal lavage in 23 patients with atypia on cytology, 13 (52%) had normal cytology on repeat lavage. They conclude that atypia may be artefactual or physiological in many instances.

Cytology may be helpful in confirming duct ectasia, especially when it is associated with periductal mastitis. Large foamy macrophages with few, if any, epithelial cells are typically seen.

In conclusion, we regard cytology of the discharge as useful in those over 35 years old, but as with other tests for malignancy, negative results should be ignored. Sometimes a positive cytology is the sole positive investigation in the assessment of a patient with serosanguineous discharge.

Occult blood testing

In most cases it is easy to determine from the fluid whether it is bloodstained or not. Where there is doubt, use of a Clinistix paper applied to the discharge will give a rapid answer.

Other biochemical tests

Tests for various enzymes and biological markers in the discharge have been described, but cannot yet be regarded as sufficiently discriminatory to enter routine clinical use. An example is that of Inaji et al.,[61] who used the combination of Erb-2 and CEA levels to detect cancer, though with some false-positive results with benign proliferative lesions. Sauter et al.[62] have developed a predictive model based on clinical findings and the results of a proteomic analysis of nipple aspirate fluid. Such an approach might be of value in those patients in whom a definitive diagnosis of the cause of nipple discharge cannot be obtained by conventional investigations.

Management

The importance of accurate assessment of the nature of the discharge cannot be overestimated, since most patients will have benign disease and can be reassured, some with and some without, investigation. Coloured, opalescent discharges are very common, and can be treated expectantly, as can any discharge which cannot be reproduced in a young woman. Similarly, most galactorrhoea can be ignored if a specific endocrine cause is excluded. Most such discharges will stop spontaneously, and firm reassurance that cancer has been excluded will be satisfactory for most patients. A minority will dislike the discharge so much that they wish to have it stopped even though it carries no serious import. The only reliable method of achieving this is complete division of the duct system, and this procedure is described in Chapter 18. We have no experience of blocking the offending ducts with fibrin as described by Hockel and Klose[63] nor can we find any further reports of this technique.

The management of the blood-related group of discharges is more contentious. If cancer can be confidently excluded then an expectant management policy can be followed. The gamut of investigations outlined above now means that diagnostic surgery is rarely required.

Treatment can thus be aimed at securing symptomatic relief.

This is a far cry from recent conventional practice and it is useful to consider the approach to management of nipple discharge from an historical perspective as the philosophy of management of serous or serosanguineous discharge has changed radically. Opinion regarding the likelihood of it being due to cancer was sharply divided early in the twentieth century. Judd,[64] in 1917, reported a 57% incidence of cancer in 100 cases at the Mayo Clinic. At about the same time, Bloodgood[65] regarded it as an innocuous symptom due to duct papilloma and not duct carcinoma. Two papers in the 1930s played an important role in influencing the vogue for mastectomy which dominated the mid-decades of the twentieth century. In 1930, Adair reported 108 cases from the Memorial Hospital,[66] with 47% malignant. In 1931, Cheatle and Cutler[67] argued strongly from pathological evidence that benign papillomas could progress to papillary carcinoma. This led to simple mastectomy being the standard treatment for blood-related discharge in many clinics.

A more conservative approach is now accepted, resulting particularly from the studies of Haagensen in the USA and Atkins and Wolff[68] in the UK, who all recognized that those patients whose discharge was due to duct papilloma were cured by removing the papilloma. Both groups recommended conservative operations; Atkins developed the operation of microdochectomy and Haagensen[6] used a procedure intermediate between the microdochectomy of Atkins and the major duct excision operation of Urban.[69]

More recent series have given a better indication of the likely pathology of these blood-related discharges. Leis's study of 560 patients undergoing breast surgery for discharge showed that only 20% of those with blood-related discharge had cancer or a premalignant condition.[10] Funderbunk and Syphax[70] give a clear breakdown of the causes of 167 cases of nipple discharge. Of 46 which were opalescent or green, none had cancer or hyperplasia; but of 121 patients with a clear, serous or bloody discharge, 11 had cancer, 11 had 'papillomatosis' (hyperplasia) and 59 had a duct papilloma. Richards et al.[71] have reported a series of 83 patients observed over a 3-year period. All patients with a pathological discharge (defined as blood-stained, serosanguineous, serous or clear) with a normal triple assessment were offered ductal surgery. Two in situ cancers were identified, neither had red blood cells in the discharge and both were over 60. The series shows a marked relationship between the incidence of cancer and increase in age, as discussed below.

More recently, nonsanguineous discharges have also become better recognized, and management of nipple discharge is now related to a number of factors, particularly the type of discharge, the age of the patient, and whether a blood-related discharge can be localized to a single duct.

General principles of management

Nature of the discharge

If the discharge is milk, look for a cause outside the breast, such as an endocrine cause or continuing mechanical stimulation.

Coloured, opalescent discharges have no serious significance. They should only be treated if causing social embarrassment. In doubtful cases, blood should be excluded by a chemical test.

Blood-related discharges cause much more concern to the patient and are associated with cancer risk. The risk is minimal in young patients but more significant with increasing age. The age of the patient is only important in decision-making

This is important only in blood-related discharges because of the cancer risk. No active treatment is necessary in young patients if the discharge ceases spontaneously. Wilson et al.[72] followed 74 young women and adolescents and found that none of them developed cancer before the age of 30. The threshold for advising surgical biopsy is clearly lower in older women but even then most women can be assessed preoperatively and be treated conservatively if they so wish. The adoption of a conservative approach to blood-related discharge is dependent on the availability of high-quality imaging and cytological assessment.

Localization

If the discharge can be localized to a single duct, microdochectomy gives satisfactory results in younger patients with minimal interference to the breast. In older patients where breastfeeding is not required, major duct excision may be preferable irrespective of whether the discharge is localized to one duct, both to avoid the inconvenience of further discharge from a different duct and to provide more comprehensive histology.

Specific details of management

The management of nipple discharge is summarized in Table 13.5 and Figure 13.9.

Blood-related discharge: serous, serosanguineous, sanguineous, watery

Under the age of 30, risk of malignancy is low, so the patient may be safely observed after full assessment as above. If discharge persists, and a solitary duct can be identified, the procedure of choice is microdochectomy (see Ch. 18). While standard descriptions of this operation suggest removing approximately 2 cm of duct, the duct excision should be extended into the breast if the duct remains distended at this level. If the discharge ceases and does not recur within a year, no further follow-up is indicated.

When surgery is indicated for patients over 45 our preferred operation is a formal excision of the major duct system (2.5 cm or as far as dilated ducts contain blood/serum) on the affected side (see Ch. 18), with urgent paraffin section. It is important to remember to mark the terminal part of the ducts immediately behind the nipple so that the pathologist can orientate the specimen. The advantages of this approach are that it is not essential to isolate a solitary offending duct; it deals with multiple papillomas if these are present and gives maximum histological information, and it deals with duct ectasia if this proves to be the cause. With well-performed surgery (and in the absence of chronic infection) there is no significant difference in the cosmesis following single or multiple duct excision.

Table 13.5 Management of milky and opalescent discharge

MILK DISCHARGE (GALACTORRHOEA)

Eliminate mechanical stimulation

Stop or change medication

Measure serum prolactin

Reassure

COLOURED OPALESCENT DISCHARGE

Exclude blood

Mammogram to exclude other pathology (over age 35 only)

Reassure

Major duct excision if socially embarrassing

Patients between 30 and 45 are suitable for either approach. In general, they may be treated as for the under-30 age group, but may be moved towards major duct excision by additional factors, e.g. strong family history of breast cancer, a particularly worried patient, or coexisting nipple inversion which the patient wants corrected.

Is it acceptable to avoid surgery in older patients with normal imaging and no mass, as has been advocated by some. The group from Nottingham[73] have advocated this approach on the basis that they only found two cases in their retrospective analysis of 97 cases that had not been already suspected on mammography. Other authors demur. For example, Leis[10] found a false-negative rate of 9.5% for mammography and 17.8% for cytology in 84 patients with cancers. Hence, we believe the emphasis should remain on surgical exploration for those judged to be at risk of cancer on the above criteria. Bauer et al.[74] reviewed the pathological findings in 277 women following surgery for spontaneous blood-related discharge; 15.5% were found to have ductal carcinoma in situ (DCIS). The discharge was bloody in 29, clear in 8 and brown in 6. Lau et al.[75] reported the results of 118 duct excisions performed between 1995 and 2002 for pathological discharge. Eleven (9.3%) cancers were found although this rose to 12.7% for postmenopausal women. Solitary duct papillomas were found in 25 patients and diffuse papillomatosis in 43. In only 7 cases were they unable to make a formal diagnosis. They too conclude that surgical exploration is advisable even in those without evidence of serious disease on clinical and imaging assessment.

We still recommend surgery in all blood-related cases defined by our criteria set out above. The operation is a minor one and the incidence of previously undiagnosed DCIS too high to be ignored. An alternative approach, at any age, is to perform an ultrasound-guided mammotome excision. This provides an adequate treatment for benign papillomas and allows rational decision-making for those with more aggressive lesions.[76] One series reported the experience of 77 patients with satisfactory results in 95%. Four patients either required a second mammotome excision or a microdochotomy. It has the added advantage that it can be performed as an office procedure.[76]

Coloured opalescent discharge

This only requires treatment if the amount of discharge is personally embarrassing, with the need to wear pads constantly. The only effective procedure is a total duct excision, and in well-selected cases is welcomed by the patient.

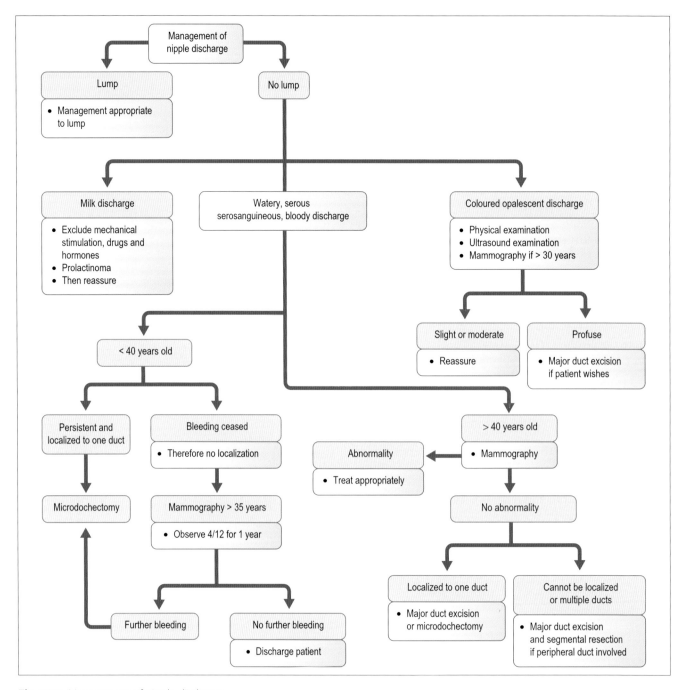

Fig. 13.9 Management of nipple discharge.

Galactorrhoea

The management is that of the underlying cause. Prolactinomas are treated by bromocriptine or cabergolamine, or surgical excision. For drug-induced galactorrhoea, an alternative medication is usually available if the galactorrhoea remains unacceptable. In cases of physiological discharge, reassurance and cessation of mechanical stimulation should prove sufficient.

Follow-up

Patients who prove to have solitary duct papilloma have insufficient increase in the risk of subsequent malignancy to justify routine follow-up. Patients with multiple papillomas, or where cytological atypia has been found, do have an increased risk[77] and should be kept under review. Because the risk is small, long-term and affecting both breasts, long-term follow-up is more appropriate than prophylactic mastectomy.

Carty et al.[78] followed a small mixed series of patients with mainly non-blood-related discharge for 5 years and showed that the discharge had resolved spontaneously in three-quarters of the women in that period.

REFERENCES

1. Gulay H, Bora S, Kilicturgay S *et al.* Management of nipple discharge. *Journal of American College of Surgeons* 1994; **178:** 472–474.

2. Cheung KL & Alagaratnam TT. A review of nipple discharge in Chinese women. *Journal of Royal College of Surgeons of Edinburgh* 1997; **62:** 179–181.

3. King EB, Chew KC, Petrakis NL *et al.* Nipple aspirate cytology for the study of breast cancer precursors. *Journal of National Cancer Institute* 1983; **71:** 1115–1121.

4. Selzer MH, Perloff LJ, Kelley RI *et al.* The significance of age in patients with nipple discharge. *Surgery, Gynecology and Obstetrics* 1970; **131:** 519–522.

5. Devitt JE. Management of nipple discharge by clinical findings. *American Journal of Surgery* 1985; **149:** 789–792.

6. Haagensen CD. *Diseases of the Breast*, 3rd edn. Philadelphia: WB Saunders; 1986.

7. Cochrane RA, Singhal H, Moneypenny IJ *et al.* Evaluation of general practitioner referrals to a specialist clinic according to the UK national guidelines. *European Journal of Surgical Oncology* 1997; **23:** 198–201.

8. The BRIDGE Study Group. The presentation and management of breast symptoms in general practice in South Wales. *British Journal of General Practice* 1999; **49:** 811–812.

9. Seltzer MH. Breast complaints, biopsies, and cancer correlated with age in 10,000 consecutive new surgical referrals. *Breast Journal* 2004; **10:** 111–117.

10. Leis HP. Management of nipple discharge. *World Journal of Surgery* 1989; **13:** 736–742.

11. Chaudary MA, Millis RR, Davies GC *et al.* Nipple discharge. The diagnostic value of testing for occult blood. *Annals of Surgery* 1982; **196:** 651–655.

12. Vorherr H. *The Breast, Morphology, Physiology and Lactation*. New York: Academic Press; 1974.

13. Webster J, Piscitelli G, Polli A *et al.* A comparison of carbergolamine and bromocriptine in the treatment of hyperprolactinaemic amenorrhoea. *New England Journal of Medicine* 1994; **331:** 904–909.

14. Scanlon MT, Peters JR, Picton-Thomas J *et al.* The management of selected patients with hyper-prolactinaemia by partial hypophysectomy. *British Medical Journal* 1986; **291:** 1547–1550.

15. Hall R, Anderson J, Smart GA *et al. Fundamentals of Clinical Endocrinology*, 3rd edn. Tunbridge Wells: Pitman Medical; 1980.

16. Ogan A, Yanardag R, Colgar U *et al.* Lipid composition of nipple discharges of women with galactorrhoea. *Gynecology and Endocrinology* 1994; **8:** 109–114.

17. Petrakis NL, Lowenstein JM, Wiencke JK *et al.* Gross cystic disease fluid protein in nipple aspirates of breast fluid in Asian and non-Asian women. *Cancer, Epidemiology, Biomarkers and Prevention* 1993; **2:** 573–579.

18. Petrakis NL, Lim MI, Miike R *et al.* Nipple aspirate fluids in adult non-lactating women – lactose content, cationic Na$^+$, K$^+$, Na$^+$/K$^+$ ratio and coloration. *Breast Cancer Research and Treatment* 1989; **13:** 71–78.

19. Petrakis NL, Miike R, King EB *et al.* Association of breast fluid colouration with age, ethnicity and cigarette smoking. *Breast Cancer Research and Treatment* 1988; **11:** 255–262.

20. Lee EH, Venta LA, Morrow M *et al.* The role of galactography in patients with post-operative nipple discharge. *Breast Journal* 1997; **3:** 74–76.

21. Lafreniere R. Bloody nipple discharge during pregnancy: a rationale for conservative treatment. *Journal of Surgical Oncology* 1990; **43:** 228–230.

22. O'Callaghan MA. Atypical discharge from the breast during pregnancy and/or lactation. *Australian and New Zealand Journal of Obstetrics and Gynaecology* 1981; **21:** 214–216.

23. Kline TS & Lash SR. The bleeding nipple of pregnancy and the post-partum period. *Acta Cytologica Philadelphia* 1964; **8:** 336.

24. Lewison EF & Chambers RG. Clinical significance of nipple discharge. *Journal of the American Medical Association* 1951; **147:** 295–299.

25. Sandison AT. An autopsy study of the human breast. *National Cancer Institute Monograph No. 8*, US Dept Health, Education and Welfare, 1962.

26. Winchester DP. ACP consensus statement. The relationship of fibrocystic disease to breast cancer. *American College of Surgeons Bulletin* 1986; **71:** 29–31.

27. Cardenosa G & Eklund G. Benign papillary neoplasms of the breast – mammographic findings. *Radiology* 1991; **181:** 751.

28. Ohuchi N, Abe R & Kasai M. Possible cancerous change of intraductal papilloma of the breast: a 3-D reconstruction study of 25 cases. *Cancer* 1984; **54:** 605–611.

29. Murad T, Contesso G & Mouriesse H. Papillary tumours of the large lactiferous ducts. *Cancer* 1981; **48:** 122–133.

30. Rosen P, Cantrell B, Mullen D *et al.* Juvenile papillomatosis (Swiss cheese disease) of the breast. *American Journal of Surgical Pathology* 1980; **4:** 3–12.

31. Rosen PP, Holmes P, Lesser ML *et al.* Juvenile papillomatosis and breast carcinoma. *Cancer* 1985; **55:** 1345–1352.

32. Rosen PP & Kimel M. Juvenile papillomatosis of the breast – a follow-up study of 41 patients diagnosed before 1979. *American Journal of Clinical Pathology* 1990; **93:** 599–603.

33. Davies JD. Pigmented periductal cells (ochrocytes) in mammary dysplasias: their nature and significance. *Journal of Pathology* 1974; **114:** 205–216.

34. Cabioglu N, Hunt KK, Singletary SE *et al.* Surgical decision making and factors determining a diagnosis of breast carcinoma in women presenting with nipple discharge. *Journal of the American College of Surgery* 2003; **197:** 697–698.

35. Heyman RB & Rauth JL. Areolar gland discharge in adolescent females. *Journal of Adolescent Health Care* 1983; **4:** 285–292.

36. Watkins F, Giacomantonio M & Salisbury F. Nipple discharge and breast lump related to Montgomery's tubercles in adolescent females. *Journal of Paediatric Surgery* 1988; **23:** 718–720.

37. Casteels-Van Daele M, Wijndaele L, Eeckels R *et al.* Nipple discharge in children and adolescents: an irritating cause. *Clinical Pediatrics* 1990; **29:** 53.

38. Rogerson T, Ingram D, Sterrett G *et al.* Areolar discharge and peri-areolar breast cysts in adolescent females. *Breast* 2002; **11:** 181–184.

39. Miller JD, Brownell MP & Shaw A. Bilateral breast masses and bloody nipple discharge in a 4-year-old boy. *Journal of Paediatrics* 1990; **116:** 744–747.

40. Hussain S & Lui DM. Ultrasound guided percutaneous galactography. *European Journal of Radiology* 1997; **24:** 163–165.

41. Baker KS, Davey DD & Stelling CB. Ductal abnormalities detected with galactography: frequency of adequate excisional biopsy. *American Journal of Roentgenology* 1994; **162:** 821–824.

42. Sardanelli F, Imperiale A, Zandrino F *et al.* Breast intraductal masses. US-guided fine-needle-aspiration after galactography. *Radiology* 1997; **204:** 143–148.

43. Vega BA, Landeras AR & Ortega GE. Intraductal placement of a Kopan's spring-hookwire guide to localise non-palpable breast lesions detected by galactography. *Acta Radiologica* 1997; **38:** 240–242.

44. Saarela AO, Kiviniemi HO & Rissanen TJ. Preoperative methylene blue staining of galactographically suspicious breast lesions. *International Surgery* 1997; **82:** 403–405.

45. Nakahara H, Namba K, Watanabe R *et al.* A comparison of MR imaging, galactography and ultrasonography in patients with nipple discharge. *Breast Cancer* 2003; **10:** 320–329.

46. Ozaki A, Ozaki M & Asaishi K. Fibreoptic ductography of the breast. *Japanese Journal of Clinical Oncology* 1991; **21:** 188–193.

47. Makiti M, Sakamoto G, Akiyama F *et al.* Duct endoscopy and endoscopic biopsy in the evaluation of nipple discharge. *Breast Cancer Research and Treatment* 1991; **18:** 179–181.

48. Pereira B & Mokbel K. Mammary ductoscopy: past, present, and future. *International Journal of Clinical Oncology* 2005; **10:** 112–116.

49. Matsuda M, Seki T, Kikawada Y *et al.* Mammary ductoscopy by helical CT: initial experience. *Breast Cancer* 2005; **12:** 118–121.

50. Moncrief RM, Nayar R, Diaz LK *et al.* A comparison of ductoscopy-guided and conventional surgical excision in women with spontaneous nipple discharge. *Annals of Surgery* 2005; **241:** 575–581.

51. Nathan M. Diagnostic precoce d'un neoplasme du sein par l'examen de son suintement hemmorragique. *Clinique, Paris* 1914; **60:** 38–39.

52. Kjellogren O. The cytologic diagnosis of cancer of the breast. *Acta Cytologica* 1964; **8:** 216–223.

53. Rimsten A, Skoog V & Stenkvist B. On the significance of nipple discharge in the diagnosis of breast disease. *Acta Chirugica Scandinavica* 1976; **142:** 513–518.

54. Groves AM, Carr M, Wadhera V *et al.* An audit of cytology in the evaluation of nipple discharge. A retrospective study of 10 years experience. *Breast* 1996; **5:** 96–99.

55. Dunn JM, Lucarotti ME, Wood SJ *et al.* Exfoliative cytology in the diagnosis of breast disease. *British Journal of Surgery* 1995; **82:** 789–791.

56. Wrensch MR, Petrakis NL, Gruenke LD *et al.* Factors associated with obtaining nipple fluid: analysis of 1428 women and literature review. *Breast Cancer Research and Treatment* 1990; **15:** 39–51.

57. Gupta RK, Gaskell D, Dowle CS *et al.* The role of nipple discharge cytology in the diagnosis of breast disease: a study of 1948 nipple discharge smears from 1530 patients. *Cytopathology* 2004; **15:** 326–330

58. Khan SA, Wolfman JA, Segal L *et al.* Ductal lavage findings in women with mammographic microcalcifications undergoing biopsy. *Annals of Surgical Oncology* 2005; **12:** 6896.

59. Fraylinger JA & Kurtzman SH. Combined ductal lavage and ductoscopy: what is the future for the intraductal approach. *Journal of Surgical Oncology* 2006; **94:** 553–554.

60. Johnson-Maddux A, Ashfaq R, Cler L *et al.* Reproducibility of cytologic atypia in repeat nipple duct lavage. *Cancer* 2005; **103**: 1129–1136.

61. Inaji H, Koyama H, Motomura K *et al.* Erb-2 protein levels in nipple discharge: role in diagnosis of early breast cancer. *Tumour Biology* 1993; **14**: 271–278.

62. Sauter ER, Shan S, Hewett JE *et al.* Proteomic analysis of nipple aspirate fluid using SELDI-TDF-MS. *International Journal of Cancer* 2005; **114**: 791–796.

63. Hockel M & Klose KJ. Treatment of non-neoplastic nipple discharge with fibrin adhesive. *Lancet* 1987; **ii**: 331–332.

64. Judd ES. Intracanalicular papilloma of the breast. *Journal Lancet* 1917; **37**: 141.

65. Bloodgood JC. Benign lesions of female breast for which operation is not indicated. *Journal of American Medical Association* 1922; **78**: 859–863.

66. Adair FE. Sanguinous discharge from the nipple and its significance in relation to cancer of the breast. *Annals of Surgery* 1930; **91**: 197–201.

67. Cheatle GL & Cutler M. *Tumours of the Breast.* Philadelphia: JB Lippincott; 1931.

68. Atkins H & Wolff B. Discharges from the nipple. *British Journal of Surgery* 1964; **51**: 602–606.

69. Urban JA. Excision of the major duct system of the breast. *Cancer* 1963; **16**: 516–520.

70. Funderbunk WW & Syphax B. Evaluation of nipple discharge in benign and malignant disease. *Cancer* 1969; **24**: 1290–1296.

71. Richards T, Hunt A, Courtner S *et al.* Nipple discharge: a sign of breast cancer? *Annals of the Royal College of Surgeons of England* 2007; **89**: 124–126.

72. Wilson M, Craner ML & Rosen PP. Papillary duct hyperplasia of the breast in children and young women. *Modern Pathology* 1993; **6**: 570–574.

73. Locker AP, Galea MH, Ellis IO *et al.* Microdochectomy for single duct discharge from the nipple. *British Journal of Surgery* 1988; **75**: 700–701.

74. Bauer RL, Eckhert KH & Nemoto T. Ductal carcinoma in situ-associated nipple discharge: a marker for locally extensive disease. *Annals of Surgical Oncology* 1998; **5**: 452–455.

75. Lau S, Kuchenmeister I, Stachs A *et al.* Pathologic nipple discharge: surgery is imperative in postmenopausal women. *Annals of Surgical Oncology* 2005; **12**: 546–551.

76. Govindarajulu S, Narreddy SR, Shere MH *et al.* Sonographically guided mammotome excision of ducts in the diagnosis and management of single duct nipple discharge. *European Journal of Surgical Oncology* 2006; **32**: 725–728.

77. Carter D. Intraductal papillary tumours of the breast – a study of 78 cases. *Cancer* 1977; **39**: 1689–1692.

78. Carty NJ, Mudan SS, Ravichandran D *et al.* Prospective study of outcome in women presenting with nipple discharge. *Annals of the Royal College of Surgeons of England* 1994; **76**: 387–389.

Infections of the breast

Introduction

Infection of the breast may occur as a localized phenomenon or as part of a systemic illness. The common acute infective conditions are usually easy to diagnose; the importance of the rarer infections of the breast lies in the similarity of their presentation to a carcinoma, a painless indurated mass. Specific infective conditions are now uncommon in the UK but are of historical interest. Tuberculosis remains important in British practice with respect to immunocompromised patients and immigrant populations, particularly from the Indian subcontinent. The other infections are mainly interesting curiosities.

Studies based on hospital experience are likely to give a distorted picture of the true incidence of breast infection. In hospital practice, nonpuerperal abscess is more common than lactational abscess,[1,2] but in general practice a survey showed 80% of infective episodes were puerperal.[3] Lactational infection remains common[4] but only a small percentage progress to abscess formation and thence hospital referral. The incidence is therefore high and is relatively underappreciated in hospital practice because the majority of cases are diagnosed early by general practitioners when treatment with appropriate antibiotics is effective.

Lactational breast infection

Epidemiology

Lactational mastitis is a common condition that has been described as occurring in up to 9% of puerperal women in the 1940s,[5] 20% in the 1990s[6] and 14% at the beginning of the twenty-first century,[4] the higher rates probably being more apparent than real because different definitions of infection were used. Our experience (Fig. 14.1) gives an indication that puerperal breast infection remains a significant problem and occurs following about 6% of pregnancies.

In a review of 966 lactating women, Kaufmann and Foxman[7] reported an incidence of 2.9% in the first 7 postpartum weeks. In a subsequent report Foxman et al.[8] studied 946 breastfeeding women in Michigan and Nebraska for three postpartum months. They found an overall incidence of 9.5% of puerperal breast infection and found both previous mastitis and sore nipples to be predictive factors. Kinlay et al[6] evaluated the risk

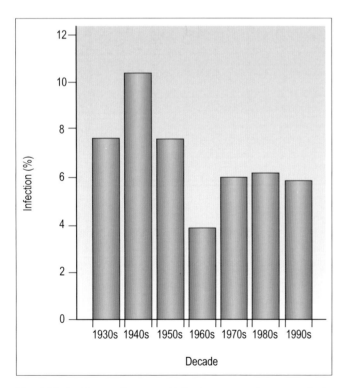

Fig. 14.1 Incidence of puerperal infection, reported retrospectively by 632 patients undergoing 1532 pregnancies between 1930 and 2000.

factors in 1075 breastfeeding women and found significant risk factors were blocked milk duct, use of nipple creams, previous mastitis, college education and cracked nipples.

A careful cohort study from Australia reported the experience of 1193 women assessed 6 months postpartum.[4] Two hundred and seven (17%) reported mastitis and five developed an abscess. The authors calculated that the incidence of breast abscess was 0.4% in those who commenced breastfeeding. Of those who commenced antibiotics for mastitis, 2.9% went on to develop an abscess.

Although puerperal breast infection is sometimes described in sporadic and epidemic forms, the pathological processes within the breast are identical. The epidemic form is seen in institutional outbreaks in which the organism is transmitted from infant to infant by cross-infection and thence to its mother.

Prophylaxis

Attention to detail in the care of the breast during pregnancy and lactation can do much to reduce the chances of developing infection. Good hygiene and avoidance of breast engorgement or cracked nipple are important. During pregnancy, daily washing will remove the dried secretions that will otherwise collect on the nipple. After feeding the infant, the nipples should be dried and any segments of the breast that have not been adequately emptied during feeding expressed. A bland moisturizing cream can then be applied. However, Kinlay et al.[6] have pointed out these creams may sometimes harbour pathogens.

Pathology and bacteriology

The organism most commonly implicated is *Staphylococcus aureus*, which gains entry via a cracked nipple. Occasionally, the infection is haematogenous. In the early stages, the infection tends to be confined to a single segment of the breast and it is relatively late that extension to other segments may occur. Milk provides an ideal culture medium, so bacterial dispersion in the vascular and distended segment is easy. The pathological process is identical to acute inflammation occurring elsewhere in the body, although the loose parenchyma of the lactating breast and the stagnant milk of an engorged segment allow the infection to spread rapidly if unchecked. The bacteria are excreted in the milk.

In the study of Goodman and Benson,[9] all the 98 hospital-acquired infections were *Staph. aureus* and, of these, only 50% had penicillin-sensitive organisms. Breast abscess associated with methicillin-resistant *Staphylococcus aureus* (MRSA) has been reported and is likely to be an increasing problem.

A wide variety of organisms may occasionally be encountered. Typhoid is a well-recognized cause of breast abscess in countries where this disease is common. This is a particularly important diagnosis to make because the organism is secreted in the milk.

Clinical features

Nursing mothers are most vulnerable to breast abscess at two stages:

- During the first month of lactation following the first pregnancy when, due to inexperience, the nipples are more likely to be damaged and hygiene inadequate. Eighty-five per cent of lactational breast abscesses occur during the first month after delivery.[10]
- At weaning, when the breasts are more likely to become engorged. An additional factor after about 6 months is that the baby's teeth increase the likelihood of nipple trauma.

The patient complains of a painful red swollen breast associated with constitutional upset and fever. The local signs of infection vary greatly with the stage of infection. In early cases, a little cellulitis or nothing at all is found; in neglected cases, a fluctuant abscess with overlying skin necrosis may be observed (Fig. 14.2).

In patients who have already had treatment, antibiotics leading to a mass without the classic signs of infection, and which may or may not be tender, may have masked the signs.

Figure 14.5 shows the sites of breast abscesses. Most lie in the parenchyma. Abscesses in the less common sites, such as the retromammary space, periareolar region or subcutaneous tissue, should alert the clinician to the possibility of an underlying pathology.

Assessment

The clinical problem may be resolved into cellulitis without pus formation and abscess. The importance of an accurate assessment of the situation cannot be overemphasized. Surgery in the early cellulitic phase is

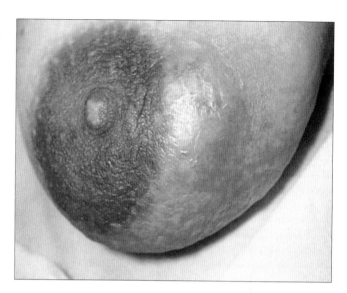

Fig. 14.2 Late typical lactational breast abscess with compromised skin.

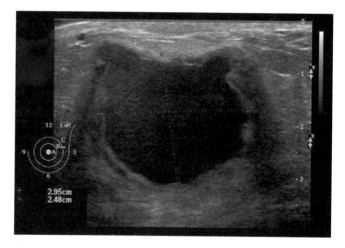

Fig. 14.3 Ultrasound showing large breast abscess; liquefied contents within irregular walled cavity; lactating patient.

meddlesome and unnecessarily destructive; continued antibiotic therapy in the presence of an abscess may lead to unnecessary tissue destruction by the disease process. Test needle aspiration of the cellulitic area, preferably preceded by ultrasound examination (Figs 14.3 and 14.4), should be performed.[11] If ultrasound shows an abscess, the needle can be guided into the cavity with ultrasound guidance. It is wrong to wait for the development of fluctuation and pointing before proceeding to drainage, because further destruction of breast tissue will occur. Even if no pus is aspirated the opportunity should be used to carry out bacteriological examination of the aspirated material.

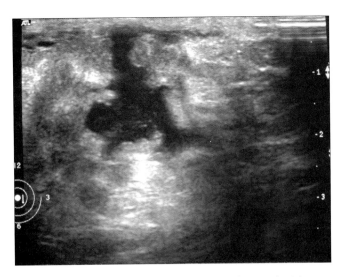

Fig. 14.4 Ultrasound image of breast abscess showing liquid matter within an ill defined cavity.

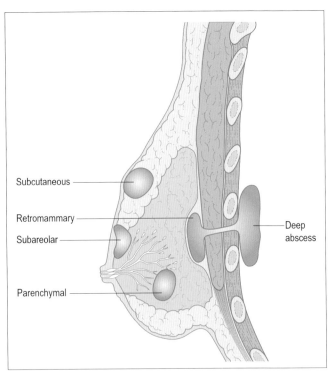

Fig. 14.5 The sites of breast abscesses.

A useful bonus of this approach is that the rare case of inflammatory carcinoma may be diagnosed on the smear, thus avoiding operation in this difficult condition (Fig. 14.6).

Treatment

Taylor and Way[12] clearly enunciated the principles of treatment: curtail infection and empty the breast. The methods of achieving this differ in the cellulitic and abscess stages.

Curtailing infection: cellulitic phase

During the cellulitic phase, treatment with antibiotics may be expected to give rapid resolution. The predominance of *Staph. aureus* allows a rational choice of antibiotic without having to wait for the results of bacteriological culture. A penicillinase-resistant antibacterial should be given; flucloxacillin 500 mg four times daily will prove satisfactory but, if the patient has penicillin sensitivity, erythromycin is a satisfactory alternative. If rapid improvement does not occur, repeated ultrasound will usually reveal the presence of pus. After 24 hours, the results of culture should give guidance to a possible change in antibiotic therapy if the lesion is not improving and no pus is found on repeat aspiration. If resolution is proceeding satisfactorily, no further action is required.

Antibiotics are secreted in milk so tetracyclines, aminoglycosides, sulphonamides and metronidazole

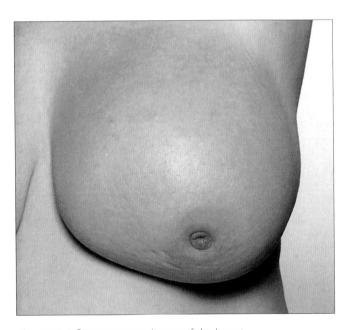

Fig. 14.6 Inflammatory carcinoma of the breast.

should be avoided because of their possible ill effects on the child. Penicillin, cephalosporins and erythromycin, however, are considered safe. Such a regimen will prove adequate in most cases but in fewer than 5% an abscess will develop.[4]

Curtailing infection: abscess phase

Once abscess formation has occurred, which is likely after 48 hours, use of antibiotics alone may cause a temporary regression of the symptoms without sterilizing the abscess and lead to a protracted illness. Newton and Newton[10] observed in the 1950s that the introduction of antibiotics led to delayed resolution of the abscess. At that time, opposition to the use of antibiotics was often vehement, on the basis that it led to chronic, thick-walled abscesses that could simulate cancer, as well as being difficult to eradicate. Such chronic indurated abscesses undoubtedly occurred at that time: they probably arose from the treatment of subareolar abscesses, and abscesses elsewhere, with antibiotics ineffective against anaerobic organisms.

In cases where the development of an abscess is uncertain, aspiration should resolve the point. The routine use of ultrasound in the evaluation of breast abscesses allows a rational approach to be developed. O'Hara et al.[13] studied 53 suspected cases of abscess, in 18 no abscess was seen and antibiotic treatment caused complete resolution in 16; one of these developed an abscess, which required drainage, the other had an inflammatory cancer.

Where an abscess has formed, aspiration of the pus, preferably under ultrasound control, has now supplanted open surgery as the first line of treatment. Antibiotics should be continued to reduce systemic infection and local cellulitis. Several series support this change in management. For example, O'Hara et al.[13] treated 22 abscesses with aspiration, 19 of which settled without surgical intervention. Further aspirations can be performed if the problem is not resolving, preferably under ultrasound guidance to ensure that all the loculi are drained. It seems to us that repeated drainage by aspiration is preferable to the placement of percutaneous drainage catheters advocated by some.[14,15] The series of O'Hara et al.[13] supports this policy of repeated aspiration. The results reported by Erylimaz et al.[16] of their controlled trial comparing incision and drainage (I&D) and aspiration reflect common experience. Seventy per cent of I&D patients (23) were unhappy with the cosmetic result; in the aspiration group, without the benefit of ultrasound, 3 resolved with a single aspiration, 10 with repeated aspirations while 9 proceeded to I&D. The patients who did not resolve had larger abscesses >5 cm diameter or presented late. Varey et al.[17] successfully treated five such refractory patients with a vacuum suction device, thus avoiding I&D in all patients. A minority of patients will require open drainage either because the aspiration approach has failed or because of late presentation when the overlying skin is already necrotic. When open drainage is indicated, our preference is for open drainage and packing but Benson and Goodman[18] have argued for a policy of immediate closure under antibiotic cover. Their study was performed before the role of aspiration had been fully evaluated so their results may not be relevant to the group of patients who now require open drainage. The selection of antibiotics should follow the guidelines given in the cellulitic phase.

Emptying the breast

This important aspect of the management of puerperal breast infection is sometimes ignored. The breast may be emptied either by suckling or by expression. Rowley[19] in 1772 described and illustrated the use of a breast pump that is similar to some still in use today. Although bacteria are present in the milk, no harm appears to be done to the infant if breastfeeding is continued.[20]

After open surgical drainage of an abscess, suckling may be difficult for a few days for mechanical reasons on the affected side, but the mother should be encouraged to feed on the unaffected side. The infected breast, however, should be emptied either by manual expression or by a pump.

Suppression of lactation

Following development of a breast abscess, patients are often advised to abandon breastfeeding. This advice is given on the grounds that the bacteria are excreted in the milk and may then infect the infant, and that continued pain makes it difficult to empty the affected breast satisfactorily, thus causing further engorgement and stasis leading to rapid spread of the infecting organisms. There is no real basis for these views, and with skilled nursing assistance the infant may be safely fed on the contralateral breast and the affected breast may be expressed by pump until such time as feeding can be recommenced.[21] Indeed, except when the presence of the cavity makes suckling impossible, there is no indication to remove the child from the affected breast. The bacteria in the milk do not appear to harm the child. A leading article in the *British Medical Journal*[22] reviewed the evidence and concluded that mothers with breast abscesses should be encouraged to continue breastfeeding.

If it is decided to abandon breastfeeding, lactation should be suppressed as quickly as possible. The most effective suppressant currently available is probably cabergolamine, which is effective as a single dose and so is preferable to bromocriptine 2.5 mg twice daily for 14 days.[23] The engorged breast should be emptied as far as possible mechanically. Fluid restriction and firm binding seem unnecessary.

Subclinical mastitis

Subclinical mastitis[24] is a well recognized entity in veterinary and agricultural practice but is relatively undiagnosed in humans, although it is probably as common as overt infection. This condition is unlikely to present in the breast clinic but may be apparent in obstetric practice. Subclinical mastitis is characterized by reversal of the normal $Na^+:K^+$ ratio and reduction in milk output. Subclinical mastitis leads to changes in the tight junctions between luminal epithelial cells, with a consequent leak of sodium.

Inflammatory cells and other mediators in milk

Normal breast milk contains 5–6 mmoL sodium; this increases to 12–20 mmoL in subclinical mastitis. Raised levels of milk sodium are also seen in colostrum, at weaning, or in milk following preterm delivery. Subclinical mastitis is thought to be unilateral in the majority of women and, as with clinical mastitis, its prevalence is reduced by the provision of active counselling and advice to promote milk expression.[25] The natural history and clinical importance of subclinical mastitis remains unclear although there are implications for the baby, especially in women with HIV.

Nonlactational breast abscess

Nonlactational abscess is more common than lactational abscess in hospital practice, but as pointed out earlier, is less common in family practice. The average age of the patients tends to be older than that for patients with lactational infections (Fig. 14.7).

It falls naturally into two main groups, subareolar and peripheral, which differ in many respects. The microbiological profile of nonlactational abscess is far more

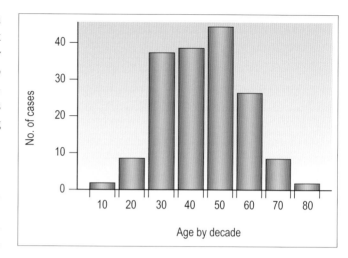

Fig. 14.7 The age distribution of 160 nonlactational abscesses in Cardiff series.

variable than that of lactational breast abscess;[26] this is particularly true of the subareolar group. In addition, there are several specific groups of abscesses, which need to be treated separately, those in immunocompromised patients, iatrogenic abscesses, factitial abscess and those in neonates.

Subareolar abscess

Subareolar abscess is seen mainly in women in their reproductive years, is mainly due to the duct ectasia/periductal mastitis (DE/PDM) complex and is associated with a mixed bacterial spectrum. Several studies have now confirmed the original observation[27] that recurrent periareolar sepsis is associated with cigarette smoking.[2,28,29] Recurrence is likely unless the underlying pathology is dealt with although even then the problem may persist.[29] This very important group of infections is dealt with fully in Chapter 11, and is not considered further here.

Peripheral abscess

This is much less common than subareolar abscess. The most typical presentation is in a postmenopausal woman who presents with a recent-onset, typical breast abscess with no underlying pathology. Standard management is effective.[13] The pathogenesis of these abscesses is uncertain. In view of the age group, it is possible that they are associated with a degree of the involutional form of DE, where mildly dilated ducts provide a focus for the proliferation of organisms frequently present in low numbers in the normal breast.[30] Whether or not this is the basis, no treatment of any underlying disorder is necessary, in contrast to subareolar abscess.

Peripheral abscesses are occasionally seen arising on the basis of gross DE (in older patients) or conspicuous histological PDM (in younger women). In such cases the underlying disease requires excision, and examples of both types are given in Chapter 11. We believe that some of these are examples of the condition also called granulomatous lobular mastitis. Whether this is a specific condition – there are many causes of granulomatous histology in the breast including PDM – is arguable. The main problem is failure to heal or recurrence after numerous excisions. In our experience, they heal if excision is carried out in continuity with the retroareolar ducts.

Treatment

Treatment of nonlactational abscesses should follow general principles. Dixon[31] has shown that the majority of such abscesses can be managed as out-patients, either aspirating the pus or draining it under a local anaesthetic. If an aspiration approach is used, multiple attempts are to be expected. The overall management is much more complex than that needed for lactational abscess with a high incidence of recurrence. Management is discussed in detail in Chapter 11. In view of the likelihood of finding anaerobic bacteria[32] it is advisable to cover such organisms when selecting antimicrobial therapy.

Infections in immunocompromised patients

These have classically occurred in patients on immunosuppressive drugs, and were sufficiently uncommon to escape detailed attention. With the advent of AIDS as a major problem, opportunistic infections have become better recognized. Whatever the underlying cause, the abscesses are found to have similar features: unusual organisms, poor host resistance and often fulminant progression.

HIV infection

Breast abscess in these patients is increasing in incidence, and presents a bewildering variety of organisms. In Nigeria 30% of breast abscesses in young women are nonlactational, and 77% of these are associated with HIV.[33] As the virus is excreted in breast milk there are implications for the baby; the risk is particularly increased if mastitis occurs.[34] There is evidence that HIV excretion is greater, as is vertical transmission of HIV, in those with subclinical mastitis.[35] Nussenblatt et al. found that 27% of HIV positive women in Malawi had at least one episode of subclinical mastitis during lactation; they grew staphylococcus in 30% of cases.

Tuberculosis is also seen as a cause of breast abscess in these patients, and may present as an apparently normal pyogenic abscess, and even be the first manifestation of HIV infection.[36] This emphasizes the need for full bacteriological and, where possible, histological assessment of all nonlactational abscesses.

Immunosuppressive drugs

Immunosuppressed patients provide similar problems. An example is an abscess due to *Nocardia asteroides* in a patient with systemic lupus erythematosus (SLE).[37] *Nocardia* infections are well recognized in immunocompromised patients, so it is not surprising that it should be found in a breast abscess. The patient was a 57-year-old woman treated with azathioprine and cyclophosphamide for SLE. She developed a 9×5-cm abscess from which *Nocardia* was isolated. It responded to appropriate antibiotics and drainage.

Iatrogenic abscess

Bacteriology of the normal breast

It has always been recognized that skin flora can often be isolated from the terminal centimetre or so of the mammary ducts, but generally considered that the central area of the breast is sterile. Thornton and et al.[30] question this assumption. They took multiple tissue samples from the breast during plastic surgical procedures and submitted them to stringent culture conditions. Fifty-three per cent of the cultures grew *Staph. epidermidis*, and the presence of these, and the other organisms grown, did not vary with the depth of the biopsy from the surface. Other common aerobic organisms were haemolytic *Streptococcus*, *Diptheroides*, *Lactobacillus* and *Enterococcus*. Anaerobic organisms cultured included *Propionobacterium acne*, *Peptostreptococcus* and *Clostridium sporogenes*. They also found some correlation between organisms grown from biopsies and subsequent postoperative infection. If this work is confirmed, it may explain some of the infections after elective surgery, but does not explain why they are not much more common.

Breast infections following breast surgery are not rare, and are diverse in origin and clinical features. Such infections range from mild superficial cellulites to deep abscess formation associated with an infected haematoma.

Abscess following lumpectomy and radiotherapy

This is more common than may be realized, and occurred in 6% of patients in one series.[38] The abscesses occurred between 1 and 8 months following treatment, at a median of 5 months. The incidence was not related to prophylactic antibiotic use, adjuvant radiotherapy or individual surgeons, but was related to large biopsy cavities, prior biopsy infection, skin necrosis and repeated seroma aspiration. Six of seven abscesses grew staphylococci, but three were coagulase negative, suggesting introduction of skin organisms into an area of reduced resistance following radiotherapy. All abscesses occurred in patients whose operation included axillary dissection, although few of the patients had not had axillary dissection. All abscesses resolved with drainage and antibiotics, but with impaired cosmesis. An interesting historical aside to this is the use of radiotherapy for treatment of lactational mastitis in the 1940s and 1950s. The subsequent risk of breast cancer was found to be dose dependent and linear.[39]

Periprosthetic breast infections

Infection around silicone prosthesis occurs in about 1% of placements, more following subcutaneous than subpectoral placement. The commonest organism is *Staph. aureus*, but a wide variety can be responsible, including *Pseudomonas*, *Staph. epidermidis* and *Mycobacterium*.[40] The *Mycobacterium fortuitum* group is particularly associated with prostheses,[41] but unless special precautions are taken in culturing the fluid, the organism is unlikely to be identified. The mammographic and computerized tomography (CT) findings in infected prosthesis have been described by Walsh et al.[42] Such infections may present in the classic way with redness, swelling and pain; others may be relatively quiescent.

Periprosthetic infection is likely to occur more frequently in patients who have primary reconstruction in association with some other procedure on the breast. Careful aseptic technique is particularly necessary in these cases. Once infection has occurred, the prosthesis is

usually removed and reinserted some months later when the infection has subsided. Even then, it is difficult to guarantee that re-infection will not occur, particularly if *Staph. aureus* was the organism. Some surgeons have recommended conservative management with antibiotics and drainage of the pus, leaving the prosthesis in situ, but this is best reserved for special situations. In our experience such an approach is seldom successful.

Pajkos et al.[43] have presented evidence that lends considerable support to the theory that capsular contraction is related to subclinical infection. Using a broth culture they were able to grow bacteria from the 17 of 19 patients with grade 3 or 4 Baker capsules but in only one of eight patients with Baker grade 0 or 1 capsules. The majority of cultures grew coagulase-negative staphylococci. It should be noted that no growth occurred on routine culture.

Retained foreign bodies

Many different surgical foreign bodies have been reported as the cause of delayed abscess, including a piece of drainage tube left at an operation for an abscess 35 years earlier, and presenting as a dense mass suggestive of cancer.[44] A similar case was due to migration of plombage material through the chest wall after 40 years; it was demonstrated on CT scan.[45] Infection associated with nipple piercing has been estimated to be as high as 10%.[46]

Following central venous catheterization

A number of reports have demonstrated that the breast may be affected if a central venous catheter leaves its intended path. In one report,[47] a late perforation of the right internal mammary vein by a catheter inserted via the left subclavian vein led to extravasation of parenteral nutrition fluid and a breast abscess. They describe three cases, all with good early function of the catheter, then chest pain and signs of inflammation in the contralateral breast. They stress the importance of promptly investigating this combination of symptoms if the complication is to be diagnosed early.

Factitial abscess

This condition should always be considered with abscesses that do not seem to fit the normal pattern, but confident diagnosis is notoriously difficult.[48] It is seen most commonly in nurses and members of other paramedical disciplines. Abscess may follow self-injection or insertion of foreign bodies. The condition is discussed more fully in Chapter 17.

Toxic shock syndrome

This has been reported a number of times in association with breast infections. It is usually mild, and especially related to periprosthetic infections or minor postoperative collections; however, deaths have been reported.[40] The sudden deterioration occurs, usually in a young woman, when an apparently innocuous collection is drained.[49] It is rare, does not seem to differ significantly from the more common occurrence with tampon use, and is managed in the same way.

Neonatal breast abscess

Neonatal breast abscess is uncommon (Fig. 14.8). Efrat et al.[50] reported 21 cases of neonatal mastitis over 8 years; half presented with mastitis and half with an established abscess. *Staphylococcus* was present in 85% of cases, and 50% resolved on antibiotics alone, usually intravenous orbenin or augmentin. Abscess was treated by needle drainage or incision, and both were effective. Stricker et al.[51] found 18 cases over 10 years. It was more common in girls, with a peak incidence in the fourth and fifth weeks.

Not all series show such a high incidence of staphylococcal infection. The detailed bacteriology has been reported in a series of 14 cases over a 10-year period.[52] In this series there were 10 girls and 4 boys, with a mean age of 13 days, range 12–28. A wide variety of organisms were recovered, more reminiscent of nonpuerperal abscess in adults than of lactational abscess. Aerobic organisms were found in 57%, anaerobic in 21% and mixed organisms in 21%. The commonest isolates were *Staph. aureus* (7), *Bacteroides* (5), *Streptococcus* group B (2), *Escherichia coli* (2) and *Peptostreptococcus* (2). No clinical differences were seen among abscesses harbouring different organisms, and no recurrence was seen after management with antibiotics and conservative drainage. If neonatal mastitis is encountered, care needs to be taken to ensure that as little tissue damage as possible is caused either by disease or surgery. It is easy to remove the whole breast disc at this stage, leading to secondary amastia. The incision should avoid the breast bud behind the nipple and no tissue should be excised, so a policy of aspiration and appropriate antibiotics should be pursued.

Specific infections of the breast

Tuberculosis (Fig. 14.9)

Experience with tuberculosis of the breast is changing rapidly, so that the subject needs to be discussed from two points of view: the classic disease is rarely seen in Western countries but still commonly occurs in developing countries; and the new disease pattern is seen in immunocompromised patients, especially those with HIV infection.

Tuberculosis is an uncommon condition in the UK today, but was more frequent in the earlier part of the twentieth century. Scott in 1904[53] reported that 1.5% of the breast cases seen at St Bartholomew's Hospital in London were due to tuberculosis. This represented one case for every 40 new cancers seen. In India it is still a relatively common condition: Rangabashyam et al.[54] reviewed 215 cases of breast disease over a 5-year period in Madras and recorded seven cases of tuberculous disease (3%), while Banerjee et al.[55] found 1.06% of all breast lesions were due to tuberculous mastitis. Murthy et al.[56] reported tuberculosis in 10 of 302 benign breast biopsies performed over a 10-year period in Papua New Guinea. Alagaratnam and Ong[57] reported that they still found one case per year in Hong Kong.

In a mammographic survey from Saudi Arabia Makanjuola et al.[58] reported that 0.52% of 1152 consecutive examinations showed evidence of tuberculosis. Shinde et al.[59] have reported 100 cases referred with a diagnosis

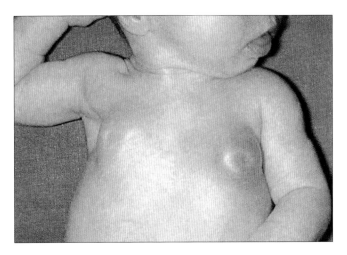

Fig. 14.8 Neonatal breast abscess.

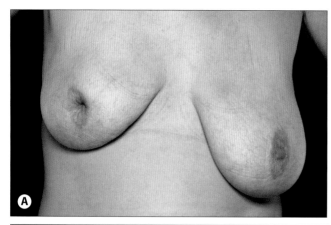

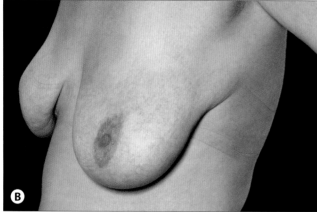

Fig. 14.9 (**A**) Nipple retraction caused by tuberculosis of the breast. (**B**) Same patient showing tuberculous abscess in the inframammary fold.

to the Tata Memorial Hospital in Mumbai. Although tuberculosis is now seen mainly in developing countries, it is still not uncommon in recent immigrants to the UK.[60] Newly diagnosed breast tuberculosis in Western populations has been reported as the first manifestation of AIDS.[36] However, not all granulomatous lesions of the breast prove to be tuberculosis. In the past, the foreign body granulomas of PDM were frequently confused with tuberculosis; every effort should be taken to identify the bacteria in the tissue or on culture.

In most patients, the diagnosis is relatively straightforward as they have evidence of tuberculosis elsewhere. However, in a few patients breast disease is the first manifestation and since on clinical grounds it can be difficult to differentiate between tuberculosis and cancer a high index of suspicion needs to be maintained. Tuberculosis in the breast may appear as one of three types: nodular, disseminated and sclerosing.[59] Each of these may be difficult to differentiate from cancer. The nodular form may

appear as a painless mass that later involves the skin, forming sinuses and ulcers. In the disseminated form multiple foci become confluent and caseate with skin ulceration and association with axillary lymphadenopathy. In sclerosing tuberculosis there is more fibrosis than caseation and nipple retraction is a common consequence. It may also be secondary to retromammary abscess, spreading through the chest wall from pleural disease. Since mammography may not show underlying chest wall disease, CT scanning should be used when mammary disease reaches the posterior aspect of the breast.[61] Jalali et al.[62] have reviewed the presenting features of 50 consecutive cases; 60% had a solitary breast lump, 26% breast lump with axillary lymphadenopathy, 8% diffuse breast swelling with axillary lymphadenopathy, 4% with breast abscess and 2% with breast lump and axillary fistula. Sixty-four per cent of the patients were already known to have tuberculosis.

The condition appears to occur more frequently during pregnancy.[63] Pathological examination of the tissue shows granulomatous reactions which are indistinguishable from those seen in other granulomatous diseases. Diagnosis is dependent on identifying the organism either in the sections or on culture. Shinde et al.,[59] however, were able to culture only 12 of their 100 patients successfully. It follows that the clinician needs to be aware of this disease and to plan the appropriate bacteriological investigations in suspected cases.

Treatment should follow general principles. The infection is controlled by a prolonged course of antituberculosis chemotherapy. For example, Jalali et al.[62] treated 50 patients with 1 year of antituberculosis chemotherapy and obtained complete resolution of the disease in 48; the remaining two had the lump excised. In the past, many patients have undergone mastectomy but this now seems unreasonable.

Other mycobacteria

Mycobacterial species other than tuberculosis also occasionally cause problems in the breast. Leprosy has been described and is usually accompanied by other manifestations of the disease.[64] Atypical mycobacteria are found in association with periprosthetic infection.[41]

Syphilis

This disease is now very rare but deserves a mention if only for historical reasons. The breast used to be regarded as a common site of extragenital chancres. Fitzwilliams[65] quoted the findings of Buckley, who described 1148 examples of nipple chancre.

Tertiary syphilis may affect the breast either as a diffuse fibrotic reaction or as a gumma. The gumma usually appears as a discrete lump that disappears when appropriate antisyphilitic treatment is instituted.

Today, these conditions are a medical curiosity, but the possibility of a primary chancre needs to be considered because early treatment is curative.

Actinomycosis and brucellosis

Actinomycosis occasionally occurs in the breast. It is not different from actinomycosis elsewhere in the body and is characterized by induration, sinus formation and excretion of sulphur granules. There is usually actinomycosis elsewhere, but sometimes the breast is the first or only part afflicted.[66] Both breast abscess and granulomatous mastitis due to brucellosis has been reported.[67]

Mycotic infections

Painful nipple during breastfeeding may be associated with thrush infection. Interestingly, *Candida* infection of the nipple is more common in those who do not breast-feed.[68] Candida may also be a problem in the inframammary fold, particularly in those with pendulous breasts.

Other mycotic infections occasionally occur and have been reviewed by Symmers.[69] Salfelder and Schwartz[70] speculated on the rarity of mycotic infection of the breast and considered that many cases were overlooked. A number of fungi have been demonstrated in the breast. Blastomycosis has been most commonly described and may be diagnosed on fine needle aspiration cytology.[71] The usual mode of presentation is of a breast mass clinically suspicious for carcinoma. Other fungi causing similar problems are *Pityrosporum*,[72] *Cryptococcus*,[73] *Aspergillus*[74] and *Histoplasma*.[71] Appropriate antifungal treatment is successful in many cases although excision may also be required. Cases of fungal infection complicating augmentation mammoplasty have been reported.[75]

Protozoan infections

These are extremely rare in the Western world. In developing countries where the appropriate conditions are common, they are met from time to time when they presumably represent metastatic septic foci. Marsden et al.[76]

have, however, described two cases of leishmaniasis of the nipple that they considered to have been directly infected, one from the mouth of her suckling child.

Helminthic infection

Filaria

This is relatively common in Asia and is clinically easily confused with carcinoma. In Madras, there were five cases in the 215 cases of benign disease described by Rangabashyam et al.[54] The pathological process appears to be confined to the superficial dermal layers and lymphatics, the glandular tissue being spared. In the early stages, appropriate antifilarial therapy is effective although, when secondary damage has occurred, simple mastectomy may be indicated in occasional patients.

Filaria is the most frequently reported infestation of the breast and may take a variety of forms. The adult worm may appear at the nipple,[77] or a granulomatous reaction may present as a mass.[78] Most of the reports emanate from Southeast Asia. The diagnosis may be made on fine needle aspirates. Kapila and Verma[79] recorded nine cases in 4714 benign breast cytological examinations reported over a 15-year period. Among the cases of filariae in breast aspirates, gravid adult females of *Wuchereria bancrofti* were seen in three cases and microfilarial larvae in four. In the remaining two cases, an intense, eosinophilic infiltrate was seen in breast aspirates, while microfilariae were identified in aspirates from draining axillary lymph nodes. Living *W. bancrofti* have been demonstrated on ultrasound.[80]

Other infestations

Hydatid disease may rarely occur in the breast in parts of the world where this is common. It was known as an entity to Sir Astley Cooper,[81] who clearly described a case in his work. Such an event occurs in less than 0.5% of patients with hydatid cysts.[82] The lesion is usually cystic and the diagnosis made on aspiration. If the possibility is considered prior to this, full appropriate precautions for dealing with hydatid cysts should be taken. Excision of the cyst should prove curative for the local disease, although it should always be assumed that it is secondary to internal hydatid disease, usually of the liver.

Cysts due to cysticercosis have also been reported.[83] The diagnosis may be made on cytological examination.[79] Guinea worm infection has also been reported. The adult

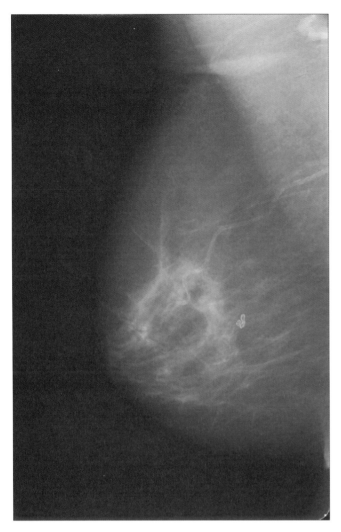

Fig. 14.10 Calcified Guinea worm in breast of African woman.

worms may be seen on mammography (Fig. 14.10).[84] Similarly, schistosomiasis may affect the breast.[85]

Viral infections

Mastitis is frequently described as a complication of mumps. The incidence is uncertain because the only symptom, swelling and tenderness of the breast, is such a common one that recognition that this is a separate condition may be difficult. Philip et al.,[86] in their study of a mumps epidemic in an isolated Eskimo population, reported that 15% of 158 women had mastitis. The ages of the affected patients ranged from 12 to 61; the incidence of mastitis was 31% of women over 15 years old. As the majority of women in this age group would be

menstrually active, it is difficult to be certain that the symptoms were not related to cyclical discomfort rather than mumps-specific mastitis. We have never seen a case that could be attributed to mumps.

A more important consideration of viruses in the breast is that some such as HIV, cytomegalovirus, hepatitis and HLTV-1 are excreted in milk and may cause infection in the infant. This topic has been reviewed by Lawrence & Lawrence.[87] Some aspects of HIV infection have been discussed in the section on lactational infection.

Infections of associated structures

Skin lesions

The breast is covered by normal skin and any cutaneous infection may occur on the breast. Perhaps the commonest of these is an infected sebaceous cyst. Furuncles and carbuncles may also occur occasionally. There is not usually any problem with diagnosis because they are clearly dermal in origin, or involving the subcutaneous tissue in the case of carbuncle.

Hidradenitis suppurativa may occur. When it occurs in association with axillary disease, diagnosis is not a problem. Isolated hidradenitis, particularly in the intermammary cleft or the inframammary fold, may cause difficulty. When this condition occurs in the skin overlying the breast, differentiation from an underlying peripheral DE with PDM may be difficult. It is dealt with more fully in Chapter 11.

Pilonidal abscess

In the series of mammary duct fistula described by Patey and Thackray,[88] it is recorded that loose hairs were found in a lactiferous sinus of one of their patients. They also record that they found loose hairs in a normal lactiferous sinus. Because there are no hair follicles in the nipple, it seems that this event is analogous to the classic pilonidal sinus. Bowers[89] has described three cases of periareolar pilonidal abscess acquired as work-related disease in sheep shearers and barbers. Gannon et al.[90] have described a patient with recurrent periareolar abscesses. Hairs from their male patients were seen to protrude from the nipple ducts and were also found within the abscess cavity. Routine questioning of hairdressers in the clinic suggests that they at least recognize this as a common problem.

REFERENCES

1. Scholefield JM, Duncan JL & Rogers K. Review of hospital experience of breast abscess. *British Journal of Surgery* 1987; **74**: 469–470.

2. Bundred NJ, Dover MS, Coley S *et al.* Breast abscesses and cigarette smoking. *British Journal of Surgery* 1992; **79**: 58–59.

3. Bates T, Down RHL, Tant DR *et al.* The current treatment of breast abscess in hospital and in general practice. *Practitioner* 1973; **211**: 541–547.

4. Amir LH, Forster D, McLachlan H *et al.* Incidence of breast abscess in lactating women: report from an Australian cohort. *British Journal of Obstetrics and Gynaecology* 2004; **111**: 1378–1381.

5. Fulton AA. Incidence of puerperal and lactational mastitis in an industrial town of some 43,000 inhabitants. *British Medical Journal* 1945; **1**: 693–696.

6. Kinlay JR, O'Connell DL & Kinlay S. Risk factors for mastitis in breastfeeding women: results of a prospective cohort study. *Australian and New Zealand Journal of Public Health* 2001; **25**: 115–120.

7. Kaufmann R & Foxman B. Mastitis among lactating women: occurrence and risk factors. *Social Science and Medicine* 1991; **33**: 701–705.

8. Foxman B, D'Arcy H, Gillespie B *et al.* Lactation mastitis: occurrence and medical management among 946 breastfeeding women in the United States. *American Journal of Epidemiology* 2002; **155**: 103–114

9. Goodman MA & Benson EA. An evaluation of current trends in the management of breast abscesses. *Medical Journal of Australia* 1970; **1**: 1034–1039.

10. Newton M & Newton NR. Breast abscess. A result of lactation failure. *Surgery, Gynecology and Obstetrics* 1950; **91**: 651–655.

11. Hayes R, Michell M & Nunnerly HB. Acute inflammation of the breast – the role of breast ultrasound in diagnosis and management. *Clinical Radiology* 1991; **44**: 253–256.

12. Taylor MD & Way S. Penicillin in treatment of acute puerperal mastitis. *British Medical Journal* 1946; **2**: 731–732.

13. O'Hara RJ, Dexter SPL & Fox JN. Conservative management of infective mastitis and breast abscesses after ultrasonographic assessment. *British Journal of Surgery* 1996; **83**: 1413–1414.

14. Pluchinotta AM & Catania S. Percutaneous drainage of peripheral nonlactational breast abscesses. *Breast Disease* 1996; **9**: 223–227.

15. Berna JD, Garcia Medina V, Madrigal M *et al.* Percutaneous drainage of breast abscesses. *European Journal of Radiology* 1996; **21**: 217–219.

16. Eryilmaz R, Sahin M, Hakan Tekelioglu M *et al.* Management of lactational breast abscesses. *Breast* 2005; **14**: 375–379.

17. Varey AH, Shere MH & Cawthorn SJ. Treatment of loculated lactational breast abscess with a vacuum biopsy system. *British Journal of Surgery* 2005; **92**: 1225–1226.

18. Benson EA & Goodman MA. Incision with primary suture in the treatment of acute puerperal breast abscess. *British Journal of Surgery* 1970; **57**: 55–58.

19. Rowley WA. *Practical Treatise on Diseases of the Breast of Women.* London: Newberry & Ridley; 1772.

20. Marshall BR, Hepper JK & Zirbell CC. Sporadic puerperal mastitis: an infection that need not interrupt lactation. *Journal of the American Medical Association* 1975; **233**: 1377–1379.

21. Applebaum RM. The modern management of successful breast feeding. *Pediatric Clinics of North America* 1970; **17**: 203–225.

22. Editorial. Puerperal mastitis. *British Medical Journal* 1976; **1**: 920–921.

23. European Multicentre Group for Cabergoline in Lactation Inhibition. Single dose cabergoline versus bromocriptine in inhibition of puerperal lactation: randomised double blind multicentre study. *British Medical Journal* 1991; **302**: 1367–1371.

24. Pyörälä S. Indicators of inflammation in the diagnosis of mastitis. *Veterinary Research* 2003; **34**: 565–578.

25. Flores M & Filteau S. Effect of lactation counselling on subclinical mastitis among Bangladeshi women. *Annals of Tropical Paediatrics: International Child Health* 2002; **22**: 85–88.

26. Walker AP, Edmiston CE Jr, Krepel CJ *et al.* A prospective study of the microflora of nonpuerperal breast abscess. *Archives of Surgery* 1988; **123**: 908–911.

27. Schafer P, Furrer C & Merillod B. An association of cigarette smoking with recurrent subareolar breast abscess. *International Journal of Epidemiology* 1988; **17**: 810–813.

28. Rahal RM, de Freitas-Junior R, Paulinelli RR. Risk factors for duct ectasia. *Breast Journal* 2005; **11**: 262–265.

29. Versluijs-Ossewaarde FN, Roumen RM & Goris RJ. Subareolar breast abscesses: characteristics and results of surgical treatment. *Breast Journal* 2005; **11**: 179–182.

30. Thornton JW. Argenta LC, McClatchy KD *et al.* Studies on the endogenous flora of the human breast. *Annals of Plastic Surgery* 1988; **20**: 39–42.

31. Dixon JM. Outpatient treatment of non-lactational breast abscesses. *British Journal of Surgery* 1992; **79**: 56–57.

32. Leach RD, Eykyn SJ, Phillips I *et al.* Anaerobic subareolar breast abscess. *Lancet* 1979; **i**: 35–37.

33. Cotton MH. Breast abscesses in Nigeria. Lactational versus non-lactational. *Journal of the Royal College of Surgeons of Edinburgh* 1997: **42**: 61.

34. John GC, Nduati RW, Mbori-Ngacha DA *et al.* Correlates of mother-to-child human immunodeficiency virus type 1 (HIV-1) transmission: association with maternal plasma HIV-1 RNA load, genital HIV-1 DNA shedding, and breast infections. *Journal of Infectious Diseases* 2001; **183**: 206–212.

35. Nussenblatt V, Lema V, Kumwenda N *et al.* Epidemiology and microbiology of subclinical mastitis among HIV-infected women in Malawi. *International Journal of STD and AIDS* 2005; **16**: 227–232.

36. Hartstein M & Leaf HL. Tuberculosis of the breast as a presenting manifestation of AIDS. *Clinical Infectious Diseases* 1992; **15**: 692–693.

37. Simpson AJH, Juma A & Das SS. Breast abscess caused by *Nocardia asteroides*. *Journal of Infection* 1995; **30**: 266–267.

38. Keidan RD, Hoffman JP, Weese JL *et al.* Delayed breast abscess after lumpectomy and radiotherapy. *American Surgeon* 1990; **56**: 440–444.

39. Shore RE, Hildreth N, Woodard E *et al.* Breast cancer among women given X-ray therapy for acute postpartum mastitis. *Journal of the National Cancer Institute* 1986; **77**: 689–696.

40. Brown SL, Hefflin B, Woo EK *et al.* Infections related to breast implants reported to the Food and Drug Administration, 1977–1997. *Journal of the Long Term Effects of Medical Implants* 2001; **11**: 1–12.

41. Clegg HW, Foster MT, Sanders WE *et al.* Infections due to organisms of the *Mycobacterium fortuitum* complex after augmentation mammaplasty: clinical and epidemiological features. *Journal of Infectious Diseases* 1983; **147**: 427–433.

42. Walsh R, Kliewer MA, Sullivan DC *et al.* Periprosthetic mycobacterial infection – CT and mammographic findings. *Clinical Imaging* 1995; **19**: 193–196.

43. Pajkos A, Deva AK, Vickery K *et al.* Detection of subclinical infection in significant breast implant capsules. *Plastic and Reconstructive Surgery* 2003; **111**: 1605–1611.

44. Hoda SA, Borgen P & Rosen PP. Unanticipated presentation of an unusual foreign body in the breast. *Breast Disease* 1994; **7**: 227–230.

45. Griffiths AA, Cooper RA & Demos TC. Breast abscess as a late complication of plombage. *Canadian Association of Radiologists Journal* 1995; **46**: 43–44.

46. Jacobs VR, Golombeck K, Jonat W *et al.* Mastitis nonpuerperalis after nipple piercing: time to act. *International Journal of Fertility and Women's Medicine* 2003; **48**: 226–231.

47. Clark KR & Higgs MJ. Breast abscess following central venous catheterisation. *Intensive Care Medicine* 1991; **17**: 123–124.

48. Rosenberg MW & Hughes LE. Artefactual breast disease: a report of three cases. *British Journal of Surgery* 1985; **72**: 539–540.

49. Tobin G, Shaw RC & Goodpasture HC. Toxic shock syndrome following breast and nasal operations. *Plastic and Reconstructive Surgery* 1987; **80**: 111–114.

50. Efrat M, Mogilner JG, Iutjman M *et al.* Neonatal mastitis – diagnosis and treatment. *Israel Journal of Medical Sciences* 1995; **31**: 558–560.

51. Stricker T, Navratil F, Sennhauser FH. Mastitis in early infancy. *Acta Paediatrica* 2005; **94**: 166–169.

52. Brooke I. The aerobic and anaerobic microbiology of neonatal breast abscess. *Pediatric Infectious Disease Journal* 1991; **10**: 785–786.

53. Scott SR. Tuberculosis of the female breast. *St Bartholomew's Hospital Reports* 1904; **40**: 97–122.

54. Rangabashyam N, Gnanaprakasam D, Krishnaraj B *et al.* Spectrum of benign breast lesions in Madras. *Journal of the Royal College of Surgeons of Edinburgh* 1983; **28**: 369–373.

55. Banerjee SN, Ananthakrishnan N, Mehth RB *et al.* Tuberculous mastitis: a continuing problem. *World Journal of Surgery* 1986; **11**: 105–109.

56. Murthy DP, Sengupta SK & Muthaiah AC. Benign breast disease in Papua New Guinea. *Papua New Guinea Medical Journal* 1992; **35**: 101–105.

57. Alagaratnam TJ & Ong GB. Tuberculosis of the breast. *British Journal of Surgery* 1980; **67**: 125–126.

58. Makanjuola D, Murshid K, Al Sulaimani S *et al.* Mammographic features of breast tuberculosis: the skin bulge and sinus tract sign. *Clinical Radiology* 1996; **51**: 354–358.

59. Shinde SR, Chandawarkar RY & Deshmukh SP. Tuberculosis of the breast masquerading as carcinoma: a study of 100 patients. *World Journal of Surgery* 1995; **19**: 379–381.

60. Jah A, Mulla R, Lawrence FD *et al.* Tuberculosis of the breast: experience of a UK breast clinic serving an ethnically diverse population. *Annals of the Royal College of Surgeons of England* 2004; **86**: 416–419.

61. Chung SY, Yang I, Bae SH *et al.* Tuberculous abscess in the retromammary region – CT findings. *Journal of Computer Assisted Tomography* 1996; **20**: 766–769.

62. Jalali U, Rasul S, Khan A *et al.* Tuberculous mastitis. *Journal of the College Physicians and Surgeons of Pakistan* 2005; **15**: 234–237.

63. McKeown KC & Wilkinson KW. Tuberculous disease of the breast. *British Journal of Surgery* 1952; **39**: 409–429.

64. Furniss AL. Leproma occurring in a female breast presenting as a carcinoma. *Indian Medical Gazette* 1952; **87**: 304.

65. Fitzwilliams DSL. *On the Breast.* London: William Heinmann; 1924.

66. Jain BK, Schgal VN, Jagdish S *et al.* Primary actinomycosis of the breast: clinical review and a case report. *Journal of Dermatology* 1994; **2**: 497–500.

67. Al Abdely HM & Amin TM. Breast abscess caused by brucellosis mellitensis. *Journal of Infection* 1996; **33**: 219–220.

68. Morrill JF, Heinig MJ, Pappagianis D *et al*. Risk factors for mammary candidosis among lactating women. *Journal of Obstetrics, Gynecology and Neonatal Nursing* 2005; **34**: 37–45.

69. Symmers WS. The breasts. In: Payling Wright G (ed.). *Systemic Pathology*, vol 1. London: Longman Green; 1966:953–955.

70. Salfelder K & Schwartz J. Mycotic 'pseudotumours' of the breast. *Archives of Surgery* 1975; **110**: 751–754.

71. Farmer C, Stanley MW, Bardales RH *et al*. Mycoses of the breast: diagnosis by fine-needle aspiration. *Diagnostic Cytopathology* 1995; **12**: 51–55.

72. Bertini B. Cytopathology of nipple discharge due to *Pityrosporum orbiculare* and cocci in an elderly woman. *Acta Cytologica* 1975; **19**: 38–42.

73. Goldman M & Pottage JC. Cryptococcal infection of the breast. *Clinical Infectious Diseases* 1995; **21**: 1166–1167.

74. Govindarajan M, Verghese S & Kuruvilla S. Primary aspergillosis of the breast. Report of a case with fine needle aspiration cytology diagnosis. *Acta Cytologica* 1993; **37**: 234–236.

75. Williams K, Walton RL & Bunkis J. Aspergillus colonisation associated with bilateral silicone mammary implants. *Plastic and Reconstructive Surgery* 1983; **71**: 260–261.

76. Marsden PD, Almeida EA, Llanos Cuentas EA *et al*. *Leishmania braziliensis* infection of the nipple. *British Medical Journal* 1985; **290**: 433–434.

77. Lahiri VL. Microfilariae in nipple secretion. *Acta Cytologica* 1975; **19**: 154.

78. Chen Y. Filarial granuloma of the female breast. A histopathologic study of 131 cases. *American Journal of Tropical Medicine and Hygiene* 1981; **30**: 1206–1210.

79. Kapila K & Verma K. Diagnosis of parasites in fine needle breast aspirates. *Acta Cytologica* 1996; **40**: 653–656.

80. Dreyer G, Branda AC, Amaral F *et al*. Detection by ultrasound of living adult *Wuchereria bancrofti* in the female breast. *Memorias do Instituto Oswaldo Cruz* 1996; **91**: 95–96.

81. Cooper A. *Illustrations of the Diseases of the Breast*. London: Longman; 1829.

82. Dew HR. *Hydatid Disease*. Sydney: Australia Medical Publishing; 1928.

83. Leggat CAC. Cysticercosis of the breast. *Australian and New Zealand Journal of Surgery* 1983; **53**: 281.

84. Stelling CB. Dracunculiasis presenting as a sterile abscess. *American Journal of Roentgenology* 1982; **138**: 1159–1161.

85. Sloan BS, Rickman LS, Blau EM *et al*. Schistosomiasis masquerading as carcinoma of the breast. *Southern Medical Journal* 1996; **89**: 345–347.

86. Philip RN, Reinhard KR & Lackman DB. Observations on a mumps epidemic in a 'virgin' population. *American Journal of Hygiene* 1959; **69**: 91–111.

87. Lawrence RM, Lawrence RA. Breast milk and infection. *Clinical Perinatology* 2004; **31**: 501–528.

88. Patey DH & Thackray AC. Pathology and treatment of mammary duct fistula. *Lancet* 1958; **ii**: 871–874.

89. Bowers PW. Roustabouts' and Barber's breasts. *Clinical and Experimental Dermatology* 1982; **7**: 445–448.

90. Gannon MX, Crowson MC & Fielding JWL. Periareolar pilonidal abscesses in a hairdresser. *British Medical Journal* 1988; **297**: 1641–1642.

CHAPTER 15

Congenital and growth disorders

Key points and new developments

1. Congenital abnormalities of the breast, relating mainly to absence, hypoplasia or ectopia, are sometimes part of wider congenital syndromes, with particular tendency to affect the urinary tract or limb girdles.

2. It is now recognized that the fetal 'milk line' is not as extensive in humans as in some animals, so most ectopic tissue is found between the axilla and epigastrium.

3. Axillary accessory breasts can be subject to all varieties of pathology seen in the breast proper, so axillary masses should be assessed individually, as well as in association with any breast mass.

4. Breast hypertrophy conforms to the ANDI concept, and can be loosely categorized as normal (the larger end of the normal spectrum), aberration (when breast weight is sufficient to cause physical symptoms as well as embarrassment) and disease (the rapid and extreme enlargement of gigantomastia, requiring urgent intervention).

5. Gigantomastia shows characteristic pathology, including excess ducts and stroma with a paucity of lobules, oestrogen receptor negative but progesterone receptor positive, but the aetiology remains obscure and treatment unsatisfactory.

Introduction

The breast, like other physical features, exhibits a wide range of appearances. There is variation in size, shape and, to some extent, position. The borderline of what is socially and cosmetically acceptable is one of perception because most variants retain normal function. Other conditions show a greater deviation from normal, arising on a congenital basis, or as an aberration of development of the breast during reproductive life. Those aspects of these conditions related to general principles of breast development, aetiology and pathophysiology are dealt with in this chapter. The details of management, particularly those involving reconstructive and cosmetic surgery, are beyond the scope of this book.

Developmental anomalies

These may be unilateral or bilateral, involve either nipple or breast or both, and be seen as absent, hypoplastic, supernumerary or ectopic structures. They may occur as isolated abnormalities, but may also be associated with a variety of other developmental abnormalities, particularly of the upper limb and urinary tract. Hypertrophy of the breast is also considered in this chapter, as an aberration of growth of uncertain aetiology, with only a few known to have an underlying genetic component.

The development of the breast has been described in Chapter 3. The fetal mammalian milk line has classically been considered to run from the base of the upper limb bud to the base of the lower limb bud, but the validity of this theory in humans is now challenged (see Ch. 3). In most adult mammals, breast tissue is confined to this milk line but, in some, breast tissue is found in other sites: either the milk line is more extensive or breast tissue migrates. Examples of these ectopic sites are the labia in whales and dolphins, the scapular region in nutria, abdominal midline in the possum, dorsal thigh in the viscaccia, and the acromion in a species of lemur. The occurrence of breastlike structures or pathology in these areas, along the milk line, has been regarded as evidence of embryological remnants of a human axilla–groin milk line. However, true congenital lesions in the human are overwhelmingly confined to the axillo-pectoral region.

Polythelia and supernumerary nipples

Some authors use these terms synonymously; others reserve polythelia for those examples of more than one nipple appearing on the same breast mound.[1] We see no benefit in the distinction and regard the terms as interchangeable.

Supernumerary nipples may occur in association with accessory glandular breast tissue or more commonly occur alone. Extra nipples are most commonly found on the lower part of the breast, chest wall and upper abdomen just below the rib margin and are often mistaken for naevi (Fig. 15.1). The reported incidence of supernumerary nipples varies greatly in the literature. Most cases are sporadic but sometimes there is a clearly demonstrable inherited predisposition.[2] Schmidt[3] examined 502 children to establish the prevalence, size, sex and side predilection of supernumerary nipples. Twenty-eight (5.6%) exhibited a supernumerary nipple. It was more common

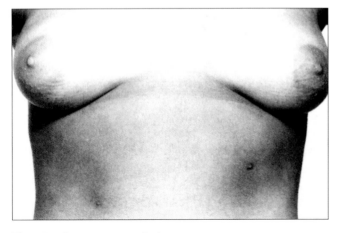

Fig. 15.1 Supernumerary nipples.

in boys than girls (20:8) and more common on the left than right.

Méhes[4] screened 4000 neonates in Hungary and found an incidence of polythelia of only 0.2% and described an association with renal abnormalities. The condition is usually considered to be more common in Oriental populations.[5]

The association with renal anomalies reported by Méhes[4] was supported by the findings of another study that found an incidence of supernumerary nipples in 16% of patients with end-stage renal failure, but only 2% of control patients.[6] Other studies have failed to confirm the findings. Robertson et al.[7] found an incidence of 1.2% in 2875 black children with no evidence of associated renal anomalies. Grotto et al.[8] found two cases of supernumerary nipples in 98 children with radiological renal tract anomalies and two in 103 with normal renal tracts. They do not consider the presence of a supernumerary nipple as adequate indication for radiological investigation of the renal tract.

The balance of evidence suggests that supernumerary nipples are common (1–2%) and associated congenital abnormalities rare.[9] However, the associations and classifications of congenital abnormalities linking breast/nipple, urinary tract and limbs are complex, and should be borne in mind when any of the abnormalities are found in the newborn.

No treatment is required for this condition except when it is accompanied by active breast tissue or if the patient finds it cosmetically unacceptable.

Athelia

Absence of the nipple is a rare event and usually is associated with absence of the breast. Athelia is usually associated with other abnormalities such as the autosomal dominant inherited scalp-ears-nipple (Finlay-Marks) syndrome,[10] although it may appear as an isolated anomaly.[11] Athelia in neonates has also been described following maternal use of carbimazole.[12] Occasional examples of imperforate nipple have been reported as a cause of failure to lactate with an engorged breast. It is difficult to be certain that these obstructed nipples were not secondary to trauma such as burns.

Nipple inversion

Nipple inversion is a common finding. There are three main causes: congenital, periductal inflammation and tumour infiltration. The last of these is beyond the scope of this text but in our series represents only a small percentage of observed nipple retraction.

The distinction between inversion and retraction is rather arbitrary: we use inversion to describe the nipple that did not protrude at the time of adolescent development and retraction for those cases in which a previously everted nipple is affected by an underlying pathological process.

Congenital

During fetal life, the nipple is represented by a central depression which persists after birth until development of the underlying breast produces elevation of the areola. Subsequent retraction of the surrounding smooth muscle leads to flattening of the mound and protrusion of the nipple.[13]

Some degree of nipple inversion in nulliparous adult women is common. The wide range of reported prevalence probably reflects different criteria for diagnosis rather than real differences in different populations. Alexander and Campbell[14] found that the incidence was almost 10%. Park et al.[15] found that 53 of 1625 (3.26%) unmarried Korean women between 19 and 25 had inverted nipples. Schwager et al.,[16] in their study of 339 breasts, found six with inversion of the nipple (a prevalence of 1.8%). They considered the cause of the inversion to be a deficiency in the supporting stroma immediately behind the nipple as there was no qualitative difference in the constituents of the areola, mammary ducts, smooth muscle or collagen. An alternative view is to regard the inversion as due to the failure of the smooth muscle bundles of Sappy (circular) and Myerholtz (radial) to relax.[17] In any event it appears that inversion is best regarded as failure of normal eversion to occur. In the established case, the ducts are shortened and deeply attached, while the normally tough musculo-fibro-collagenous tissue behind the nipple is replaced by a potential hollow cavity into which the nipple retracts.

The findings are usually bilateral, but often to different degrees, and it is not rare to find one side completely inverted and the other normal. The true incidence of congenital nipple inversion is hard to determine because such women are more disposed to periductal inflammation, the second most common cause of nipple inversion.

Problems related to inverted nipples are functional (associated with breastfeeding) and cosmetic.

Inverted nipples and breastfeeding

The problems associated with breastfeeding have been reviewed by Inch.[18] Waller[19] found that nearly 40% of young women in their first pregnancy had at least a minor degree of failure of normal protrusion of the nipple, but maintained that this should not be considered a contraindication to breastfeeding, as so many maintain. He recommended a 'pinch test' to assess protrusion, and patients failing this test were given a glass (Woolwich) shield to wear during pregnancy, the purpose of which was gradually to stretch and loosen the nonprotractile nipple. Of patients with poorly protractile nipples treated in this way, only 44% were deemed to have breastfed successfully. Alexander et al.[20] found no intervention to be as effective as shells or Hoffman's exercises. Hytten[21] found that only 14% of 2461 primiparae had unsatisfactory nipples, and only 16% of these had breastfeeding problems as a direct result (2.2% of the whole group). Of those with normal nipples, 3.5% had similar problems. Thus, although antenatal examination of the nipples might have some predictive value, most patients with poor nipples will have no related problems with breastfeeding.[22] Our advice to nulliparous women with inverted nipples is that there is no contraindication in them attempting to breastfeed, and that post lactation the situation may have improved spontaneously.

These findings may be explained by cineradiographic[23] and ultrasound studies[24] of breastfeeding, which show that the nipple itself plays a relatively small part in the anatomical aspects of suckling. The infant makes a 'teat' from the surrounding breast tissue as well as the nipple, in a ratio of about 3:1. Thus, mothers with inverted nipples should be encouraged to ensure that the baby has an adequate mouthful of breast to form the teat, and be reassured that the contribution of the nipple is relatively small. Correct positioning during feeding is perhaps the most important factor and the patient should be given skilled help from a midwife before starting to breastfeed.

Inverted nipples and cosmesis

Treatment consists of reassurance that there is no serious underlying disease and, when the cosmetic defect is severe (or the patient very concerned about it), consideration of surgical correction. Park et al.[15] found that only nine of their 53 patients thought that it required correction. Problems can arise if the inversion interferes with cleansing, giving retained secretions, although this is more commonly seen in retraction due to duct ectasia (DE) in older women.

It is said that inversion can be improved by repeated massage, although there are few data from controlled studies to support this. In severe cases surgical correction may be requested. In general, a procedure involving excision of the shortened ducts, with core nipple excision if there is a persisting tendency to reinversion (as described for DE in Chapter 18), gives good long-term results, but is much too radical a procedure to be appropriate for most young girls.

Pitanguy[17] has described a procedure of dividing the muscle bundles without damaging the lactiferous tissues – an important consideration in young women who may still wish to feed their children. However, the large number of procedures described for congenital inverted nipple suggests that none of them is ideal. There is considerable doubt about the efficacy of procedures which do not divide the ducts, although new procedures continue to be recommended. Strombeck reported a 23% recurrence rate in his own unit, even after completely dividing the ducts.[25] The uncertain long-term outcome of any lesser procedure should be explained to the patient if surgery is advised. Our own views on surgical management are given in Chapter 18.

Retracted nipples following periductal inflammation

Periductal inflammation is discussed more fully elsewhere. While congenital inversion predisposes to inflammatory complications of periductal mastitis, and the associated secondary nipple retraction may give rise to problems of cosmesis, management needs to be directed towards the inflammatory process, and so is dealt with in Chapters 11, 14 and 18.

Supernumerary breasts (accessory breasts, axillary breasts)

The incidence of supernumerary breasts, defined as structures that produce milk under appropriate hormonal influences, remains uncertain although the condition has been recorded since antiquity. Statues of both Artemesia and Diana of Ephesus represent these ancients as having supernumerary breasts. Fitzwilliams[1] gave a good account of many of the earlier, and often colourful, descriptions. Darwin was clearly aware of the existence of polymastia and used the condition as an illustration of an atavistic phenomenon in 'the descent of man'. Most accessory breasts develop along the milk line, and of these the great majority occur in the axilla. Indeed, we have not seen one occurring outside the axillo-pectoral area.

Ectopic milk-producing structures have been described at all the ectopic sites that occur in the mammals described above, but the commoner examples used to justify an extensive milk line in humans, such as mammary-like tumours of the groin and labia, are now recognized to arise in glands (mammary-like glands) related to eccrine sweat glands occurring in that region. Thus, the widely quoted concept of a milk line extending to the groin in humans is now questioned.[26] Supernumerary breasts may rarely be found anywhere on the body; outside the so-called milk line, these too may be better regarded as mammary-like glands rather than true breasts. The commonest site of accessory breasts is the axilla, although still quite rare as Down et al.[27] estimated that the incidence was about 0.5% of referrals. It is remarkable how often these remain unnoticed until the second or third pregnancy (Fig. 15.2).These accessory glands do not always have nipples and may be quite troublesome during pregnancy and lactation. It is presumably because of hormonal stimulation that accessory breasts are more frequently recorded in women than in men (there being no embryological reason to suppose a difference).

The most important aspect of axillary breasts, apart from the discomfort associated with pregnancy and lactation, arises from the fact that axillary breasts are subject

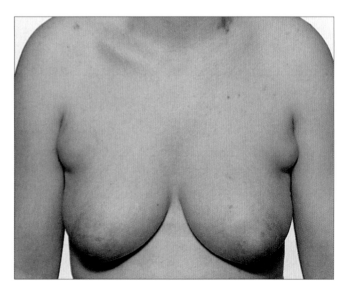

Fig. 15.2 Accessory (axillary) breasts. First noticed at time of lactation following first pregnancy.

to all the pathological processes seen in the breast, and as such can give rise to diagnostic errors. An example is the occurrence of nodularity of aberrations of normal development and involution (ANDI) (fibroadenosis) in an accessory breast suggesting metastatic lymph nodes in a patient with breast cancer.[28] Conditions as diverse as fibromatosis, phyllodes tumour, and hamartoma and primary cancer have been described. This reinforces the need for histological diagnosis of axillary as well as breast lesions, and considerable accuracy can be achieved in cytological assessment of lesions in axillary breast tissue.[29]

Treatment is only indicated if the accessory breast proves troublesome to the patient, the treatment then being surgical excision. Down et al.[27] reviewed the experience in Manchester. They found the overall incidence was 0.5%, more common on the right side and in Asian women. Twenty-eight of their 35 patients chose to undergo surgery; 11 of these had complications such as intercostobrachial nerve injury, poor scars, residual breast tissue and seromas. Many examples of accessory breast remain undiagnosed until removed with a clinical diagnosis of lipoma that is found to contain mammary tissue.

Accessory breast tissue may be isolated or may be connected to an accessory nipple. In the former case, the breast will involute soon after parturition; in the latter, an active secreting gland may produce sufficient milk to sustain the infant.

Amastia and hypoplasia

Amastia is a rare condition and is presumably due to failure of the milk line to develop, or to complete its involution. It is not surprising that such an obvious abnormality was recorded in biblical times (Song of Solomon, viii 8). The condition is quite uncommon, however, and is usually unilateral. Some cases have an associated absence of the pectoral muscles and associated syndactyly (a condition known as Poland's syndrome following his description in 1841). In spite of its popular eponym, this condition was apparently first described in 1839 by Floriep. The terminology has been challenged and, although Ravitch[30] has argued that the term should be abandoned, descriptions of Poland's syndrome persist. The familial nature of this condition was first remarked upon in 1894 by Whyte and, more recently, it has been established that it is transmitted as an autosomal dominant feature,[31] so is as common in boys as girls.

Mild, partial forms of Poland's syndrome are commoner than the full picture, and frequently go undiagnosed when they consist only of breast asymmetry and a horizontal anterior axillary fold due to partial absence of the pectoralis muscle (Fig. 15.3).[32] Spear et al.[33] regard this as a separate entity that they call anterior thoracic hypoplasia in which the nipple–areola complex lies superior and the pectoralis muscle is normal.

Poland's syndrome is the best known of a number of rare inherited disorders of breast development. The Pallister ulnar-mammary syndrome (UMS) is an example; the common manifestations of a very varied clinical picture include limb deficiencies and failure of breast development. This condition may also be inherited.[34]

Hypoplastic breasts of a lesser degree are not uncommon and there is some evidence of an association with mitral valve prolapse. Patients attending for breast augmentation have a higher incidence of mitral valve prolapse; patients with a diagnosis of mitral valve prolapse have been found to have smaller breasts than controls, the putative defect occurring during a time of mesenchymal development in the sixth week.[35]

Asymmetry

Minor degrees of breast asymmetry are very common and the patient may be reassured. When the discrepancy is great (Fig. 15.4), surgical correction may be indicated to equalize the breasts. Augmentation of the smaller breast, reduction of the larger breast, or both procedures, may be required to obtain a satisfactory result.

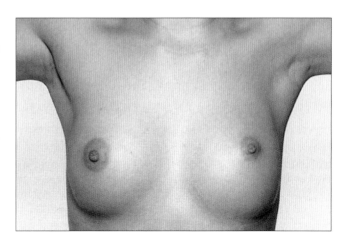

Fig. 15.3 Partial degree of Poland's syndrome (left), with a horizontal axillary fold due to hypoplasia of pectoral muscles, and asymmetry of nipple and areola.

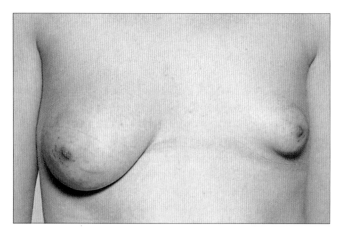

Fig. 15.4 Marked asymmetry of breasts for which plastic surgery is indicated.

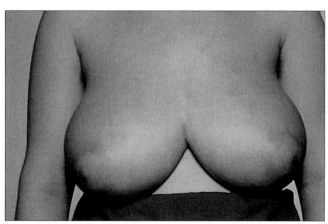

Fig. 15.5 Fused breasts.

More severe cases may be partially expressed examples of Poland's syndrome or follow trauma (usually burns or surgery) in childhood when the breast bud is damaged. Thoracotomy by the anterolateral or posterolateral route in prepubertal girls may result in ipsilateral hypoplasia of moderate degree and the thoracotomy technique should be modified appropriately to avoid this.[36]

Tubular breasts (trunk breast)

This is a distressing developmental abnormality where the areola is of excessive size relative to the rest of the breast.[37] Most of the spectrum lies within a normal or acceptable degree, but in severe examples the breast is elongated from a narrow base to take a sausage-shaped contour, with a disproportionately large and protuberant areola and nipple. The breast parenchyma may herniate into the large areola. Management requires skilled plastic surgery; a standard augmentation procedure merely accentuates the protrusion of the narrow breast. Mandrekas et al.[38] consider a key step is to divide the constricting ring at the base of the breast before resecting the excess areola tissue.

Fusion of the breasts

There is a wide variation of normality in the placing of the breasts on the chest wall. With one extreme, the breasts are fused in the midline (Fig. 15.5). This can cause difficulty and discomfort with clothing, and we have found it worthwhile separating the breasts by the simple plastic procedure shown in Figure 15.6.

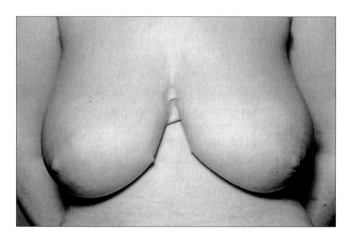

Fig. 15.6 Postoperative result of patient in Figure 15.5.

Premature breast development

An otherwise normal breast may enlarge for no discernible reason at several stages in childhood and adolescence. This excludes those cases due to excessive hormone production in childhood, e.g. from tumours, and in none of the conditions described below has any abnormality of circulating hormones been demonstrated.

Neonatal enlargement

Reference has already been made to neonatal hyperplasia in Chapter 3. It is normal to have some palpable breast tissue at birth and for this to disappear by the age of 6 months, although it tends to remain longer in girls than boys.[39]

Prepubertal (premature) thelarche

The normal development of the breast is described in Chapter 3. Premature breast development (thelarche) may occur as an isolated occurrence, usually a constitutional deviation from normal, or as a part of precocious puberty. This is defined as occurring before the age of 8 years in girls, since it is not uncommon to see breast development at about this age. This is often unilateral. Premature thelarche is not common. Zukauskaite et al.[40] only found one (0.6%) case in 225 7-year-old Lithuanian girls. The clinical appearances are of a firm discoid lesion behind the nipple, not unlike that found in the pubertal boy with gynaecomastia. The importance of the lesion is in recognizing it for what it is – normal breast tissue! Surgical removal of the mass is a disaster because it represents the whole of the developing breast. Removal will result in secondary amastia on the affected side. In a review of the natural history of this condition in 46 cases, 32% regressed completely over a 2-year period, 57% remained unchanged and 11% underwent progressive enlargement.[41]

Breast development before the age of 8 years requires full endocrine assessment, although in most cases no cause can be discovered and the prognosis is benign.[42] Verroti reported a long-term follow-up of 46 girls to see if those with isolated thelarche could be differentiated from those who would develop the full process of precocious puberty.[43] Endocrine assessment gave similar results in the two groups, but the age of onset was important; those showing thelarche between the age of 2 and 8 years were more likely to develop precocious puberty, while breast development before the age of 2 was more likely to regress.

Precocious breast development is one of the greatest causes of psychological upset in these girls. However, one-third can expect to have reversion of breast development to normal or near normal following treatment with a long-acting gonadotrophin-releasing hormone (GnRH) agonist such as triptorelin.[44]

Pubertal asymmetry

The breasts do not always develop synchronously and parents sometimes seek advice about a unilateral lump.

The same considerations apply to this condition as to the prepubertal variety – biopsy and excision must be avoided. Asynchronous development is not uncommon in normal pubescent girls.

Hypertrophic abnormalities of the breast

Large breasts range across a wide spectrum, from the 'well-endowed' who may consider their breasts a boon or an embarrassment depending on their individual outlook, through a size where discomfort, back and neck pain and interference with normal activities are added to embarrassment, to extreme enlargement (usually of sudden onset and rapid progression) where breast size may be life-threatening through ulceration and bleeding. This division fits well into the ANDI concept, the first being normal, the second an aberration and the third, disease (see Ch. 4).

The three degrees are also useful with regard to management, following the general approach to benign processes fitting the ANDI concept (normal, aberration, disease). Surgery should be approached with reluctance in the first group, where there is a high chance that the patient will consider the scarring and any complications as a poor exchange; in the second, surgery may be welcomed because of improvement in physical symptoms as well as relief from embarrassment; and surgery is imperative in the third group, at least until an effective pharmacological control becomes available.

Equally, it is useful to use precise nomenclature for the three groups, even though they merge and overlap: large breasts for the first, hypertrophy (virginal, gravid or involutional) for the second, and gigantomastia for the third. The retention of such an inelegant term as gigantomastia is justified by the necessity to recognize this as a specific condition that may require urgent and radical treatment.

Division into the three groups is a subjective exercise, although objective guidelines have been proposed by Lalardrie and Jouglard based on frontal projection and height of the breast (Table 15.1).[45] A useful clinical guide is to examine the depth to which the bra straps have indented the shoulder.

Clearly, such measurements must be assessed in relation to general habitus, obesity and the patient's own perception. Changes in body weight tend to be reflected

Table 15.1 Objective assessment of breast size

1	Ideal	250–300 cc
2	Moderate hypertrophy	400–600 cc
3	Rather significant	600–800 cc
4	Significant	800–1000 cc
5	Gigantomastia	>1500 cc

Adapted from Lalardrie and Jouglard.[45]

in the breasts. Strombeck has calculated that a gain of 1 kg of body weight gives 20 g enlargement of each breast, so that a weight gain of 7–8 kg is equivalent to prostheses of 150 g.[25]

The grosser degrees of hypertrophy occur most commonly in young adolescents, less commonly during pregnancy, and least commonly as an involutional phenomenon. The latter is probably a different condition, with a greater proportion of fat to stroma than in younger women, although the proportion of fat to parenchyma varies considerably in all groups. Because of the rarity of extreme cases, histological and endocrine analysis using recent techniques is based mainly on individual cases, but adolescent and pregnancy cases appear to have common features. In one series of 41 cases, 32 were juvenile, 7 gravid and 2 involutional.[46] A family history was frequent, and two cases in monozygotic twins were recorded.

Macroscopically, the tissue is pale grey with a uniform rubbery consistency, and a variable amount of fat. The histology is distinctive, with abundant, large ducts and stroma contrasting with the lack of lobules; the atrophy or destruction of lobular units is associated with extensive fibrosis. The stroma is often of the loose connective tissue type seen in gynaecomastia. 'Juvenile units', consisting of ramified new ducts proceeding to atrophy, are sometimes seen in all types and, when seen in association with atrophic lobular units, are diagnostic of this condition.[46]

Equally characteristic is the absence of oestrogen receptors but presence of progesterone receptors, found also in reduction mammoplasties for less severe degrees of hypertrophy. It is difficult to explain this finding when there is much clinical evidence for a local hyper-responsiveness to oestrogen; the most plausible suggestion is that oestrogen acts through an intermediary substance, not directly on the oestrogen receptor.[47]

The pathology of the 'second-degree group', the average patient seeking reduction mammoplasty, is similar, with relatively more ductal tissue and stroma than lobular tissue. The relative amounts of fat and parenchyma, relevant to the use of suction lipectomy as an adjuvant to reduction, varies greatly.[48] It can be assessed preoperatively more accurately by magnetic resonance imaging (MRI) than by mammography.[49] The amount of 'abnormal' pathology found in reduction mammoplasty does not vary from what would be expected in the general population.[50] The majority of findings are manifestations of ANDI. For example, Pitanguy et al.,[50] in their analysis of the histopathological findings in 2488 reduction mammoplasties, found changes of ANDI in over 80%. Two per cent had fibroadenomas and 0.5% had malignant disease.

There have been a number of studies of the psychological factors motivating women to seek breast reduction surgery. In general, they are more concerned with physical limitations and discomfort (and increasing confidence) than the concern for femininity and womanliness that motivate many women seeking breast augmentation. Symptoms complained about most frequently include body discomfort (97%) and difficulty buying clothes (96%), while more than three-quarters complain of local, back and neck pain. There is an excess of single and cohabiting women among those seeking reduction compared with a control obstetric population.[51]

Outcome studies have shown that patients report a high degree of satisfaction with competently performed reduction surgery. In a study of 363 consecutive patients treated at the Mayo Clinic, 90% responded to a questionnaire, and of these 90% regarded the procedure as very or completely successful, against 1.5% taking the opposite view.[52] Miller and colleagues found similar results, but were unable to find a formula for predicting which patients would, or would not, benefit from surgery.[53]

There has been much interest in whether breast reduction surgery might reduce the incidence of subsequent breast cancer. It has been hypothesized that reducing the mass of glandular tissue at risk would provide a corresponding reduction, or that a decreased epithelial mass might be at risk of greater stimulation by circulating hormones, etc. Observational studies have given conflicting results, but a study from Denmark gives some support to both concepts.[54] In a long-term study of 7720 women undergoing breast reduction surgery, breast cancer incidence was reduced overall by 50%, but only in women over 40 years of age at the time of surgery, and particularly those over 50.

Adolescent (virginal) hypertrophy

The normal development of the breast occasionally continues unchecked so that huge breasts result (Fig. 15.7).

Gigantomastia is the most acute and extreme end of the spectrum. This condition, first reported in 1669,[55] is almost invariably bilateral but occurs as a unilateral disease sufficiently often to imply that it is due, at least in some cases, to local factors rather than a hormonal imbalance. No hormonal problem has been identified in these patients except possibly a rather high rate of infertility.[5] Sometimes there is a familial component: Govrin-Yehudain et al.[56] have reported a family in which there was an association with anonychia. However, episodes of epidemic breast enlargement which seem to be caused by exogenous steroids rather militate against the view that hypertrophy is not a hormonal event. Epidemics of breast enlargement attributed to steroids present in chicken meat have been reported from Italy[57] and Puerto Rico.[58] Other compounds such as the 'parabens' found in cosmetics may also possess oestrogenic activity.[59] Gigantomastia may also occasionally be induced by drugs such as D-penicillamine,[60] or occur immediately after starting the contraceptive pill,[47] presumably in a patient who was constitutionally predisposed to the condition.

As the breasts enlarge and become pendulous, the nipple and areola may stretch to an extent where they are recognized with difficulty. The superficial veins enlarge and palpation reveals general firmness with a varying degree of nodularity, sometimes minimal, sometimes very marked. The weight results in back pain, the characteristic grooving of the shoulders by the brassiere straps, and even orthopnoea. Once a significant degree of hypertrophy has become established, regression does not seem to occur.[5]

Multiple giant fibroadenomas can enlarge rapidly in adolescent girls and cause confusion with virginal hypertrophy (see Ch. 7).

When the enlargement of the breast occurs rapidly, medical treatment with danazol[60] and bromocriptine[61,62] may be tried but insufficient data exist to give clear guidelines as to their use. Dihydrogesterone has also been recommended, both before and for 6 months after surgery.[63] Tamoxifen has been used as an adjuvant after reduction mammoplasty for gross cases.[64] On the whole, surgery is at present the only reliable method of control, even then retained breast tissue may cause further problems. It is usually advised that the operation is deferred to the age of 17, but this is purely arbitrary and in the most severe forms surgery cannot be delayed.

Modest degrees of hypertrophy are much more common than the gross examples, and in this age group psychological reactions are particularly distressing. Taunts and ridicule from peers may take the situation out of perspective, increasing the difficulty of making a decision about reduction mammoplasty.

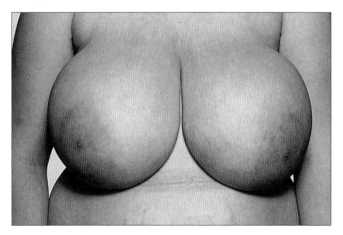

Fig. 15.7 Adolescent hypertrophy. This degree of enlargement causes great psychological and physical embarrassment. It may be more severe and acute than shown here.

Hypertrophy in pregnancy (gravid hypertrophy)

Very occasionally, bilateral or unilateral gross hypertrophy occurs in relation to pregnancy, usually the former. The aetiology is uncertain, but there is an increased incidence of a maternal family history, and in some cases there appears to be a paternal element, in that it has occurred in the first pregnancy following remarriage. Beischer et al. report three cases and give a helpful review of the literature.[65] It occurs in about 1 : 100 000 pregnancies. It may not occur in the first or second pregnancy, but once it occurs it is very likely to recur with subsequent pregnancies. It may arise very early, becoming obvious before the first period is missed. The breasts always lose the ability to produce milk, as would be expected with the defective lobular formation.

Treatment of this condition should follow the same guidelines as adolescent hypertrophy, although it may progress to the stage where ulceration or infarction may occur. Medical treatment is not usually effective; in one case reported tamoxifen, bromocriptine and steroids were ineffective.[66] In some of the more extreme cases occurring in pregnancy, more than one resection may be needed if further progression occurs.[5] Usually a combination of antihormone therapy and surgery is required to curtail the problem and the patient should be warned that a similar event might occur in subsequent pregnancies. Some authors suggest that the appropriate treatment is bilateral total mastectomy with reconstruction.[67] In such a case occurring in the first 12 weeks of the third pregnancy, bilateral total mastectomy was performed (removing 6.5 and 7 kg, respectively) and the pregnancy carried to a successful conclusion.[68]

In less severe cases, regression can be expected postpartum, although not necessarily complete. There is a high probability of recurrence (perhaps more severe) in subsequent pregnancies.

Elevation of parathyroid-related protein and hypercalcaemia has been reported in association with mammary hypertrophy.[69] In this context it is worth noting that Liapis et al.[70] found evidence that parathyroid-like protein is involved in normal breast differentiation.

Excessive postlactational involution

Women not uncommonly complain that after pregnancy and lactation, their breasts involute excessively and are much smaller than before. This is to be regarded as physiological. If the involution is marked and the psychological distress is great, augmentation mammoplasty is well justified. It is usually performed by submammary or subpectoral silicone implants (Fig. 15.8).

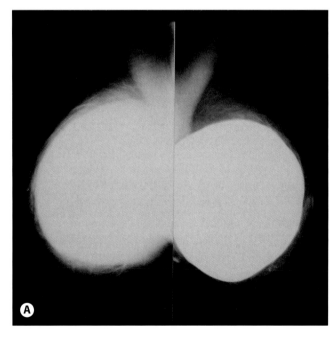 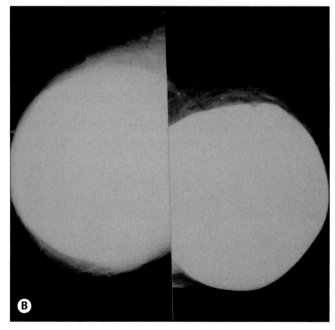

Fig. 15.8 (A) Bilateral silicone breast augmentation; **(B)** detail of underlying breast tissue is severely limited.

Genetic abnormalities involving the breast

A number of genetic abnormalities involve the breast in addition to those arising as disorders of development. They may cause clinical and imaging problems, and lead to unnecessary or inappropriate biopsy if not recognized. An example is the Carney syndrome, where multiple breast fibroadenomas or ductal adenomas may be part of a multisystem disorder.[71] They are dealt with in parts of this book appropriate to the individual condition.

Surgical treatment

Details of surgical treatment are beyond the scope of this text and the reader is referred to the plastic surgery literature. In general hypoplastic breasts may be considered for augmentation mammoplasty with prosthesis insertion. Patients undergoing such procedures need to be aware of the risks with relation to difficulties with later imaging (see Figs 15.9–15.11), capsular contraction and infection. For those of childbearing age, concern has been expressed at possible effects on the fetus.[72] Patients with large breasts may be considered for reduction mammoplasty, and procedures have been described to correct deformities such as tubular and fused breasts.

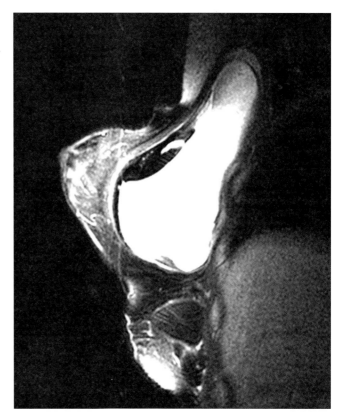

Fig. 15.10 Sagittal MRI showing inframammary leak of silicone in a woman with implants.

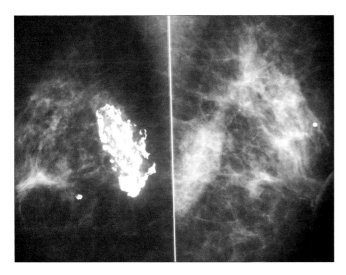

Fig. 15.9 Mammographic images following removal of silicone implants; right side shows resultant heavily calcified focus with scarring.

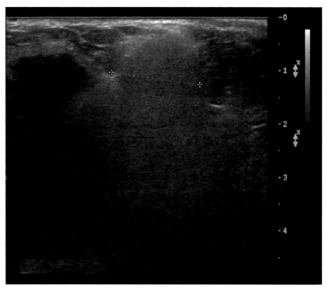

Fig. 15.11 So called 'snow storm' sonographic appearance of leaked silicone in a patient with implants.

REFERENCES

1. Fitzwilliams DCL. *On the Breast.* London: William Heinemann; 1924.

2. Galli-Tsinopoulou A, Krohn C & Schmidt H. Familial polythelia over three generations with polymastia in the youngest girl. *European Journal of Pediatrics* 2001; **160**: 375–377.

3. Schmidt H. Supernumerary nipples: prevalence, size, sex and side predilection – a prospective clinical study. *European Journal of Pediatrics* 1998; **157**: 821–823.

4. Méhes K. Association of supernumerary nipples with other anomalies. *Journal of Pediatrics* 1979; **95**: 274–275.

5. Haagensen CD. *Disease of the Breast,* 3rd edn. Philadelphia: WB Saunders; 1986.

6. Matesanz R, Teniel JL, Garcia-Martin F *et al.* High incidence of supernumerary nipples in end stage renal failure. *Nephron* 1986; **44**: 385–386.

7. Robertson A, Sale P & Sathyanarayan. Lack of association of supernumerary nipples with renal anomalies in black infants. *Journal of Pediatrics* 1986; **109**: 502–503.

8. Grotto I, Browner-Elhanan K, Mimouni D *et al.* Occurrence of supernumerary nipples in children with kidney and urinary tract malformations. *Pediatric Dermatology* 2002; **19**: 463–464.

9. Lewis EJ & Crutchfield CE. Accessory nipples and associated conditions. *Pediatric Dermatology* 1997; **14**: 333–334.

10. Baris H, Tan WH, Kimonis VE. Hypothelia, syndactyly, and ear malformation – a variant of the scalp-ear-nipple syndrome? Case report and review of the literature. *American Journal of Medical Genetics* 2005; **134**: 220–222.

11. Ishida LH, Alves HR, Munhoz AM *et al.* Athelia: case report and review of the literature. *British Journal of Plastic Surgery* 2005; **58**: 833–837.

12. Foulds N, Walpole I, Elmslie F *et al.* Carbimazole embryopathy: an emerging phenotype. *American Journal of Medical Genetics* 2005; **132**: 130–135.

13. McFarland J. Residual lactation acini in the female breast. Their relation to chronic cystic mastitis and malignant disease. *Archives of Surgery* 1922; **5**: 1–12.

14. Alexander JM & Campbell MJ. Prevalence of inverted and non-protractile nipples in antenatal women who intend to breast feed. *Breast* 1997; **5**: 88–89.

15. Park HS, Yoon CH & Kim HJ. The prevalence of congenital inverted nipple. *Aesthetic Plastic Surgery* 1999; **23**: 144–146.

16. Schwager RG, Smith JW, Gray GF *et al.* Inversion of the human female nipple, with a simple method of treatment. *Plastic and Reconstructive Surgery* 1974; **54**: 564–569.

17. Pitanguy I. Reconstruction of congenital nipple deformities. In: Chang WHJ & Petry JJ (eds). *The Breast, an Atlas of Reconstruction.* Baltimore: Williams and Wilkins; 1984:355–361.

18. Inch S. Inverted nipples and breast feeding. In: Chalmers I, Enkin M & Kierse M (eds). *Effective Care in Pregnancy and Childbirth.* Oxford: Oxford University Press; 1989.

19. Waller H. The early failure of breast feeding. A clinical study of its causes and their prevention. *Archives of Disease in Childhood* 1946; **21**: 1–12.

20. Alexander JM, Grant AM & Campbell MJ. Randomised controlled trial of breast shells and Hoffman's exercises for inverted and non-protractile nipples. *British Medical Journal* 1992; **304**: 1030–1032.

21. Hytten F. Clinical and chemical studies in human lactation: IX Breast feeding in hospital. *British Medical Journal* 1954; **2**: 1447–1452.

22. L'Esperance CM. Pain or pleasure. The dilemma of early breast feeding. *Birth and the Family Journal* 1980; **7**: 21–26.

23. Ardran GM, Kemp FH & Lind J. A cineradiographic study of breast feeding. *British Journal of Radiology* 1958; **31**: 156–162.

24. Weber F, Woolridge MW & Baum JD. An ultrasonographic analysis of suckling and swallowing in new born infants. *Pediatric Research* 1984; **18**: 806.

25. Strombeck JO. In: Strombeck JO & Rosato FE (eds). *Surgery of the Breast.* Stuttgart: Verlag; 1986.

26. Van der Putte SC. Mammary-like glands of the vulva and their disorders. *International Journal of Gynecological Pathology* 1994; **13**: 150–160.

27. Down S, Barr L, Baildam AD *et al.* Management of accessory breast tissue in the axilla. *British Journal of Surgery* 2003; **90**: 1213–1214.

28. Kitamura K, Kuwano H, Kiyomatsu K *et al.* Mastopathy of the accessory breast in the bilateral axillary regions occurring concurrently with advanced breast cancer. *Breast Cancer Research and Treatment* 1995; **35**: 221–224.

29. Das DK, Matthew SU, Sheikh ZA *et al.* Fine needle aspiration cytologic diagnosis of axillary accessory breast tissue, including its physiological changes and pathologic lesions. *Acta Cytologica* 1994; **38**: 130–135.

30. Ravitch MM. Poland's syndrome – a study of an eponym. *Plastic and Reconstructive Surgery* 1977; **59**: 508–512.

31. Nelson MM & Cooper CKN. Congenital defects of the breast – an autosomal dominant trait. *South African Medical Journal* 1982; **61**: 434–436.

32. Aznar JMP, Urbano J, Laborda EG *et al.* Breast and pectoralis muscle hypoplasia – a mild degree of Poland syndrome. *Acta Radiologica* 1996; **37**: 759–762.

33. Spear SL, Pelletiere CV, Lee ES *et al.* Anterior thoracic hypoplasia: a separate entity from Poland syndrome. *Plastic and Reconstructive Surgery* 2004; **113**: 69–77.

34. Bamshad M, Root S & Carey JC. Clinical analysis of a large kindred with the Pallister ulnar-mammary syndrome. *American Journal of Medical Genetics* 1966; **65**: 325–331.

35. Rosenberg CA, Derman GH, Grubb WC *et al.* Hypomastia and mitral valve prolapse. Evidence of a linked embryologic and mesenchymal dysplasia. *New England Journal of Medicine* 1983; **309**: 1230–1232.

36. Cherup LL, Siewers RD & Futrell JW. Breast and pectoral muscle maldevelopment after anterolateral or posterolateral thoracotomies in children. *Annals of Thoracic Surgery* 1986; **41**: 492–497.

37. Seitler D & Beller FK. The trunk breast (protrusion of the breast). *Breast Disease* 1988; **1**: 121–127.

38. Mandrekas AD, Zambacos GJ, Anastasopoulos A *et al.* Aesthetic reconstruction of the tuberous breast deformity. *Plastic and Reconstructive Surgery* 2004; **113**: 2231–2232.

39. McKiernan JK & Hull D. Breast development in the newborn. *Archives of Diseases of Childhood* 1981; **56**: 525–529.

40. Zukauskaite S, Lasiene D, Lasas L *et al.* Onset of breast and pubic hair development in 1231 preadolescent Lithuanian schoolgirls. *Archives of Diseases of Childhood* 2005; **90**: 932–936.

41. Mills JL, Stolley PD, Davies J *et al.* Premature thelarche. Natural history and etiologic investigation. *American Journal of Diseases of Children* 1981; **135**: 743–745.

42. Midyett LK, Moore WV & Jacobson JD. Are pubertal changes in girls before age 8 benign? *Pediatrics* 2003; **111**: 47–51.

43. Verrotti A, Ferrarri M, Morgese G *et al.* Premature thelarche: a long-term follow-up. *Gynecological Endocrinology* 1996; **10**: 214–217.

44. Xhrouet-Heinrichs D, Lagrou K, Heinrichs C *et al.* Longitudinal study of behavioural and affective patterns in girls with central precocious puberty during long-acting triptorelin therapy. *Acta Paediatrica* 1997; **86**: 808–815.

45. Lalardrie JP & Jouglard JP. *Plasties mammaires pour hypertrophie et ptose.* Paris: Masson; 1973.

46. Anastassiades OT, Choreftaki T, Ioannovich J *et al.* Megalomastia: histological, histochemical and immunohistochemical study. *Virchows Archiv – A, Pathological Anatomy and Histopathology* 1992; **420**: 337–344.

47. Hugh JC, Friedman MH, Danyluk JM *et al.* Absence of oestrogen receptors in a case of virginal hypertrophy of the breasts related to oral contraception. *Breast Disease* 1993; **6**: 143–148.

48. Lejour M. Evaluation of fat in breast tissue removed by vertical mammaplasty. *Plastic and Reconstructive Surgery* 1997; **99**: 386–393.

49. Lee NA, Rusinek H, Weinreb J *et al.* Fatty and fibroglandular tissue volumes in the breasts of women 20-83 years old: comparison of X-ray mammography and computer-assisted MR imaging. *American Journal of Radiology* 1997; **168**: 501–506.

50. Pitanguy I, Torres E, Salgado F *et al.* Breast pathology and reduction mammoplasty. *Plastic and Reconstructive Surgery* 2005; **115**: 729–734.

51. Birtchnell S, Whitfield P & Lacey JH. Motivational factors in women requesting augmentation and reduction surgery. *Journal of Psychosomatic Research* 1990; **34**: 509–514.

52. Schnur PL, Schnur DP, Petty PM *et al.* Reduction mammoplasty: an outcome study. *Plastic and Reconstructive Surgery* 1997; **100**: 875–883.

53. Miller AP, Zacher JB, Berggren RB *et al.* Breast reduction for symptomatic macromastia: can objective predictors for operative success be identified? *Plastic and Reconstructive Surgery* 1995; **95**: 77–83.

54. Boice JD Jr, Friis S, McLaughlin JK *et al.* Cancer following breast reduction surgery in Denmark. *Cancer Causes and Control* 1997; **8**: 253–258.

55. Durston W. Concerning a very sudden excessive swelling of a woman's breasts. *Philosophical Transactions for Anno 1669.* London Royal Society; 1670.

56. Govrin-Yehudain J, Kogan L, Cohen HI *et al.* Familial juvenile hypertrophy of the breast. *Journal of Adolescent Health* 2004; **35**: 151–155.

57. Fara GM, Del Corvo G, Bernuzzi S *et al.* Epidemic of breast enlargement in an Italian school. *Lancet* 1979; **ii**: 295–297.

58. Bongiovanni AM. An epidemic of premature thelarche in Puerto Rico. *Journal of Pediatrics* 1983; **103**: 245–246.

59. Golden R, Gandy J, Vollmer G. A review of the endocrine activity of parabens and implications for potential risks to human health. *Critical Review of Toxicology* 2005; **35**: 435–458.

60. Taylor PJ. Successful treatment of D-penicillamine induced breast gigantism with danazol. *British Medical Journal* 1981; **282**: 362–363.

61. Kullander S. Effect of 2Br alpha ergocryptin (CB134) on serum prolactin and clinical picture in a case of gigantomastia in pregnancy. *Annales Chirugiae et Gynaecologie Fenniae* 1976; **65**: 227–233.

62. Hedberg K, Karlsson K & Lindstedt A. Gigantomastia during pregnancy: effect of a dopamine agonist. *American Journal of Obstetrics and Gynecology* 1979; **133**: 928–931.

63. Mayl N, Vasconez LO & Jurkiewicz MJ. Treatment of macromastia in the actively enlarging breast. *Plastic and Reconstructive Surgery* 1974; **54**: 6–12.

64. Baker SB, Burkey BA, Thornton P *et al.* Juvenile gigantomastia: presentation of four cases and review of the literature. *Annals of Plastic Surgery* 2001; **46**: 517–525.

65. Beischer NA, Hueston JH & Peperell RJ. Massive hypertrophy of the breast in pregnancy – report of 3 cases and review of literature. *Obstetrical and Gynecological Survey* 1989; **44**: 234–243.

66. Abid SU, Gutman M, Herman O *et al.* Massive breast hypertrophy during pregnancy: failure of medical treatment. *The Breast* 1995; **4:** 153–155.

67. Stavides S, Hacking A, Tiltman A *et al.* Gigantomastia in pregnancy. *British Journal of Surgery* 1987; **74:** 585–586.

68. Gogas JC, Markopovlos M, Gogas HJ *et al.* Gigantomastia developing in post-partum period and exacerbated by subsequent therapy. *Breast Disease* 1994; **7:** 231–234.

69. Khosla LS, van Heerden JA, Charib H. Parathyroid related protein and hypercalcaemia secondary to mammary hyperplasia. *New England Journal of Medicine* 1990; **322:** 1157.

70. Liapis H, Crouch EC, Grosso LE *et al.* Expression of parathyroid-like protein in normal, proliferative, and neoplastic human breast tissues. *American Journal of Pathology* 1993; **143:** 1169–1178.

71. Courcoutsakis NA, Chow CK, Shawker TH *et al.* Syndromes of spotty pigmentation, myxomas, endocrine overactivity and schwannomas (Carney complex). Breast imaging findings. *Radiology* 1997, **205:** 221–227.

72. Brown SL, Todd JF, Cope JU *et al.* Breast implant surveillance reports to the U.S. Food and Drug Administration: maternal-child health problems. *Journal of Long Term Effects of Medical Implants* 2006; **16:** 281–290.

The male breast

1. Gynaecomastia is the only common condition affecting the male breast.

2. Careful assessment is required to exclude rare cases of male breast cancer.

3. An underlying cause should be considered.

4. Drug treatment is problematic.

5. Surgical treatment needs careful consideration.

6. Atypical infective episodes should raise the possibility of HIV infection. Men seek advice for similar reasons to women; either they fear cancer or the symptoms themselves may be troublesome. The characteristic presentations of ANDI are rare but do occur occasionally. Many of the non-ANDI conditions described in this text are seen nearly as frequently in men as women.

Development of the male breast

Before puberty, breast development is similar in males and females; in neonates the incidence and behaviour of mastitis neonatorum is identical. The incidence of absent breast or nipple and presence of supernumerary nipples is similar to that found in the female. At puberty, the male breast develops ductal structures but, in the absence of oestrogenic stimulation, lobular structures are not formed. It follows that the majority of male breast pathology relates to ductal structures but in the presence of long-term oestrogen stimulation pathology related to lobular structures may occur.

Gynaecomastia

Gynaecomastia is the commonest condition affecting the male breast. The term was used by Galen to describe the changes that would now be described as pseudogynaecomastia although Paulus Aegina had described surgery for gynaecomastia in the first century AD. The term appears to have been reintroduced in the 1860s.[1,2] The alternative term of gynaecomazia is now regarded as obsolete.

Gynaecomastia is defined as an enlargement of the ductal and stromal tissue of the male breast, which is palpably and histologically different from the surrounding subcutaneous fat. It may range in size from a small retroareolar button of tissue to enlargement indistinguishable from the normal female breast. The ratio of fat to fibrous stroma is variable.

Gynaecomastia may be either primary (physiological) or secondary (to a defined extramammary stimulus). It requires careful distinction from pseudogynaecomastia, a condition sometimes referred to as lipomastia, in which the external appearance suggests the presence of breast tissue, but palpation (and histology) reveals that the swelling is all fat with no increase in breast tissue.

Clinical presentation

The patient usually presents with a swelling of the breast, often unilateral (Fig. 16.1), which is frequently tender. He may be concerned about the tenderness itself, cosmetic appearance or the possibility of underlying malignancy. In many cases, especially in secondary gynaecomastia, changes are asymptomatic and are noted by the attending physician. Rarely, nipple discharge may be associated with gynaecomastia. Kapil & Verma.[3] found only nine cases in 22 years of studying cytology from patients with gynaecomastia.

Examination reveals a firm disc of retroareolar tissue, which is mobile and often tender. There is usually a clear, but not sharp, demarcation of the firm, often slightly tender, breast tissue from softer surrounding fat. It needs to be distinguished from carcinoma of the male breast and pseudogynaecomastia, retroareolar fat deposition in obesity. The hallmark of gynaecomastia is its concentricity, if an eccentric mass is found an alternative diagnosis should be considered and fine needle aspiration (FNA) and/or core biopsy performed. At the initial assessment careful examination is needed to decide whether the enlarged breast is due to breast tissue, fat or muscle. In cases where clinical examination leaves doubt, mammography or ultrasound will allow quantification of the amount of fat and breast parenchyma. Hypertrophy of the pectoral muscles may simulate or accentuate gynaecomastia. Such changes are particularly likely in weightlifters, who may have gynaecomastia from steroid use, so the pectoral contribution should be assessed separately.

Histology

The histological pattern of gynaecomastia progresses from an early, active phase to, eventually, an inactive senescent phase. This progression occurs no matter what the aetiology, and is even seen when the hormonal stimulus continues. In the active or florid phase there is proliferation of ducts with active epithelial proliferation and hyperplasia of the periductal stromal tissue. Multiplication, branching and elongation of the ducts may accompany the ductal proliferation. There is also periductal, or more widespread, infiltration by plasma cells, lymphocytes, and large mononuclear cells (Fig. 16.2).[4] When the inactive stage has been reached there is atrophy of the ductal epithelium with prominent stromal fibrosis. As the process passes into the inactive phase, breast enlargement may diminish, although dense fibrous tissue means that the gynaecomastia is unlikely to regress completely. Kono et al.[5] studied the role of Ki-67 during the development of gynaecomastia and found that early in gynaecomastia the levels of expressed Ki-67 were raised but falling off in the fibrous stage. They consider that gives some indication of the likelihood of a response to hormonal manipulation.

Lobular formation seems to occur only after long-term oestrogen treatment or in Klinefelter's syndrome[6] although Anderson and Gram[7] described six cases of focal lobular formation in a series of 76 surgical resections in which they failed to identify a source of oestrogens and so concluded that oestrogenic stimulation was unnecessary for acinar formation. In view of the obscure source of some

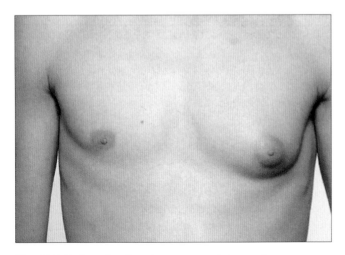

Fig. 16.1 Unilateral, pubertal gynaecomastia in a male.

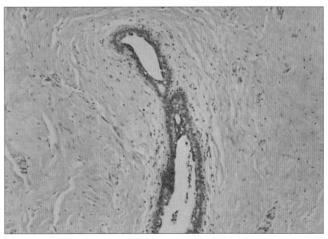

Fig. 16.2 Typical histological features of gynaecomastia.

exogenous oestrogens,[8] this view must remain unproven. Azzopardi[9] has commented on the lack of periductal elastic tissue in these patients in comparison to the female.

Cytology

Cytology of gynaecomastia shows considerable variation. Kapil and Verma[10] reported a study of 389 cases seen over 22 years. Florid gynaecomastia with ductal and stromal proliferation often with focal cytological atypia and numerous background naked myoepithelial nuclei was noted in 134 (34%). Columnar cells, apocrine cells and foam cells were also seen in some of the samples. The remaining 255 cases showed benign ductal cells. In a second study, Kapil and Verma[3] found similar changes in nipple discharge from male breasts. In another study of 100 men, Amrikachi et al.[11] reported cytological findings as: cohesive sheets of cells containing 20–1000 cells (98%); scattered, single, bipolar cells (78%); spindle cells (68%); ductal epithelial atypia (26%); apocrine metaplasia (8%); and foamy histiocytes (12%). In nine cases the atypia was marked, and in two of them the possibility of malignancy could not be ruled out.

The cytopathology of gynaecomastia is so variable that in the past a mistaken diagnosis of breast cancer has been made. A number of series now suggest that given appropriate experience this is no longer the case. For example Siddiqui et al.[12] reported their findings in 614 male breast samples over 10 years. They claimed a sensitivity of 95.3% and a specificity of 100%. They commented on the relatively high rate of inadequate samples. Westenend and Jobse[13] from the Netherlands reviewed 153 FNA samples in male patients and, after excluding 13% inadequate samples, were able to claim 100% sensitivity and 89% specificity. They had no false positives based on either histological specimens or follow-up on a national database. These studies suggest that the cytological changes of gynaecomastia are now so well known that false positives should be avoided.

Incidence

The histological incidence of gynaecomastia at autopsy has been estimated by Sandison[6] as 4% and by Anderson and Gram[14] as 55%. However, Anderson and Gram[14] described three phases of gynaecomastia: active, inactive and intermediate. Only a few (7%) of the cases were active or intermediate so that there is less discrepancy

than is immediately apparent. Williams,[15] in her autopsy study of 447 cases, found 38 (8%) to have florid gynaecomastia, 140 (31%) to have the more indolent form and the remaining 269 to have no histological evidence of gynaecomastia. She found associations with prostatic disease even after patients receiving oestrogen therapy had been excluded. She also found correlations with cirrhosis, and adrenal and testicular changes.

A review of the literature reveals conflicting information on the prevalence and significance of gynaecomastia. Specialist endocrinologists who see a selected group of patients may consider the development of gynaecomastia to be of sinister significance. In one series it was considered that 27 out of 46 cases had endocrine causes susceptible to, or curable by, endocrine therapy.[16] It is unusual to find a defined endocrinological cause in patients referred to a surgical clinic.

Mild forms of gynaecomastia are very common although presentation as a clinical complaint is far less frequent. Nydick et al.[17] showed in their study of 1855 Boy Scouts, that the overall incidence between the ages of 10 and 16 was 38%; this reached a maximum of 65% in the 14-year-old boys, which had dropped to 14% in those of 16 years. Nuttall,[18] in his study of 306 men showed that an incidence of 17% in youths in their late teens gradually increased in the following decades so that the incidence was 57% in those over 50 years. The overall incidence was 36% and in the vast majority bilateral disease existed. Figure 16.3 combines the findings of Nydick et al.[17] and Nuttall.[18] Georgiadis et al.[19] found 40.5% of 954 healthy men aged 18–26 to have

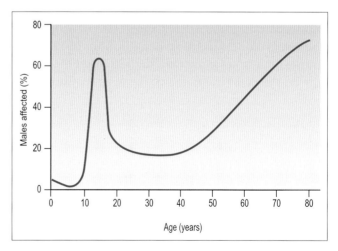

Fig. 16.3 The age incidence of gynaecomastia found on routine examination. (Derived from Nydick et al.[17] and Nuttal.[18], by permission.)

gynaecomastia. The majority of these were bilateral but 14% were unilateral. They also established a relationship with obesity in this age group, as did Ersoz et al.[20]

The literature, however, provides conflicting information on the laterality of gynaecomastia; for example, in his study of the radiology of 40 patients with this condition Dershaw[21] found 28 had unilateral disease, 4 had symmetrical involvement and 8 had bilateral but asymmetrical involvement. In another radiological study, 63% of 94 patients had bilateral but usually asymmetrical involvement.[22] The variations in these reports probably reflect referral patterns, as diagnostic doubt is likely to be increased when the condition is unilateral.

Primary gynaecomastia is usually considered under the headings neonatal, pubertal and senescent, although, as can be seen from the foregoing, it would be better to regard it as a continuum with a peak at puberty, which falls in the late teens to be followed by steadily increasing incidence with age, as illustrated in Figure 16.3.

Aetiology

Because of the clear relationship between the incidence of gynaecomastia and hormonal events, the role of an endocrine abnormality in gynaecomastia needs to be seriously considered.

Androgen physiology

The major androgen in the adult human male is testosterone produced by the testes; the normal adrenal gland produces an insignificant amount of this hormone. The active hormones are dihydrotestosterone, produced peripherally from testosterone at its site of action, and androstenedione, which is derived from the adrenal cortex. Both testosterone and androstenedione may be converted to oestrogens by peripheral aromatization.

Hormonal defect in gynaecomastia

The putative hormonal defects in gynaecomastia have been well studied. Prolactin appears to have no influence on the development of gynaecomastia.[23,24] A number of studies have shown a relative alteration in circulating sex steroids in patients with gynaecomastia. Lee[25] prospectively studied 29 boys, 20 of whom subsequently developed gynaecomastia. Those who did so had a transient increase in oestrogen levels before the gynaecomastia became clinically apparent. Moore et al.[24] studied 30

pubertal boys with gynaecomastia and 20 without and demonstrated a lower d[4]-androstenedione/oestrone and oestradiol ratio (the testosterone/oestrone ratio remaining normal) in the affected boys and postulated that the cause was peripheral conversion of adrenal androgens to oestrone and oestradiol. Ersoz et al.[20] evaluated patients with idiopathic gynaecomastia. They found an increased body mass index in the patients that correlated with a reduced testosterone and luteinizing hormone level. Oestradiol was unchanged. They postulated that increased peripheral aromatization was a likely explanation.

Pirke and Doerr[26] have shown that the androgen:oestrogen ratio falls with increasing age, an observation that fits well with the observation of increasing incidence of gynaecomastia with age.[18] Despite these somewhat inconsistent results, it seems likely that the development of gynaecomastia is the result of a relative increase in the levels of circulating oestrogens with respect to androgens and that in most cases of primary gynaecomastia this is the operative mechanism. It seems likely that examples of secondary gynaecomastia, except those related to drugs, are due to a similar perturbation of hormonal equilibrium. The mechanisms by which these changes may occur have been reviewed by Wilson et al.[27] Unilateral gynaecomastia presumes an end-organ factor, presumably related to hormone receptors or local hormone conversion, but which remains an endocrinological enigma.

Physiological gynaecomastia

Infantile

A small percentage of male neonates have noticeable breast enlargement due to circulating maternal hormones. This resolves by the age of 4 months. It is usually bilateral but may be unilateral. No treatment beyond reassurance of the mother is required.

Adolescence

This is a common age to develop gynaecomastia. Nydick et al.,[17] in their study of 1855 Boy Scouts aged between 10 and 16, found a 38% incidence of gynaecomastia. They have shown that the majority resolved within 6 months, although 27% of cases persisted for 2 years and 8% for 3 years. In 25% of cases, the disease was unilateral but, when bilateral, the sides were usually affected to different degrees and the onset was usually asynchronous.

Rarely, pubertal gynaecomastia may be familial. In one such family, elevated oestrone levels were detected.[28]

Adult

Asymptomatic gynaecomastia in the adult usually persists unless a reversible underlying cause is found. When symptomatic, it runs a variable course and often undergoes spontaneous remission, although examination will reveal persisting enlargement of the breast disc. Psychological stress has been postulated as a possible cause of intermittent gynaecomastia.[29]

Secondary gynaecomastia

A number of disparate conditions are associated with gynaecomastia as summarized in Table 16.1. When the clinical sign of gynaecomastia is so common in healthy men, care needs to be taken in ascribing such findings to underlying pathology or medication. A number of well-described associations do, however, merit some discussion.

Table 16.1 Causes of secondary gynaecomastia

DECREASED ANDROGENS
Reduced production
Congenital anorchia
Chromosomal abnormalities, e.g. Klinefelter's syndrome
Bilateral cryptorchidism
Viral orchitis
Bilateral torsion
Granulomatous disease
Renal failure
Androgen resistance
Testicular feminization
INCREASED OESTROGENS
Increased secretion
Testicular tumours
Carcinoma lung
Increased peripheral aromatization
Adrenal disease
Liver disease
Starvation re-feeding
Thyrotoxicosis
DRUG INDUCED
See Table 16.3

Tumours

A number of tumours that secrete hormones may be associated with gynaecomastia. Both teratomas and seminomas of the testis may secrete sufficient oestrogens to produce gynaecomastia. In a study of 636 patients with testicular tumour, 10% presented with extratesticular complaints and gynaecomastia or mastalgia was the second most common of these. Many of these patients had inappropriate treatment, although the correct diagnosis should have been suggested by abnormal testicular findings, raised serum markers or cryptorchidism.[30] Bronchogenic carcinoma is a well-recognized source of ectopic hormone production and may also produce hormones with oestrogenic activity. Tumours of the pituitary adrenal and hypothalamus may also produce gynaecomastia, presumably mediated via the testis by gonadotropic hormones.

Klinefelter's syndrome

This chromosomal anomaly, when an apparent male has an XXY karyotype, is due to nondisjunction of the parental sex chromosomes. The clinical features of the syndrome are testicular atrophy, eunuchoid habitus with female hair distribution and gynaecomastia. Confirmation of the diagnosis depends on chromosomal examination. The gynaecomastia in this condition is unusual in that the patient may develop lobular structures,[6] and is associated with an increased incidence of carcinoma.[31]

Secondary testicular failure

Testicular damage from any cause may result in decreased testosterone production and a change in the androgen : oestrogen ratio. The absolute levels of oestrogen do not need to be raised for gynaecomastia to occur. Viral orchitis, most commonly due to mumps, is the most frequent cause of testicular atrophy but a variety of causes should be considered. Leprosy is a common cause in relevant geographical areas. One in five cases of lepromatous leprosy has gynaecomastia due to testicular involvement, which in turn is due to the preference of the organism for cooler parts of the body.[32]

Liver failure

With the exception of drug-induced changes, this is probably the commonest cause of secondary gynaecomastia. The failing liver fails to eliminate androstenedione, which is then available for peripheral conversion to oestrogens by aromatization.[33]

Starvation re-feeding

The mechanism by which this occurs is probably related to the fatty liver change that occurs in such patients. Originally described in liberated prisoners of war,[34] it may also be seen in patients who have been severely ill on intensive care units.

Drugs

A large number of drugs have been implicated in the development of gynaecomastia (Table 16.2). When the finding of gynaecomastia is as common as it appears to be, isolated case reports need to be treated with scepticism. Thompson and Carter[35] have reviewed the literature on drug-induced gynaecomastia. They conclude that calcium channel blockers, cancer chemotherapeutic agents, histamine$_2$ receptor blockers, ketoconazole and spironolactone may cause gynaecomastia. They consider the evidence regarding digitalis, neuroleptic agents and marijuana as inconclusive. These changes are produced either by a relative increase in oestrogenic activity or inhibition of androgenic activity. Administration of female sex hormones, for example stilboestrol in treatment of prostatic cancer, not surprisingly lead to increased breast development. Perhaps more surprising is that enough oestrogen may be absorbed from topical preparations to cause gynaecomastia.[36–40]

Some drugs have antiandrogenic effects either as part of their intended therapeutic action, e.g. cyproterone used for prostatic cancer, or as an unwanted and unexpected effect as seen with cimetidine or spironolactone (Fig. 16.4). The gynaecomastia of spironolactone, almost universal when used for treating hepatic ascites, may be avoided by administration of its active metabolite, sodium canrenoate.[41]

Rodriguez and Jick[42] studied a population of 81 000 men receiving anti-ulcer drugs to quantify the incidence of gynaecomastia. Cimetidine carried a relative risk of some seven times. The risk was dose related, so that current users on a dose of 1000 mg had a risk of 40 times non-users, and was highest 7–12 months after starting cimetidine. Misoprostol, omeprazole and ranitidine carried no significant risk. Spironolactone and verapamil carried a risk equivalent to cimetidine.

A current fashion among weightlifters to take anabolic steroids with tamoxifen to counteract the resulting gynaecomastia can produce histological changes suggestive of premalignancy, though we have not yet seen a case of invasive cancer from this combination.

The mechanisms by which drugs produce the changes of gynaecomastia vary. In broad theoretical terms they

Table 16.2 Drugs associated with gynaecomastia

Drug	Mechanism
Androgens	? Peripheral aromatization
Cyproterone	Antiandrogens
Spironolactone	
Digitalis	Bind to oestrogen receptors and oestrogenic activity
Cannabis	
Griseofulvin	
Phenothiazines	Disturbance of gonadotrophin control
Reserpine	
Tricyclics	
Cimetidine	
Methyldopa	
Isoniazid	
Metoclopramide	

After Hall et al.

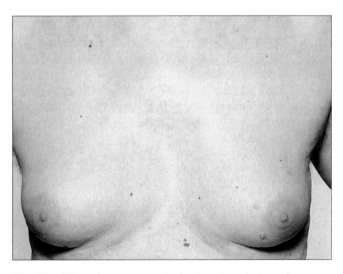

Fig. 16.4 Bilateral gynaecomastia due to spironolactone therapy.

could act by inhibiting testosterone production, by increasing peripheral aromatization or by direct stimulation of the oestrogen receptors in breast tissue. Satoh et al.[43] systematically evaluated the effect of 29 drugs known to be associated with gynaecomastia and found no changes in either the aromatase or sulphatase pathways at clinical concentrations. The known mechanisms of action are indicated in Table 16.3.

Assessment of gynaecomastia

Clinical

In the majority of patients, history and examination will reveal the likely cause of the gynaecomastia. The age of onset, relation to drug ingestion and underlying ill health are the main pointers from the history. As drugs are a potent cause of gynaecomastia, a careful drug history is essential. While most causes are obvious, it is worth remembering that dermal oestrogens may cause gynaecomastia in both children[38,39] and adults.[36,37,40] In this last study, an epidemic of gynaecomastia in Haitian refugees was found to be due to phenthrin used as a delousing agent.

Examination of the liver, testes and chest as well as the gynaecomastia itself is clearly important.

Investigation

Investigation should be confined to liver function tests and a chest radiograph in the older patient, unless there is reason to think that there is an underlying endocrine abnormality, when more sophisticated investigations may be indicated.

Exclusion of malignancy

Confirmation of the diagnosis, with imaging and tissue diagnosis, should be sought in those patients at an age where cancer is a possibility. This is particularly important in the absence of a well-defined cause, in unilateral disease and when the palpable mass is eccentric instead of having the usual concentricity.

Dershaw[21] has reviewed the role of mammography in the male breast. Gynaecomastia appears as a flame-shaped opacity extending into the surrounding fat. It is possible to distinguish those patients on oestrogens when the breast takes on the appearance of the female. Cases of pseudogynaecomastia can be readily identified by the absence of breast tissue. Malignancy can usually be diagnosed by mammography. For example, Evans et al.[44] showed an overall accuracy of 90% in distinguishing benign from malignant change in the male breast

Table 16.3 Drugs that induce gynaecomastia by known mechanisms

Oestrogen-like, or binds to oestrogen receptor	Stimulate oestrogen synthesis	Supply aromatizable oestrogen precursors	Direct testicular damage	Block testosterone synthesis	Block androgen action	Displace oestrogen from SHBG
Oestrogen vaginal cream	Gonadotropins	Exogenous androgen	Busulfan	Ketoconazole	Flutamide	Spironolactone
Oestrogen-containing embalming cream	Growth hormone	Androgen precursors (i.e. androstenedione and DHEA)	Nitrosurea	Spironolactone	Bicalutamide	Ethanol
Delousing powder			Vincristine	Metronidazole	Finasteride	
Digitalis			Ethanol	Etomidate	Cyproterone	
Clomiphene					Zanoterone	
Marijuana					Cimetidine	
					Ranitidine	
					Spironolactone	

in 104 cases in which histological confirmation was available.

The value of ultrasound is in defining focal abnormalities in dense fibrotic breast tissue (Fig. 16.5). MRI has not been systematically evaluated but may help to distinguish true from lipomatous gynaecomastia in patients on treatment for HIV.

Fine needle aspiration cytology and core biopsy

We prefer core biopsies to aspiration cytology in any case of doubt. The older concerns about the reliability of cytology have been addressed (see above) so with an experienced cytologist this investigation can be pursued with confidence.

Treatment

Two premises govern the management of gynaecomastia. First, most cases are due to minor hormonal imbalances or to drugs and carry no serious significance. Second, a serious cause should be considered in each case and, in the older patient, breast cancer excluded. In the majority of cases reassurance that this is a benign self-limiting condition that is not premalignant will suffice. A minority of patients will require treatment for either tenderness or cosmesis.

Treatment of the secondary gynaecomastia

If a cause for the gynaecomastia is identified, it will resolve with treatment of the underlying abnormality or with-

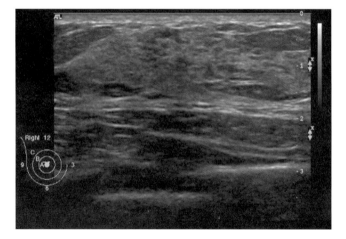

Fig. 16.5 Male breast ultrasound image showing florid gynaecomastia; well-developed glandular breast tissue beneath the areola.

drawal of the offending drug. If, for some reason, the disease is not amenable to treatment or, if continuation of a drug is essential and treatment of gynaecomastia is still considered necessary, the plan for treatment of primary gynaecomastia may be followed with advantage.

Treatment of primary gynaecomastia

For the minority of patients in whom firm reassurance proves inadequate a number of options are open.

Drug therapy

A hormonal basis for gynaecomastia is widely accepted so it is not surprising that attempts have been made to correct the putative abnormality. What is surprising is that no agent has been studied in a systematic manner. Initially, drugs such as testosterone and clomiphene were used. Testosterone has been reported to be of variable value but occasionally produces a dramatic effect;[45] paradoxically, the gynaecomastia may get worse because of the peripheral aromatization of the testosterone. Eberle et al.[46] treated four pubertal patients with dihydrotestosterone heptanoate, which does not undergo peripheral aromatization, and claimed good results. The clinical improvement was associated with falls in circulating oestradiol, luteinizing hormone (LH), follicle-stimulating hormone (FSH) and free testosterone. There had been no return of symptoms during a follow-up period ranging between 5 and 15 months. Dobs et al.[47] compared transdermal testosterone with intramuscular testosterone to treat hypogonadal men. Gynaecomastia resolved more frequently during transdermal treatment (4 of 10 patients) than with i.m. treatment (1 of 9 patients). Beveniste et al.[48] used topical dihydrotestosterone to treat four patients with antiretroviral-induced gynaecomastia and claimed that all had complete relief of symptoms.

Clomiphene citrate, which appears to act locally as an antioestrogen[49] has been used in prepubertal gynaecomastia. Leroith et al.[49] used a dose of 100 mg with a 64% response rate in 22 boys. Stephanas et al.[50] reported that 18 of 19 patients responded to clomiphene 50 mg daily whereas Plourde et al.[51] found a similar dose unsatisfactory in a group of 12 patients.

It is not surprising that tamoxifen has been tried in men with gynaecomastia, although it is not licensed for this indication. The earliest report dates from 1979.[52] Parker et al.[53] reported a crossover study of 10 men between the ages of 54 and 80. Seven regressed, one of whom recurred after cessation of treatment. No patient responded to the placebo. McDermott et al.[54] reported a crossover trial in six men with painful gynaecomastia; five of six men responded to the tamoxifen and one of six during the placebo phase. There was a significant rise in luteinizing hormone and total oestradiol during tamoxifen treatment. The largest series reported is that of Alagaratnam,[55] who treated 61 Chinese men with idiopathic gynaecomastia with an 80% complete regression. Dosage was 40 mg tamoxifen daily for 2 months, and sometimes to 4 months. He noticed no untoward side effects with follow-up in excess of 3 years. Symptomatic response was seen in 2 weeks, although swelling took longer to resolve. Khan et al.[56] reported their results in 36 men using 20 mg tamoxifen daily. Patients with fatty gynaecomastia were less successfully treated than those with 'lump' gynaecomastia who all derived benefit. Derman et al.[57] treated 37 boys with pubertal gynaecomastia without noting any long-term toxicity although two relapsed after cessation of treatment. Novoa et al.[58] evaluated the effect of tamoxifen in 25 pubertal boys and found changes in lipids and coagulation that mirrored those found in women but were quantitatively less marked. Tamoxifen is used by men taking anabolic steroids to prevent the development of gynaecomastia. Evans[59] reviewed the experience of 100 male steroid users in Cardiff, UK, and found significant use of tamoxifen to control the symptoms of gynaecomastia.

Buckle[60] reported the results of danazol treatment in 42 patients: 25 had marked regression of the gynaecomastia and 10 moderate regression. The dosage used in adults was 100 mg three times daily increased to 200 mg three times daily if no response was seen, continued for between 4 and 6 months, followed by maintenance at the lower dose for 4 months. In adolescents the dosage used was 100 mg twice daily. Side effects were acceptable and no patient stopped treatment on account of these. The levels of testosterone fell during treatment, as did the levels of gonadotrophins; oestrogen levels were not measured. Daniels & Layer[61] reviewed 175 consecutive male patients referred with breast symptoms over a 7-year period. Of these, 127 were considered to have gynaecomastia. Twenty were treated with danazol with a satisfactory response in 16. Three subsequently had surgery.

Jones et al.[62] have reported a randomized study of danazol, which confirms its safety and the therapeutic benefit. Our own experience in 18 cases is that half of them obtain useful relief of symptoms. Tenderness disappears rapidly in those who are going to respond but there has been slower change in the patients whose main complaint is cosmetic. We have used varying doses between

100 mg and 200 mg three times daily with no definable side effects. A typical course is 100 mg three times daily for 4 weeks then 100 mg twice daily for 8 weeks. Age of onset and duration of symptoms were not predictive of those who were going to respond, although a good response would not be expected in longstanding fibrotic cases. We have reviewed our own experience of danazol in 18 patients with a median age of onset of 21 years (range 12–54). It was unilateral in 11, painful in 14, focal in 5 and diffuse in 13. Seven patients had a complete response and three a partial response. Treatment failed in six patients and two failed to take the tablets. There were no side effects. The time to response was 6–12 weeks, and there was no recurrence at a median follow-up of 8 months, extending to 18 months. A review of 13 of our recent patients with painful gynaecomastia confirmed that this is effective.[63]

Ting et al.[64] have performed a randomized study that directly compared tamoxifen with danazol in 68 patients. The response rate in the tamoxifen group was higher (78% vs 40%) but was more often associated with relapse once the treatment was stopped.

It has been postulated that aromatase inhibitors may be useful in gynaecomastia,[65,66] but although there are sporadic reports of the use of early aromatase inhibitors[65] none of the new generation of aromatase inhibitors appears to have been studied in the context of gynaecomastia.

There is thus no clear consensus on the optimum medical treatment of gynaecomastia for the small number of patients who require it. Gynaecomastia is not a recognized indication for any of these treatments and long-term side effects have not been adequately evaluated. Until such time as results from formal trials are available, tamoxifen 20 mg daily seems to be the best documented of the available treatments. Apart from the need to consider drug interactions, these comments are pertinent to secondary gynaecomastia.

Prevention of gynaecomastia

Gynaecomastia is such a frequent consequence of treatment of prostatic cancer with bicalutamide that four randomized trials have been reported of attempts to alleviate this problem. Boccardo et al.[67] compared the effect of tamoxifen and anastrazole in 114 patients: 73% of patients with bicalutamide alone developed gynaecomastia reduced to 10% with those who had tamoxifen 20 mg daily and 51% in those who had anastrazole 1 mg daily.

Similar results were reported by Saltzstain et al.[68] Perdona et al.[69] reported on 150 on bicalutamide either alone or in combination with tamoxifen 10 mg daily or with radiotherapy. The gynaecomastia rates were 68%, 8% and 34%, respectively. Fradet et al.[70] found a dose-dependent protective effect of tamoxifen in bicalutamide-treated patients with prostatic cancer. Only 8.8% patients on 20 mg tamoxifen per day developed gynaecomastia. In none of these trials was any detrimental effect on tumour response detected.

It seems from the results of these studies that tamoxifen is more effective in preventing gynaecomastia than either the aromatase inhibitor or radiotherapy. It also suggests that end-organ changes are at least as important as changes in circulating hormones in the genesis of gynaecomastia. Furthermore, Perdona et al.[69] found tamoxifen effective in those in the original control group who developed gynaecomastia.

Radiotherapy

Prophylactic irradiation therapy of breast tissue to prevent the gynaecomastia that regularly accompanies the hormonal treatment of prostatic cancer is effective.[71] Widmark et al.[72] evaluated patients with prostatic cancer in a Scandinavian trial in which prophylactic radiotherapy was given as a single fraction of 12–15 grays. The incidence of gynaecomastia symptoms fell from 81% in controls to 28% in those treated. The use of radiotherapy in prevention of gynaecomastia has been reviewed by Dicker.[73] Later reports such as that by Van Poppell et al.[74] suggest that the benefit once the gynaecomastia has developed is much smaller.

Surgery

When reassurance is inadequate, and drug treatment either inappropriate or unsatisfactory, surgical removal of the breast tissue is indicated. Although the operation is usually described as a subcutaneous mastectomy, it is important to leave a small area of subareolar breast tissue, as overzealous resection will replace the cosmetic deformity of a swelling with one of a hollow. In obese patients particularly, the cosmetic benefit may be marginal, and the patient should appreciate the difficulty in judging the right amount of tissue. Too much or too little removed from the obese is likely to leave a dissatisfied patient. In other cases, the gynaecomastia may merge with firm subcutaneous fat rather than form a localized protrusion and these cases are also unlikely to

get a satisfactory cosmetic result from surgery. In general, the overall results of surgery are disappointing, so much so that some purchasing groups are very restrictive in their indications for surgery. Recurrence arising from ductal tissue under the areola is well recognized; tamoxifen has been suggested as a possible treatment of such recurrence.

It is useful to be able to grade the degree of gynaecomastia in assessment and planning treatment, as well as for comparing results. A three-stage grading was proposed by Simon and colleagues.[75] Their classification is as follows:

- Grade I: Minor but visible breast enlargement without skin redundancy.
- Grade IIa: Moderate breast enlargement without skin redundancy.
- Grade IIb: Moderate breast enlargement with minor skin redundancy.
- Grade III: Gross breast enlargement with skin redundancy and ptosis so as to simulate a pendulous female breast.

With Grade I, IIa and IIb, treatment will leave the nipple approximately in its correct position. With Grade III, mastectomy will leave unsightly skin folds and the nipple much lower than normal. To overcome this, Ward and Khalid[76] have proposed an operation in which the nipple–areolar complex is left mounted on a vertical deepithelialized pedicle, which can be folded on itself to leave the nipple at its correct position.

Beckenstein et al.[77] studied 100 normal males to identify the ideal parameters of nipple position and areolar diameter to assist the cosmetic outcome in these Grade III patients. They found that the nipple lies 20 cm from the sternal notch and 18 cm from the midclavicular line with an ideal nipple-to-nipple distance of 21 cm. The average areolar diameter is 2.8 cm.

Liposuction has established a place in the management of gynaecomastia. It is particularly useful when there is much fatty tissue and is more effective when used with ultrasound guidance.[78] Fruhstorfer and Malata reviewed their results and found that a wide armamentarium of surgical procedures is necessary to produce a good result[78]. Some patients will need open resection and/or reduction of the skin envelope. Boljanovic et al.[79] combined liposuction and surgical resection of the residual glandular tissue under local anaesthetic. They reported that 80% of their 21 patients were satisfied with the results. Iwuagwu et al.[80] used a mammotome, with ultrasound guidance, a technique that may be more appropriate for very fibrotic examples of gynaecomastia.

On the basis of our early experience with a combination of liposuction for the fatty tissue and mammotomy for the residual fibroglandular tissue it seems to us likely that this minimally invasive approach will become the standard surgical approach.

Details of the surgical procedures will be found in Chapter 18.

Other male breast disease

Any other disease of the male breast is uncommon. However, most diseases of the breast that afflict women have also been reported in men from time to time. Not surprisingly, lesions that have their origin in lobular tissue are excessively rare but may occur in XXY phenotypes and in patients with longstanding raised oestrogen levels.

Fibroadenoma

In his postmortem study Sandison[6] records that one of his subjects had a localized fibroadenoma, a surprising finding in view of the absence of lobular activity in the male. Fibroadenomas require oestrogen stimulation so it is not surprising that most examples that have been recorded in males have mainly occurred in patients receiving oestrogen treatment for prostatic cancer; and even then the doses used have been in excess of those normally recommended.[81] Davies and Wallace[82] described a phenotypic male with complete androgen insensitivity who developed a fibroadenoma. Phyllodes tumours have also been described in men with gynaecomastia,[83,84] indeed most recorded cases of male fibroadenomas are associated with gynaecomastia.[85] Ansahboatene and Tavassoli[86] have reviewed the experiences of the US Armed Forces and described five cases all of whom also had gynaecomastia. A condition equivalent to fibroadenomatoid hyperplasia of the female breast has also been described in a 69-year-old man on spironolactone.[87]

Duct ectasia

This is a rare clinical entity, but Sandison[6] in his postmortem study of 500 men found that 6% of the specimens had histological evidence of duct ectasia. Anderson and Gram[7,14] found 30 examples of ectatic ducts in 100 consecutive male autopsies but in only seven of these was it diffuse. In none of these patients was there periductal inflammation; there were no clinical associations and they considered that the findings were different from duct ectasia of the female breast. Tedeschi and McCarthy[88] described periductal mastitis in a male. Haagensen[89] describes a patient with nipple discharge, which was attributed to androgens, although the description of the pathological findings in this case suggests that he had at least some degree of duct ectasia with periductal inflammation. The patient was clearly endocrinologically hypogonadal, following mumps orchitis at the age of 4. We have seen a number of cases in the male, some of which have been previously reported.[90] The patients have shown all the features of the condition as seen in women with nipple inversion, nipple discharge, abscess and fistula formation (Fig. 16.6). Whatever the underlying cause, treatment is by excision of the duct system as performed in postmenopausal women.

Not all periareolar infections in men are due to duct ectasia. More commonly, inflammatory masses around the nipple in men are due to retention cysts or infection in adjacent skin structures (Fig. 16.7).

HIV and the male breast

There are two facets to the development of breast swellings in men who are HIV positive. Firstly, the incidence

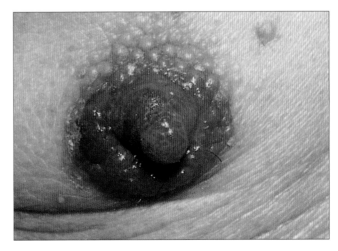

Fig. 16.6 A male patient with nipple discharge due to duct ectasia resulting in inflammation of the areolar skin.

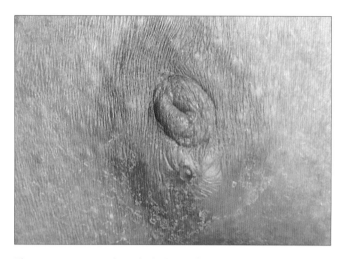

Fig. 16.7 Young male with discharge from a retention cyst of an areolar gland; treated by local excision.

of duct ectasia is increased in HIV-positive males who have a propensity to develop subareolar abscesses.[91,92]

Breast infections and abscesses are being seen more commonly in HIV-positive and otherwise immunocompromised males. The bacteriology is often unusual and should arouse suspicion. In general, wide drainage and excision of necrotic material has been needed to obtain resolution.

Secondly, antiretroviral treatment is one of the recognized causes of gynaecomastia. Careful evaluation of these patients is required because some of them will have lymphomas of the breast tissue. For example, Evans et al.[93] evaluated 13 men with breast enlargement who were HIV seropositive. Nine had gynaecomastia, one lipomastia and three lymphoma. Allen et al.[94] found that gynaecomastia could be reliably diagnosed by FNA in this group of patients. Thirteen of 15 patients in their study were on retroviral drugs known to be associated with gynaecomastia. The pathology of the breast associated with HIV infection has been reviewed by Pantanowitz and Connolly.[95]

Epithelial hyperplasia

Sandison[6] in his review of 500 postmortems in men records that 11 had significant epithelial hyperplasia, in three of whom it was associated with ectatic ducts. The clinical significance of this finding is uncertain. Anderson and Gram[14] found seven cases of epithelial hyperplasia in their postmortem series. Waldo et al.[96] reported a case of florid papillomatosis, a recognized premalignant condition in women, in a man taking diethylstilboestrol. Carcinoma in situ is rare in the male breast. Cutuli et al.[97] reported 31 cases treated in 19 French Regional Cancer Centres over 21 years, but this represented 5% of all male breast cancers treated. Eleven patients had gynaecomastia and three had a family history of breast cancer. Forty per cent presented with a bloody discharge, 48% with a mass and 12% with both. The left breast was affected twice as commonly as the right. One case was bilateral, and several patients had received long-term treatment for gynaecomastia.

Half the patients had axillary node dissection and none was positive, so total mastectomy seems appropriate if it is clear that there is no invasion.

Local excision was followed by recurrence and sometimes invasive cancer, so this approach is to be condemned.

Nipple discharge

Detraux et al.[98] performed galactography in seven males with unilateral nipple discharge. The lesions causing discharge were two papillomas, two carcinomas, two cases of duct ectasia and one breast abscess.

Treves et al.[99] collected 42 male patients with a serosanguineous discharge in 23 years and estimated that about 2% of male breast disease had nipple discharge as a symptom. Of their 42 cases, 18 were found to have benign disease and in many cases the discharge had been present for several years. The underlying causes in these cases were duct papilloma or gynaecomastia, all instances of bloodstained nipple discharge occurring with papilloma. An unusual case of bloodstained nipple discharge in an infant, associated with gynaecomastia,[100] is probably a variant of mastitis neonatorum; the case described by Miller et al.[101] is harder to categorize.

Reid-Nicholson et al.[102] reported the experience from Sloan Kettering: 11 cases of papillary lesions in the male breast were seen in an 8-year period. The lesions ranged from papillary hyperplasia in gynaecomastia to invasive papillary carcinoma. All of the patients had a periareolar mass; only two had nipple discharge.

The galactocele described by Boyle et al.[103] is also probably a variant of mastitis neonatorum.

Diabetic mastopathy

Diabetic mastopathy is well recognized in young women with longstanding insulin-dependent diabetes type I, and a similar picture may be seen in male diabetics with apparent gynaecomastia. The histological picture is one of marked perivascular and periductal round cell infiltration with predominance of B lymphocytes, together with focal fibrosis. This histological picture of diabetic mastopathy is different from gynaecomastia, with which it is likely to be confused clinically.[104]

Fat necrosis

As with many other conditions, this occasionally is recorded in men.[105]

Adenoma of the nipple

Azzopardi[9] mentions seven male patients with this condition in the world literature, and records a case of his own. It behaves identically to the same lesion in women.

Mondor's disease

We have seen only one example of this condition (Fig. 16.8) although Oldfield[106] considers that at least a third of the cases occur in men.

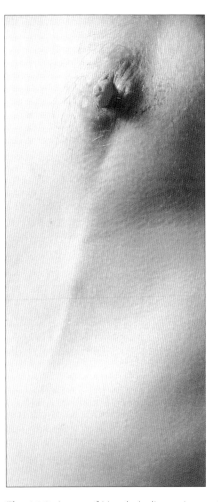

Fig. 16.8 A case of Mondor's disease in a male; the appearance is similar to that seen in women.

REFERENCES

1. Foot H. Remarks on gynaecomazia. *Dublin Quarterly Journal of Medical Sciences* 1866; **XLI**: 451–453.

2. Gruber F. Uber die gynaecomastie. *Memoires de l'academi du Science de St Petersburg* 7th series t 10, 1866.

3. Kapila K & Verma K. Cytology of nipple discharge in florid gynecomastia. *Acta Cytologica* 2003; **47**: 36–40.

4. Karsner HT. Gynecomastia. *American Journal of Pathology* 1946: **22**: 235–315.

5. Kono S, Kurosumi M, Simooka H et al. Immunohistochemical study of the relationship between Ki-67 labeling index of proliferating cells of gynecomastia, histological phase and duration of disease. *Pathology International* 2006; **56**: 655–658.

6. Sandison AT. *An Autopsy Study of the Human Breast*, Monograph No. 8, National Cancer Institute, US Dept Health, Education and Welfare, 1962.

7. Anderson JA & Gram JB. Gynecomasty: histological aspects in a surgical material. *Acta Pathologica et Microbiologica Scandinavia Section A: Pathologica* 1982; **90**: 185–190.

8. Miller RW & Sharpe RM. Environmental oestrogens and human reproductive cancers. *Endocrine related cancer* 1998; **5**: 69–96.

9. Azzopardi J. *Problems in Breast Pathology*. Philadelphia, WB Saunders; 1979:14.

10. Kapila K & Verma K. Cytomorphological spectrum in gynaecomastia: a study of 389 cases. *Cytopathology* 2002; **13**: 300–308.

11. Amrikachi M, Green LK, Rone R et al. Gynecomastia: cytologic features and diagnostic pitfalls in fine needle aspirates. *Acta Cytologica* 2001; **45**: 948–952.

12. Siddiqui MT, Zakowski MF, Ashfaq R *et al.* Breast masses in males: multi-institutional experience on fine-needle aspiration. *Diagnostic Cytopathology* 2002; **26**: 87–91.

13. Westenend PJ, Jobse C. Evaluation of fine-needle aspiration cytology of breast masses in males. *Cancer* 2002; **96**: 101–104.

14. Andersen JA & Gram JB. Male breast at autopsy. *Acta Pathologica et Microbiologica Scandinavia Section A: Pathologica* 1982; **90**: 191–197.

15. Williams MJ. Gynecomastia. Its incidence, recognition and host characterization in 447 autopsy cases. *American Journal of Medicine* 1963; **34**: 103–112.

16. Burke CW. Gynaecomastia. *Practitioner* 1982; **226**: 1403–1410.

17. Nydick M, Bustos J, Dale JH *et al.* Gynaecomastia in adolescent boys. *Journal of the American Medical Association* 1961; **178**: 449–457.

18. Nuttall FQ. Gynaecomastia as a physical finding in normal men. *Journal of Clinical Endocrinology and Metabolism* 1979; **48**: 338–340.

19. Georgiadis E, Papandreou L, Evanglopoulou C *et al.* Incidence of gynaecomastia in 954 young males and its relationship to somatometric parameters. *Annals of Human Biology* 1994; **21**: 579–587.

20. Ersoz H, Onde ME, Terekeci H *et al.* Causes of gynaecomastia in young adult males and factors associated with idiopathic gynaecomastia. *International Journal of Andrology* 2002; **25**: 312–316.

21. Dershaw DD. Male mammography. *American Journal of Roentgenology* 1986; **146**: 127–131.

22. Kapdi CC & Parekh NJ. The male breast. *The Radiological Clinics of North America* 1983; **21**: 137–148.

23. Turkington RW. Serum prolactin levels in patients with gynaecomastia. *Journal of Clinical Endocrinology and Metabolism* 1972; **34**: 62–66.

24. Moore DC, Schlaepfer LV, Paunier L *et al.* Hormonal changes during puberty vs transient pubertal gynaecomastia and abnormal androgen estrogen ratios. *Journal of Clinical Endocrinology and Metabolism* 1984; **58**: 492–499.

25. Lee PA. The relationship of concentrations of serum hormones to pubertal gynaecomastia. *Journal of Pediatrics* 1975; **86**: 212–215.

26. Pirke KM & Doerr P. Age related changes and interrelationships between plasma testosterone, oestradiol and testosterone-binding globulin in normal adult males. *Acta Endocrinologica* 1973; **74**: 792–800.

27. Wilson JD, Aiman J & MacDonald PC. The pathogenesis of gynaecomastia. *Advances in Internal Medicine* 1980; **25**: 1–32.

28. Binder G, Iliev DI, Dufke A *et al.* Dominant transmission of prepubertal gynecomastia due to serum estrone excess: hormonal, biochemical, and genetic analysis in a large kindred. *Journal of Clinical Endocrinology and Metabolism* 2005; **90**: 484–492.

29. Gooren LJG & Daantje CRE. Psychological stress as a cause of intermittent gynaecomastia. *Hormone Metabolism Research* 1986; **18**: 424.

30. Cespedes RD, Caballero RL, Peretsman SJ *et al.* Cryptic presentation of germ cell tumours. *Journal of the American College of Surgeons* 1994; **178**: 261–265.

31. Swerdlow AJ, Schoemaker MJ, Higgins CD *et al.* UK Clinical Cytogenetics Group. Cancer incidence and mortality in men with Klinefelter syndrome: a cohort study. *Journal of the National Cancer Institute* 2005; **97**: 1204–1210.

32. Stacey-Clear A. Gynaecomastia. *British Journal of Surgery* 1992; **79**: 182–183.

33. Gordon GG, Olivo J, Rafii F *et al.* Conversion of androgens to estrogens in cirrhosis of the liver. *Journal of Clinical Endocrinology and Metabolism* 1975; **40**: 1018–1026.

34. Jacobs EC. Effects of starvation on sex hormones in the male. *Journal of Clinical Endocrinology* 1948; **8**: 227–232.

35. Thompson DF & Carter JR. Drug induced gynaecomastia. *Pharmacotherapy* 1993; **13**: 37–45.

36. Gabrilove J & Luria M. Persistent gynecomastia resulting from scalp inunction of estradiol: a model for persistent gynaecomastia. *Archives of Dermatology* 1978; **114**: 1672–1673.

37. Rissanen TJ, Makarainen HP, Kallioinen MJ *et al.* Radiography of the breast in gynaecomastia. *Acta Radiologica* 1992; **33**: 110–114.

38. Edidin DV & Levitsky LL. Prepubertal gynecomastia associated with estrogen-containing hair cream. *American Journal of Diseases in Children* 1982; **136**: 587–588.

39. Felner EI & White PC. Prepubertal gynecomastia: indirect exposure to estrogen cream. *Pediatrics* 2000; **105**: E55.

40. Brody SA & Loriaux DL. Epidemic of gynecomastia among Haitian refugees: exposure to an environmental antiandrogen. *Endocrine Practice* 2003; **9**: 370–375.

41. Bellati G & Ideo G. Gynaecomastia after spironolactone and potassium canrenoate. *Lancet* 1986; **i**: 626.

42. Rodriguez LA & Jick H. Risk of gynaecomastia associated with cimetidine, omeprazole and other anti-ulcer drugs. *British Medical Journal* 1994; **308**: 503–506.

43. Satoh T, Itoh S, Seki T *et al.* On the inhibitory action of 29 drugs having side effect gynecomastia on estrogen production. *Steroid Biochemistry and Molecular Biology* 2002; **82**: 206–209.

44. Evans GF, Anthony T, Turnage RH *et al.* The diagnostic accuracy of mammography in the evaluation of male breast disease. *American Journal of Surgery* 2001; **181**: 96–100.

45. Myhre SA, Ruvalcaba RHA, Johnson HR *et al.* The effects of testosterone treatment in Klinefelter's syndrome. *Journal of Pediatrics* 1970; **76**: 267–276.

46. Eberle AJ, Sparrow JT & Keenan BS. Treatment of persistent pubertal gynaecomastia with dihydrotestosterone heptanoate. *Journal of Pediatrics* 1986; **109**: 144–149.

47. Dobs AS, Meikle AW, Arver S *et al.* Pharmacokinetics, efficacy, and safety of a permeation-enhanced testosterone transdermal system in comparison with bi-weekly injections of testosterone enanthate for the treatment of hypogonadal men. *Journal of Clinical Endocrinology and Metabolism* 1999; **84**: 3469–3478.

48. Benveniste O, Simon A & Herson S. Successful percutaneous dihydrotestosterone treatment of gynecomastia occurring during highly active antiretroviral therapy: four cases and a review of the literature. *Clinical Infection and Disease* 2001; **33**: 891–893.

49. LeRoith D, Sobel R & Glick SM. The effect of clomiphene citrate on pubertal gynaecomastia. *Acta Endocrinol (Copenh)* 1980; **95**: 177–180.

50. Stephanas AV, Burnet RB, Harding PE *et al.* Clomiphene in the treatment of pubertal adolescent gynaecomastia: a preliminary report. *Journal of Pediatrics* 1977; **90**: 651–653.

51. Plourde PV, Kulin HE & Santner SJ. Clomiphene in the treatment of adolescent gynecomastia. *American Journal of Diseases of Children* 1983; **137**: 1080–1082.

52. Jeffreys DB. Painful gynaecomastia treated with tamoxifen. *British Medical Journal* 1979; **i**: 1119–1120.

53. Parker LN, Gray DR, Lai MK *et al.* Treatment of gynecomastia with tamoxifen: a double blind cross-over study. *Metabolism* 1986; **35**: 705–708.

54. McDermott MT, Hofeldt FD & Kidd GS. Tamoxifen therapy for painful idiopathic gynecomastia. *Southern Medical Journal* 1990; **83**: 1283–1285.

55. Alagaratnam TT. Idiopathic gynaecomastia treated with tamoxifen. A preliminary report. *Clinical Therapeutics* 1987; **9**: 483–487.

56. Khan HN, Rampaul R & Blamey RW. Management of physiological gynaecomastia with tamoxifen. *Breast* 2004; **13**: 61–65.

57. Derman O, Kanbur NO & Kutluk T. Tamoxifen treatment for pubertal gynecomastia. *International Journal of Adolescent Medical Health* 2003; **15**: 359–363.

58. Novoa FJ, Boronat M, Carrillo A *et al.* Effects of tamoxifen on lipid profile and coagulation parameters in male patients with pubertal gynecomastia. *Hormone Research* 2002; **57**: 187–191.

59. Evans NA. Gym and tonic: a profile of 100 male steroid users. *British Journal of Sports Medicine* 1997; **31**: 54–58.

60. Buckle R. Danazol therapy in gynaecomastia; recent experience and indications for therapy. *Postgraduate Medical Journal* 1979; **55**(suppl 5): 71–78.

61. Daniels IR & Layer GT. How should gynaecomastia be managed? *Australian and New Zealand Journal of Surgery* 2003; **73**: 213–216.

62. Jones DJ, Holt SD, Surtees P *et al.* A comparison of danazol and placebo in the treatment of adult idiopathic gynaecomastia: results of a prospective study in 55 patients. *Annals of the Royal College of Surgeons of England* 1990; **72**: 296–298.

63. Hanvadi S, Banerjee D, Monypenny IJ *et al.* The role of tamoxifen in the management of gynaecomastia. *Breast* 2006; **15**: 276–280.

64. Ting AC, Chow LW & Leung YF. Comparison of tamoxifen with danazol in the management of idiopathic gynecomastia. *American Surgeon* 2000; **66**: 38–40.

65. Braunstein GD. Aromatase and gynaecomastia. *Endocrine Related Cancer* 1999; **6**: 315–324.

66. Miller WR & Jackson J. The therapeutic potential of aromatase inhibitors. *Expert Opinion in Investigative Drugs* 2003; **12**: 337–351.

67. Boccardo F, Rubagotti A, Battaglia M *et al.* Montefiore evaluation of tamoxifen and anastrozole in the prevention of gynecomastia and breast pain induced by bicalutamide monotherapy of prostate cancer. *Journal of Clinical Oncology* 2005; **23**: 587–592.

68. Saltzstein D, Sieber P, Morris T *et al.* Prevention and management of bicalutamide-induced gynecomastia and breast pain: randomized endocrinologic and clinical studies with tamoxifen and anastrozole. *Prostate Cancer and Prostatic Disease* 2005; **8**: 75–83.

69. Perdona S, Autorino R, De Placido S *et al.* Efficacy of tamoxifen and radiotherapy for prevention and treatment of gynaecomastia and breast pain caused by bicalutamide in prostate cancer: a randomised controlled trial. *Lancet Oncology* 2005; **6**: 295–300.

70. Fradet Y, Engerdie B *et al.* Tamoxifen as a prophylaxis for prevention of gynaecomastia and breast pain associated with bicalutamide 150mg monotherapy in patients with prostate cancer: a randomized placebo-controlled, dose response study. *European Urology* 2007; **52**: 106–114.

71. Malis I, Cooper JF & Wolever THS. Breast radiation in patients with carcinoma of the prostate. *Journal of Urology* 1969; **102**: 336–340.

72. Widmark A, Fossa SD, Lundmo P *et al.* Does prophylactic breast irradiation prevent antiandrogen-induced gynaecomastia? Evaluation of 253 patients in the randomized Scandinavian trial SPCG-7/SFUO-3. *Urology* 2003; **61**: 145–151.

73. Dicker AP. The safety and tolerability of low-dose irradiation for the management of gynaecomastia caused by antiandrogen monotherapy. *Lancet Oncology* 2003; **4**: 30–36.

74. Van Poppel H, Tyrrell CJ, Haustermans K *et al.* Efficacy and tolerability of radiotherapy as treatment for bicalutamide-induced gynaecomastia and breast pain in prostate cancer. *European Urology* 2005; **47**: 587–592.

75. Simon BE, Hoffman S & Khan S. Classification and surgical management of gynaecomastia. *Plastic and Reconstructive Surgery* 1973; **51**: 48–52.

76. Ward CM & Khalid K. Surgical treatment of Grade III gynaecomastia. *Annals of the Royal College of Surgeons of England* 1989; **71**: 226–228.

77. Beckenstein MS, Windle BH & Stroup Jr RT. Anatomical parameters for nipple position and areolar diameter in males. *Annals of Plastic Surgery* 1996; **36**: 33–36.

78. Fruhstorfer BH & Malata CM. A systematic approach to the surgical treatment of gynaecomastia. *British Journal of Plastic Surgery* 2003; **56**: 237–246.

79. Boljanovic S, Axelsson CK & Elberg JJ. Surgical treatment of gynecomastia: liposuction combined with subcutaneous mastectomy. *Scandinavian Journal of Surgery* 2003; **92**: 160–162.

80. Iwuagwu OC, Calvey TA, Ilsley D *et al.* Ultrasound guided minimally invasive breast surgery (UMIBS): a superior technique for gynecomastia. *Annals of Plastic Surgery* 2004; **52**: 131–133.

81. Soonso IN, Rashid A & Skidmore FD. Fibroadenoma arising in the axilla of a male patient. Effect of high dose diethylstilboestrol. *The Breast* 1996; **5**: 265–266.

82. Davis SE, & Wallace AM. A 19 year old with complete androgen insensitivity syndrome and juvenile fibroadenoma of the breast. *Breast Journal* 2001; **7**: 430–433.

83. Hilton DA, Jameson JS & Furness PN. A cellular fibroadenoma resembling a benign phyllodes tumour in a young male with gynaecomastia. *Histopathology* 1991; **18**: 476–477.

84. Bartoli C, Zurrida SM & Clemente C. Phyllodes tumour in a male patient with bilateral gynaecomastia induced by oestrogen therapy for prostatic cancer. *European Journal of Surgical Oncology* 1991; **17**: 215–217.

85. Uchida T, Ischii M & Motomiya Y. Fibroadenoma associated with gynaecomastia in an adult man. *Scandinavian Journal of Plastic and Reconstructive Surgery and Hand Surgery* 1993; **27**: 327–329.

86. Ansahboatene Y & Tavassoli FA. Fibroadenoma and cystosarcoma phyllodes of the male breast. *Modern Pathology* 1992; **5**: 114–116.

87. Nielsen BB. Fibroadenomatoid hyperplasia of the male breast. *American Journal of Surgical Pathology* 1990; **14**: 774–777.

88. Tedeschi LG & McCarthy PE. Involutional mammary duct ectasia and periductal mastitis in a male. *Human Pathology* 1974; **5**: 232–236.

89. Haagensen CD. *Diseases of the Breast*. Philadelphia, WB Saunders; 1986.

90. Mansel RE & Morgan WP. Duct ectasia in the male. *British Journal of Surgery* 1979; **66**: 660–662.

91. Downs AMR, Fisher M, Tomlinson D *et al.* Male duct ectasia associated with HIV infection. *Genitourinary Medicine* 1996; **72**: 65–66.

92. Higgins SP, Stedman YF, Bundred NJ *et al.* Periareolar breast abscess due to *Pseudonas aeroginosa* in an HIV antibody positive male. *Genitourinary Medicine* 1994; **70**: 147–148.

93. Evans DL, Pantanowitz L, Dezube BJ *et al.* Breast enlargement in 13 men who were seropositive for human immunodeficiency virus. *Clinical and Infectious Disease* 2002; **35**: 1113–1119.

94. Allen EA, Parwani AV, Siddiqui MT *et al.* Cytopathologic findings in breast masses in men with HIV infection. *Acta Cytologica* 2003; **47**: 183–187.

95. Pantanowitz L & Connolly JL. Pathology of the breast associated with HIV/AIDS. *Breast Journal* 2002; **8**: 234–243.

96. Waldo ED, Sidhu GS & Hu AW. Florid papillomatosis of the male breast after diethyl stilboestrol therapy. *Archives of Pathology and Laboratory Medicine* 1975; **99**: 364–366.

97. Cutuli B, Dilhuydi JM, DeLaFontan B *et al.* Ductal carcinoma in situ in the male breast. Analysis of 31 cases. *European Journal of Cancer* 1997; **33**: 35–38.

98. Detraux P, Benmussa M, Tristant H *et al.* Breast disease in the male: galactographic evaluation. *Radiology* 1985; **154**: 605–606.

99. Treves N, Robbins GF & Amoroso WL. Serous and serosanguineous discharge from the male nipple. *Archives of Surgery* 1956; **90**: 319–329.

100. Olcay I & Gokoz A. Infantile gynecomastia with bloody nipple discharge. *Journal of Pediatric Surgery* 1992; **27**: 103–104.

101. Miller JD, Brownell MD & Shaw A. Bilateral breast masses and bloody nipple discharge in a 4-year-old boy. *Journal of Paediatrics* 1990; **116**: 744–747.

102. Reid-Nicholson MD, Tong G, Cangiarella JF *et al.* Cytomorphologic features of papillary lesions of the male breast: a study of 11 cases. *Cancer* 2006; **108**: 222–230.

103. Boyle M, Lakhoo K & Ramani P. Galactocoal in a male infant: case report and review of the literature. *Pediatric Pathology* 1993; **13**: 305–308.

104. Steinbach BG, Steinbach JJ & Zander DS. Bilateral breast masses in a man. *Military Medicine* 1993; **158**: 356–357.

105. Bahal V & Mansel RE. Mondor's disease secondary to breast abscess in a male. *British Journal of Surgery* 1986; **73**: 931.

106. Oldfield MC. Mondor's disease. A superficial thrombophlebitis of the breast. *Lancet* 1962; **i**: 994–996.

CHAPTER 17

Miscellaneous conditions

Introduction

This chapter brings together a number of conditions that do not conveniently fit elsewhere. Although individually uncommon, their main importance lies in their presentation that often clinically mimics carcinoma. These conditions are mostly outside the concept of aberrations of normal development and involution (ANDI) and often reflect local manifestations of systemic disease although some are important in their own right as a source of morbidity. When the disease is already diagnosed, resolution of the problem is straightforward. When it is the first, or only, manifestation then diagnostic difficulty may be encountered. Adherence to the principles of triple assessment coupled with an awareness of possible diagnoses will usually allow the problem to be identified without recourse to surgery. In the past, many such diagnoses have only been made on histological sectioning of the mastectomy specimen; the more rational approach to breast disease that now appertains means the diagnosis should be made before such a tragedy occurs. Hoda and Rosen[1] have provided a useful review of some of the common pitfalls for the pathologist meeting unusual lesions.

Apart from glandular elements and supporting fibrous stroma, lesions may arise from blood vessels, nerves, fat and lymphatics. Lesions of the skin and underlying musculoskeletal tissue are often of concern to patients but can usually be identified as being outwith the breast by careful clinical assessment.

Trauma

The breast is relatively infrequently damaged in trauma. The commonest injuries are blunt chest wall trauma and burns, although quite trivial trauma to the developing breast bud may cause marked asymmetry.[2]

Burns

Burns of the chest wall are not uncommon in children, usually as a result of scalds.[3] The resulting scars are unsightly and, if the nipple is involved, there may be subsequent problems with breastfeeding. Partial-thickness burns may be disturbing but are otherwise of little importance. Full-thickness burns may lead to failure of breast development, although in one series all 28 patients with significant thermal injury involving the nipple–areola complex developed breasts in adolescence.[4] However, stimulation of viable breast tissue growth subsequent to thermal injury can be inhibited by the tight burn scar in the overlying breast envelope. Such scarring can adversely affect the development, contour and positioning of the breast as well as the cosmetic appearance of the skin surface. If the scarring is severe, plastic surgery may play a useful role in management and pressure garments may help to minimize scarring. Complex procedures may be required to correct the deformity and are best delayed until growth is complete.[5] Young girls may require corrective surgery many years after the injury.[6]

Seatbelt injury

In adult life, blunt trauma is the most usual form. Even a clear history of injury, such as that obtained in car accidents with bruising, does not exclude the possibility of an underlying carcinoma. The introduction of seatbelt legislation has led to a number of reports of breast injury due to seatbelts, sometimes sufficient to cause complete disruption of the breast.[7] The injury is caused by a combination of compression between the seatbelt and the rib cage, and shearing stresses associated with torsion of the body.

The typical injury in a severe case is a furrowed deformity in the line of the seatbelt. This may be masked initially by haematoma and soft tissue oedema, but as this resolves the defect in the breast may be seen and palpated. The architectural disturbance may be revealed on mammography, ultrasonography and magnetic resonance imaging: in particular lipid cysts and parenchymal calcification occurring in a bandlike distribution.[8] In less severe cases, the clinical features of fat necrosis are evident, but beware the possibility that the accident may only have served to draw attention to a pre-existing carcinoma, so formal evaluation is mandatory.

Fat necrosis

The most common sequel to trauma that gives rise to clinical problems is fat necrosis. This is one of those uncommon lesions that is perversely known to all medical students as a condition that simulates cancer. In spite of the universal teaching that fat necrosis may simulate cancer, procrastination with cancer still occurs because doctors accept a history of trauma from the patient and accept the possibility of a condition so familiar to them.

It would be better if the condition were unknown, for it is sufficiently rare in its classic form that no one would be disadvantaged if the condition were unrecognized without formal cytological or histological diagnosis. Breast cancer is 40 times more common than traumatic fat necrosis in Haagensen's experience.[9] The situation would have been very different in 1920 when Lee and Adair[10] first reported it, for radical mastectomy was then commonly performed on clinical appearance alone. Sandison[11] found evidence of fat necrosis in only two of his 800 autopsies.

It is now clear that fat necrosis may appear as a complication of surgery on the breast. Mandrekas et al.[12] reported an incidence of 1% following 300 reduction mammoplasties. A more worrying scenario for the patient is the appearance of painful lumps in the region of scars following treatment for breast cancer. We have seen this in transverse rectus abdominis myocutaneous (TRAM) flaps used for postmastectomy reconstruction[13] and after breast-conserving surgery with postoperative radiotherapy. A number of reports now exist of fat necrosis developing in a breast treated by local excision and radiotherapy. In one study, 27% of 300 women developed clinical evidence of fat necrosis after wide local excision and brachytherapy.[14] The incidence of fat necrosis after breast-conserving treatment in breast cancer is usually under 5%. When a new problem occurs, be it clinical or radiological, it is wise to formally re-evaluate the breast before assuming that this represents recurrent cancer; for example, Chaudary et al. re-evaluated 17 patients, out of 214 having breast conservation, with suspicious lesions but only seven were found to be due to breast cancer.[15]

Clinical features

Two distinct forms of fat necrosis occur: one simulates cancer; the other simulates simple cysts, although differing from uncomplicated cysts in having an added symptom of a dull, aching pain.

The first form is more common in elderly patients, perhaps because the involuted breast tissue is less able to absorb a sudden blow. The diagnosis is aided by the presence of bruising or redness of the skin, although this is not always present. The actual lump is usually small and attached to surrounding tissue. Later, a more florid, inflammatory picture may produce skin fixity and oedema, resembling both cancer and the chronic form of periductal mastitis (PDM). Mammography in this group may show features consistent with carcinoma with spiculation and linear calcification, but usually with a radiolucent centre.

The mammographic and ultrasound appearances of fat necrosis have been reviewed by Baillie and Mok[16] and are quite variable. Ultrasound-guided biopsy is indicated; the typical findings are of necrotic fat cells associated with macrophages. In fat necrosis, section shows a small cavity with thick necrotic material and often white fat necrosis on the edge of the cavity. Other cases merge into a picture of haematoma with some fat necrosis around the edge.

The pathology is that of a chronic inflammatory reaction with marked histiocytic reaction and peripheral fibrosis, which increases with time. The diagnosis should not be made without core biopsy for we have seen several cases where fat necrosis and cancer have been adjacent to each other. Mammography and cytology may both be helpful but needle biopsy is mandatory.

If there is a good history of trauma accompanied by bruising and typical fat necrosis seen on core biopsy, an expectant treatment plan may be pursued. If the lesion resolves no further action is required. If the lesion persists or enlarges, a rare event in our experience, operative intervention may be indicated to confirm the diagnosis and to remove necrotic material. The series reported by

Pullyblank et al.[17] illustrate some of the problems that may be encountered when treating patients with apparent fat necrosis. The second type of fat necrosis has been seen in our experience in women who present with tender swellings some time after quite severe trauma such as a car accident. Nothing is noted on inspection, but palpation reveals one or more tender cystic structures, which feel like ordinary cysts but with a sensation of slight thickening around the wall. Ultrasound may show cystic areas (Fig. 17.1) and mammograms may show calcification (Fig. 17.2).

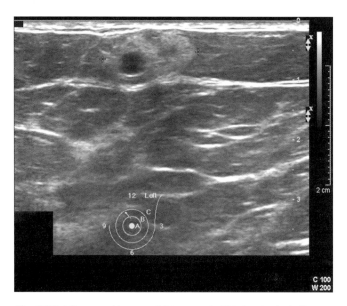

Fig. 17.1 Ultrasound image of fat necrosis. This is a typical oil cyst caused by leakage of fat from damaged cells.

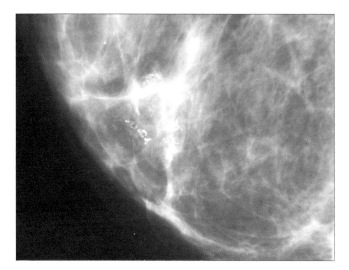

Fig. 17.2 Magnified mammographic image of partly calcified fat necrosis.

Aspiration produces a typical oily fluid (Fig. 17.3) and is curative. Occasionally the cysts may be multiple.

The mammographic and ultrasound features of fat necrosis have been reviewed by Bilgen et al.[18] In general, the imaging allows a likely diagnosis of fat necrosis to be made, but confirmation by aspirating oil cysts and a core needle biopsy for those cases where solid tissue predominates.

Paraffinoma and silicone reactions

Early attempts at augmentation using injections of silicone and paraffin had disastrous results with chronic discharging lesions which may appear at sites remote from the breast.[19] The diagnosis is not always immediately apparent because an interval of up to 35 years may occur between the injection and re-presentation.[19] Although such procedures have long been abandoned, reports of late complications continue to appear in the literature[20,21] and, given the mobility of populations, may occur anywhere. Alagaratnam and Ong[19] recognized two modes of presentation: a painless hard mass clinically resembling cancer and hard masses with ulceration or sinus formation usually associated with lymphadenopathy. A further aid to diagnosis is the mammographic finding of a characteristic honeycomb appearance. Ho et al. have delineated the magnetic resonance imaging (MRI) features of this condition.[20]

In the first group, treatment is by local excision without entering the paraffinoma; the paraffin remains liquid and, if spilt, will lead to recurrence of the problem. The cosmetic deformity may be considerable but is preferable

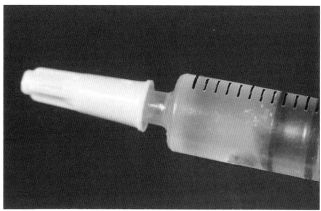

Fig. 17.3 The oily fluid aspirated from a cyst.

to a simple mastectomy. When the skin ulceration is extensive, simple mastectomy may become necessary although, in less severe cases, excision of the secondarily infected mass may be sufficient. In one series from Hong Kong, Alagaratnam and Ng[22] had to perform a mastectomy in 30 of 43 patients. Migratory masses should be removed in continuity with the breast mass. Some patients will request further reconstructive surgery. Those who have experience of this problem advise that reconstruction should be delayed until it is clear that the original problem will not recur.

Although breast augmentation has largely been replaced by silicone gel prostheses, Christensen et al.[23] have reported the continuing use of polyacrylamide hydrogel as a method of breast reconstruction. They found that polyacrylamide hydrogel was well tolerated by the breast and did not give rise to severe fibrosis, pain, or capsule shrinkage. It is stable over time, nondegradable, confined to the breast and does not appear to migrate. However, Zhao et al.[24] reviewed the histology from 31 patients who had requested that the polyacrylamide gel be removed. They compared the findings with archival material related to silicone removal. They found more foreign body giant cells but fewer lymphocytes in the polyacrylamide than the silicone group. They concluded that the difficulty of removing the material, breast pain and inflammatory changes limited its use in breast augmentation.

The use of paraffin has been superseded by the use of silicone gel-filled envelopes. Apart from unsatisfactory cosmesis, the two main problems of such prostheses are capsule formation and rupture of the envelope. If the envelope ruptures, when the silicone remains confined within the capsule it causes, little tissue reaction occurs. If it leaks outside the capsule, silicone granulomas occur and silicone migrates to the lymph nodes. Austad[25] has reviewed the literature on silicone granulomas associated with breast prostheses. The clinical awareness of these events causes considerable concern to the patient. Evaluation of breast disease may be difficult as needle biopsy carries with it the risk of breaking the envelope of a prosthesis that is still intact. MRI may be helpful in elucidating difficult cases of painful breasts in patients with previous augmentation mammoplasty. If a combination of MRI, computerized tomography (CT) scan and ultrasound fails to elucidate the problem, exploration of the pocket and direct visualization of the prosthesis are indicated. In spite of the publicity that has surrounded such events, there is no substantive evidence that this is associated with systemic diseases such as arthritis.

The problems of rupture of silicone gel breast implants have been well reviewed by Brown et al.[26] The main conclusions of their review of the published literature are that envelope rupture is more common than generally supposed, and that trauma is a rare cause of rupture which is more often associated with the age of the prosthesis. Prostheses that have been in situ for over 8 years have a higher incidence of rupture. This is due to a combination of maturing of the material and a fold flaw. In many cases the rupture remains asymptomatic but may cause pain. If the capsule as well as the envelope is breached, migration of the silicone may cause granuloma formation in the surrounding tissues and lymph nodes. Occasionally, the silicone may be discharged through the nipple. Investigation should be confined to symptomatic patients; best specificity and sensitivity is obtained using MRI with a dedicated breast coil. Symptomatic ruptured prostheses should be removed but there is debate about optimal management of localized leaks retained within the capsule.

Lipoma

It is not surprising that lipomas are sometimes found in the breast. Haagensen[9] describes a series of 186 patients with a mean age of 45. Variant lipomas with brown fat,[27] spindle cells[28] and angiolipomas[29] have all been described. The clinical features are those of lipoma elsewhere: a smooth, slightly lobulated mobile mass. Their main importance lies in distinguishing them from a clinical variant of carcinoma: the pseudolipoma. This condition is produced by shortening of Cooper's ligaments as a carcinoma infiltrates. The intervening fat lobules are compressed and 'bunched up', so that they take on a lobulated form as seen in lipoma, at the same time concealing the small underlying cancer. As lipomas occur in the cancer age group, they require formal triple assessment.

The mammographic and ultrasound features are typical, producing a circumscribed translucent area compressing the surrounding structures (Fig. 17.4). Although some consider that the features are so distinctive that a biopsy is unnecessary,[30] our view is that it is prudent to perform a core biopsy. This view is reinforced by the observations of Lanng et al.[31] who found that 27 of 108 (25%) clinically diagnosed lipomas were incorrect but recommended that provided no adverse features were seen on mammography, ultrasound and with a needle or

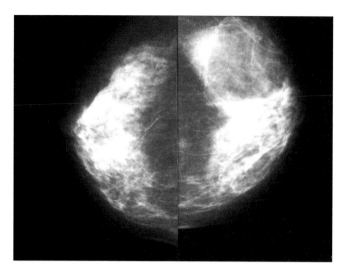

Fig. 17.4 Mammographic image of large lipoma left outer breast.

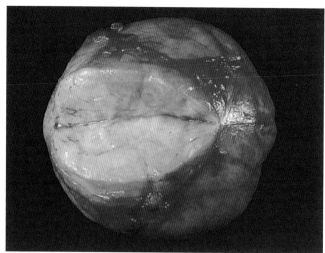

Fig. 17.5 Fibroadenolipoma of the breast.

core biopsy containing fat that an expectant treatment could be followed. These authors also pointed out that only a minority of cases showed the typical features of lipoma on either mammography or ultrasound. If there is any doubt about the diagnosis, the lesion is better removed.

Hamartoma (adenolipoma)

Haagensen[9] and Azzopardi[32] both regard this as a variant of lipoma that has incorporated epithelial elements. An alternative view is to regard these lesions as hamartomas, as argued by Arrigoni et al.,[33] since they meet the criteria for this condition: the presence of normal components of a tissue but abnormal in proportions and arrangement. This assumes that they arise from embryonic rests, now the most widely accepted theory. These lesions are uncommon; Crothers et al.[34] recorded only eight cases in 20 000 mammograms.

This lesion tends to occur at an earlier age group than lipoma, usually in the fifth decade, but can occur over a very wide age range. Clinically, they resemble lipomas, appearing as soft, circumscribed, mobile masses, which feel harder if there is a large proportion of fibrous tissue. They are usually a few centimetres in diameter, but may reach 10 cm, and growth may vary with pregnancy or lactation.[35]

Mammographically, they have a typical appearance of a smooth mass with a fat halo,[34] although in detail the appearances can be very variable. With larger masses, the

trite description is 'a breast within a breast'. Park et al.[35] have analyzed the mammographic and sonographic features and describe a typical compressibility of the lesion on ultrasound when round lesions become ovoid.

Core biopsy and cytology have no characteristic features and any of the changes of ANDI may be encountered. At operation, they appear well encapsulated although no capsule is found on histology (Fig. 17.5).

Problems can arise with pathological diagnosis, since the normal appearance of the tissues may lead a pathologist to report a biopsy as 'normal breast tissue' or 'no pathological diagnosis' which is at variance with the obvious clinical lesion. A useful feature is the presence of both ducts and lobules, since lobules are absent or rare in a fibroadenoma. The epithelial elements may contain the whole spectrum of ductal and lobular involution.

Davies et al. carried out a detailed dissecting microscope study of thick sections, together with conventional study of thin sections.[36] This led them to define a distinctive combination of features to allow a precise histological diagnosis, without relying on clinical and radiological features for confirmation.

Oedema of the breast

The breast may become oedematous due to heart failure and inanition. The changes in the skin of the breast are those of peau d'orange, which may progress to ulceration, so a provisional diagnosis of carcinoma is made even though no mass is palpable. General examination usually reveals evidence of generalized oedema due to either heart failure[37] or the nephrotic syndrome. The so-called nursing home breast represents another variant of this problem,[38] where the unilateral localization of the oedema results from the patient being left on one side, with that breast continually dependent. A history from the attendants will usually reveal that the patient nearly always lies on the same side.

We have seen a case in which the cardiac failure went unrecognized, a clinical diagnosis of carcinoma was made and the patient treated with tamoxifen in spite of negative biopsies. Mammography revealed skin oedema but no focal lesion. The clinical and radiographic signs of malignancy resolved upon appropriate treatment of her heart failure.

The mammographic findings of this condition differ from diffuse inflammatory carcinoma. The skin oedema is thicker, there is a prominent reticular parenchymal pattern, and nipple retraction is absent.[39]

The commonest situation in which an oedematous breast occurs is following breast-conserving surgery for breast cancer. Most often, this occurs after both axillary surgery and radiotherapy. In large breasts it may pose a significant discomfort but its real anxiety lies in the difficulty of ensuring that the changes do not represent a recurrence of the carcinoma. Post-treatment breast oedema is commoner after nodal clearance than after sentinel node biopsy but Ronka et al.[40] found that even then nearly one in four patients had appreciable breast oedema.

The post-irradiated breast

Radiotherapy is often used in the management of malignant breast disease. Lower doses of radiation were used during a vogue for treating mastalgia with radiation between the 1920s and the 1950s.[41] The doses used in these patients are unlikely to produce local tissue damage but there are obvious implications for the induction of malignant change.

Over half the patients presenting with early breast cancer are now suitable for conservation therapy so it is pertinent to review the problems apart from recurrent cancer that may occur in the post-irradiated breast. Patients with conserved breasts following breast cancer treatment who develop new breast symptoms pose difficulties in management. Psychologically, they are stressed; the scarring from previous surgery and the changes associated with radiotherapy make evaluation more difficult.

When a new problem arises, be it clinical or radiological, it is wise to formally re-evaluate the breast before assuming that this represents recurrent cancer; for example, Chaudery et al.[15] re-evaluated 17 patients with new lumps out of 214 having breast conservation and only seven were found to be due to breast cancer. The clinician needs to be aware of the changes that can occur in the breast after such treatment. Skin thickening, oedema and fat necrosis are common causes for concern to the patient. Although the time sequence usually suggests the diagnosis, later change needs to be regarded more circumspectly. One interesting phenomenon is the delayed noninfective cellulites seen in patients who have had breast conserving treatment.[42] It is usually attributed to obstructed lymphatics. There is no specific treatment; in particular, antibiotics are ineffective; it usually resolves over a period of weeks rather than days. Interestingly, we have seen a similar problem confined to the skin of a TRAM flap, which resolved over a 6-week period, having developed 9 months after surgery. This could also be satisfactorily explained on the basis of lymphatic obstruction. The histological changes induced by therapeutic radiation have been reported by Moore et al;[43] they assessed stromal vascular and fibroblastic changes and epithelial cell changes of the terminal duct lobular unit and extralobular ducts as well as terminal duct lobular unit fibrosis/atrophy. This group found all these parameters were altered from the pre-radiation findings and did not change with time.

Most ulcerating lesions that occur after radiotherapy for breast cancer will prove to be due to recurrent disease, but this requires histological confirmation because some of these will be due to radionecrosis. The patient has usually had radical surgery and radiotherapy, often some years previously. The presentation is of a clinically discharging ulcer, most frequently on the medial half of the chest wall (Fig. 17.6). Examination will usually reveal necrotic underlying costal cartilage. Occasionally, severe bleeding will occur from the internal mammary artery.

The only satisfactory treatment is surgical with debridement of the ulcer and removal of the underlying necrotic costal cartilage. It is impracticable to excise the whole of the irradiated area, so skin and subcutaneous tissue need only be excised until good bleeding is seen. Because of their poor blood supply, the whole of the involved, and infected, costal cartilage will need to be removed. The underlying pleura are usually markedly thickened and the pathology lends itself to excisional surgery and reconstruction.[44] Any form of reconstruction should be with

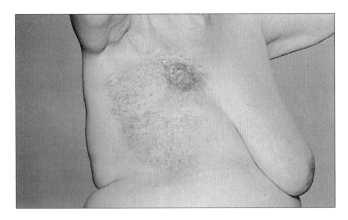

Fig. 17.6 Radiation necrosis of the chest wall. There is no recurrent tumour in this case, in spite of the malignant appearance of the ulcer.

unirradiated tissue and bring with it a new blood supply. The defect may be covered by a variety of means but, if available, a latissimus dorsi myocutaneous flap will provide not only skin cover but also an excellent new blood supply to facilitate healing.

Fibrous disease of the breast

This is a rarely recognized clinical entity without a clear pathological basis. In this way it resembles painful nodularity and indeed parallels this condition in a number of ways. It is a reflection of exaggerated normal physiological processes proceeding to excess, in this case the involutional replacement of lobules by dense fibrous tissue (see Chs 1 and 4). This proceeds to an excessive degree in one area of the breast, presenting clinically as a mass, yet the pathological changes are no different from those occurring during involution in a clinically inconsequential breast.

The clearest description is that of Haagensen[9] and we have a small parallel experience of this as a clinical entity. It is uncommon in Haagensen's experience, one case for every 10 carcinomas. We recognize it considerably less commonly. All but a few of Haagensen's patients were premenopausal, although ranging in age from 24 to 72 (average 42). Our experience is mainly of patients in the fifth and sixth decades. It is difficult to explain its occurrence in the young patients, yet involutional changes are normally evident by the age of 35 and can sometimes occur earlier. One can only speculate that such changes occur earlier than usual in a particular part of the breast,

perhaps a further putative example of local idiosyncratic end-organ response to hormonal stimulation, which may ultimately prove to be the cause of much obscure breast disease.

Haagensen described marked lymphocytic infiltration of the mammary lobule associated with the lobular sclerosis and atrophy. More recently, Schwartz and Strauchen highlighted this feature, categorized the lymphocytes as predominantly B cells, and suggested this might be an autoimmune disease of the breast analogous to that seen in the thyroid and salivary glands.[45]

It presents as a painless, well-defined mass but without a clear edge; it merges into surrounding breast tissue. It is usually in the upper, outer quadrant and firm rather than hard. This consistency (there is no suggestion of cragginess at all) does not raise an expectation of cancer in an experienced examiner. The modest degree of fixity to the breast tissue and the absence of skin retraction also help in the differentiation. Aspiration is possible, but an attempt at Trucut needle biopsy produces a characteristic result – bending of the cutting obturator, although the newer spring-loaded needles may do better. If resected, the tissue is dense white with an abnormally tough consistency, in fact, exactly the finding in involutional nodularity but to a more marked degree. Like this condition, it is diffuse, merging gradually with surrounding breast tissue. Hence, excision, if carried out, must be based on preoperative palpatory assessment of the extent of disease and not on the macroscopic appearance of the breast tissue. Ignoring this will lead to a subcutaneous mastectomy.

The clinical management of this condition raises a problem, for clearly it is best if excision can be avoided. Our approach is to leave the condition if investigation convincingly excludes malignancy, as is often the case in the older patient. Where malignancy cannot be excluded, biopsy must be carried out, and the decision between incisional and excisional biopsy is made according to individual circumstances.

Fibromatosis (desmoid tumour)

Fibromatosis of the breast needs to be considered in the differential diagnosis of fibrous disease. Rosen and Ernsberger[46] collected 22 cases. The condition is analogous to desmoid tumour of the abdominal wall and, like that condition, can be seen in association with colonic polyps in cases of Gardner's syndrome, although this is unusual. The disease process is much more extensive than in fibrous disease and fixes the breast to underlying tissues, such as the pectoral muscle. It can be recognized on mammography[47] but the stellate picture seen can also resemble that of cancer.

A useful study is that of Wargotz et al.[48] who describe the clinical and pathological findings of 28 examples of fibromatosis of the breast not involving the deep fascia or chest wall. This condition can occur in all age groups. Patients often give a history of surgery or trauma at the site. Five of the 20 lesions treated by local excision recurred, usually within a few months but in one case after 6 years. Rosen and Ernsberger[46] had a similar recurrence rate in their patients. The lesions that recurred had been inadequately excised initially because surgical margins showed fibromatosis. Histological features such as cellularity, atypia and mitotic figures did not help in predicting recurrence. Wide local excision appeared to have been adequate in the majority of patients, stressing the importance of documentation of free tissue margins. Although abdominal desmoid tumours sometimes express hormone receptors, paradoxically this did not seem to occur in 33 tumours arising in the breast reported by Devouassoux-Shisheboran et al.[49]

We have seen two cases of bilateral asynchronous fibromatosis in young women below 20 years of age which required mastectomy, including an emergency mastectomy for fungation (see Fig. 17.7).

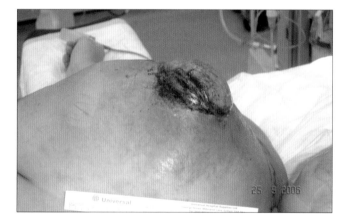

Fig. 17.7 Preoperative view of a huge fibromatosis of the right breast with fungation requiring emergency mastectomy. The tumour weighted over 2.5 kg. Patient's head is to the right of the picture.

Nodular fasciitis

This may occur in the breast as a primary lesion, when it will behave in the same way as those in the more commonly situated soft tissue locations. It is typically a small lesion with a history of rapid growth over a few weeks, important because it may simulate malignancy, although prolonged follow-up has demonstrated it to be benign. Cases have been reported of spontaneous resolution.[50]

Diabetic mastopathy

This condition was first described as recently as 1984 by Soler and Khardori as a variant of fibrosis in the breast associated with autoimmune thyroiditis and arthropathy of the hands.[51] Their incidence was 13% in patients with insulin-dependent diabetes mellitus (IDDM), but overall it constitutes less than 1% of all benign breast disorders. The palpable mass is reminiscent of cancer but awareness of this condition and the criteria required for its diagnosis should prevent the unnecessary surgery that has been performed in the past. The criteria suggested for making the diagnosis are: early onset, longstanding (usually >10 years), insulin-dependent diabetes in a premenopausal patient.[52] There is usually a hard, painless, irregular discrete mobile mass, usually multiple and often bilateral (synchronous or metachronous) but sometimes solitary. The lesions are markedly resistant to fine needle aspiration (FNA) because of the dense fibrous tissue; a specimen can be obtained in only 50%, but cells obtained will be benign.

The mass may be found clinically or on mammogram; the latter shows dense glandular tissue, and there is marked acoustic shadowing on ultrasound.

If all the above criteria are met, it is now suggested that the condition can be managed conservatively to prevent multiple and repeated biopsies.

Formal histology shows dense, keloid-like fibrosis, B-lymphocytic infiltrates around ducts and lobules, lymphocytic vasculitis and epithelioid fibroblasts in the stroma. Perivascular lymphocytes may be confused with lobular carcinoma or lymphoma.

The relationship of diabetes to lymphocytic lobulitis has been carefully evaluated by Kudva et al.[53] who found a clear relationship to type I diabetes and a correlation with retinitis and neuropathy but found no correlation with subsequent malignancy. Interestingly, they also found a weak correlation with autoimmune thyroiditis. Tomaszewski et al.[54] studied eight patients and compared them with short-term insulin-diabetic patients with 'fibrosis and chronic mastitis'. They described cells, which they designated 'epithelioid fibroblasts', that did not appear in other situations. These cells were found in a keloid-like matrix and were accompanied by a B-cell lymphocytic infiltration around the lobules and ductules. They concluded that diabetic mastopathy may be an immune reaction to abnormal matrix. When lymphocytic mastitis occurs in non-IDDM patients, it shows a more heterogeneous pattern with less inflammation and fibrosis.

In males, the condition simulates gynaecomastia.

Idiopathic granulomatous mastitis (non-specific granulomatous disease)

Granulomatous mastitis is a diagnosis of exclusion. A histological appearance of an inflammatory process with granuloma formation may be seen with a number of specific conditions, infections such as TB, leprosy and fungi; with systemic granulomatous diseases such as sarcoid; and as a reaction to lipid material, as occurs with fat necrosis and duct ectasia/periductal mastitis (DE/PDM). It has also been reported in association with vaccination. Al-Suliman et al.[55] reviewed the histology of all patients diagnosed with granulomatous disease and found 14 with evidence sufficient to allow the diagnosis of vaccination granuloma. In 8 of these there was a clear history of tetanus immunization. The histological diagnosis was supported by the demonstration of aluminium in the sections.

In 1972, Kessler and Wolloch described a granulomatous condition of the breast which appeared to be unassociated with any infective process or specific granulomatous disease.[56] Fletcher et al.[57] reported a further seven cases and gave a description of the clinical features and histology. The condition was seen in young parous women within 6 years of the last pregnancy and presented as a painful, peripheral mass that could simulate malignancy. Axillary lymphadenopathy may be found. Histologically, a granulomatous inflammation closely related to the lobules was seen. They speculated on the aetiology, and came down in favour of an immunological process analogous to autoimmune thyroiditis. A report of nine cases[58] confirmed the above features, and confirmed management problems reported

in other series with a protracted course after excision, and a high incidence of wound infection, delayed healing and recurrence.

Is the condition related to DE/PDM? Most authors (e.g. Going et al.[58]) admit an overlap between this condition and PDM, but still believe granulomatous mastitis to be a specific entity, usually stating that PDM has been excluded 'on clinical and histological grounds'. What constitutes these grounds is not spelt out, but appears to be the peripheral location of the mass, the tendency to persistence and recurrence, and the perilobular location of the inflammation. See Figure 17.8.

Going et al.[58] specifically addressed this question, comparing nine cases of granulomatous mastitis with 10 cases of DE/PDM. In most respects the cases were identical: all the DE/PDM cases were granulomatous in the sense that histological granulomas were present. The only two differences were age – the DE patients were older – and

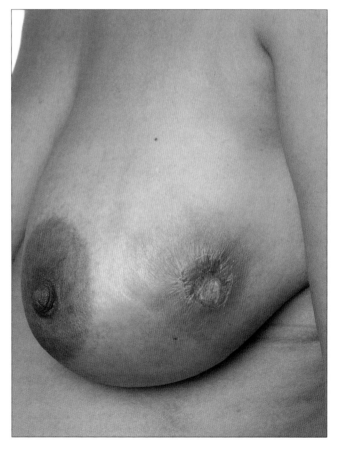

Fig. 17.8 A putative case of granulomatous mastitis. Pathology shared florid granuloma formation but no underlying cause could be identified.

histological location of inflammation – predominantly perilobular rather than periductal. The first difference must be due to selection, and while the 'secretory disease' aspect of DE is seen in older patients, the periareolar inflammation is seen over a wide age range. The perilobular distribution of the inflammation is encompassed by the broader spectrum of the DE/PDM complex that we have always put forward on the basis of our experience. It would appear that none of these patients had the surgical procedure that we recommend, and which has been successful in our practice (see Ch. 11). Tse et al.[59] reported a series of 23 cases of idiopathic granulomatous mastitis. Four (15%) showed evidence of associated duct ectasia. Interestingly, 19 cases were subjected to polymerase chain reaction (PCR) for tuberculosis and one of these was positive, thus raising the possibility of occult tuberculous infection. They consider that granulomatous mastitis is a heterogeneous group of diseases.

Another paper gives further evidence of confusion, where it is believed that granulomatous mastitis can be diagnosed cytologically, without consideration of the cytological similarities of PDM.[60] In fact, this author describes duct dilatation with central suppuration in the confirmatory histology. We have seen patients with a clinical and histological picture identical to that described above which recurred after local excision but resolved completely and permanently when re-excised in continuity with the central (but clinically silent) ectatic ducts. There is an erroneous belief that PDM is only found in a juxta-areolar position, whereas it can extend from the nipple to the periphery of the breast segment, as described in Chapter 11.

Azzopardi[32] described the centrifugal progression of this condition within a segment, and also pointed out that as the process extends, the more central ducts may lose their obvious ectasia by a process of sclerosis. He made the interesting observation: 'Duct ectasia is the prime example of a truly segmental disease.'

With a condition as rare as this it is not possible to be dogmatic regarding all cases. Hence, we cannot claim that all non-specific granulomatous mastitis is unrecognized peripheral PDM, but we believe this to be the case sufficiently frequently that the mass should be locally excised in continuity with a central duct excision under appropriate antibiotic control, before patients are put on prolonged high-dose steroid medication, or subjected to ever wider surgical excision because of repeated recurrence. In the past, some cases of PDM were misdiagnosed as

tuberculosis. Now some are being misdiagnosed as 'idiopathic granulomatous mastitis'.

Treatment

In a condition that is probably a common response to a wide range of underlying conditions it seems unlikely that all will behave in the same way and require the same treatment. In the past, treatment with high-dose steroids has been advocated.[60] A more conservative approach should be considered in light of the results reported by Lai et al.[61] In a series of nine cases, one underwent a local excision with no recurrence. The remaining eight had no specific treatment. In four, the lesion regressed and in the remainder it remained static. We advocate an expectant approach after core needle biopsy diagnosis, using local excision if the lesion continues to be symptomatic and reserving steroids for those with recurrent disease.

Sarcoid

Sarcoid is rarely recorded in the breast. Its importance lies not in the disease itself but because, like many other unusual conditions in the breast, it mimics carcinoma in its presentation. Haagensen[9] documents three cases from the literature, two from the UK and one from Denmark, and mentions two further cases, one his own and another from Australia. Ojeda et al.[62] reviewed the literature and found 45 case reports between 1921 and 1997. The mammographic, ultrasound and MRI findings were reviewed in 1997.[63]

Amyloid

Amyloid deposits, mimicking the clinical presentation of cancer, have been recorded on about 14 occasions.[64] The cases usually present with a lump that clinically and radiologically appears to be a carcinoma. Extensive amyloid deposits may be found elsewhere and usually antedate the breast lesion. The amyloid deposits are more often of the kappa than the lambda light chain.[65] We have seen a case in which an isolated deposit of amyloid adjacent to the scar mimicked a local recurrence of carcinoma following mastectomy where there was no evidence of systemic amyloid.

Blood vessels

Vasculitis

It is not surprising that multifocal arteritis should occasionally afflict the breast, but it is perhaps surprising that it seems to be such a rare occurrence. The clinical manifestations mimic carcinoma, which is a particular problem if the breast is the first site of disease to present. Giant cell arteritis,[66] polyarteritis nodosa[67,68] and Wegener's granulomatosis[69] have all been reported, but even together there are less than 20 cases reported in the literature.

Gateley and Foster[70] reported two cases of pyoderma gangrenosum. In one case the diagnosis was straightforward because the patient had a known underlying disease which predisposed to pyoderma gangrenosum. In the second case, with no known predisposing cause, diagnosis was delayed and artefactual disease was considered during a prolonged period of failed wound healing. Considerable deformity remained after healing had been induced by steroid therapy. The histological features are non-specific, making clinical consideration of the diagnosis important. The marked degree of pain experienced, often apparently out of proportion to the appearance, should raise the possibility of pyoderma. Steroids are often effective if given in high dosage, reducing rapidly as the symptoms come under control. Selva et al.[71] described a case in which the only evidence of systemic disease was the presence of lupus anticoagulant.

Haemangioma

Clinically significant haemangiomas of the breast are rare. Both capillary and cavernous haemangiomas have been reported.[72] One large cavernous haemangioma appears to have been related to hormone replacement therapy.[73] Most are incidental, perilobular structures seen only on histology in biopsies for unrelated conditions.

Atherosclerosis and aneurysm

Artherosclerotic changes are seen as incidental findings on mammograms. Kemmeren et al.[74] reviewed 12 239 women in a mammographic screening programme. Nine per cent had evidence of arterial calcification which was associated with an increased risk of cardiovascular death of 40%. The risks were even greater in diabetic patients and the calcification was also more common in such patients. These authors conclude that mammographically demonstrated arterial calcification is an independent prognostic variable for heart disease (Fig. 17.9). This conclusion is supported by a study from Cambridge in which vascular calcification was a predictor for coronary disease that did not correlate with other predictive factors for heart disease.[75] A single case of an aneurysm of a vessel within the breast has been reported.[76] The diagnosis was made by auscultation and confirmed by Doppler flowmetry of the lump. It was successfully treated by local excision. Davies and Kulke[77] have drawn attention to the phenomenon of false aneurysms associated with FNA or core biopsy of complex sclerosing lesions. Such lesions appear to be confined to lesions over 10 mm in diameter. Dixon and Enion[78] have reviewed the literature regarding pseudoaneurysm following core needle biopsy.

Mondor's disease

Superficial thrombophlebitis over an area of the breast was described several times before Mondor's paper in 1939;[79] the earliest appears to be that of Fagge in 1869,[80] but Mondor's name is now firmly attached to the condition. It is one of those rather rare conditions that every doctor has heard about as a medical student, and this carries two risks. The rarity of the condition may lead to

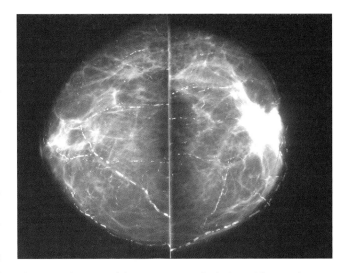

Fig. 17.9 Craniocaudal mammogram displaying widespread arterial calcification bilaterally.

unnecessary biopsy to avoid missing cancer or in the desire to recognize a condition long known about but never encountered; alternatively, an atypical cancer may be described as Mondor's disease. The latter is much the more serious error, for cancer is common but Mondor's disease is rare. Haagensen[9] reported that one in 125 consultations were for Mondor's disease, although our experience in Cardiff, UK, is that it is much less frequent: we have seen five cases in 5 years with an annual referral rate of about 3500 patients.

Clinical features

Females are affected considerably more commonly than males.[81] The patient develops a dull aching pain over the breast or hypochondrium and notices a tender, elongated mass in the region (Fig. 17.10).

Palpation reveals a tender narrow cord just below the skin. This is the thrombosed vein attached to the skin so that elevation of the arm produces a narrow furrow over the vein, accentuated by traction from either end. The furrow is more obvious over the breast. It contracts to a bowstring if the thrombosed vein extends across the submammary fold to the epigastrium. The vein usually affected is the thoraco-epigastric vein which runs from the hypochondrium up across the lateral aspect of the breast to the anterior axillary fold; although Bejanga[81] reported that it occurred more frequently in the lateral thoracic vein.

As with spontaneous thrombophlebitis elsewhere, any vein may be affected; less rare examples are a vein from the

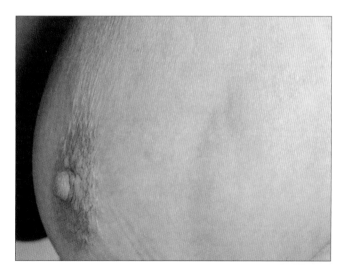

Fig. 17.10 Mondor's disease, with skin retraction simulating dimpling due to cancer.

epigastrium over the lower medial quadrant of the breast and one extending vertically down from the nipple.

The thrombophlebitis follows a similar pattern to that elsewhere. The pain settles over 10 days or so, a process accentuated by rest. The tender cord resolves more slowly, taking from 2 to 12 weeks until finally no evidence remains of the lesion.

An important variant is when a short segment of vein is affected, giving local dimpling which may suggest a cancer. Of greater importance is the fact that a wedge-shaped area of ductal cancer may suggest the diagnosis of Mondor's disease to an inexperienced observer.

The imaging findings have been reviewed by Shetty and Watson[82] who considered the combination of a tubular structure on mammography and a superficial vessel, with or without an intraluminal thrombus and without flow on Doppler imaging diagnostic.

Pathology and pathogenesis

The pathology was well described by Hughes.[83] It shows the typical stages of thrombophlebitis: a thrombosed thickened area with surrounding thrombosis.

Many cases appear to be spontaneous, a situation analogous to thrombophlebitis elsewhere. A variety of aetiological factors have been described. Unusual exercise usually involving the arms above the head is commonest. Direct trauma is of greater importance in males.[84] There also appears to be a trend for the condition to be associated with high parity and large breasts.[85] Operative trauma is well recognized (Fig. 17.11), the condition developing distal to the scar 2 or 3 weeks after biopsy of a benign condition.

Mondor's disease is occasionally the presenting symptom of underlying malignancy although Catania et al.[86] found a cancer incidence of 10.2% in 70 cases. We have seen two patients who had no obvious cancer at initial presentation who represented with breast cancer in the area of the previous phlebitis within 2 years.

Treatment

Provided the clinician is familiar with the condition and the clinical features are classic, the patient may be treated conservatively. If there is the slightest doubt, mammography should be performed. Because of our experience with two patients, we now recommend review with mammography at 1 year.

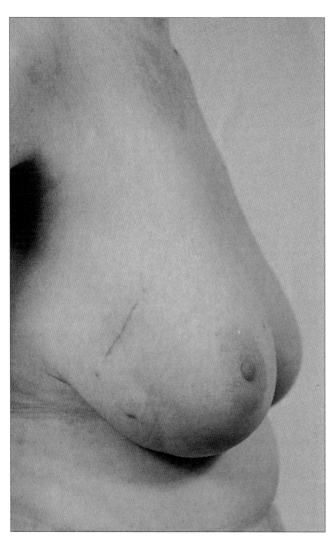

Fig. 17.11 Mondor's disease following excision of a breast mass.

The condition will resolve spontaneously without treatment, but symptomatic relief can be obtained with general measures appropriate to the management of thrombophlebitis: rest to the arm and support for the breast. Simple analgesics are inadequate; phenylbutazone is effective. Anticoagulants are not necessary.

Some authors have recommended introducing active approaches to management. Abramson[85] recommended disruption of the cord by forcible distraction from the ends. Millar[87] divided the cords under local anaesthesia and found symptoms relieved immediately. We have no experience of such methods but they are worth consideration in particularly painful cases.

Infarction

The breast may occasionally undergo infarction, an event first described in 1894.[88] An important review of this subject is that of Robitaille et al.,[89] who divide such events into those that mimic carcinoma and those that do not. Infarction of fibroadenoma has been previously described in Chapter 7, and infarction of duct papilloma in Chapter 13.

Spontaneous mammary infarction is a rare event usually occurring in pregnant (third trimester) or lactating women.[90] The clinical finding is of a tender nodule in the breast rather suspicious of lactational cancer, a diagnosis which may appear to be confirmed on frozen section.[32] It is treated by local excision, with milk fistula a possible complication.

When infarcts occur in the elderly, cancer is even more likely to be diagnosed. Infarcts have also been reported in association with diabetes and carbon monoxide poisoning. Rashid et al.[91] have reported a case of breast infarction following harvest of the internal thoracic artery. The subsequent histology of the breast showed changes consistent with calciphylaxis.

Haemorrhagic necrosis complicating anticoagulant therapy

Since the first report by Flood et al.[92] in 1943, there has been a steady flow of papers reporting single cases of this syndrome. It may occur with any of the oral anticoagulants of the coumarin group. The sequence of events is obscure. It usually starts within a few days of commencing therapy, as a markedly painful erythematous patch with petechiae, soon turning black (sometimes within hours) with a surrounding erythematous blush. The final picture is of aseptic ischaemic necrosis with local venous and arterial thrombosis of small and medium-sized vessels, and evidence of vasculitis. The sharply demarcated necrosis is established by 48 hours, and if untreated, separates around 2 weeks later. Extensive calcification may later develop in the breast, giving a dramatic mammogram.

Haematological consultation is urgent, both in relation to stopping coumarin therapy and replacing it with heparin to maintain control of the underlying thrombotic condition, and also because it has been suggested that prompt administration of heparin may lessen the amount of necrosis. Recently, an association with protein C or protein S deficiency has been recognized.[93]

Treatment is by debridement of the affected tissue; if the subsequent cosmetic defect is severe, secondary plastic surgery may be indicated if the underlying condition permits.

Spontaneous haematoma

Although concealed trauma or factitial disease cannot be excluded with certainty, there is no reason to question a patient's claim that a haematoma has appeared spontaneously (Fig. 17.12).

Our cases have been followed by slow but uneventful resolution. Mammography is always performed to exclude an underlying carcinoma.

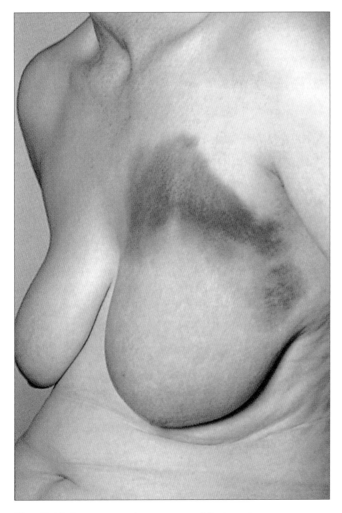

Fig. 17.12 Spontaneous haematoma of the breast; no cause found.

Skin-related conditions

Lesions arising in the skin cause concern to patients but usually do not cause any serious difficulty in distinguishing them from lesions deep in the breast. Sebaceous cysts are not infrequently encountered. Perhaps more significant is the inclusion dermoid cyst that may follow core needle biopsy and may be confused with squamous metaplasia of either benign or malignant breast lesions.[94]

Hidradenitis suppurativa of the breast

Apocrine sweat glands are found predominantly in the axilla and inguinoperineal regions but are described in a number of other sites. In relation to the breast, they are described in the areola and in the chest wall, particularly in the inter- and inframammary folds.[95] Hidradenitis has been described as involving the breast, in most series only one or two cases, but in a series from the Mayo Clinic it was reported in 8% of 177 women with the disease.[96] We have not been able to find a paper which details the site of the disease, but most papers suggest it is the areola. Our experience is different. We have seen it mainly in the inter- and inframammary folds, usually in obese patients. In an experience of over 150 patients requiring surgery for hidradenitis, and many more with mild disease, we have not seen a single case involving the areola. We suspect that the reported cases reflect misdiagnosis of recurrent subareolar abscesses (see Ch. 11) because these reports arose at a time when this condition was not widely recognized.

Patients with extensive hidradenitis elsewhere will sometimes have an individual or a few lesions scattered on the lower part of the breast (Fig. 17.13).

However, severe and extensive disease in the inter- and particularly the inframammary folds is well described in obese patients, and especially in those who are also cigarette smokers. These patients often have scattered lesions on the lower half of the breast, although it is sometimes difficult to differentiate these from cystic acne; the two conditions frequently coexist. The distribution of the true hidradenitis lesions suggests that pressure is an aetiological factor. The worst lesions are seen under the strap of the brassiere and on the skin surfaces where the undersurface of the breast and the chest wall are in contact and rub together.

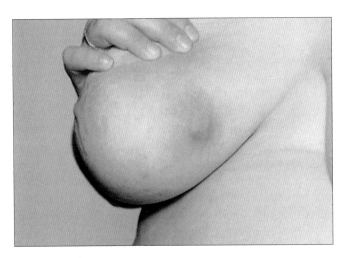

Fig. 17.13 Localized lesion of hidradenitis suppurativa of the breast, in a patient with the disease elsewhere.

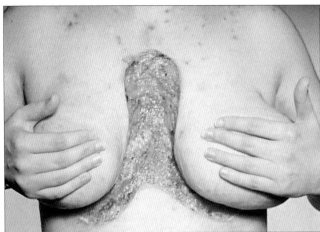

Fig. 17.15 Radical excision of extensive hidradenitis of the inter- and inframammary fold.

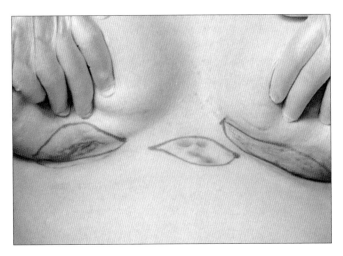

Fig. 17.14 Local clusters of lesions are best treated by local excision, followed by conservative therapy for recurrence.

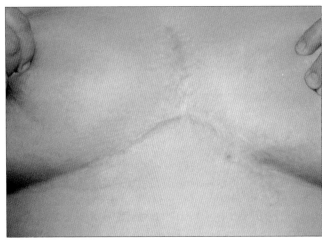

Fig. 17.16 The wound was allowed to heal by granulation and gave a satisfactory scar.

Treatment is unsatisfactory, in contrast to surgical excision of hidradenitis in other sites.[97] Patients are urged to lose weight and cease smoking, but in our experience are rarely willing to act on such advice. We recommend conservative excision for local areas of disease, recognizing that recurrence is very likely (Figs 17.14–17.17).

Since local pressure and sweating play a role in hidradenitis, it is possible that reduction mammoplasty might help in those who are particularly obese and have pendulous breasts. Reduction mammoplasty can be tailored to excise the area of skin in the inframammary fold most commonly involved by hidradenitis, at the same time as reducing the effects of obesity. We have used this approach with satisfactory results.[98] Some patients with recurrent disease benefit from conservative therapy with an

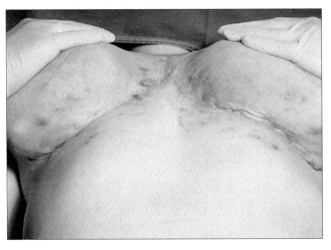

Fig. 17.17 Same patient as Figure 17.16. Within 2 years there were multiple recurrent lesions of hidradenitis.

antiandrogen/oestrogen combination, such as cyproterone acetate and ethinyloestradiol, as used for severe acne. There are no reports as yet of properly controlled trials of this combination in hidradenitis with adequate follow-up. In our experience, about half the patients benefit but are more likely to do so if they have mild disease, or the worst affected areas are first excised surgically.

Tumours of nerve origin

Such tumours are identical to those occurring elsewhere. They are reported surprisingly infrequently.[99]

Granular cell tumour (myoblastoma)

This rare tumour occurs in both men and women, and approximately 6% are found over or in the breast. The granules giving its name are believed to be intracellular myelin, and it is considered most likely that the tumour is of Schwann cell origin. Adeniran et al.[100] reported on 17 cases and reviewed the literature.

Clinically and mammographically it can mimic malignancy very closely, in fact more so than any other benign condition. It occurs as a solitary (usually), progressively growing lump, hard and painless, fixed to the skin, or in the case of the breast, the underlying pectoral fascia. Size can vary from very small to 10 cm in diameter, and larger ones can ulcerate, while occasionally adjacent similar nodules may also suggest malignancy, in spite of the young age of the patient. The fixity is due to gross fibrosis and an infiltrative margin, both features also seen on histology. Pseudo-epitheliomatous hyperplasia of the overlying skin can further cloud the clinical picture.

Diagnosis is difficult on cytology so biopsy is preferred; again, the hard, white cut surface can suggest malignancy. The histology is the same as with those tumours occurring more commonly in the skin. Immunocytochemistry may be helpful; the cells stain positive for S100, negative for cytokeratin, epithelial membrane antigen and myoglobin. Complete local excision is necessary to avoid local recurrence, taking any attached fascia, and confirming clearance margins.

Artefactual disease of the breast

Artefactual or factitial disorders are ones which are created by the patient, often through complicated and repetitive actions. All reviews in the literature refer only to hospitalized patients. It is impossible for us to estimate the number of patients who have artefactual illnesses who are never suspected or who are treated as out-patients. Such disorders involving the female breast have only rarely been reported even though recognized by Hippocrates: 'It is a sign of madness when blood congeals on a woman's nipples.'[101] Sampson[102] described a case of dermatitis artefacta in which the woman had her left nipple excised for intermittent profuse bleeding. One month later she had a large tender hard mass above the incision which was found to be a pocket containing multiple small stones, gravel and sand.

General reviews of dermatitis artefacta sometimes include cases affecting the nipple (Figs 17.18 and 17.19).[103-105] We have reported three patients with this condition[106] and have seen others since. One complained of intermittent bleeding from her right nipple which eventually led to simple mastectomy. She was then referred to us because of bleeding which soon started from the opposite breast (Fig. 17.20).

A second case was one of persistent eczema of the nipple and a third was a woman who had recurrent breast abscesses resistant to all the standard methods of treatment for DE and PDM (Fig. 17.21).

The organisms grown were faecal in nature, suggesting deliberate infection. After a number of years, a period in hospital with occlusion of the breast led to healing, only to be followed after discharge by a similar problem appearing on the opposite side. The patient was dis-

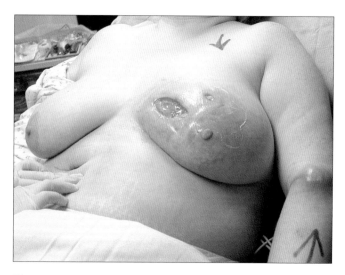

Fig. 17.18 Dermatitis artefacta. Several breast abscesses, epigastric scar and left arm lesion.

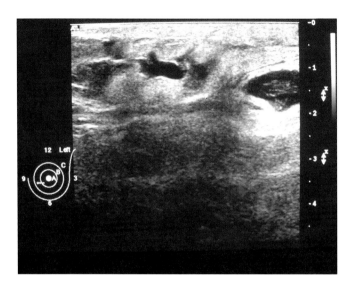

Fig. 17.19 Dermatitis artefacta. Multiple abscess foci, not interconnecting.

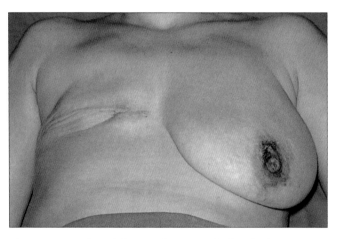

Fig. 17.20 Artefactual disease. The patient had multiple operations on the right breast for recurrent severe bleeding from the right nipple, culminating in a simple mastectomy. The condition promptly occurred on the left side and has all the hallmarks of artefactual injury.

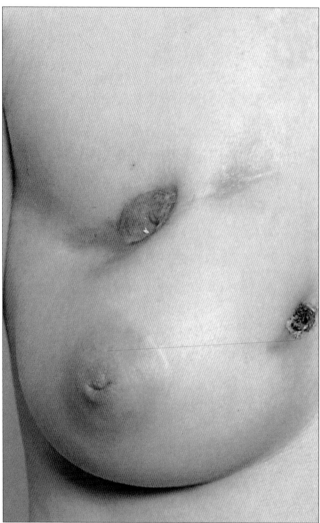

Fig. 17.21 Artefactual disease. This nursing assistant had multiple operations for recurrent persistent sepsis in the right breast. Typical bowel organisms were grown from the discharge.

charged with the advice that no active therapy would be effective, but that the lesions would eventually heal. Her local physician confirmed that this occurred, with no further problem during the following 5 years.

Such patients have usually had many investigations and operations before the nature of the underlying mechanism is recognized. Even so, establishing the diagnosis may be difficult and time consuming. Although the self-induced nature of the problem may be suspected, it is usually difficult to prove. The disorders may extend over a long period of time, may be recurrent and may result in long-term disability or cosmetic problems from tissue destruction; they are occasionally life threatening. The patients are usually young to middle-aged women, often in medically related employment.[104] They are often pleasant and cooperative and do not appear to be bizarre or psychologically disturbed, but they tend to be immature and to have problems with their sexuality. A husband who appears to be unusually (excessively) concerned may hide underlying marital stress, but this is hardly specific to artefactual disease.

Sometimes, as in two of our cases, patients will actively and without appropriate effect seek mastectomy. This should alert the clinician to the possibility of artefactual disease. The diagnosis is difficult to establish but artefactual disease should be considered where the clinical situation does not conform to common appearances or pathological processes. Unusual infections need to be considered such as tuberculosis, fungal infection or chronic subareolar abscess. A number of cases where self-injury has been suspected have cleared satisfactorily when appropriate attention was paid to this latter diagnosis.

It is difficult to give specific recommendations regarding treatment. Psychiatric consultation is often helpful in elucidating a personality disorder consistent with a diagnosis of artefactual breast disease. Direct confrontation of the patient is probably not worth while but may be considered in association with psychiatric help. These problems are difficult to manage and may extend over a long period of time. They tend to resolve if the patient is strongly reassured and attention withdrawn. Unnecessary and repetitive surgery must be avoided.

In the longer term, most factitious disorders are self-limiting and have an excellent prognosis.[107]

Foreign bodies

Occasionally, foreign bodies are found in the breast. Often they are incidental findings on mammography; less commonly they are responsible for ongoing infective episodes. Consideration has to be given to the possibility of non-accidental injury and deliberate introduction of such materials, a specific type of factitious disease as described above.

Iatrogenic materials such as catheters, localization wires and sponges have all been described and have been reviewed by Barzilai et al.[108] The advent of MRI scanning of the breast has revealed that small metal fragments from biopsy needles cause considerable artefacts. Leakage of CSF from abdomino-ventricular shunts has been described as a cause of breast cysts that contain CSF.[109]

A retained surgical swab (also known as 'gossypiboma') is extremely rare following breast surgery with only two cases reported in the English literature. We were recently referred a young woman who detected a breast mass following bilateral breast augmentation using silicone gel implants in a private clinic outside the UK. Clinical examination revealed a mass in the upper outer quadrant adjacent to the implant. It was difficult to establish the diagnosis preoperatively, but, at surgery a retained surgical swab was revealed to be the cause of this mass (Fig.

17.22). We are not aware of any other similar cases in the setting of breast augmentation surgery.

Mammalithiasis

In his postmortem series, Sandison[11] noted four examples (0.5%) of laminated concretions in the breast which were either intramammary or intraductal. The nature of this rare condition is obscure, and we have not seen an example.

Phantom breast syndrome

The presence of sensations related to a removed breast – phantom breast – has long been recognized, although it has not received nearly so much attention as the similar condition after limb amputation. About 39% of postmastectomy women experience this symptom which is more common in those who had previous breast pain. One study looked at 97 patients who had undergone mastectomy, and found some phantom sensations in 29, with

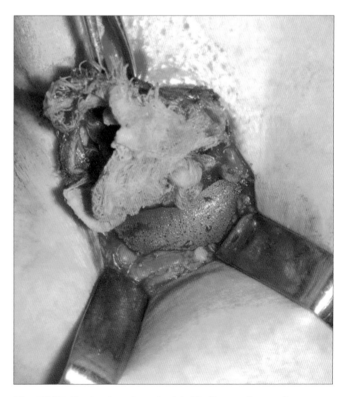

Fig. 17.22 Retained swab embedded in fibrous tissue adjacent to implant (lower part of figure) used for augmentation of the breast.

symptoms persisting more than 4 years in about half. The sensation was sited in the nipple in half, with total breast involvement in only four. The intensity was usually mild (the characteristics being itching, throbbing, paraesthesia or pressure), being described as a pain in only three; the rest described the sensation as no more than discomfort.[110] Kudel et al. found that patients with phantom breast were likely to have other types of postmastectomy pain syndromes.[111]

Mammary mucocele-like lesion

This lesion (MML), which is analogous to similar lesions in the minor salivary glands, consists of a mass of cystic spaces filled with mucin and requires differentiation from a mucinous carcinoma. It also needs differentiation from cystic hypersecretory hyperplasia. Rosen described six cases in 1986,[112] and at that time they were considered always to be benign. It is now recognized that a wider spectrum occurs, with malignant forms being perhaps as common as the benign.[113] Recently, cases have been reported associated with atypical ductal hyperplasia.[114]

In its benign form, the lesion consists of a mass of mucus-containing cysts, 1–4 cm in diameter. It occurs across a wide age group, and can simulate cancer clinically and radiologically. The cystic spaces are lined by benign epithelium with some focal hyperplasia, so that diagnosis can be difficult on cytology or frozen section, and is best made on paraffin section.

Complete local excision is adequate for the benign lesions, and at present there is no evidence that the malignant ones should be treated differently from other cancers.

Breast tumour of pregnancy (lactating adenoma)

This uncommon tumour is customarily called lactating adenoma, in spite of the fact that it is usually discovered during pregnancy, rather than lactation. Equally, there is no good evidence that it is an adenoma, in the tumour sense. Hence, James et al. make a plea that it be called 'breast tumour of pregnancy'.[115]

Patients usually present with a 2–4-cm mass in the second or third trimester, and are typically young, in the third decade. On histology, the mass shows the normal constituents of the pregnant breast, but varies in the degree of 'pregnant' change, and is out of step with the stage of pregnancy.

Lactating adenoma can be diagnosed on aspiration cytology or core biopsy. Conservative management is advocated because spontaneous resolution is likely.[116]

Collagenous spherulosis of the breast

This is a histological finding in breast biopsies with intraluminal clusters of eosinophilic spherules within areas of benign epithelial hyperplasia.[117] The condition is mainly of interest to histopathologists, because it may lead to a mistaken diagnosis of malignancy. The histological details are given in the paper cited above.

Gynaecomastia-like lesions in women

This rare condition has been reported in eight of 3951 surgical breast biopsies in two reported series.[118–119] It presents as a mass lesion in the breast and may be associated with a non-specific mammographic density. Histologically, it appears as the florid form of gynaecomastia with ductal hyperplasia and periductal stromal fibrosis or oedema. Typically, it occurs in the fourth decade. No particular association with hormonal abnormalities or medication has been identified in the reported cases. The finding of other benign breast change in adjacent breast tissue suggests that this condition is likely to be a manifestation of ANDI.

REFERENCES

1. Hoda SA & Rosen PP. Observations on the pathologic diagnosis of selected unusual lesions in needle core biopsies of breast. *Breast Journal* 2004; **10**: 522–527.

2. Jansen DA, Stoetzel R & Leveque JE. Premenarchal athletic injury to the breast bud as the cause for asymmetry: prevention and treatment. *Breast Journal* 2002; **8**: 108–111.

3. Burvin R, Robinpour M, Milo Y et al. Female breast burns: conservative treatment with a reconstructive aim. *Israel Journal of Medical Sciences* 1996; **32**: 1297–1301.

4. McCauley RL, Beraja V, Rutan RL et al. Longitudinal assessment of breast development in adolescent female patients with burns involving the nipple–areolar complex. *Plastic and Reconstruction Surgery* 1989; **83**: 676–680.

5. MacLennan SE, Wells MD, Neale HW. Reconstruction of the burned breast. *Clinical Plastic Surgery* 2000; **27**: 113–119.

6. Foley P, Jeeves A, Davey RB et al. Breast burns are not benign: long-term outcomes of burns to the breast in pre-pubertal girls. *Burns* 2008; **34**: 412–417.

7. Dawes RFH, Smallwood JA & Taylor I. Seat belt injury to the female breast. *British Journal of Surgery* 1986; **73**: 106–107.

8. Dipiro DJ, Meyer JE, Frenna TH et al. Seat belt injuries of the breast. Findings on mammography and sonography. *American Journal of Roentgenology* 1995; **164**: 317–332.

9. Haagensen CD. *Disease of the Breast*, 3rd edn. Philadelphia: WB Saunders; 1986.

10. Lee BJ & Adair FE. Traumatic fat necrosis of the female breast and its differentiation from carcinoma. *Annals of Surgery* 1920; **37**: 189.

11. Sandison AT. An autopsy study of the human breast. *National Cancer Institute Monograph No. 8*, US Dept Health, Education and Welfare, 1962.

12. Mandrekas AD, Assimakoloulos GI, Mastorakos DP et al. Fat necrosis following breast reduction. *British Journal of Plastic Surgery* 1994; **47**: 560–562.

13. Patel RT, Webster DJT, Mansel RE et al. Is immediate reconstruction safe in the long term? *European Journal of Surgical Oncology* 1993; **19**: 372–375.

14. Wazer DE, Lowther D, Boyle T et al. Clinically evident fat necrosis in women treated with high-dose-rate brachytherapy alone for early-stage breast cancer. *International Journal of Radiation, Oncology, Biology and Physiology* 2001; **50**: 107–111.

15. Chaudary MM, Girling A, Girling S et al. New lumps in the breast following conservation treatment for early breast cancer. *Breast Cancer Research and Treatment* 1988; **11**: 51–58.

16. Baillie M & Mok PM. Fat necrosis in the breast: review of the mammographic and ultrasound features, and a strategy for management. *Australasian Radiology* 2004; **48**: 288–295.

17. Pullyblank AM, Davies JD, Basten J et al. Fat necrosis of the female breast – Hadfield re-visited. *Breast* 2001; **10**: 388–391.

18. Bilgen IG, Ustun EE & Memis A. Fat necrosis of the breast: clinical, mammographic and sonographic features. *European Journal of Radiology* 2001; **39**: 92–99.

19. Alagaratnam TT & Ong GB. Paraffinoma of the breast. *Journal of the Royal College of Surgeons of Edinburgh* 1983; **28**: 260–263.

20. Ho WS, Chan AC & Law BK. Management of paraffinoma of the breast: 10 years' experience. *British Journal of Plastic Surgery* 2001; **54**: 232–234.

21. Chen JS, Liu WC, Yang KC et al. Reconstruction with bilateral pedicled TRAM flap for paraffinoma breast. *Plastic and Reconstructive Surgery* 2005; **115**: 96–104.

22. Alagaratnam TT & Ng WF. Paraffinomas of the breast: an oriental curiosity. *Australian and New Zealand Journal of Surgery* 1996; **66**: 138–140.

23. Christensen LH, Breiting VB, Aasted A et al. Long-term effects of polyacrylamide hydrogel on human breast tissue. *Plastic and Reconstructive Surgery* 2003; **111**: 1883–1890.

24. Zhao Y, Qiao Q, Yue Y et al. Clinical and histologic evaluation of a new injectable implant: hydrophilic polyacrylamide gel. *Annals of Plastic Surgery* 2004; **53**: 267–272.

25. Austad ED. Breast implant-related silicone granulomas: the literature and the litigation. *Plastic and Reconstructive Surgery* 2002; **109**: 1724–1730.

26. Brown SL, Silverman BG & Berg WA. Rupture of silicone-gel implants: causes, sequelae and diagnosis. *Lancet* 1997; **350**: 1531–1537.

27. Gardner-Thorpe D, Hirschowitz L & Maddox PR. Mammary hibernoma. *European Journal of Surgical Oncology* 2000; **26**: 430.

28. Mulvany NJ, Silvester AC & Collins JP. Spindle cell lipoma of the breast. *Pathology* 1999; **31**: 288–291.

29. Darling ML, Babagbemi TO, Smith DN et al. Mammographic and sonographic features of angiolipoma of the breast. *Breast Journal* 2000; **6**: 166–170.

30. Pui MH & Movson IJ. Fatty tissue breast lesions. *Clinical Imaging* 2003; **27**: 150–155.

31. Lanng C, Erikson B & Hoffman J. Lipoma of the breast: a diagnostic dilemma. *Breast* 2003; **13**: 408–411.

32. Azzopardi J. *Problems in Breast Pathology*. London: WB Saunders; 1979.

33. Arrigoni MG, Docherty MB & Judd ES. The identification and treatment of mammary hamartoma. *Surgery, Gynecology and Obstetrics* 1971; **133**: 577–582

34. Crothers JG, Butler NF, Fortt RW et al. Fibroadenolipoma of the breast. *British Journal of Radiology* 1985; **58**: 119–120.

35. Park SY, Oh KK, Kim EK et al. Sonographic findings of breast hamartoma: emphasis on compressibility. *Yonsei Medical Journal* 2003; **44**: 847–854.

36. Davies JD, Kulke J & Mumford AD. Hamartomas of the breast – six novel diagnostic features in 3-dimensional thick sections. *Histopathology* 1994; **24**: 161–168.

37. McElligott G & Harrington MG. Heart failure and breast enlargement suggesting cancer. *British Medical Journal* 1986; **292**: 446.

38. Kaufman SA. Nursing home breast. *Archives of Surgery* 1984; **119**: 615.

39. Keller RJ & Hermann G. Unilateral edema simulating inflammatory carcinoma of the breast. *Breast Disease* 1990; **3**: 61–74.

40. Ronka RH, Pamilo MS, von Smitten KA *et al.* Breast lymphedema after breast conserving treatment. *Acta Oncologica* 2004; **43**: 551–557.

41. Mattsson A, Ruden BI, Palmgren J *et al.* Dose- and time-response for breast cancer risk after radiation therapy for benign breast disease. *British Journal of Cancer* 1995; **72**: 1054–1061.

42. Zippel D, Siegelmann-Danieli N, Ayalon S *et al.* Delayed breast cellulitis following breast conserving operation. *European Journal of Surgical Oncology* 2003; **29**: 327–330.

43. Moore GH, Schiller JE & Moore GK. Radiation-induced histopathologic changes of the breast: the effects of time. *American Journal of Surgical Pathology* 2004; **28**: 47–53.

44. Hughes LE. Repair of the chest wall defects after irradiation for breast cancer. *Annals of the Royal College of Surgeons of England* 1976; **58**: 140–143.

45. Schwartz IS & Strauchen JA. Lymphocytic mastopathy. An autoimmune disease of the breast? *American Journal of Clinical Pathology* 1990; **93**: 725–730.

46. Rosen PP & Ernsberger D. Mammary fibrosis. A benign spindle cell tumour with a significant risk for local recurrence. *Cancer* 1989; **63**: 1363–1369.

47. Hermann G & Schwartz IS. Focal fibrous disease of the breast: Mammographic detection of an unappreciated condition. *American Journal of Roentgenology* 1983; **140**: 1245–1246.

48. Wargotz ESM, Norris HJ, Austin RM *et al.* Fibromatosis of the breast. A clinical and pathological study of 28 cases. *American Journal of Surgical Pathology* 1987; **11**: 38–45.

49. Devouassoux-Shisheboran M, Schammel MD, Man YG *et al.* Fibromatosis of the breast: age-correlated morphofunctional features of 33 cases. *Archives of Pathology and Laboratory Medicine* 2000; **124**: 276–280.

50. Brown V & Carty NJ. A case of nodular fasciitis of the breast and review of the literature. *Breast* 2005; **14**: 384–387.

51. Soler NG & Khardori R. Fibrous disease of the breast, thyroiditis, and cheiroarthropathy in type I diabetes mellitus. *Lancet* 1984; **i**: 193–194.

52. Morgan MC, Weaver MG, Crowe JP *et al.* Diabetic mastopathy: a clinicopathologic study in palpable and nonpalpable breast lesions. *Modern Pathology* 1995; **8**: 349–354.

53. Kudva YC, Reynolds CA, O'Brien T *et al.* Mastopathy and diabetes. *Current Diabetic Reports* 2003; **3**: 56–59.

54. Tomaszewski JE, Brooks JS, Hicks D *et al.* Diabetic mastopathy: a distinctive clinicopathological entity. *Human Pathology* 1992; **23**: 780–786.

55. Al-Suliman NN, Grabau DA, Kiaer H *et al.* A tumour in the breast: vaccination granuloma as a differential diagnosis. *European Journal of Surgical Oncology* 1999; **25**: 34–37.

56. Kessler E & Wolloch Y. Granulomatous mastitis: a lesion clinically simulating carcinoma. *American Journal of Clinical Pathology* 1972; **58**: 642–646.

57. Fletcher A, McGrath IM, Riddell RH *et al.* Granulomatous mastitis: a report of seven cases. *Journal of Clinical Pathology* 1982; **35**: 941–945.

58. Going JJ, Anderson TJ, Wilkinson S *et al.* Granulomatous lobular mastitis. *Journal of Clinical Pathology* 1987; **40**: 535–540.

59. Tse GM, Poon CS, Ramachandram K *et al.* Granulomatous mastitis: a clinicopathological review of 26 cases. *Pathology* 2004; **36**: 254–257.

60. Salam IMA, Alhausi MF, Daniel MF *et al.* Diagnosis and treatment of granulomatous mastitis. *British Journal of Surgery* 1995; **82**: 214.

61. Lai EC, Chan WC, Ma TK *et al.* The role of conservative treatment in idiopathic granulomatous mastitis. *Breast Journal* 2005; **11**: 454–456.

62. Ojeda H, Sardi A & Totoonchie A. Sarcoidosis of the breast: implications for the general surgeon. *American Surgeon* 2000; **66**: 1144–1148.

63. Kenzel PP, Hadijuana J, Hosten N *et al.* Boeck sarcoidosis of the breast: mammographic, ultrasound, and MR findings. *Journal of Computer Assisted Tomography* 1997; **21**: 439–441.

64. Deolekar MV, Larsen J & Morris JA. Primary amyloid tumour of the breast: a case report. *Journal of Clinical Pathology* 2002; **55**: 634–635.

65. Rocken C, Kronsbein H, Sletten K *et al.* Amyloidosis of the breast. *Virchows Archives* 2002; **440**: 527–535.

66. Stephenson TJ & Underwood JCE. Giant cell arteritis: an unusual cause of palpable masses in the breast. *British Journal of Surgery* 1986; **73**: 105.

67. McCarthy DJ, Imbrigia J & Hung JK. Vasculitis of the breasts. *Arthritis and Rheumatism* 1968; **11**: 796–801.

68. Ng WF, Chow LT & Lam PW. Localized polyarteritis nodosa of breast – report of two cases and a review of the literature. *Histopathology* 1993; **23**: 535–539.

69. Paterson AG, Fortt RW & Webster DJT. Wegener's granulomatosis. An unusual cause of a breast lump. *Journal of the Royal College of Surgeons of Edinburgh* 1985; **30**: 332–335.

70. Gateley CA & Foster ME. Pyoderma gangrenosum of the breast. *British Journal of Clinical Practice* 1990; **44**: 713–714.

71. Selva A, Ordi J, Roca M *et al.* Pyoderma-gangrenosum-like ulcers associated with lupus anticoagulant. *Dermatology* 1994; **189**: 182–184.

72. Rosen PP, Jozefczyk MA & Boram LH. Vascular tumors of the breast. IV. The venous haemangioma. *American Journal of Surgical Pathology* 1985; **9**: 659–665.

73. Mesurolle B, Wexler M, Halwani F et al. Cavernous hemangioma of the breast: mammographic findings and follow-up in a patient receiving hormone-replacement therapy. *Journal of Clinical Ultrasound* 2003; **31**: 430–436.

74. Kemmeren JM, Beijerinck D, van Noord PA et al. Breast arterial calcifications: association with diabetes mellitus and cardiovascular mortality. *Radiology* 1996; **201**: 75–78.

75. Kataoka M, Warren R, Luben R et al. How predictive is breast arterial calcification of cardiovascular disease and risk factors when found at screening mammography? *American Journal of Roentgenology* 2006; **187**: 73–80.

76. Dehn RB & Lee ECG. Aneurysm presenting as a breast mass. *British Medical Journal* 1986; **292**: 140.

77. Davies JD & Kulke J. Traumatic arterial damage after fine needle aspiration cytology in mammary sclerosing lesions. *Histopathology* 1996; **28**: 65–70.

78. Dixon AM & Enion DS. Pseudoaneurysm of the breast: case study and review of literature. *British Journal of Radiology* 2004; **77**: 694–697.

79. Mondor H. Tronculite sous-cutanee subaigue de la paroi thoracique antero-laterale. *Memoires Academies de Chirurgie* 1939; **65**: 1271.

80. Fagge CH. Remarks on certain cutaneous affections. *Guys Hospital Reports* 1869; **15**: 295–364.

81. Bejanga BI. Mondor's disease: analysis of 30 cases. *Journal of the Royal College of Surgeons of Edinburgh* 1992; **37**: 322–324.

82. Shetty MK & Watson AB. Mondor's disease of the breast: sonographic and mammographic findings. *American Journal of Roentgenology* 2001; **177**: 893–896.

83. Hughes ESR. Sclerosing peri-angiitis of the lateral thoracic wall. *Australian and New Zealand Journal of Surgery* 1952; **22**: 17–24.

84. Oldfield MC. Mondor's disease. A superficial phlebitis of the breast. *Lancet* 1962; **i**: 994–996.

85. Abramson DJ. Mondor's disease and string phlebitis. *Journal of the American Medical Association* 1966; **196**: 1087.

86. Catania S, Zurrida S, Veronesi P et al. Mondor's disease and breast cancer. *Cancer* 1992; **69**: 2267–2270.

87. Millar DM. Treatment of Mondor's disease. *British Journal of Surgery* 1967; **54**: 76–77.

88. Schneck J. A case of gangrenous necrosis of the mammary gland. *Journal of the American Medical Association* 1894; **23**: 181.

89. Robitaille Y, See Mayer TA, Thelmo WL et al. Infarction of the mammary region mimicking carcinoma of the breast. *Cancer* 1974; **33**: 1183–1189.

90. Hasson J & Pope C. Mammary infarcts associated with pregnancy presenting as breast tumours. *Surgery* 1961; **49**: 313–316.

91. Rashid A, Basheer M & Khan K. Breast necrosis following harvest of internal mammary artery. *British Journal of Plastic Surgery* 2004; **57**: 366–368.

92. Flood EP, Redish MH, Bociek SJ et al. Thrombophlebitis migrans disseminata: report of a case in which gangrene of a breast occurred. *New York State Journal of Medicine* 1943; **43**: 1124.

93. Chan W, Chan D, Copplestone JA et al. Necrosis of the female breast: a complication of oral anticoagulation in patients with protein S deficiency. *The Breast* 1994; **3**: 116–118.

94. Davies JD, Nonni A & D'Costa HF. Mammary epidermoid inclusion cysts after wide-core needle biopsies. *Histopathology* 1997; **31**: 549–551.

95. Craigmyle MBL. *The Apocrine Glands and the Breast.* Chichester: John Wiley & Sons; 1984.

96. Jackman RJ & McQuarrie HB. Hidradenitis suppurativa: its confusion with pilonidal disease and anal fistula. *American Journal of Surgery* 1949; **77**: 349–351.

97. Harrison BJ, Mudge M & Hughes LE. Recurrence after surgical treatment of hidradenitis suppurativa. *British Medical Journal* 1987; **294**: 487–489.

98. Williams EV, Drew PJ, Douglas-Jones AG et al. Combined wide excision and mastopexy/reduction mammoplasty for inframammary hidradenitis: a novel and effective approach. *Breast* 2001; **10**: 427–431.

99. Uchida N, Yokoo H & Kuwano H. Schwannoma of the breast: report of a case. *Surgery Today* 2005; **35**: 238–242.

100. Adeniran A, Al-Ahmadie H, Mahoney MC et al. Granular cell tumor of the breast: a series of 17 cases and review of the literature. *Breast Journal* 2004; **10**: 528–531.

101. Radice B (ed.) *Hippocractic Writings.* Harmondsworth: Penguin Classics; 1983:225.

102. Sampson D. An unusual self-inflicted injury of the breast. *Postgraduate Medical Journal* 1975; **51**: 116–118.

103. Carney MWP & Brown JP. Clinical features and motives among 42 artefactual illness patients. *British Journal of Medical Psychology* 1983; **56**: 57–66.

104. Reich P & Gottfried LA. Factitious disorders in a teaching hospital. *Annals of Internal Medicine* 1983; **99**: 240–247.

105. Sneddon I & Sneddon J. Self-inflicted injury. A follow-up study of 43 patients. *British Medical Journal* 1975; **3**: 527–530.

106. Rosenberg MW & Hughes LE. Artefactual breast disease: a report of three cases. *British Journal of Surgery* 1986; **72**: 539–541.

107. Masterton G. Factitious disorders and the surgeon. *British Journal of Surgery* 1995; **82**: 1588–1589.

108. Barzilai M & Roisman I. Foreign bodies in the breast. *Breast Disease* 1995; **8**: 179–183.

109. Kalra N, Mani NB, Jain M et al. Cerebrospinal fluid pseudocyst of the breast. *Australasian Radiology* 2002; **46**: 76–79.

110. Poma S, Varenna R, Bordin G et al. Phantom breast syndrome. *Revista Clinica Espanola* 1996; **196**: 299–301.

111. Kudel I, Edwards RR, Kozachik S et al. Predictors and consequences of multiple persistent postmastectomy

pains. *Journal of Pain Symptom Management* 2007 Jul 13 [Epub ahead of print].

112. Rosen PP. Mucocele-like tumors of the breast. *American Journal of Surgical Pathology* 1986; **10**: 87–101.

113. Hamela-Bena D, Cranor ML & Rosen PP. Mammary mucocele-like lesions. *American Journal of Surgical Pathology* 1996; **20**: 1081–1085.

114. Duun S & Rank F. Mucocele-like tumours of the breast associated with atypical ductal hyperplasia. *Breast Disease* 1996; **9**: 71–73.

115. James K, Bridger J & Anthony PP. Breast tumours of pregnancy ('lactating adenoma'). *Journal of Pathology* 1988; **156**: 37–44.

116. Choudhury M, Singal MK. Lactating adenoma – cytomorphologic study with review of literature. *Indian Journal of Pathology and Microbiology* 2001; **44**: 445–448.

117. Clement PB, Young RH & Azzopardi JG. Collagenous spherulosis of the breast. *American Journal of Surgical Pathology* 1987; **11**: 411–417.

118. Umlas J. Gynecomastia-like lesions in the female breast. *Archives of Pathology and Laboratory Medicine* 2000; **124**: 844–847.

119. Kang Y, Wile M & Schinella R. Gynecomastia-like changes the female breast. *Archives of Pathology and Laboratory Medicine* 2001; **125**: 506–509.

CHAPTER 18

Operations

Introduction

The detailed indications for various operations have been outlined in previous chapters dealing with individual conditions. The general indications, detailed technique and complications of each operation are gathered together in this chapter.

Tissue diagnosis in the clinic

The majority of breast abnormalities should be diagnosed in the clinic preoperatively. Diagnostic open biopsy is now an unusual event in symptomatic patients and is also used infrequently in the screening clinic. The two preoperative diagnostic techniques are cytological examination and core needle biopsy for histology. Sampling may be clinical or image guided.

Breast samples for cytological examination may be obtained by aspiration cytology or by exfoliative cytology of nipple discharge or by imprint cytology of ulcerated lesions of the breast or nipple.

Two forms of needle biopsy need to be differentiated: fine needle aspiration for cytology and core needle biopsy for definitive histology.

Fine needle aspiration (FNA) cytology is simple, causes little discomfort and can be used to sample lesions of all sizes. It does not spread tumour cells or lead to implantation along the needle track. Accurate interpretation, however, is critically dependent on the availability of a skilled, experienced cytologist.

Core needle biopsy is easily performed under local anaesthesia, and with spring-loaded techniques is probably less painful than FNA. An adequate core can provide definitive histology equivalent to that from an open biopsy.

With both techniques, the benefit lies only in obtaining a positive diagnosis, and little credence should be placed on a negative result unless sampling error can be excluded with certainty.

Fine needle aspiration

The first description of aspiration cytology was made by Martin and Ellis,[1] who described the technique and the results in 65 patients (six breast) with cancer. Stewart[2] described the results in 500 breast lumps and gave clear descriptions of both benign and malignant breast lesions. He recognized many of the pitfalls of this technique and showed how they might be avoided. In spite of the advantages of the technique described by these authors it was not used very much until popularized in Europe at the Karolinska Institute in Sweden.[3] Webb was the first to report a series in Britain in 1970, and did much to establish the value of this approach.[4] Bates et al.[5] showed that the introduction of aspiration cytology led to a reduced open biopsy rate. The benign:malignant ratio dropped from 1.9 to 0.7 without an increase in the number of patients who subsequently developed cancer.

Indications

Aspiration cytology may be used to take samples from very small mobile lesions which cannot be biopsied and can also be used to obtain cells in very small screen-detected lesions. If there is no palpable lump, then two techniques for obtaining tissues may be considered: ultrasound- and stereotactic-guided aspiration cytology. Ultrasound-guided biopsy is obviously suitable for those mass lesions which can be identified sonographically. As it is unusual to be able to detect microcalcification on ultrasound, stereotactic-guided techniques are appropriate for microcalcification and those masses not visible on ultrasound. These two techniques are described below.

Important principles

- Ensure that the patient does not have any form of internal mammary prosthesis.
- Make sure the technique used is that approved by one's cytologist.
- Interpret the result in the light of the other components of triple assessment (see Ch. 5).

Technique

The equipment necessary for making satisfactory smears should be available (Fig. 18.1; Table 18.1).

No anaesthetic is required. The skin is cleansed with a spirit-based antiseptic and a 21-gauge needle attached to a syringe is inserted into the lump which is steadied between two fingers of the second hand. A special syringe holder (CAMECO) is available to facilitate one-handed manipulation but many prefer the more direct feel obtained by holding the syringe. Considerable information can be acquired in this way, as the consistency of the breast tissue, and of the lump in particular, is 'sensed' with the needle point: the lack of resistance of fat, the toughness of fibrous tissue, the characteristic gritty sensation of cancer, and the firmness followed by a sudden 'give' as the needle enters a cyst.

If the lesion proves to be a cyst, a record should be made of the site, colour and quantity of the aspirate. Cytology is not indicated. Measurement of electrolyte content[6] has given some indication of likelihood of recurrence, but is not used routinely. Cysts may be deeper than suggested by palpation, so if no cyst is located on the first needle-pass, it is worthwhile exploring a little deeper or using ultrasound guidance. After withdrawing the needle, the area is palpated to ensure that the lump has disappeared completely. The use of ultrasound in the clinic allows precise localization of cysts and eliminates most of these uncertainties.

If the lesion proves to be solid, the needle should be moved in and out of the mass in several directions while maintaining modest negative pressure until material appears in the hub of the needle. Fifteen or 20 passes may be necessary. Care is taken to enter the lesion in a plane parallel to the chest wall to reduce the risk of penetrating the underlying pleura. The negative pressure is released before removing the needle from the lump; failure to do this results in the sample becoming splattered around the barrel of the syringe rather than being retained in the needle. The needle is disconnected, the syringe filled with air and the needle replaced to expel the contents onto a labelled microscope slide. Expulsion should be repeated several times before it is assumed that no specimen is present; a completely dry aspirate is rare.

Gross blood contamination interferes with cytology so that, if a blood vessel is hit, it is usually best to repeat the procedure later. Some authorities pass the needle without using suction, maintaining that this gives specimens that are just as satisfactory but with a much reduced incidence of bleeding. A cottonwool ball is then held firmly over the entry point to reduce the chance of a haematoma,

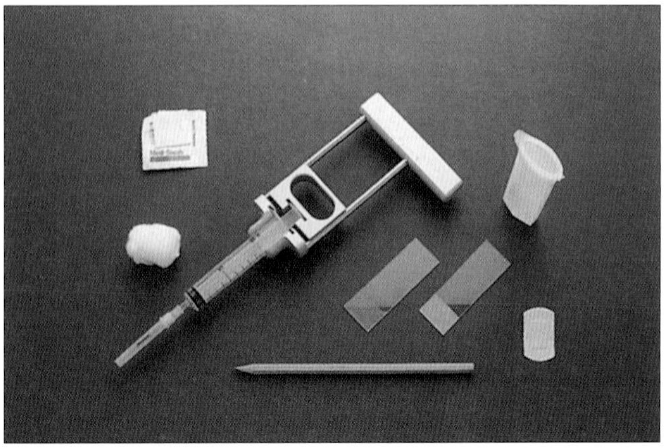

Fig. 18.1 The instruments and equipment needed for FNA.

Table 18.1 Equipment for aspiration cytology

21-gauge needle
10-mL syringe
Mediswab
Slides with ground glass end
Fixative
Pencil
Cottonwool ball
Adhesive dressing (Airfix)
±Syringe holder

more common in the relatively vascular cancers, before covering it with an adhesive dressing.

The exact technique and the method of fixing the specimen should be discussed with the cytologist. The specimens may be fixed immediately in alcohol or air-dried prior to fixation. The results of cytological assessment are graded as shown in Table 18.2.

Contraindications and complications

There are no real contraindications to performing aspiration cytology, although it is better avoided in very uncooperative and restless patients. Occasionally, patients will not give consent to this procedure.

Pneumothorax is a well-recognized complication of FNA and it is important that those using the technique are aware of it. There have been a number of reports since Gateley et al. first described seven cases in 1991.[7] They estimated the frequency of this complication to be 1 per 1000 FNA procedures. The clinical picture is similar in most cases, although varying in severity. The patient typically complains of some pain at the time of the procedure, and further pain in the chest after a period of a few minutes to a few hours. There is frequently mild distress, but shock or other severe symptoms are not usually seen. The patient rapidly recovers. The suggested mechanism is a Valsalva manoeuvre by an apprehensive patient at the time of needle insertion, with the lung expanded under pressure against the parietal pleura.

A second paper from Italy[8] reported 19 cases from 201 000 aspirations carried out in 48 institutions. This gives an incidence of 0.01%, but as it is a retrospective survey, it probably underestimates the frequency. Kaufman et al.[9] also found an incidence of 1:417; all procedures were carried out by experienced personnel. It is now clear that this complication can occur with the most experienced operators, and is seen more commonly in thin women and in peripheral or axillary needlings, where the thickness of the breast is least, although it has been seen with lumps in all sites and breasts of all configurations. If suspected, a chest X-ray will show a small to moderate pneumothorax, which usually resolves spontaneously over 7–10 days.

While some patients have been treated aggressively by insertion of a chest drain, especially when admitted on a thoracic service, most cases resolve quickly without active interference. If suspected, the patient should be observed for a few hours (or occasionally overnight) to ensure stabilization. If the pneumothorax is large enough to cause respiratory distress, simple aspiration of the air should be sufficient.

One serious complication has been reported[10] in a patient who developed a haemopneumothorax after FNA. This required insertion of a chest drain, transfusion and an emergency thoracotomy. The problem was thought to be due to disruption of a vascular adhesion when a pneumothorax developed after the FNA.

This serious complication is very rare. Diagnosis is dependent on awareness of the complication and knowledge of those situations where it is most likely to occur: thin, restless patients and a needle passed directly into a peripherally sited lump, at right angles to the chest wall.

Other complications

The most common complication of aspiration cytology is a haematoma. This is undesirable for a number of reasons: it is uncomfortable for the patient; if the lesion proves to be malignant there is the theoretical risk of spreading cancer cells further in the breast; it may become infected; and it may make further evaluation of the lesion, clinically or by imaging, more difficult. Sometimes a cyst will become painful after aspiration, either from infection or more often when cyst contents leak into the surrounding breast.

Horobin et al.[11] have examined the effect of fine needle biopsy on subsequent mammograms. Fifty-two women had mammograms before and 3–4 days after fine needle biopsy. In 10 cases there were differences in the mammographic appearance but none was sufficient to lead to a change in radiological diagnosis. In seven of these, cystic lesions became less obvious; in three cases an increased density was noted and the authors expressed

Table 18.2 Grading of biopsy (B) and cytology (C) reports

Grading	Interpretation
B1 / C1	Inadequate[a]
B2 / C2	Benign
B3 / C3	Probably benign
B4 / C4	Probably malignant
B5 / C5	Malignant

[a]Inadequate, no epithelial cells. If the aspirate contains inflammatory cells such as macrophages or lymphocytes appropriate deductions may be made in the clinical context.

concern that a malignant lesion might have been over-looked or that haematoma around a benign lesion might be misread as having features of malignancy; in consequence they recommend performing mammography before aspiration cytology or waiting for 1 week afterwards. Provided the radiologist has the information that aspiration has been performed, these rules need not be absolute.

One further situation in which caution should be urged is the patient with augmentation mammoplasty. The silicone prosthesis may be close to the lump and perforation of the envelope must be avoided. In this situation, ultrasound-guided aspiration may reduce the chance of inadvertent damage to the prosthesis.

Core needle biopsy

Core needle biopsy is easily performed under local anaesthesia, but can cause some discomfort. The development of an automated spring-loaded firing device permits biopsy of subclinical lesions visualized on ultrasonography and mammography. An adequate core can provide definitive histology equivalent to that from an open biopsy.

Indications

Today, a core biopsy is usually taken in preference to an FNA from any solid mass and indeterminate calcifications with imaging control. Needle biopsy can cause sufficient tissue oedema to obscure mammographic detail so mammography should preferably precede core biopsy in triple assessment. If the purpose of mammography is to screen the rest of the breast after a dominant mass has been assessed by image-guided biopsy, there is no need to defer mammography.

While most patients readily tolerate needle biopsy, some find that it causes considerable pain, so it should be used with discretion for tender masses or those deep to the areola.

Important principles

- Ensure that the patient does not have any form of internal mammary prosthesis.
- Use local anaesthetic but avoid this form of biopsy if the lump is particularly painful.
- Develop a one-hand technique for needle manipulation so the other hand can stabilize the lump.

- Insert the closed needle up to, but not into, the lump as the spring-loading mechanism carries both trocar and sheath into the lump.
- Ensure that the direction of the instrument allows for a 2-cm throw without encountering any vital structure.
- Apply pressure after biopsy for at least 5 minutes, to minimize early and late bleeding.

Technique

The equipment necessary for the procedure (Fig. 18.2) should be available and a no-touch technique used.

A number of biopsy needles are available. Our preference for breast biopsy is a spring-loaded instrument with a short (3 inch; 7.6 cm) needle because short needles are easier to control. An instrument with a 2-cm throw will give the best biopsy specimens (Fig. 18.3).

Our impression accords with that of McMahon et al.[12] that the spring-loaded device for automatic sampling is less painful than the hand-held procedure. After cleansing the skin, a small intradermal weal of local anaesthetic (1% lidocaine) is raised at the biopsy site (Fig. 18.4).

The proposed line of the needle should also be infiltrated down to the lesion to be biopsied, but excessive infiltration is to be avoided because it will obscure the position of the underlying mass. Using a sterile technique, a small nick is made in the skin and through to the subcutaneous fat with a pointed disposable scalpel blade (No. 11 or 15; Fig. 18.5), and the closed needle, held in the spring-loaded gun, is inserted through this until it abuts the lesion (Fig. 18.6).

The gun allows the needle to be manipulated with one hand, leaving the second hand free to steady and

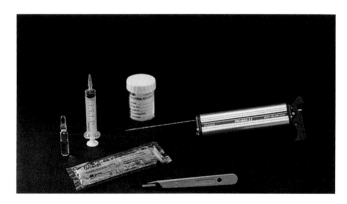

Fig. 18.2 The instruments and equipment needed for core needle biopsy using a spring-loaded needle carrier.

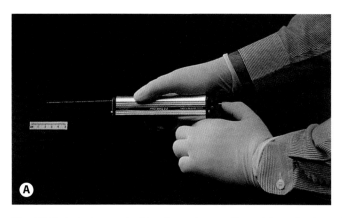 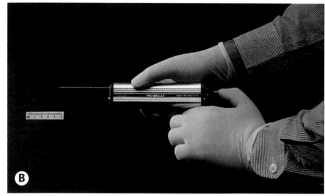

Fig. 18.3 An instrument with a 2-cm throw will provide optimal specimens.

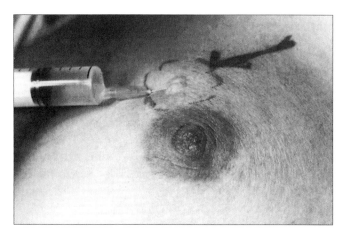

Fig. 18.4 Infiltration of skin and underlying tissues with local anaesthetic.

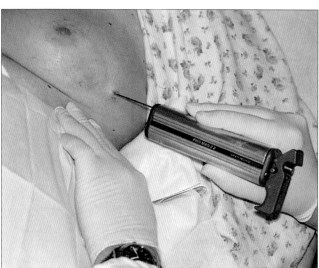

Fig. 18.6 The needle is inserted up to, but not into, the mass.

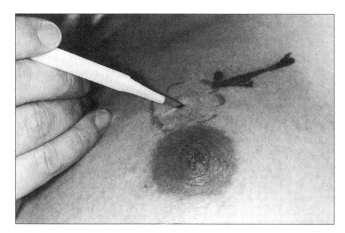

Fig. 18.5 A small stab incision is made through the skin and subcutaneous tissue with a fine-pointed scalpel.

manipulate the mass or hold the ultrasound probe. The safety catch on the gun is then released and the gun fired. The needle is withdrawn in the closed position and the core of tissue placed straight into formalin. If necessary, further cores of tissue can be taken until a satisfactory specimen is obtained (Fig. 18.7).

A general guide to the nature of the specimens can be obtained by examining the cores. If these float on the formalin they are likely to be fat only. If they sink, they are likely to be breast tissue (Fig. 18.8).

Bleeding is not uncommon, so haemostasis is secured by firm digital pressure over the area for several minutes. The small skin incision is then covered with an occlusive dressing.

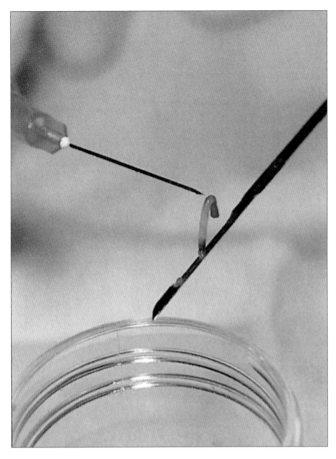

Fig. 18.7 A satisfactory specimen.

Complications

The contraindications and complications of needle biopsy are similar to those of aspiration cytology but bruising is noticeably commoner. Roberts et al.[13] reported a 37% incidence of bruising, although none of these was described as a haematoma. A haematoma may occur when a vascular lesion has been biopsied or a subcutaneous vein punctured and moderate bruising is common, hence the need for local pressure for at least 3 or 4 minutes. Extensive bruising is more common in patients on aspirin or anticoagulants such as warfarin (Fig. 18.9), when special precautions should be taken.

Image-guided needle biopsy

Ultrasound-guided biopsy

This technique is used for impalpable lesions that can be defined ultrasonically and for palpable lumps to improve accuracy. A study has shown that two accurately placed cores are usually sufficient to make a diagnosis.[14] A 7.5–13 Mhz linear probe is used. The technique is similar to the method used for palpable lumps except that the operator holds the ultrasound head with one hand while guiding the needle with the other. The lesion and the needle are both apparent to the operator so very accurate localization can be achieved. The major advantages of this method are that it is quick and without radiation exposure.

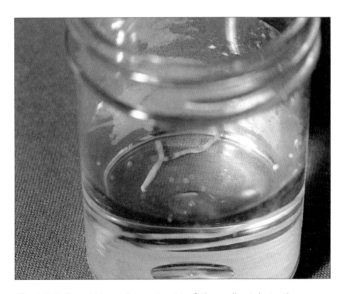

Fig. 18.8 Breast tissue (in contrast to fat) usually sinks to the bottom of the fluid.

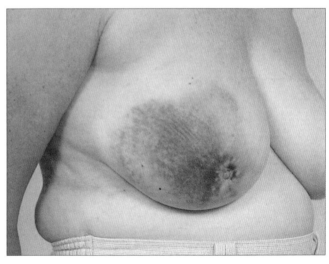

Fig. 18.9 Extensive haematoma of the breast following core needle biopsy in a woman on warfarin.

Stereotactic biopsy

Stereotactic biopsy can be used where a lesion is not visible on ultrasound. It is useful in performing both localized aspiration cytology and core needle biopsy, and provides very accurate localization of microcalcifications (see Ch. 6).

Mammotome or vacuum-assisted biopsy

A mammotome takes tissue biopsies using a vacuum-assisted approach. It can be guided by ultrasound or stereotactic methods. As for core biopsies, the skin is infiltrated with local anaesthetic and a small incision is made in the skin. The needle (11-gauge) is guided to the biopsy site by ultrasound or X- ray imaging. A vacuum gently draws and collects some breast tissue into a small collecting chamber. This allows multiple biopsies to be taken without having to remove and reinsert the probe. This technique is used for diagnostic procedures and occasionally for removal of known benign lesions as it takes larger pieces of tissue than a conventional core biopsy. If the biopsy is being done for diagnostic purposes, it may be necessary to leave a 'gel marker' at the site of the biopsy in order to guide future definitive surgery if required later. After the biopsy, the probe is removed and a dressing is applied to the small cut. Patients may experience mild discomfort following the procedure and there may be some bruising for a few days, but it is generally well tolerated.[15,16]

Open biopsy procedures

Open biopsy covers a number of procedures, including excision biopsy, incision biopsy, removal of a fibroadenoma and biopsy under radiological control. Each procedure carries different indications and requires a special technique.

Local anaesthesia

Small, superficial, mobile fibroadenomas can be satisfactorily removed under local anaesthesia. A problem of local anaesthesia is that occasionally the lesion is less readily palpable after the anaesthetic has been introduced. Lidocaine 1% without adrenaline is infiltrated along the line of the proposed incision. Usually, the procedure is painless but there is some discomfort if too much traction is placed on the breast tissue during mobilization of the lump. A further injection of local anaesthetic deep to the lump will usually solve this problem. Diathermy haemostasis is safe. The use of a long-acting local anaesthetic such as bupivacaine in combination with lidocaine can assist pain control with outpatient procedures. Many women prefer the discomfort of local anaesthesia to the experience of recovery from a general anaesthetic.

General anaesthesia

This is an elective procedure, but in general can be carried out on an outpatient (day case) basis. The patient is starved and as muscle relaxation is not required endotracheal intubation is unnecessary. A laryngeal mask technique is safe and satisfactory.

Indications

Open biopsy is only indicated for removal of any persistent undiagnosed discrete lump or after previous biopsies have given B3 or B4, i.e. are inconclusive, or for removal of previously diagnosed benign lumps at the patient's request, as outlined in Chapter 5.

Wounds in young girls may be complicated by hypertrophic scars and this is particularly frequent and noticeable in the upper inner quadrant of the breast, and close to the sternum. Before recommending removal of lumps in young girls, patients should be warned about this as it is unpredictable.

Important principles

- Think carefully before excising breast lumps under local anaesthetic, especially in young girls, where breast tissue is dense and deep lumps may feel superficial.
- Never remove a lump without triple assessment.
- Define the lump carefully before operation. Avoid the temptation to keep removing fibrotic breast tissue which looks and feels 'abnormal' at operation; this can lead to inadvertent subcutaneous mastectomy.
- Be careful with haemostasis; vessels in fibrotic breast tissue are difficult to control.
- Mark the site of the lump before operation with the patient in the position in which she will be placed on the operating table and mark the position of the incision with the patient sitting up preoperatively.

Technique

It is customary for the patient to lie supine but occasionally it is helpful to rotate the patient a little if the breast is large and the planned incision lies laterally. Periareolar incisions are preferred for all masses within 5 cm of the areola, and curved incisions parallel to the circumference for more peripheral masses (Fig. 18.10).

Incisions close to, but parallel to, the areolar margin are to be avoided, as the double line can give an unsightly appearance (Fig. 18.11).

In general, the blood supply to the breast is so profuse that ischaemia need not cause concern except in extensive periareolar incisions. The blood supply of the breast and its implications for biopsy are discussed by Robertson.[17] Where cancer is suspected, the incision should be planned to take into account subsequent treatment. In re-excising a biopsy wound for malignancy, the whole of the wound and contaminated tissue should be removed without re-entering the original wound, so a badly orientated biopsy wound may necessitate excessive sacrifice of skin at the second procedure (Fig. 18.12).

The skin at the selected site of incision is held under slight tension by the assistant and a slightly curved inci-

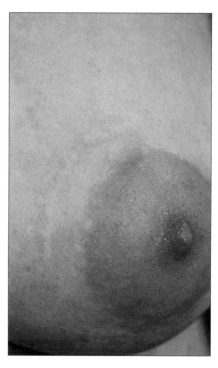

Fig. 18.11 Scar resulting from an excision through a close periareolar incision, giving an unnecessarily obvious scar.

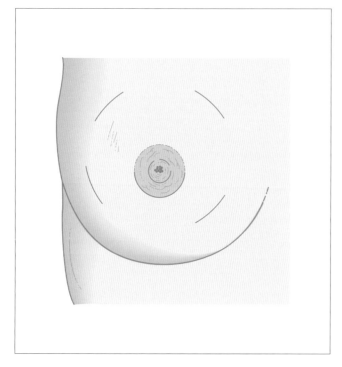

Fig. 18.10 Incisions for breast biopsy for benign conditions. Where the mass lies within 5 cm of the areola, a periareolar incision is used. For more distant masses, a curved incision parallel to the areola is used.

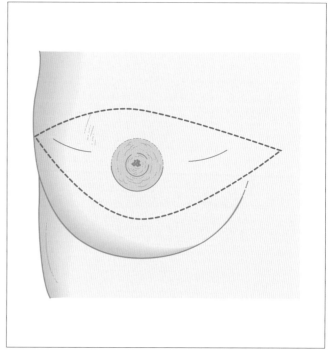

Fig. 18.12 In patients of the cancer age group, biopsy incisions should be sited in such a way as to be readily re-excised within the skin island of a mastectomy wound, should this be necessary.

sion made with a number 10 blade. The incision is deepened throughout its length into the subcutaneous fat and veins divided and diathermied. A self-retaining retractor will allow good exposure of the lesion while giving excellent haemostasis from the sometimes troublesome superficial vessels.

The incision is deepened until the breast disc is encountered. In young patients this is easily identified; in the postmenopausal involuted breast it may be represented by a few strands of fibrous tissue. The lesion should now be palpated and the decision to perform either excision or incision biopsy confirmed or occasionally revised. The mass is grasped with an Allis forceps and excised with a combination of scissors and diathermy. Bleeding is often troublesome because the small vessels lie embedded in the dense fibrous tissue. This can be tedious as tumours are often vascular and the vessels bleed easily; meticulous haemostasis now will be rewarded by a low incidence of subsequent bleeding and haematoma formation. Diathermy is usually sufficient, but occasionally suture transfixion of vessels in fibrous tissue is used, and the wound is carefully inspected for bleeding prior to closure.

These days, open diagnostic biopsies are performed rarely. If they are, the defect in the breast tissue is not closed. If the diagnosis is subsequently that of malignancy, further surgery will be needed. The skin should be closed with a subcuticular absorbable suture.

Complications

The common complications of breast biopsy are confined to persistent bleeding from the wound and haematoma formation. Haemostasis at the time of surgery is the most important preventive measure. Wound infections are rare except as a complication of a haematoma.

Painful haematomas occurring in the first 48 hours are best managed by opening the wound and evacuating the clot rather than allowing spontaneous resolution. After ensuring haemostasis, the wound should be closed with antibiotic cover. Allowing natural resolution may take some time, may cause considerable pain both early and late and may make subsequent assessment of the breast more difficult. Haematomas presenting late after liquefaction may be managed by repeated aspiration through a wide-bore needle.

One situation where special care needs to be taken is in the irradiated breast. The use of breast-conserving treatments for early breast cancer makes the need to evaluate such patients important. Pezner et al.[18] reported that 30%

of patients having open biopsies had wound-healing problems with significant deterioration in the cosmetic appearance of the biopsied breast. Complications were more common in women with large breasts. They reported no complications in a small number of women who had needle biopsies of irradiated breasts, so image-guided biopsy should be used as often as possible.

Postoperative care

Most patients will be able to go home on the same day, with adequate provision of analgesia. Pathology results should be reviewed at a multidisciplinary meeting to decide whether any further management is required.

Incision biopsy

Incision biopsy is rarely required these days and should be avoided if at all possible. It is an important rule that a diagnosis should be made before definitive treatment is planned for large masses of obscure aetiology, benign or malignant. This will prevent unsatisfactory procedures such as a poorly planned excision of a large phyllodes tumour, which may make it impossible to ensure an adequate excision margin at a secondary procedure. In the rare instances where preoperative diagnosis has not been made, it is better to perform an incision biopsy than to do a wide excision for a lump which may prove to be no more than fibrous tissue.

Removal of a fibroadenoma

The early stages of the operation are the same as those described under open biopsy. However, fibroadenomas in young women usually lie within a well-defined capsule and can be enucleated easily. The pedicle may require ligation or diathermy (Fig. 18.13) and the base of the pedicle may require excision if this is broad because there may be some extension of fibroadenomatous tissue into the area of the capsule (Fig. 18.14).

Bleeding is minimal and a drain should not be inserted into the cavity. The parenchyma of the breast is hardly disturbed, so there is no need to close the defect in the breast tissue, as it will soon disappear.

In older women, a fibroadenoma usually presents as a dominant mass in an involuting breast. These fibroadenomas often do not enucleate satisfactorily and are best removed by the technique of excision biopsy described earlier.

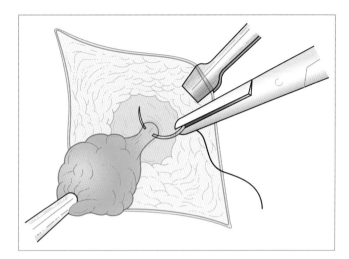

Fig. 18.13 Removing a fibroadenoma. The blood supply comes only through the pedicle so this should be diathermied or ligated if it is substantial.

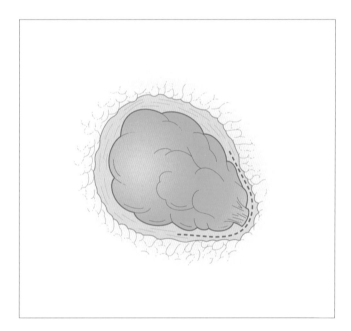

Fig. 18.14 There is sometimes extension of fibroadenomatous tissue in the pedicle so that, where this is broad, an area adjacent to the base should be removed to minimize recurrence.

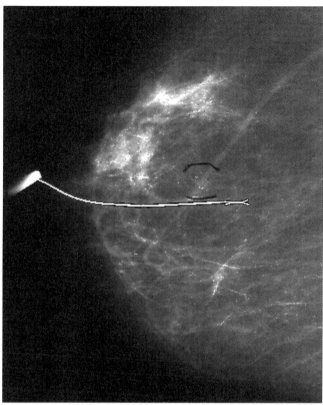

Fig. 18.15 A subclinical radiological lesion has been localized with a wire inserted into the breast.

Image-controlled biopsy

Indications

This procedure is indicated to remove a lesion seen on mammography but which cannot be felt clinically. The commonest indication is a small area of microcalcification or trabecular distortion for which the differential diagnosis usually lies between early carcinoma (in situ or invasive), radial scar and sclerosing adenosis. Because these conditions cannot be safely differentiated radiologically, excision biopsy may be indicated if image-guided core biopsy has not given a conclusive result (see Ch. 6).

Important principles

- Close cooperation is required between surgeon, radiologist and pathologist.
- The radiological abnormality is localized by the radiologist in the radiology department (Fig. 18.15).
- Excision biopsy is performed by the surgeon under general anaesthetic.
- Immediate specimen radiology is carried out to confirm that the area in question has been removed.
- Further tissue excision is performed if the abnormal area was not located in this specimen.

Techniques: wire localization

This technique is the most widely practised in localizing nonpalpable breast lesions. A hooked wire enclosed within a needle is placed in the breast under ultrasound guidance or stereotactic techniques. Further mammographic views are taken and the relationship of the tip of the needle to the lesion ascertained. Multiple wires may be used to delineate large or multiple lesions, such as extensive areas of microcalcification. The needle is removed, leaving the wire in situ, which is then taped to the skin while the patient is transferred to the operating theatre.

Fixation of the wire should be secure, but migration may occur, especially in large and fatty breasts. Although some surgeons report that the subsequent search of the breast can be satisfactorily done under a local anaesthetic, most patients prefer this under general anaesthetic. There are a number of different wires available. The general conduct of the operation is as for an open biopsy, with either a periareolar incision or one related to the wire entry point. After the incision has been made, a mosquito forceps is placed on the wire to allow the assistant to keep the wire steady while its track is followed through the fat into the breast tissue. A pair of Allis forceps is placed on either side of the wire in a plane opposite to the side of the lesion, so that if the wire lies inferior and lateral to the lesion the forceps are placed in this quarter. The Allis forceps are then lifted to bring the breast tissue to the incision, the breast tissue is divided along the wire in this plane for a short distance and haemostasis secured.

The Allis forceps are now repositioned adjacent to the place where the wire disappears into the tissue and the process is repeated. Gentle palpation will eventually reveal the hook on the wire. When this is found, the suspicious area can be defined and excised; a palpable abnormality may or may not be apparent. Gentle handling of the wire is required at this stage so as not to dislodge it.

The tissue is excised and imaged using a Faxitron to confirm that the correct area has been removed (Fig. 18.16). The remainder of the operation proceeds as for biopsy of a palpable lump.

Careless excision can result in large defects with unnecessary cosmetic deformity from benign lesions, so emphasis should be placed on accurate localization. The document entitled 'Guidelines for surgeons in the management of screen-detected breast disease in the United

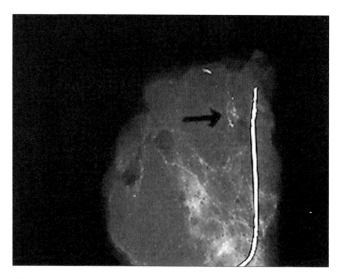

Fig. 18.16 The specimen radiology confirms the presence of the lesion.

Kingdom'[19] recommends that, as a quality outcome measure, >90% of diagnostic biopsies which subsequently prove to be benign should weigh less than 20 g and that the surgeon should ensure that the biopsy is weighed by the pathologist.

An alternative technique that is used in some institutions for localization is injection of radioisotope (technetium labelled colloidal albumen) into the area of concern under imaging and subsequent use of a gamma counter to identify the abnormality.[20]

Complications of localization biopsy

Helvie et al.[21] reported the immediate complications of localization and needle aspiration in 370 cases while still in the radiology department. Vasovagal attacks occurred in 7% and four patients developed syncope. They also recorded prolonged bleeding in three patients and severe pain in two. Rappaport et al.[22] examined the complications following localization biopsy in 144 consecutive patients. They reported an infection rate of 1.2% and cases of diathermy burns of the skin.

Problems may occur with the wire, including total migration into the breast, possibly requiring a second localization to remove it, migration outside the breast (into the pleural cavity has been recorded), and accidental transsection of the wire during dissection, with loss of the deep portion.

Removal of giant fibroadenoma and phyllodes tumour

In a young patient (<20 years)

A giant fibroadenoma is usually defined as a lesion more than 5 cm in diameter. These lesions may lie close to the surface of the breast and may then be removed in the same way as a smaller fibroadenoma. Larger lesions tend to lie deeper in the breast and are best approached from behind through a submammary incision which will give a better cosmetic result than one located on the breast.

Technique

A submammary incision (Fig. 18.17) is taken down to the fascia over the serratus anterior and pectoralis major muscles and dissection is carried upwards in this largely avascular, retromammary plane (Fig. 18.18).

The fibroadenoma is then pushed through the posterior aspect into the wound, the capsule incised (Fig. 18.19) and the tumour shelled out in the usual way.

A suction drain is inserted into the retromammary space and the wound closed with subcuticular absorbable sutures. This approach to the back of the breast through the submammary fold was described by Gaillard–Thomas in 1882.[23]

It is important that more radical procedures are avoided in young girls, that no attempt is made to close the cavity, and that no complex reconstructive procedures are used.

In an older patient

Giant fibroadenomas and phyllodes tumours in older patients differ from those in young girls in a number of ways. They vary in the degree of malignancy and may not shell out from the surrounding involuting breast tissue. Hence, they are best managed by core needle biopsy to provide definitive histological assessment before planning management, which is usually by a wide local exci-

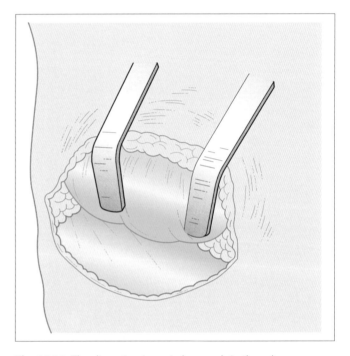

Fig. 18.18 The dissection is carried upwards in the submammary plane at the level of the pectoral fascia.

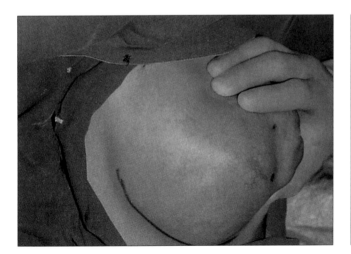

Fig. 18.17 The Gaillard–Thomas incision for giant fibroadenoma.

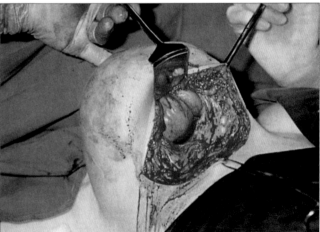

Fig. 18.19 The fascial layer on the posterior aspect of the breast is incised and the fibroadenoma enucleated and delivered through the wound.

sion or by simple mastectomy if it is a large phyllodes tumour with malignant potential.

Where a 1-cm clearance is required, as is usually the case with phyllodes tumour, this should be measured around the whole surface. This is done most satisfactorily by the surgeon placing the fingers of his left hand on the tumour, and cutting outside his finger. The details of the technique do not differ from those of the operations described above; the all-important principles are considered in Chapter 7.

Microdochectomy

Indications

This operation is indicated for bloodstained or serous discharge from a solitary duct when the opening of the affected duct on to the nipple can be identified. We use this operation for patients under the age of 40, preferring the operation of major duct excision for bloodstained nipple discharge in patients over this age (see Chs 11 and 12), but opinion differs. Burton et al.[24] reviewed a series of 52 cases of single duct nipple discharge treated by microdochectomy and reported that papilloma was the most frequent diagnosis above and below the age of 50 years so a microdochectomy is safe for women over 50 years. Another series reviewed 86 patients with nipple discharge and normal cytology, imaging and clinical examination and found that only two had malignancy, one with ductal carcinoma in situ (DCIS) and one with lobular carcinoma in situ (LCIS).[25] Other ways for investigating and treating these symptoms now include breast duct microendoscopy and brush cytology[26] and ultrasound-guided mammotome excision of ducts[27] but these are not widely available.

Important principles

- Avoid expressing fluid for a few days before operation.
- Radial or periareolar incisions are both satisfactory, the latter preferable in younger women.
- Identify the duct with a lacrimal probe.
- Excise all dilated parts of the duct system if operating for blood-related discharge.

Operative technique

The orifice of the affected duct is identified by squeezing the nipple to express a drop of discharge. A lacrimal probe is inserted into the duct and passed as far into the breast tissue as possible (Fig. 18.20).

This should be done gently to avoid creating a false passage. The probe will frequently pass only 1–2 cm because passage along the duct may be blocked by little pockets which tend to occur as the duct dilates around a papilloma. This distance is sufficient to demonstrate the direction of the duct and, after making the incision, the dark fluid in the dilated duct is usually visible.

Using the direction of the lacrimal probe as a guide, a racquet-shaped incision is made to enclose the immediate termination of the duct with a minimal amount of surrounding nipple tissue and carried radially across the areola and on to the breast skin for a total distance of 5 cm (Fig. 18.21).

The skin flaps are raised over a short distance and the whole of the affected duct and its branching system dissected out in segmental fashion for a distance of at least 5 cm from its orifice (Fig. 18.22).

The main portion of the duct can usually be identified for about 2.5 cm. It is dissected carefully to interfere as little as possible with surrounding ducts, although if a central duct is affected, some damage to the adjacent ducts is inevitable. A further segmental area of breast

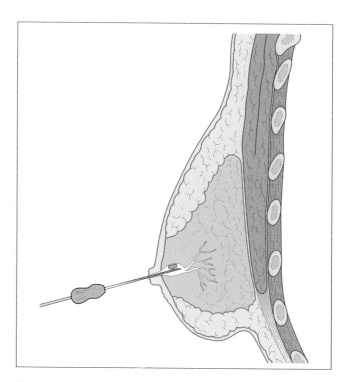

Fig. 18.20 A lacrimal probe is passed into the affected duct to find its direction within the breast. It often will not go very far because it catches in small pockets of the dilated duct.

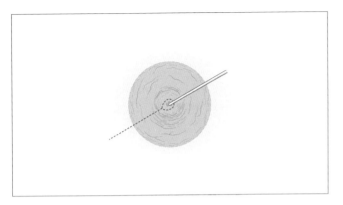

Fig. 18.21 The racquet-shaped incision for microdochectomy. The skin surrounding the terminal duct is removed in continuity within the duct.

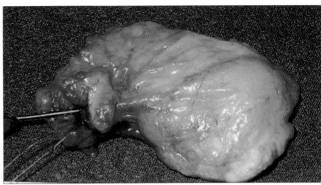

Fig. 18.23 A typical specimen following microdochectomy from a large breast.

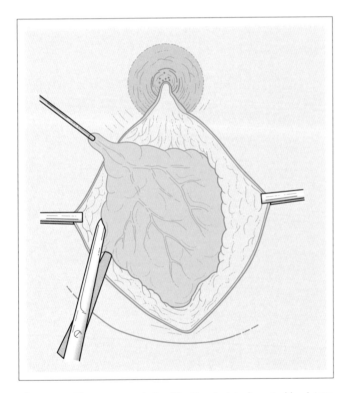

Fig. 18.22 The segment drained by the duct is dissected back into the breast for a distance of 2–3 cm, but further if the ducts remain dilated at this level.

tissue about 2.5 cm long is removed in continuity with the duct (Fig. 18.23).

A length of 5–6 cm of the duct system will usually remove any papillomas present because these are lesions of the large ducts.

However, if the duct remains dilated beyond 5 cm, it should be followed further towards the periphery of the breast. Normally a duct is only dilated between the papilloma and the nipple. So, if peripheral ducts are dilated, peripheral papillomas – benign or malignant – should be anticipated and a segmental resection of the breast carried out to encompass all dilated, blood-filled ducts.

Peripheral dilatation of ducts is particularly seen in older patients with multiple 'discrete' papillomas occupying a single ductolobular system. Such papillomas tend to be benign or of very low-grade malignancy, and complete excision of that system should be curative.

Haemostasis is secured and the specimen removed. The terminal portion of the duct is marked with a suture to help the pathologist orientate the tissue. Macroscopic papillomas are found in only about half of the cases, others being due to duct ectasia (DE). The skin is closed with subcuticular sutures.

Variations of technique

Several variations have been described for this procedure. The tissues around the duct may be infiltrated with saline containing 1 : 300 000 adrenaline solution to help maintain haemostasis and allow more exact dissection. The use of binocular magnifying loupes will also help precise dissection.

Some surgeons (e.g. Haagensen) preferred to use a periareolar incision, dissecting the flap upwards in the same manner as described under major duct excision. The dilated duct is then dissected to its entry on to the nipple. The peripheral flap is raised to allow segmental excision of the duct drainage area. Haagensen advocates this incision on cosmetic grounds, although we find a radial incision usually gives a satisfactory cosmetic result. The radial incision has the advantage that it can more readily be extended where this is necessary, so is particularly appropriate in the older patient. In contrast, a periareolar incision is to be preferred in younger women since a hypertrophic scar, although rare, is more likely with radial incisions (Fig. 18.24).

Excision of mammary duct fistula

Indications

- Established duct fistula with a single opening.
- A localized abscess which always presents at the same spot.

Important principles

- Conservative drainage or aspiration of a periareolar abscess as an acute procedure if the fistula is not established.
- The central (nipple) opening of the duct must be excised.
- Healing by granulation has proved a reliable method of obtaining a satisfactory result but the wound must be well shaped and managed correctly.
- Primary closure under antibiotic cover may be appropriate.

Fistulotomy or fistulectomy?

In his original description, Atkins[28] simply laid the fistula open and allowed it to granulate (fistulotomy). This is

probably a satisfactory procedure, but fistulectomy is preferred because it ensures that the central portion of the duct is excised (important in minimizing recurrence), removes some of the ductal system and leaves healthy tissue to granulate. This operation is described, but similar principles apply to fistulotomy. A probe is passed into the external opening of the fistula and passes easily out of the duct opening on to the nipple (Fig. 18.25).

The skin incision encompasses the fistula and an ellipse of skin is removed which need be only about 1 cm wide at its maximum (Fig. 18.26).

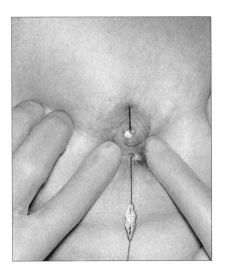

Fig. 18.25 A probe is passed through the duct fistula and out through the nipple.

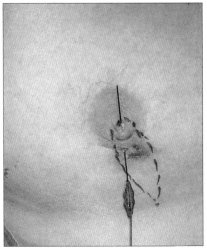

Fig. 18.26 The skin excision for mammary duct fistula.

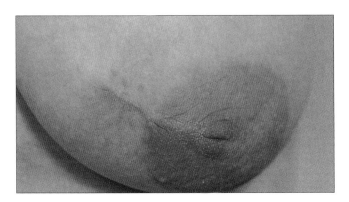

Fig. 18.24 An obvious scar from a radial incision in a young woman.

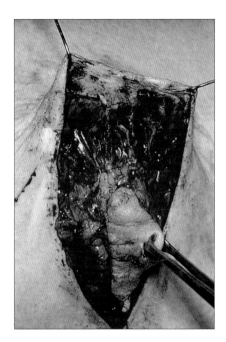

Fig. 18.27 The underlying tissue is excised conservatively.

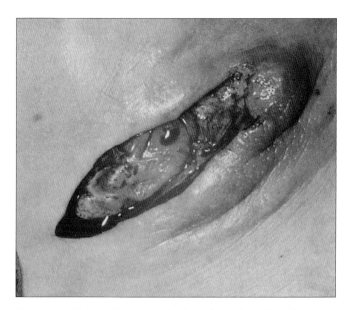

Fig. 18.28 The resulting wound is boat shaped – as broad as it is deep – so that it will heal from below.

More important is that the incision includes the whole of the affected lactiferous sinus and the opening on to the nipple; this is the portion of terminal duct lined by squamous epithelium. The ellipse and underlying tissue also include a centimetre or two of the duct system distal to the fistula. The incision is deepened through subcutaneous fat into the breast tissue just below the affected duct (Fig. 18.27).

If the wound is allowed to granulate, healing will be rapid and certain, provided the wound is well shaped (Fig. 18.28) and does not close prematurely.

If non-adherent cavity dressings are used, these cause no pain on dressing change and can be managed by the patient at home. An alternative is to close the wound primarily under antibiotic cover. A review of a series of 35 patients concluded that a simple fistula should be treated by fistulectomy, primary closure and antibiotic cover but total duct excision should be reserved for a complex fistula.[29] Lannin, in a personal series, reported excellent cosmesis and low long-term recurrence with fistulectomy and primary closure.[30]

Major duct excision (Adair/Urban/Hadfield)

This important procedure has an interesting history. It was first reported in 1960 by Hadfield,[31] based on 31 cases, and in the UK the operation is commonly referred to as Hadfield's procedure. In his paper, he paid tribute to Adair and Urban of the Memorial Hospital, New York, for having taught him the operation. Three years later, Urban described his technique,[32] reporting 167 operations. Hence, the operation is also frequently known as Urban's duct excision, although in his own paper, Urban assigns his own precedence to Adair, whose first operation preceded Urban's by 2 years, although Adair published no account of his technique.

Indications (see Chapters 11 and 13 for details)

- Blood-related discharge in a patient over the age of 40 years. Here it is preferred to microdochectomy because of the more generous pathological material provided in a patient with a significant risk of cancer. Urban[32] found 41 unsuspected cancers in 434 duct excision operations, mainly in the older age groups. Major duct excision gives more certain control of symptoms should the symptoms prove to be due to duct ectasia.
- Non-blood-related discharge sufficiently copious to be an embarrassment to the patient. If the discharge is milky, prolactinoma should first be excluded.
- Subareolar abscess, selected according to the criteria discussed in Chapter 11, or a peripheral mass or abscess with central major DE, when the mass and major ducts can be excised in continuity.

Important principles

The areolar flap, confined to one-third of the circumference, is dissected in a plane deep to the venous plexus to avoid ischaemia.

The undersurface of the nipple is bared completely to remove all terminal duct tissue and to ensure that no ducts are missed at the back of the duct cone. The central portion of the nipple is removed if the nipple does not evert easily. Peripheral dilated ducts are ignored. All excised tissue is submitted for histological assessment.

Technique: incision

The ducts are approached through a periareolar incision extending for 30–40%, and no further than 50%, around the circumference. It is usually based inferiorly but may be centred anywhere towards localized pathology. It should be placed accurately at the areolar margin to obtain maximum cosmetic benefit (Fig. 18.29).

Urban[32] recommended a radial incision removing an ellipse of skin stopping short of the nipple. He found it easier to repair the oval-shaped defect in the breast tissue.

This approach may be helpful where there is severe scarring from periareolar sepsis, because it allows easy entry to the subareolar plane through relatively normal tissue, instead of through dense scar tissue. Srivastava et al.[33] advocate the use of an incision that is only one-third of the areolar circumference and does not raise an areolar flap. In their series of 17 cases, nipple sensation was preserved and there was one case of recurrent discharge on early follow-up.

Technique: dissection

The incision is deepened until the prominent radially running subcutaneous veins are reached (Fig. 18.30). By preserving the vascular plexus of the areola, the viability of nipple and areola is assured. The penalty for neglecting this careful definition of tissue planes is shown in Figure 18.31.

The areolar flap is dissected in this plane until about one-third of the areola has been elevated and the cone of fibroductal tissue passing to the nipple is reached. A sub-areolar tunnel is then developed behind the ductal cone by blunt dissection with a haemostat working from each

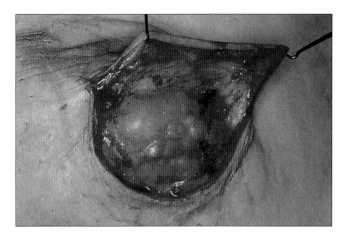

Fig. 18.30 The areolar flap is elevated in the subvenous plane.

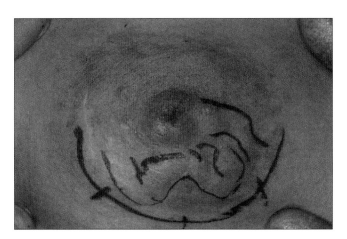

Fig. 18.29 Incision for major duct excision, exactly at the areolar margin.

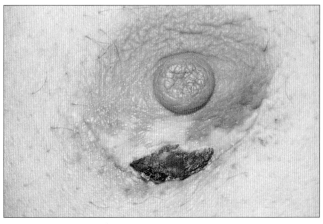

Fig. 18.31 Partial areola necrosis and depigmentation due to dissection of the flap in too superficial a plane.

side (at 3 o'clock and 9 o'clock, respectively) to meet in the middle behind the ducts (Fig. 18.32).

This can be done in the correct plane without great difficulty because both the ductal tissue and the skin of the areola are tough structures and the subcutaneous fat represents the path of least resistance.

The core of ductal tissue is grasped by a forceps passed through the subareolar tunnel. The ducts are divided on the forceps to ensure that an inverted nipple is not damaged by this manoeuvre (Fig. 18.33).

With retraction on the forceps, the ductal mass is dissected back into the breast for a distance of 3 cm or so and then transsected. During this process, any bleeding vessels should be caught and diathermied before they retract back into the breast substance.

It is not uncommon for ducts to remain dilated at the site of transsection. Attention is drawn to the undersurface of the nipple to ensure that the terminal ducts are removed completely. The nipple is fully inverted and stretched over the tip of the index finger and the remaining duct tissue excised with scissors (Fig. 18.34).

This manoeuvre also ensures that no ducts are missed, as can happen if the tunnelling traverses the duct mass rather than the subcutaneous plane, leaving some ducts at the far side of the incision.

If dissection is complete, the nipple will usually resume the everted position. If there is any tendency to re-invert, a further examination should be made to ensure that all ductal tissue has been excised, and a loose purse-string with a fine absorbable suture may be placed around its base (a tight purse-string suture may produce nipple ischaemia).

Sometimes, the centre of a deeply inverted nipple is thickened, keratotic and contains dilated terminal ducts, and cannot be everted satisfactorily after duct division. It may then be best to excise, in a conservative fashion, the central portion of the nipple and close the defect with one or two fine sutures. This central portion needs to be only 5 mm or so in diameter; the tough fibromuscular layer of the nipple with overlying skin maintains the shape of the nipple and gives a satisfactory result.

Drainage and closure

In the absence of infection, the wound is closed with a 4-0 subcuticular suture. Some authors recommend obliteration of the subareolar cavity by a series of approximat-

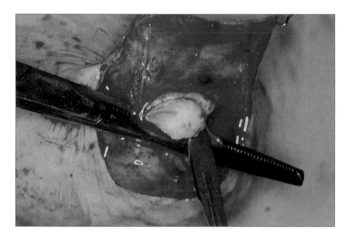

Fig. 18.33 The ducts are divided immediately below the nipple by cutting on to the forceps.

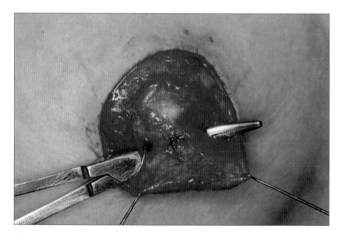

Fig. 18.32 A subareolar tunnel is formed behind the ducts by blunt dissection, and a forceps passed through the tunnel to grasp the ducts.

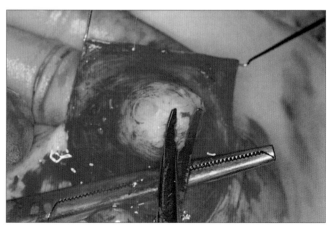

Fig. 18.34 Any residual terminal duct tissue is removed after inverting the nipple over the index finger.

ing purse-string sutures but we omit this step and have not found it to be a disadvantage. The cosmetic result of this operation is excellent when there has been little or no tissue destruction before surgery (see Fig. 11.21). When the operation is performed after extensive sepsis the cosmetic result is likely to be less satisfactory.

In the presence of overt or recent infection, the wound should not be closed, primarily because of a considerable risk of postoperative infection. This predisposes to nipple necrosis or chronic infection leading to sinus formation. It is best to pack the wound with a non-adherent dressing. In some situations, where extensive sepsis extends into the breast, it may be satisfactory to close the periareolar portion of the incision and leave a radial portion of the incision open for counter-drainage.

There is evidence for a role for bacterial infection in these abscesses. This raises the question of whether they may be safely closed primarily in the presence of adequate antibiotic therapy. If this is done, the minimum spectrum of cover should be that of anaerobic organisms and Gram-positive cocci. Metronidazole and flucloxacillin or Augmentin® seem to be satisfactory regimens. Where the infection has been well controlled by antibiotics and prior drainage so that only a track remains, we close the wound after excision of this track under antibiotic cover. Hence, our preference is for two-stage management of abscesses where possible: preliminary conservative drainage, followed by major duct excision later with primary closure under antibiotic cover.

There does not seem to be any carcinogenic risk from leaving the peripheral ducts in situ. Urban found only seven cancers developing in his 434 patients having duct excision and followed for 2–14 years. Three were in situ and four infiltrating.

Drainage of a lactational breast abscess

This is indicated when repeated percutaneous aspiration has not given rapid resolution, or when the overlying skin is compromised. It should be performed under general anaesthetic. Antibiotic cover is given if there is surrounding widespread cellulitis; otherwise, it is unnecessary. In the vast majority of cases, a curvilinear incision parallel to the areola should be made over the area of maximum tenderness after confirmation of the presence of pus by ultrasound or needle aspiration (Fig. 18.35).

The abscess is usually multilocular and these loculi will need to be broken down with the finger but without

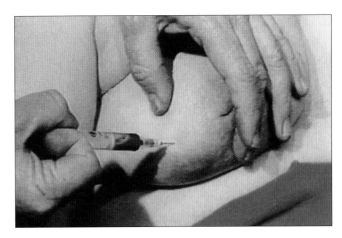

Fig. 18.35 The presence of pus should always be confirmed by needle aspiration or ultrasound before proceeding to open drainage of an abscess.

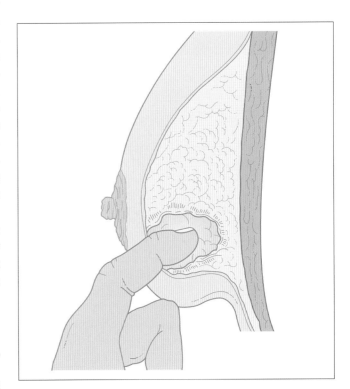

Fig. 18.36 All loculi must be broken down with an exploring finger.

unnecessary disturbance of the uninvolved breast tissue (Fig. 18.36).

The skin incision should be adequate – at least three-quarters of the diameter of the abscess (Fig. 18.37). The cavity is then lightly packed with a non-adherent dressing. Tight packing must be avoided as it interferes

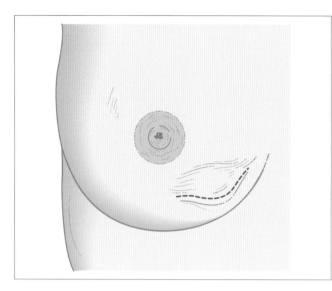

with drainage. After a day, the pack should be replaced. The cavity rapidly fills and healing is usually complete by 2–3 weeks provided the incision is generous and the wound is pyramidal shaped. Treated in this way there is surprisingly little deformity of the breast.

Subcutaneous mastectomy in male patients

This is indicated in a minority of patients with gynaecomastia, where gross degrees of breast enlargement are causing cosmetic and psychological trauma, and in cases where there is no underlying correctable cause and which have not responded to hormone therapy (see Ch. 16).

Important principles

- Submammary incision should be used for very large volumes of breast tissue.
- Periareolar incisions are preferred for moderate gynaecomastia.
- Splitting the breast tissue down to the pectoral fascia gives mobility which facilitates dissection.
- Leave a modest amount of subcutaneous fat and breast tissue adherent to the areola with closure as a separate layer beneath the nipple.

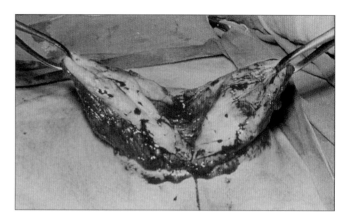

Fig. 18.38 Excision of gynaecomastia through a periareolar incision is facilitated by splitting the breast tissue cone into two (or four) pieces.

- It is not easy to obtain a good cosmetic result, especially with grosser and dependent examples of gynaecomastia. For this reason, adjuvant liposuction[34] and more complex plastic procedures are being used.

Technique

A periareolar incision is made around the lower half of the circumference. It is often necessary to extend this laterally for a short distance to achieve adequate haemostasis. Alternatively, an inframammary incision may be used, although this is cosmetically less satisfactory, especially in young patients who have a greater tendency to keloid formation. In practice, the periareolar incision is best in young patients and a submammary incision in elderly, obese patients with dependent breast tissue.

The nipple is elevated with much greater difficulty than is the case in the female breast because the fibroglandular tissue of gynaecomastia is adherent to the areola. A small amount of subcutaneous fat and adherent breast tissue is left behind the nipple, both to avoid damage to the nipple (much more easily done than might be thought) and to improve the cosmetic result by preserving normal nipple protrusion. The amount of tissue left behind the nipple is a matter of judgement and experience.

The flaps are dissected only a small distance upwards and downwards in a deep subcutaneous plane, so that a considerable thickness of subcutaneous fat is retained. The breast cone is then grasped and split transversely down to the pectoral fascia. (Fig. 18.38)

Upper and lower halves are dissected from the pectoral fascia upwards and downwards, respectively, so that the flap dissection is completed with a much more mobile breast cone. With very marked gynaecomastia, the breast cone can be quartered rather than halved and this further facilitates dissection through a small periareolar incision. It is important to dissect superficial to the pectoral fascia, as its preservation ensures that the skin retains its mobility. Haemostasis is obtained as the dissection proceeds because it is difficult to obtain adequate access to the periphery of the depth of the wound once the tissues have retracted after the breast has been removed.

Haematomas are a common complication of this procedure[35,36] when done through a periareolar incision and, in cases where haemostasis is excessively difficult, a lateral extension of the wound should be made to give adequate access (Fig. 18.39) and lighted retractors used. Other complications include seromas, infections, sensory changes and poor cosmesis. A suction drain is usually inserted and the wound closed with a subcuticular absorbable suture. Drains appear to be associated with increased morbidity.[36] The drain can be removed as soon as drainage is reduced to a small quantity, usually on the first postoperative day.

Subcutaneous mastectomy or skin sparing mastectomy in women

Important principles

- Think carefully about the validity of the indications for the operation.
- Accept the risk of skin or nipple necrosis where many previous biopsy scars are present.

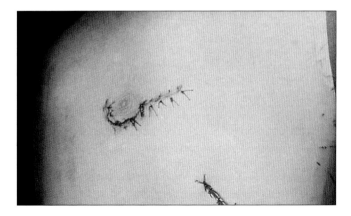

Fig. 18.39 A lateral extension to a periareolar wound impairs cosmesis, but may be necessary to give adequate access.

- Use an incision which will allow removal of all breast tissue, including the axillary tail and central nipple ducts.

Technique

This operation is very rarely indicated for non-malignant conditions. It should not be undertaken lightly. It is, however, being used increasingly as a treatment for women who need a mastectomy for widespread ductal carcinoma in situ and as prophylactic treatment for women with genetic abnormalities, i.e. carriers of BRCA1 and BRCA2 mutations. It is a difficult procedure to perform and guarantee complete removal of breast tissue with minimal complications. Only a basic account of operative detail is given here.

There are many possible complications, especially in a breast scarred by numerous previous biopsies. Incision needs to be planned to take account of these scars which may predispose to skin necrosis. A circumareolar incision or submammary incision is used most commonly. However, it should be recognized that total excision of the breast tissue (especially the axillary tail) is not achieved through a small submammary incision. For this reason, we prefer a periareolar incision with a lateral extension because it is important that all breast tissue be excised, particularly when the operation is being carried out for preinvasive conditions or prophylaxis.

The procedure differs from the operation in the male in that the nipple–areola complex and all the tissue behind the nipple needs to be removed to eliminate the terminal ducts. If the nipple–areola complex is preserved, the areola can be elevated without difficulty in the female. This is, however, a controversial area if the surgery is being performed for prophylaxis. The plane between the subcutaneous tissue and the breast tissue is usually dissected with scissors or diathermy. It is important that all the breast tissue is removed and this extends further medially, superiorly and laterally than may be anticipated.

The most troublesome part of the dissection is the axillary tail, and breast tissue is very often left in this region. The axillary tail is best defined by blunt dissection and its limit defined by palpation. A curved haemostat should be placed around the axillary tissue at its upper level. Meticulous haemostasis is especially important to avoid haematoma; lighted retractors help in achieving this. It is advisable to insert at least two suction drains at the completion of this procedure. In appropriate cases, a tissue expander may be inserted into a subpectoral pocket for reconstruction or this may be combined with a myocutaneous flap such as a latissimus dorsi flap or transverse rectus abdominis myocutaneous flap (TRAM). The skin is closed with a subcuticular suture.

Complications

The main complication of subcutaneous mastectomy is haematoma formation, resulting from inadequate haemostasis associated with the use of small incisions. Skin flap or nipple necrosis is not uncommon, particularly in patients who have had multiple previous biopsies.

The inevitable consequence of leaving ductal tissue under the nipple is the risk of cancer developing in the major ducts, a risk which is not just theoretical.[37] Similarly, the development of late cancer due to residual breast tissue left in the periphery of the breast can be a problem.[38] Where the operation is being done for prophylaxis against the development of cancer, this possibility should be considered carefully at the time of surgery. Total removal of breast tissue is necessary but not easily achieved through conventional cosmetic incisions, and should usually be combined with removal of the nipple–areola complex.

In spite of these problems, a modest result is often satisfactory to the patient, although individual patients will react very differently to similar cosmetic results.

Operations for inverted nipples

A surgeon setting out to correct congenital inverted nipples, or secondarily inverted nipples, has a wide variety of procedures from which to choose, and new approaches continue to appear in the literature in large numbers.

Such a wide choice makes it difficult to choose any individual technique and also suggests that no particular method is satisfactory. This is confirmed by the paucity of papers reporting large series of cases with long-term follow-up.

On general principles, one would expect that a successful procedure would need to deal with the underlying pathology, which is poor development or fibrotic shortening of the major ducts. This can only be corrected by transecting the ducts completely.

Reported techniques fall into two main groups:

1. Those which correct by pulling on the ducts and attempt to hold them out, by sutures or by providing an underlying buttress of tissue.
2. Those that divide the ducts completely and then use one of the methods in (1) to hold the nipple everted.[39,40] Although these reports are of small numbers with little follow-up, they at least meet the basic principles.

In our experience, major duct excision, combined if necessary with excision of the central core of the nipple, will cure inverted nipples without any additional buttressing procedures. Hence, our recommendation is that this operation, performed as described earlier in this chapter, is the procedure of choice, provided the patient is aware that she will be unable to breastfeed following this procedure.

In the absence of long-term follow-up, those procedures which do not divide the ducts must be considered unproven. It is also possible that some conservative procedures divide the ducts without recognizing it, so details of subsequent breastfeeding should accompany long-term results of operation for nipple inversion.

REFERENCES

1. Martin HE & Ellis EB. Biopsy by needle puncture and aspiration. *Annals of Surgery* 1930; **92**: 169–181.
2. Stewart FW. The diagnosis of tumours by aspiration. *American Journal of Pathology* 1933; **9**: 801–808.
3. Franzen S & Zajicek D. Aspiration biopsy in diagnosis of palpable lesions of the breast: critical review of 3479 consecutive biopsies. *Acta Radiologica* (Therapy) 1968; **7**: 241–262.
4. Webb AJ. The diagnostic cytology of breast carcinoma. *British Journal of Surgery* 1970; **57**: 259–264.
5. Bates AT, Bates T, Hastrich DJ *et al.* Delay in the diagnosis of breast cancer. The effect of the introduction of fine needle aspiration cytology to the breast clinic. *European Journal of Surgical Oncology* 1992; **18**: 433–437.
6. Dixon JM, Scott WN & Miller RW. Natural history of cystic disease: the importance of cyst type. *British Journal of Surgery* 1985; **72**: 190–192.
7. Gateley CA, Maddox PR & Mansel RE. Pneumothorax: a complication of fine needle aspiration of the breast. *British Medical Journal* 1991; **303**: 627–628.

8. Catania S, Veronesi P, Marassi A *et al.* Risk of pneumothorax after FNA of the breast: Italian experience of more than 200,000 aspirations. *The Breast* 1993; **2:** 246–247.

9. Kaufman Z, Shpitz B, Shapiro M *et al.* Pneumothorax: a complication of FNA of breast tumours. *Acta Cytologica* 1994; **38:** 737–738.

10. Whitaker IS, Elmiyeh B, Siddiqui MN *et al.* Haemopneumothorax after fine needle aspiration of the breast. *Journal of the Royal Society of Medicine* 2003; **96:** 555–556.

11. Horobin JM, Matthew BM, Preece PE *et al.* Effects of fine needle aspiration on subsequent mammograms. *British Journal of Surgery* 1992; **79:** 52–54.

12. McMahon AJ, Lufty AM, Matthew A *et al.* Needle core biopsy of the breast with a spring-loaded device. *British Journal of Surgery* 1992; **79:** 1042–1045.

13. Roberts JG, Preece PE, Bolton PM *et al.* The Trucut biopsy in breast cancer. *Clinical Oncology* 1975; **1:** 287–303.

14. de Lucena CE, Dos Santos JL Jr, deLima Resende CA *et al.* Ultrasound-guided core needle biopsy of breast masses: How many cores are necessary to diagnose cancer? *Journal of Clinical Ultrasound* 2007; **30:** 363–366

15. Mathew J, Crawford DJ, Lwin M *et al.* Ultrasound-guided vacuum assisted excision in the diagnosis and treatment of clinically benign breast lesions. *Annals of the Royal College of Surgeons of England* 2007; **89:** 494–495.

16. Plantade R, Hammou JC, Gerard F *et al.* Ultrasound-guided vacuum assisted biopsy: review of 382 cases. *Journal of Radiology* 2005; **86:** 1003–1015.

17. Robertson JLA. The choice of incision for biopsy in large breasted women. *South African Journal of Surgery* 1980; **18:** 9–12.

18. Pezner RD, Lorant JA, Terz J *et al.* Wound healing complications following biopsy of the irradiated breast. *Archives of Surgery* 1992; **127:** 321–324.

19. Guidelines for surgeons in the management of screen-detected breast disease in the United Kingdom (1995).

20. Thind CR, Desmond S, Harris O *et al.* Radio-guided localization of clinically occult lesions (ROLL): a DGH experience. *Clinical Radiology* 2005; **60:** 681–686.

21. Helvie MA, Ikeda DM & Adler DD. Localization and needle aspiration of breast lesions: complications in 370 cases. *American Journal of Roentgenology* 1991; **157:** 711–714.

22. Rappaport W, Thompson S, Wong R *et al.* Complications associated with needle localization biopsy of the breast. *Surgery, Gynecology and Obstetrics* 1991; **172:** 303–306.

23. Thomas JG. *New York Medical Journal* 1882; **XXV:** 337.

24. Burton S, Li WY, Himpson R *et al.* Microdochectomy in women aged over 50 years. *Annals of the Royal College of Surgeons of England* 2003; **85:** 47–49.

25. Richards T, Hunt A, Courtney S and Umeh H. Nipple discharge: a sign of breast cancer? *Annals of the Royal College of Surgeons of England* 2007; **89:** 124–126.

26. Beechey-Newman N, Kulkarni D, Kothari A *et al.* Breast duct microendoscopy in nipple discharge: microbush improves cytology. *Surgical Endoscopy* 2005; **12:** 1648–1651.

27. Govindarajulu S, Nareddy SR, Shere MH *et al.* Sonographically guided mammotome excision of ducts in the diagnosis and management of single duct nipple discharge. *European Journal of Surgical Oncology* 2006; **32:** 725–728.

28. Atkins HJB. Mammillary fistula. *British Medical Journal* 1955; **2:** 1473–1474.

29. Hanavadi S, Pereira G & Mansel RE. How mamillary fistulas should be managed. *Breast Journal* 2005; **11:** 254–256.

30. Lannin DR. Twenty-two year experience with recurring subareolar abscess and lactiferous duct fistula treated by a single breast surgeon. *American Journal of Surgery* 2004; **188:** 407–410.

31. Hadfield GJ. Excision of the major duct system for benign disease of the breast. *British Journal of Surgery* 1960; **47:** 472–477.

32. Urban JA. Excision of the major duct system of the breast. *Cancer* 1963; **16:** 516–520.

33. Srivastava A, Griwan MS, Samaiyar SS *et al.* A safe technique of major mammary duct excision. *Journal of the Royal College of Surgeons of Edinburgh* 1995; **40:** 35–37.

34. Hodgson EL, Fruhstorfer BH & Malata CM. Ultrasonic liposuction in the treatment of gynaecomastia. *Plastic and Reconstructive Surgery* 2005; **116:** 646–653.

35. Gabra HO, Moarbito A, Bianchi A *et al.* Gynaecomastia in the adolescent: a surgically relevant condition. *European Journal of Paediatric Surgery* 2004; **14:** 3–6.

36. Steele SR, Martin MJ & Place RJ. Gynaecomastia: complications of the subcutaneous mastectomy. *American Surgeon* 2002; **68:** 210–213.

37. Srivastava A & Webster DJT. Isolated nipple recurrence 17 years after subcutaneous mastectomy for breast cancer – a case report. *European Journal of Surgical Oncology* 1987; **13:** 459–461.

38. Sacchini V, Pinotti JA, Barros AC *et al.* Nipple sparing mastectomy for breast cancer and risk reduction: oncologic or technical problem. *Journal of the American College of Surgeons* 2006; **203:** 704–714.

39. Hartrampf CR & Schneider WJ. A simple direct method for correction of inversion of the nipple. *Plastic and Reconstructive Surgery* 1976; **58:** 678–679.

40. Broadbent TR & Woolf RM. Benign inverted nipple. Trans nipple areola correction. *Plastic and Reconstructive Surgery* 1976; **58:** 673–677.

CHAPTER 19

Psychological aspects of benign breast disease

Key points and new developments

1. Patients presenting to breast clinics have a high degree of anxiety. This is related mainly to fear of cancer and resolves when a benign diagnosis is found.

2. Attending for breast screening is associated with short-term anxiety.

3. Patients presenting with moderate to severe mastalgia fall into two broad groups: those accepting reassurance and those requesting treatment. The first group have scores for anxiety and depression similar to controls. The second group have cyclical variation in anxiety and depression scores, reaching pathological levels in the luteal period. It is not clear whether these luteal phase changes are the result of the pain or the cause.

4. Dermatitis artefacta of the breast is an uncommon expression of an underlying psychological problem.

Introduction

Following the recognition in the 1970s that breast cancer treatment was associated with significant psychosocial morbidity, an extensive body of literature has developed on a variety of psychological aspects related to breast cancer. In contrast, the literature on the psychological aspects of benign breast disease is scanty. Benign breast disease (BBD) cases are studied purely to act as 'normal' controls for the cancer cases.

A complex relationship exists between an individual's psychological state, physical well-being and underlying personality. Presented with an anxious patient complaining of breast symptoms, it can be difficult to decide whether the primary problem is somatic or psychological. Three areas have been regarded as contributing to the psychological dimensions of benign breast disease: personality, stress and mood.

The earliest suggestion that a breast condition could result from psychological causes came from Sir Astley Cooper, who described women who suffered from cyclical breast pain as being 'of an irritable and suggestive nature'.[1] Atkins considered that 'chronic mastitis' was the result of endocrine factors, neuralgic factors and psychological factors.[2] He felt that endocrine factors were the least important and postulated that the 'seed of psychological pain' lay in the woman's awareness of the breast as a common site for cancer. In 1949, Patey rejected the concept of chronic mastitis and classified benign breast disease as 'cystic diseases of the breast' and the 'pain syndrome'.[3] The latter he felt to be a 'subjective disorder' resulting from an exaggeration of the normal premenstrual feeling of engorgement and sensitivities of the breast. He, too, thought that the fear of cancer played a major role in the aetiology of the disorder but felt that a small proportion might be purely psychological in origin and might result from the patient being 'sexually maladjusted with her husband'. The view that breast pain had a psychological origin was commonly held until 1978 when Preece et al.[4] measured the neuroticism scores in women presenting with cyclical mastalgia using the

Middlesex Hospital Questionnaire (MHQ). They found no difference between women with cyclical mastalgia and women presenting at the varicose veins clinic, although both were significantly different from female psychiatric out-patients. They concluded that there was no evidence of psychological abnormality in women with breast pain.

More recent studies have examined the patient's mood or the external stress which she is experiencing. These latter studies have the advantage of examining clearly definable parameters. Studies on the interrelationship of psychological factors and breast disease now use well-accepted, independently validated measurement instruments.[5] It is then clearer that there are definite patterns of psychological morbidity associated with benign breast disease.

Psychological problems resulting from presenting with breast problems

The commonest interaction between benign breast disease and the psychological state is the development of anxiety as a result of breast symptoms. Patients presenting to breast clinics have a high level of anxiety irrespective of their subsequent diagnosis.[6] While most studies do not specifically explore the reasons for that anxiety, it is apparent that most patients are worried that they might have breast cancer. This may in fact delay a woman presenting to her doctor. One study has shown that women of younger age, lower income, with less education and a fatalistic view of developing breast cancer may delay seeking help.[7] Other characteristics of women who delay referral are: the absence of a lump, a lower perceived risk, not wanting to think about breast symptoms.[8] People who are more likely to seek advice have a negative view of delay and are feeling fearful.[7]

These days, most diagnostic procedures are performed in the out-patient clinic and most do not need surgical intervention. Ubhi et al. in 1996 measured the levels of anxiety in those women receiving immediate or delayed results of fine needle aspiration cytology (FNAC).[9] This study showed that both groups had high anxiety levels initially but if the result was subsequently benign there was a greater fall in the anxiety score if the result was received at the same visit. If the result was malignant then there was no difference in the anxiety score between receiving results immediately or delayed for a few days. A similar study looked at women attending a breast clinic

where core biopsies were done so results were received 3 days later.[10] Women with an initially low level of anxiety tended to sustain that until results were received. Those with moderate and high levels of anxiety had sustained anxiety, depression, uncertainty and confusion until the results were received. Coping was done by 'emotion focused' strategies such as 'diversion' and 'social support'. Qualitative data suggested that a delayed-result clinic structure may facilitate psychological preparation for the results, especially if they were malignant.

The anxiety levels of women who undergo open surgical biopsy for benign breast disease remain high until the results of the biopsy are known, at which time they fall to the expected levels for the general population.[11] In one study, women waiting for breast biopsy were compared with a group of women waiting for cholecystectomy. The highest levels of anxiety were found in women who subsequently were found to have benign breast disease. The women with breast cancer had the same levels of anxiety as the cholecystectomy group.[12] A similar finding was noted in a retrospective study of women who had had a breast biopsy for benign disease up to 2 years previously.[13] Fifty-eight per cent recalled severe amounts of anxiety during the period between discovery of an abnormality and the final diagnosis. The mean length of time from discovery to diagnosis was 35 days. Curiously, there was no relationship between the length of delay from discovery to diagnosis and the level of anxiety experienced. Andrykowski et al.[14] showed that in a group of women undergoing a diagnostic biopsy, breast cancer specific distress was greater at baseline compared with normal healthy controls and although it declined after a benign diagnosis was made it remained elevated compared with controls 8 months later. The longer-term effects of this period of anxiety are unknown and it seemed reasonable to try to shorten this period of uncertainty as much as possible. This was the main justification for the introduction of rapid diagnosis clinics.

Witek-Janusek et al.[15] found that as well as changes to stress, anxiety and mood, women undergoing a breast biopsy also had immunological changes such as a decrease in natural killer cell activity and cytokine dysregulation which persist for at least a month after the procedure.

Women undergoing a breast biopsy, either in a clinic or in theatre, have information needs. The most important question is a need to know when they will receive the result and the next need is for information about their risk of developing breast cancer.[16] Some women, however, are not reassured even after a benign biopsy. These women tend to have higher levels of health anxiety, perceived stress, a fear of breast cancer treatments and general anxiety. They are also more likely to have school education only, to have presented with symptoms of a change of shape or dimpling and be found to have breast pain or a benign cyst.[17]

Of women recalled for further assessment from breast screening programmes, a study showed that 46% had borderline or clinically significant anxiety which decreased significantly in a few days if the diagnosis was normal or benign. Distress remained relatively high if a surgical biopsy was needed.[18] In these cases, the anxiety is generated by concerns about cancer and not by any underlying psychological problem, and it does not give rise to long-term morbidity. Some patients, however, are put on 'early recall', for review in a few months for an abnormality which is probably benign. There is more anxiety associated with this compared to routine recall in 3 years[19] but there is less stress associated with 'early recall' with mammographic review compared with having a biopsy performed.[20] It can be argued that short-term morbidity which resolves rapidly after the confirmation of a benign diagnosis is of little importance, but such patients do have a persistent increased awareness of the possibility of developing breast cancer.[21,22] After women have been screened once, they are usually more positive about screening and are more likely to attend again, but if the experience has not been satisfactory then they are less likely to re-attend.[23]

There is some evidence of a permanent behaviour change following benign breast biopsy.[24] Women who have undergone benign biopsies are more likely to carry out regular breast self-examination than the general population, suggesting a higher level of specific anxiety. Another study, however, showed contrasting results of a decrease in breast self-examination (BSE) but this was particularly evident for younger women, those who lacked confidence in how to do BSE and women who had discovered their initial lump by self-examination.[25]

Psychological abnormality as a cause of benign breast disease

Cyclical mastalgia

Cyclical breast pain is common. In population surveys, more than 60% of women report that they have experienced cyclical mastalgia which they grade as severe.[26,27]

Despite the findings of Preece et al.,[4] there are difficulties in accepting the organic explanation as the entire explanation for the syndrome. Only 3–10% present for treatment, which raises the question of what precipitates that presentation. Some are concerned that the symptom is a sign of underlying disease. Such women can be reassured by clinical assessment and an explanation of the reason for their symptoms. Other women remain adamant that they need treatment. No difference between the two groups can be detected in the severity of the pain and an alternative explanation must be sought.

One study examined two groups of women presenting to the breast pain clinic complaining of cyclical mastalgia.[28] Both groups had moderate to severe mastalgia. One group was reassured by their examination at the clinic and did not require any treatment, but the other group requested treatment despite being told they had no serious condition affecting their breasts. Both groups were compared with a control group of similar age who did not have any breast symptoms.

All the women completed a series of questionnaires in the follicular and luteal phases of the menstrual cycle. The women who had cyclical mastalgia but did not want treatment had results for anxiety and depression similar to those for the control group of women. Their results for state anxiety, trait anxiety and depression were within the limits expected for the general population and did not alter significantly with their cycle. In contrast, the women who requested treatment had a marked cyclical variation in their levels of anxiety and depression and in the luteal phase these levels were in the pathological range. Similar levels of anxiety were found by Ramirez et al. in their study, but they did not look for cyclical variation.[29] The patients' psychosocial adjustment was assessed using the Psychosocial Adjustment to Illness Scale (PAIS). This showed a marked impairment of social functioning which improved in those women responding to therapy, suggesting that at least some of the distress is a result of the pain rather than a cause. However, both Downey and Ramirez found that effective pain relief (using goserelin) did not result in elimination of anxiety.[28,29]

It is not clear, therefore, whether the mood disturbance is the primary problem or whether it is secondary to an underlying hormonal disorder. It appears that the majority of women regard cyclical mastalgia as normal and it only becomes a problem when it is associated with mood disturbance.

Dermatitis artefacta

Occasionally, patients present with persistent ulceration of the breast which defies diagnosis. Biopsy reveals chronic inflammation without any specific features and local measures fail to alleviate the problem. Even excision of the lesion with primary closure is followed by further breakdown. In these circumstances a diagnosis of dermatitis artefacta should be considered.[30,31] The ulcer often has a bizarre and atypical shape but there is no specific diagnostic feature other than the failure to respond to therapy. Features that may raise suspicion are: presence of foreign material within the wound and an early request for mastectomy without apparent concern. It is usually a diagnosis after exclusion of other pathologies. Total occlusion by dressings may result in temporary healing but recurrence is common.

When there are grounds for suspecting a diagnosis of dermatitis artefacta, the opinion of a clinical psychologist or psychiatrist should be sought. The condition can often be cured by directly challenging the patient with the possibility that she is producing the injury herself. Almost always, the patient will deny this but will stop aggravating the lesion, which will rapidly heal. Unfortunately, if it proves impossible to deal satisfactorily with the underlying psychological problem, she is likely to re-present with other psychosomatic problems.

REFERENCES

1. Cooper, Sir Astley. *Illustrations of Diseases of the Breast.* London: Longmans; 1823:(part 1)3, 78–79.

2. Atkins HJB. Chronic mastitis. *Lancet* 1938; **1**: 707–712.

3. Patey DH. Two common non-malignant conditions of the breast. The clinical features of cystic disease and the pain syndrome. *British Medical Journal* 1949; **1**: 96–99.

4. Preece PE, Mansel RE & Hughes LE. Mastalgia: psychoneurosis or organic disease? *British Medical Journal* 1978; **1**: 29–30.

5. Leinster SJ. How to measure psychological morbidity in women with benign breast disease. In: *Proceedings of the 4th International Symposium of Benign Breast Disease.* Casterton: Parthenon; 1991:191–195.

6. Heim E, Augustiny KF, Blaser A *et al.* Coping with breast cancer – a longitudinal prospective study. *Psychotherapy and Psychosomatics* 1987; **48**: 44–59.

7. Facione NC, Dodd MJ, Hozemer W *et al.* Helpseeking for self-discovered breast symptoms. Implications for early detection. *Cancer Practice* 1997; **54**: 220–227.

8. Friedman LC, Kalidas M, Elledge R *et al.* Medical and psychological predictors of delay in seeking medical consultation for breast symptoms in women in a public sector setting. *Journal of Behavioural Medicine* 2006; **29**: 327–334.

9. Ubhi SS, Shaw P, Wright S *et al.* Anxiety in patients with symptomatic breast disease: effects of immediate versus delayed communication of results. *Annals of the Royal College of Surgeons of England* 1996; **78**: 466–469.

10. Poole K, Hood K, Davis BD *et al.* Psychological distress associated with waiting for results of diagnostic investigations for breast disease. *Breast* 1999; **8**: 334–338.

11. Ashcroft JJ, Slade PD & Leinster SJ. Psychological aspects of breast cancer treatment. In: Karras E (ed.). *Current Issues in Clinical Psychology,* vol 3. New York: Plenum; 1986.

12. Hughson AV, Cooper AF, McArdle CS *et al.* Psychosocial morbidity in patients awaiting breast biopsy. *Journal of Psychomatic Research* 1988; **32**: 173–180.

13. Benedict S, Williams RD & Baron PL. Recalled anxiety: from discovery to diagnosis of a benign breast mass. *Oncology Nursing Forum* 1994; **21**: 1467–1475.

14. Andrykowski MA, Carpenter JS, Studts JL *et al.* Psychological impact of benign breast biopsy: a longitudinal comparative study. *Health Psychology* 2002; **21**: 485–494.

15. Witek-Janusek L, Gabram S & Mathews HL. Psychologic stress, reduced NK cell activity and cytokine dysregulation in women experiencing diagnostic breast biopsy. *Psychoneuroendocrinology* 2007; **32**: 22–35.

16. Deane KA & Degner LF. Information needs, uncertainty and anxiety in women who had a breast biopsy with benign outcome. *Cancer Nursing* 1998; **21**: 117–126.

17. Meecham GT, Collins JP, Moss-Morris RE *et al.* Who is not reassured following benign diagnosis of breast symptoms? *Psychooncology* 2005; **14**: 239–246.

18. Gram IT, Lund E & Slenker SE. Quality of life following a false positive mammogram. *British Journal of Cancer* 1990; **62**: 1018–1022.

19. Ong G, Austoker J & Brett J. Breast screening: adverse psychological consequences one month after placing women on early recall because of a diagnostic uncertainty. A multicentre study. *Journal of Medical Screening* 1997; **4**: 158–168.

20. Lindfors KK, O'Connor J, Acredolo CR *et al.* Short-interval follow-up mammography versus immediate core biopsy of benign breast lesions: assessment of patient stress. *American Journal of Roentgenology* 1998; **171**: 55–58.

21. Bull AR & Campbell MJ. Assessment of the psychological impact of a breast screening programme. *British Journal of Radiology* 1991; **64**: 510–515.

22. Lampic C, Thurfjell E, Bergh J *et al.* Short and long term anxiety and depression in women recalled after breast screening. *European Journal of Cancer* 2001; **37**: 463–469.

23. Drossaert CH, Boer H & Seydel ER. Does mammographic screening and a negative result affect attitudes towards future breast screening? *Journal of Medical Screening* 2001; **8**: 204–212.

24. Benedict S, Williams RD & Baron PL. The effect of benign breast biopsy on subsequent breast cancer detection practices. *Oncology Nursing Forum* 1994; **21**: 1467–1475.

25. Beacham AO, Carpenter JS & Andrykowski MA. Impact of benign breast biopsy upon breast self-examination. *Preventative Medicine* 2004; **38**: 723–731.

26. Leinster SJ, Whitehouse GH & Walsh PV. Clinical mastalgia: clinical and mammographic observations in a screened population. *British Journal of Surgery* 1987; **74**: 220–222.

27. Maddox P & Mansel R. The treatment of mastalgia. *Breast News* 1988; **2**: 4–6.

28. Downey HM & Leinster SJ. Mood changes – an explanation why women request treatment for clinical mastalgia. In: Mansel RE (ed.). *Recent Developments in the Study of Benign Breast Disease.* London: Parthenon; 1993:117–132.

29. Ramirez AJ, Jarrett SR, Hamed H *et al.* Psychosocial distress associated with severe mastalgia. In: Mansel RE (ed.). *Recent Developments in the Study of Benign Breast Disease.* London: Parthenon; 1993:109–116.

30. Puig L, Perez M, Llaurado A *et al.* Factitial dermatosis of the breast: a possible dermatologic manifestation of Munchausen's syndrome. *Cutis* 1989; **44**: 292–294.

31. Farrier JN & Mansel RE. Dermatitis artefacta of the breast: a series of case reports *European Journal of Surgical Oncology* 2002; **28**: 189–192

CHAPTER 20

Risk assessment and management

Gareth Evans

Summary

We have not previously discussed the issue of familial breast cancer risk in this text, but there have been so many new findings in this area since the discovery of primary cancer predisposing genes, and the increasing importance of features such as breast density, that are related to benign breast disease that the editors have felt it important to include a full chapter on this topic.

The last 16 years has seen the burgeoning development of genetic risk assessment and 'family history' clinics to deal with the ever increasing demand for service by women at increased risk by virtue of their family history. While these clinics were originally based in a few major centres, the demand is such that management of moderate-risk women needs to be carried out in local units. A system of triage has developed in the UK with average-risk women being reassured in primary care, moderate-risk women receiving assessment in local units and high-risk women being referred to the regional cancer genetics centre. While mammography and MRI screening continue to be evaluated in the moderate- and high-risk categories, genetic testing for a minority of high-risk women is now in routine practice and surgical management options have gained validity. Much research is still necessary to improve early detection and develop non-surgical means of prevention.

Breast cancer: the disease

Breast cancer is the commonest cancer affecting women. One in 10 women will develop the disease in their lifetime in the UK and as many as one in eight in the USA. Every year 44 000 women develop the disease in England and Wales and 13 000 die from it (Cancer Research UK statistics). The UK used to have a poor record on survival compared to the rest of Europe and the USA. However, this has improved, with the UK one of the first to show a downward trend in breast cancer mortality. This has been followed by similar dramatic improvements in survival in Europe and North America. Nonetheless there has been little improvement in the mortality figures from breast cancer any where else in the world over the last 30 years. Two factors which have had some impact are the introduction of mammography screening, and thus early detection, and the advent of adjuvant chemotherapy.

There do appear to be racial and cultural elements in breast cancer predisposition. The disease is much less common in Chinese and other Asian groups. (Therefore a family history may be more significant here.) However, there is little evidence for increased inherited breast cancer risk according to race/ethnicity outside the rare founder populations such as the Jewish Ashkenazi and Icelandic BRCA mutations.

Risk factors

Family history

Family history can be by far the most significant factor in predisposition. While at extremes of age the relative risk can be huge, the relative risk in a woman who carries a *BRCA1/2* mutation aged 35 is higher than the risk for a 75-year-old, compared to the same 35-year-old in the general population. About 4–5% of breast cancer is thought to be due to inheritance of a high-risk dominant cancer predisposing gene.[1,2] Hereditary factors play a part in a proportion of the rest (up to 27% of breast cancer from twin studies[3,4]), but these are harder to pin down. Nonetheless, lower-risk genes are now being identified from association studies. There are no external markers of risk (no phenotype) to help identify those who carry a faulty gene, except in very rare cases such as Cowden's disease.[5] In order to assess the likelihood of there being a predisposing gene in a family, it is necessary to assess the family tree. Inheritance of a germline mutation or deletion of a predisposing gene causes the disease at a young age and often if the individual survives cancer in the contralateral breast. Some gene mutations may give rise to susceptibility to other cancers, such as ovary, sarcomas and colon.[6–10] Multiple primary cancers in one individual or related early-onset cancers in a pedigree are, therefore, suggestive of a predisposing gene. To illustrate the importance of age, it is thought that over 25% of breast cancer under 30 years is due to a mutation in a high-risk dominant gene, whereas less than 1% of the disease over 70 years is so caused.[2] The important features in a family history are therefore:

1. Age at onset
2. Bilateral disease
3. Multiple cases in the family (particularly on one side)
4. Other related early onset tumours
5. Number of unaffected individuals (large families are more informative).

There are very few families where it is possible to be certain of dominant inheritance, but where four first-degree relatives have early onset or bilateral breast cancer, the risk of inheriting a susceptibility gene for a sister or daughter is close to 50%. Epidemiological studies have shown that about 80% of mutation carriers develop breast cancer in their lifetime. Therefore, unless there is significant family history on both sides of the family, the maximum risk suggested at counselling is 40–45%. Breast cancer genes can be inherited through the father and a dominant history on the father's side of the family would give at least a 20–28% lifetime risk to his daughters.

Other risk factors

The main emphasis here is on hormonal and reproductive factors. Essentially, a woman is most protected by never ovulating. Breast cancer is, therefore, very uncommon in Turner's syndrome. The next best protection is proffered by ovulating as few times as possible before a first pregnancy. A late menarche and early first pregnancy is most protective. Pregnancy transforms breast parenchymal cells into a more stable state, where proliferation in the second half of the cycle is less. There is now good evidence that current use of the oral contraceptive and for 10 years after use there is around a 24% increase in risk.[11] The oestrogen and progesterone element of the pill, although suppressing ovulation, will still stimulate the breast cells. With a greater number of women delaying their first pregnancy by using the pill, particularly in professional classes, who may in any case be more predisposed, breast cancer incidence continues to climb. An early menopause is protective, again probably by reducing the exposure of the breast to oestrogen and progesterone. Other factors such as the number of pregnancies and breastfeeding may have a small protective effect. Hormone replacement is another area under intense debate at present. Long-term treatment (>10 years) after the menopause is associated with a significant increase in risk. However, shorter treatments may still be associated with risk to those with a family history.[12] In a large meta-analysis, the risk appeared to increase cumulatively by 1–2% per year, but disappear within 5 years of cessation.[13] It is becoming clear that the risk from combined oestrogen/progesterone hormone replacement therapy (HRT) is greater than for oestrogen only.[14–16] Interestingly the effects are less in overweight women, but these women are likely to already be at increased risk from endogenous hormone production with a relative risk of 2-fold for women who have gained 20 kg or more since aged 18 years.[17,18]

It is important to emphasize that these factors do not have an all-or-nothing effect on the breast, but may alter risks by a factor of two at the extremes.[19] Many women who have all these factors unfavourable will not develop breast cancer and some, particularly if they have a germline mutation, will develop the disease even if all are favourable. Diet may also play a part, with those on a diet low in animal fats from dairy produce and red meat being marginally less likely to develop the disease. Perhaps the greatest risk is attached to women who on biopsy are found to have proliferative disease such as atypical ductal hyperplasia.[20,21]

Risk estimation

Where there is not a dominant family history, risk estimation is based on large epidemiological studies, which give 1.5–3-fold risks with family history of a single affected relative.[1,2] Clinicians must be careful to differentiate between life time and age-specific risks. Some studies quote 9-fold or greater risk associated with bilateral disease in a mother or proliferative breast disease on biopsy. However, if these at-risk individuals are followed up for many years the risk returns toward normal levels.[20] Clearly, if one uses these risks and multiplies them on a lifetime incidence of 1 in 9–12, some women will apparently have a greater than 100% chance of having the disease. The risks do not multiply and may not even add. Perhaps the best way to assess risk is to take the strongest risk factor, which in our experience is nearly always family history. If risk is assessed on this alone, minor adjustments can be made for other factors. It is arguable whether these other factors will have a large effect on an 80% penetrant gene other than to speed up or delay the onset of breast cancer. Therefore, we can only really assume an effect on the non-hereditary element of the risk. Although studies do point to an increase in risk in family history cases associated with some factors, these may just represent an earlier expression of the gene. Generally, therefore, we will arrive at risks between 40% and 8–10%, although lower risks are occasionally given. Higher risks are only applicable when a woman at 40% genetic risk is shown to have a germline mutation, to have inherited a high-risk allele or to have proliferative breast disease.

Several methods based on currently known risk factors have been devised in order to predict risk of breast cancer in the clinic and in the general population.[22] Some depend on family history alone (e.g. the Claus and Ford models) and others depend upon hormonal and reproductive factors in addition to family history (e.g. the Gail and Tyrer-Cuzick models). Outside of risk assessment clinics where most women have sufficiently strong family histories to have a probability of harbouring mutations in BRCA1, BRCA2 and TP53 genes, it is likely that models where as many risk factors as possible are combined may be preferable. After all, only 10% of breast cancer occurs in the context of a first-degree family history of breast cancer. The Gail model accurately predicted the number of cancers in the Nurses Health Study,[23] but in our clinic, the Tyrer-Cuzick model, which depends on extent of family history and several endocrine factors, showed a better prediction than those that used fewer risk factors (Table 20.1).[24] Our own clinical assessment tool was, nonetheless, as good as Tyrer-Cuzick and significantly better than the other computer-based models.[24] Although these models have reasonably good predictive power for the number of cancer cases likely to be seen in a population, they have low discriminatory accuracy in that they

cannot positively identify which particular woman will develop breast cancer.[22,24] This is not surprising given that most of the inherited component of at least 27% from twin studies[3,4] would not be identified from family history, and the risk model cannot predict who has and has not inherited any genetic factors in a particular family. At present, most of the known non-family history risk factors are not included in risk models. In particular, perhaps the greatest factor apart from age, mammographic density,[25] is not yet included. Further studies are in progress to determine whether inclusion of additional factors into existing models, such as mammographic density, weight gain[17] and serum steroid hormone measurements,[26] will improve prediction. These are not straightforward additions, as there may be significant interactions between risk factors. Although breast density is an independent risk factor for BRCA1 and BRCA2 cancer risk[27] the density itself may be heritable and not increase risk in a similar way in the context of family history of breast cancer alone.

The breast cancer genes

There is now no doubt that there are numerous genes which will be found to predispose to breast cancer.[28] Attention thus far has been focused on the two high-risk predisposing genes; one on the long arm of chromosome 17 (BRCA1)[6] and another BRCA2[7] on the long arm of chromosome 13 (Table 20.2). They are thought to account for over 80% of highly penetrant inherited breast cancer (population frequency of approximately 0.2%).[29] It appears that the vast majority of families with breast and ovarian cancer are linked to BRCA1 and that mutations in this gene are the cause of the disease. However, breast/ovary families are not always caused by BRCA1, as up to 20% are due to mutations in BRCA2.[29] The vast majority, if not all, breast/ovarian predisposition is due to mutations in BRCA1 or BRCA2.[29] Nonetheless, if there are two or more cases of epithelial ovarian cancer in a family, that is strong evidence, in itself, that BRCA1 is likely to be involved. There is also now increasing evidence that families with BRCA1 and BRCA2 involvement have differing risks of susceptibility to ovarian cancers, although the overall cumulative lifetime risk across all the linked families is 85% for breast and 40–60% for ovarian cancer in BRCA1,[29,30] and 85% and 10–20%, respectively, for BRCA2.[31] It may well be that so-called site-specific ovarian cancer families are in fact virtually all caused by

Table 20.1 Known risk factors and their incorporation into existing risk models

	RR at extremes*	Gail	Claus	BRCAPRO Ford	Tyrer-Cuzick	BOADICEA
PREDICTION						
Amir et al.[24] validation study [E/O]		0.48	0.56	0.49	0.81	Not assessed
95% confidence interval[24]		0.54–0.90	0.59–0.99	0.52–0.80	0.85–1.41	Not assessed
PERSONAL INFORMATION						
Age (20–70)	30	Yes	Yes	Yes	Yes	Yes
Body mass index	2	No	No	No	No	No
Alcohol intake (0–4 units) daily	1.24	No	No	No	No	No
HORMONAL/REPRODUCTIVE FACTORS						
Age of menarche	2	Yes	No	No	Yes	No
Age of first live birth	3	Yes	No	No	Yes	No
Age of menopause	4	No	No	No	Yes	No
HRT use	2	No	No	No	Yes	No
OCP use	1.24	No	No	No	No	No
Breastfeeding	0.8	No	No	No	No	No
Plasma oestrogen	5	No	No	No	No	No
PERSONAL BREAST DISEASE						
Breast biopsies	2	Yes	No	No	Yes	No
Atypical ductal hyperplasia	3	Yes	No	No	Yes	No
Lobular carcinoma in situ	4	No	No	No	Yes	No
Breast density	6	No	No	No	No	No
FAMILY HISTORY						
First-degree relatives	3	Yes	Yes	Yes	Yes	Yes
Second-degree relatives	1.5	No	Yes	Yes	Yes	Yes
Third-degree relatives	No	No	No	No	Yes	Yes
Age of onset of breast cancer	3	No	Yes	Yes	Yes	Yes
Bilateral breast cancer	3	No	No	Yes	Yes	Yes
Ovarian cancer	1.5	No	No	Yes	Yes	Yes
Male breast cancer	3–5	No	No	Yes	No	Yes

E/O, expected over observed cancer ratio (all models assessed underestimated cancer occurrence).
OCP, oral contraceptive pill.
*E.g. age at menarche 9 v age at menarche 16; age at menopause 58 v age at menopause 40.

BRCA1 mutations.[32,33] Supportive evidence for this comes from the long-term follow-up of apparently site specific families,[32] new cancers in families from the UKCCCR familial ovarian cancer study[33] and linkage[34] and mutation analysis in the families.[35] Controversy still exists over the true lifetime risk associated with mutations in BRCA1/2, with population studies apparently showing risks as low as 40%,[36] but more recent large scale studies are in keeping with high levels of risk for both genes.[37]

The TP53 gene on 17p is also known to predispose to early breast cancer[8] and it is possible to look for germline mutations of this, which account for over 70% of cases of the Li Fraumeni syndrome (see Table 20.2).[38] The risk of breast cancer <30 years is higher than for BRCA1, and

Table 20.2 Hereditary conditions predisposing to breast cancer

Gene	Other tumour susceptibility	Population frequency	Proportion of breast cancer	Proportion of HPHBC	Proportion of familial breast cancer risk	Lifetime risk in women (RR)
BRCA1 AD	Ovary/prostate Colorectal	0.1%	1.5%	40%	5–10%	60–85%
BRCA2 AD	Ovary/prostate Pancreas HoZ-Fanconi (AR)	0.1%	1.5%	40%	5–10%	50–85%
TP53 LFS AD	Sarcoma, Glioma Adrenal	0.0025%	0.02%	2%	0.1%	80–90%
PTEN Cowden's AD	Thyroid Colorectal	0.0005%	0.004%	0.3%	0.02%	25–50%
CHEK2	Colorectal, prostate	0.5%	0.5%	0%	2%	18–20% (2.0)
ATM AD & AR	Lymphoma, HeZ, leukaemia, HoZ	0.5% 0.5%	0.5%	0%	2%	20%
STK11 AD	Colorectal	0.001%	0.001%	0.6%	0.04%	50%
BRIP1	HoZ-Fanconi (AR)	0.1%	0.1%	0%	0.4%	20% (2.0)
PALB2	HoZ-Fanconi (AR)	0.1%	0.1%	0%	0.4%	20% (2.0)
5 SNPs Ref 46		25-46%	0.5%	0%	2%	11–13% (1.1–1.3)
Totals		80% for any	5%	83%	27%	

AD, Autosomal dominant; AR, autosomal recessive; HoZ, homozygous; HeZ, heterozygous; HPHBC, highly penetrant hereditary breast cancer (e.g. >3 affected relatives); LFS, Li Fraumeni syndrome.

mutation carriers also have a very substantially increased risk of sarcomas, brain malignancy and other tumours. The overall impact of Li Fraumeni syndrome on breast cancer incidence is probably quite small. Carriers of the ataxia telangectasia (ATM) gene were thought to be at a 5-fold risk of breast cancer,[39] but although the carrier frequency was thought to be up to 2%, this was based on five complimentation groupings and the disease is now known to be caused by a single gene on 11q.[40] While initial studies were conflicting as to whether ATM was a major gene in breast cancer predisposition, careful large-scale association studies have assessed a relative risk of around 2-fold for pathogenic mutations.[41] The Cowden disease gene has also been identified as PTEN on chromosome 10,[5] but this gene does not appear to account for high-risk families. Additionally, after a substantial lull in identifica-

tion of susceptibility genes, further moderate risk but relatively rare genes (population frequency 0.1–2%) are now being identified.[41-47] These genes and single nucleotide polymorphisms (SNPs) are likely to account for the fact that women who test negative for a BRCA1/2 mutation in their family still appear to be at increased risk.[48] The location of further genes is being sought by genome-wide association studies and the likelihood is that there will be many more genes still to be identified.[47] The current known genetic conditions and locations of genes is shown in Table 20.2.

For the vast majority of women, we will only currently be able to come to an estimate of lifetime risk, which will eventually depend on whether or not there are susceptibility genes in the family and whether they have been inherited. In a few cases it will be possible to modify risk enormously by finding or excluding a germline mutation in the individual. The risk can only be significantly reduced if the individual is shown not to have inherited the known family mutation.[48]

Communication of risk

Risk can be expressed as a lifetime risk or a risk over a period of time. A woman from a young-onset breast cancer family may have a lifetime risk of 40%, but if she is 60 years old she only has a 25% risk of carrying the gene as >60% would have developed the disease and only a 10% chance of having a breast cancer related to an inherited gene mutation in her remaining life. This reflects the gradual equalizing of risk to normal after 60 years in those with a family history. Imparting risk has to cover some conception of when the risk is present (in old age in the general population) and how much risk remains. Some women may prefer to know their risk per year. In a dominant family this may approximate to 1% per year from the late twenties for someone at 50% risk of inheriting the gene.

Options

The options for a woman with a significantly increased risk are limited. She may bury her head in the sand and not present to a doctor, or be encouraged to seek interventions by enthusiastic doctors, which may cause more problems than it solves. While it is still not possible to be sure that screening of young women is effective in reducing mortality and morbidity we must be circumspect about advocating it to all women at risk. However, many women prefer to meet the potential problem head on and this group is likely to benefit very much from what can be offered.

Options to be considered include:

1. No action
2. Try to reduce risks (self-controlled)
   a. plan family early
   b. avoid OCP and HRT
   c. good diet
   d. exercise
   e. interventions
      i. delaying menarche
      ii. artificial early menopause (oophorectomy or treatment with goserelin)
      iii. anti-oestrogen therapy (tamoxifen, raloxifene)

Identification of a group of women at high risk provides the possibility of obtaining sufficient events (development of breast cancer) to make prevention trials worthwhile. Four major trials of prevention with tamoxifen have now published.[49-52] Tamoxifen had already been shown to reduce the risk of contralateral breast cancer in affected women and the large American NSABP trial was the first to show a reduction in risk of breast cancer in asymptomatic women (at increased lifetime risk) by 40–50%.[50] Tamoxifen is by and large well tolerated, although hot flushes and other menopausal symptoms are common and there are increased risks of thrombo-embolic events and endometrial cancer.[50-52] The IBIS1 study showed a 30–40% reduction in breast cancer risk, but a rise in all-cause mortality.[52] As a result, tamoxifen is not currently licensed for prevention in the UK and Europe but does have a licence in North America. A study comparing tamoxifen with raloxifene in America (the STAR trial) showed no overall difference in prevention between the two drugs.[53] Other studies underway involve reduction in fat intake in Canada, administration of retinoids in Italy and a number of diet and exercise trials in the Manchester centre. A high-risk trial, RAZOR, has been piloted in the UK involving switching off the ovaries with Zoladex (Goserelin) and protecting the bones (and breasts) with raloxifene. Variations of this are being undertaken in the USA and mainland Europe. Recruitment to these trials in high-risk women has been disappointing and this may be due to a reluctance to be randomized to placebo.[54]

An alternative strategy, particularly in *BRCA1* carriers, is to opt for early risk reducing Bilateral Salpingo-Oophorectomy (BSO) at about 40 years of age. This can reduce breast cancer risk by around 50%[55] and indeed earlier oophorectomy may well reduce the risk further. Nonetheless, the effects of an early menopause and doubts over long-term HRT have to be considered if the primary purpose is breast cancer prevention.

3. Try to pick up tumours early (screening)
   a. regular self examination.
   b. annual mammography screening from 35 years or 5 years before earliest cancer in family. This may be partly replaced by:
   c. annual ultrasound
   d. MRI scanning

It is likely that annual screening will identify over 60% of cancers in young women,[56] but interval cancers do occur. The young breast is denser and more difficult to interpret. However, as relative risk to the general population at age 35 may be 40-fold, this group needs to be treated as a special case. Although the first evidence for a significant survival advantage has emerged for the general population under 50 years,[57,58] the frequency of disease is probably too low to justify screening on economic grounds. However, our own work has shown that impalpable small lesions are detected in the 35–49 year age group and that similar detection rates to the NHSBSP are attainable by targeted screening.[59] There are also the first signs of a mortality benefit, although this may not be the case for *BRCA1* carriers, who appear to have a worse prognosis.[60,61] Mammography may eventually be replaced by other more sensitive techniques such as magnetic resonance imaging (MRI) in *BRCA1/2* mutation carriers,[62] but the costs and scarcity of scanners may make MRI unviable outside a very-high-risk group. Currently, MRI screening is recommended in the UK for *BRCA1/2* and *TP53* mutation carriers aged 30–49 as well as for individuals without mutations who are at very high risk (www.nice.org.uk). The very small dose of radiation involved with mammography has only a small theoretical risk of inducing a breast cancer.[63] Even cumulatively, this is unlikely to cause more than an extra breast cancer in one in every 10 000 women. This is not really comparable to a 40% lifetime risk. However, known carriers of *TP53* and *ATM* gene mutations should probably not be screened with mammography and there is now some doubt about carriers of *BRCA2*. *BRCA2* interacts with a protein involved in DNA repair and, as such, carriers may be more susceptible to radiation-induced damage. Women screened for breast cancer may undergo fine needle aspiration or open biopsy for screen-detected lumps which are entirely benign. This will be associated with at least a small degree of psychological and physical morbidity, but in experienced hands the risks of unnecessary biopsy are small.[64]

4. Remove the risk
   a. risk reducing mastectomy (RRM)

This is considered by many a drastic measure, which until recently has been carried out far more in the USA than in the UK. It is reasonable and indeed recommended to at least mention it when a woman's risks are high.[65] The most acceptable operation to women is a skin-sparing mastectomy which may spare the nipple and, therefore, some breast tissue; it is, therefore, not totally preventative.[66] The cosmetic results with implants are not always desirable and if any tissue is left under them this will mask a tumour, although this is unlikely if the dissection

is taken down to the pectoral fascia. Some women will, nevertheless, opt for a full mastectomy, and a total mastectomy without sparing the nipple is considered more appropriate by some clinics. Nonetheless, evidence has emerged from a study of nearly 1000 women at the Mayo Clinic in the USA that breast cancer risk is very substantially reduced (by 90%) even with subcutaneous mastectomy.[67] This has now been confirmed in *BRCA1* and *BRCA2* mutation carriers.[68,69] It is also not understood whether there are long-term sequelae of preventative surgery. Some women may be psychologically unprepared for the outcome and cosmetic results may not always be as good as a woman expects. The general anaesthetic and surgical risks also need to be taken into account. Nonetheless, reports have shown significant benefit to women who choose the option compared to those who do not in terms of anxiety and cancer-related worry.[70] It is nonetheless important that a comprehensive protocol for preparing women is in place, including a psychological assessment.[65,71] Increasingly, women at high risk in the UK are opting for risk-reducing mastectomy. This is likely to increase further when genetic testing is more widely available and women at 80–90% lifetime risk of breast cancer are identified. Two recent reports from Manchester and the Netherlands show an uptake of around 50% in unaffected mutation carriers.[71,72] Indeed, somewhat paradoxically, high-risk women are more likely to choose RRM than prevention trials.[55]

The genetic testing programme

The population which could benefit from presymptomatic genetic testing is difficult to define. Potentially, any person could undergo mutation testing for *BRCA1* or *BRCA2* or both. However, there would be little benefit to anyone unless there was at least some chance that they were at risk of such a gene fault in the first place. Individuals without a family history of breast or ovarian cancer would, therefore, have no alteration to their lifetime risk of these cancers from a negative screen. There would also be no benefit to the healthcare system, as these women would not be in screening programmes outside the National Breast Screening Programme (from 50 years of age in the UK). Even those with one or two relatives may not benefit that much in terms of reassurance. Currently, the target population would be at-risk relatives in families with four or more cases of breast cancer under 60 years or ovarian cancer at any age, where a living affected relative could be screened for mutations. The National

Institute for Clinical Excellence (NICE) in the UK has now set a threshold of at least a 20% likelihood of a mutation (in either *BRCA1* or *BRCA2*) in the affected individual tested in a family.[65] This likelihood can now be assessed using a simple scoring system (Table 20.3).[73] This is as accurate as more-involved computer programmes at predicting the likelihood of a mutation,[73] but newer programmes are being developed and may improve accuracy of prediction (see Table 20.1: Boadicea).[74] Testing may eventually be widened to allow for analysis of much smaller aggregations of breast cancer. Currently, probably only one in 1000 people come from families suitable for testing and a maximum of only 3% of breast cancer cases could be prevented by testing in this way for *BRCA1* and *BRCA2*. However, there could be possible cost saving from withdrawing women who test negative from existing screening.

In the main part, research laboratories will be testing those families or affected individuals with a high probability of a *BRCA1* mutation. This could be because the family is linked to *BRCA1*, has many cases of breast and/or ovarian cancer or that an individual has developed either disease at a young age or has a double primary.

Table 20.3 Manchester scoring system for identification of a pathogenic *BRCA1/2* mutation

	BRCA1	BRCA2
FBC <30	6	5
FBC 30–39	4	4
FBC 40–49	3	3
FBC 50–59	2	2
FBC>59	1	1
MBC <60	5 (if *BRCA2* tested)	8
MBC >59	5 (if *BRCA2* tested)	5
Ovarian cancer <60	8	5 (if *BRCA1* tested)
Ovarian cancer >59	5	5 (if *BRCA1* tested)
Pancreatic cancer	0	1
Prostate cancer <60	0	2
Prostate cancer >59	0	1

FBC, female breast cancer; MBC, male breast cancer.
Scores for each cancer in a direct lineage are summated. A score of 10 is equivalent to a 10% chance of identifying a mutation in each gene. A combined score of 20 points would qualify for NHS testing at the 20% threshold.

Once a mutation has been found this will usually be passed on to a service laboratory for verification and to allow a test to be offered to the extended family. Early indications were that around 60% of women offered a *BRCA1* test will take up the option.[75-76] This comes from population surveys and a clinic survey.[77-79] The actual uptake in tested families is still much lower than predicted from prior surveys and needs to be extended to families who have not been contaminated by being involved in large-scale research. A more recent audit of service testing shows variation in uptake between the Northwest of England and London with around 50% of women in Manchester opting for presymptomatic testing, but only around 30% in London.[80] Uptake in men was only around 15%. The long-term outcomes of predictive testing in women who receive appropriate genetic counselling are very satisfactory with very few adverse sequelae.[81,82]

Molecular techniques such as gene sequencing combined with an analysis for large rearrangements such as Multiple Ligation Dependant Probe Amplification (MLPA) will detect 90–95% of *BRCA1* and *BRCA2* mutations. Commercial laboratories in the USA (MYRIAD) currently charge US$2980 for a complete screen of *BRCA1/2*, and their UK subsidiary, Lab 21, UK£2113. As such, an unaffected woman can opt for testing outside the NHS as long as she has appropriate counselling and interpretation of a result. However, once a mutation is identified, subsequent tests per individual in the family can be undertaken on the NHS. Screening for the three common Jewish mutations (185 del AG, 5382 ins C and 6174 del T) cost the NHS only around UK£80. These mutations are carried by around 2.5% of the Ashkenazi population and account for around 95% of *BRCA1/2* involvement. As such, a negative test has good negative predictive value, particularly in a family with both breast and ovarian cancer.[83] It can, therefore, be seen that testing in the Jewish population could be very cost-effective, even in unaffected women with no known family mutation.

Conclusion

There have been huge advances in our knowledge of hereditary breast cancer over the last 10–12 years. While it is now possible to offer definitive testing in a few high-risk families, much is still to be learnt about the remaining genes which confer low to moderate elevations in risk. In the meantime, further evidence has to be gathered as to the efficacy of screening and preventive options. Guidelines for the appropriate management have recently been published for the UK[65] and similar approaches are being used in other parts of Europe and in North America.

REFERENCES

1. Newman B, Austin MA, Lee M *et al*. Inheritance of human breast cancer: Evidence for autosomal dominant transmission in high-risk families. *Proceedings of the National Academy of Science USA* 1988; **85**: 3044–3048.

2. Claus EB, Risch N & Thompson WD. Autosomal dominant inheritance of early onset breast cancer. *Cancer* 1994; **73**: 643–651.

3. Lichtenstein P, Holm NV, Verkasalo PK *et al*. Environmental and heritable factors in the causation of cancer analyses of cohorts of twins from Sweden, Denmark, and Finland. *New England Journal of Medicine* 2000; **343**(2): 78–85.

4. Peto J & Mack TM. High constant incidence in twins and other relatives of women with breast cancer. *Nature Genetics* 2000; **26**: 411–414.

5. Liaw D, Marsh DJ, Li J *et al*. Germline mutations of the PTEN gene in Cowden disease, an inherited breast and thyroid cancer syndrome. *Nature Genetics* 1997; **16**(1): 64–67.

6. Miki Y, Swensen J, Shattuck-Eidens D *et al*. A strong candidate for the breast and ovarian cancer gene BRCA1. *Science* 1994; **266**: 66–71.

7. Wooster R, Bignell G, Lancaster J *et al*. Identification of the breast cancer susceptibility gene BRCA2. *Nature* 1995: **378**; 789–792.

8. Malkin D, Li FP, Strong LC *et al*. Germline TP53 mutations in cancer families. *Science* 1990; **250**: 1233–1238.

9. Scott RJ, McPhillips M, Meldrum CJ *et al*. Hereditary nonpolyposis colorectal cancer in 95 families: differences and similarities between mutation-positive and mutation-negative kindreds. *American Journal of Human Genetics* 2001; **68**: 118–127.

10. Meijers-Heijboer H, Wijnen J, Vasen H *et al*. The CHEK2 1100delC mutation identifies families with a hereditary breast and colorectal cancer phenotype. *American Journal of Human Genetics* 2003; **72**(5): 1308–1314.

11. Breast cancer and hormonal contraceptives: collaborative reanalysis of individual data on 53,297 women with breast cancer and 100,239 women without breast cancer from 54 epidemiological studies. *Lancet* 1996; **347**: 1713–1727.

12. Steinberg KK, Thacker SB, Smith J *et al*. A meta-analysis of the effect of estrogen replacement therapy on the risk of breast cancer. *Journal of the American Medical Association* 1991; **265**: 1985–1990.

13. Collaborative group on hormonal factors in breast cancer. Breast cancer and hormone replacement therapy: collaborative reanalysis of data from 51 epidemiological studies of 52,705 women with breast cancer and 108,411 women without breast cancer. *Lancet* 1997; **350**: 1047–1059.

14. Ross RK, Paganini-Hill A, Wan PC *et al*. Effect of hormone replacement therapy on breast cancer risk: estrogen versus estrogen plus progestin. *Journal of the National Cancer Institute* 2000; **92**: 328–332.

15. Schairer C, Lubin J, Troisi R *et al*. Menopausal estrogen and estrogen-progestin replacement therapy and breast cancer risk. *Journal of the American Medical Association* 2000; **283**: 485–491.

16. Beral V. Breast cancer and hormone-replacement therapy in the Million Women Study. *Lancet* 2003; **362**(9382): 419–427.

17. Huang Z, Hankinson SE, Colditz GA *et al*. Dual effects of weight gain on breast cancer risk. *Journal of the American Medical Association* 2000; **278**: 1407–1411.

18. Harvie M, Hooper & Howell A. Central obesity and breast cancer risk: a systematic review. *Obesity Review* 2003; **4**(3): 157–173.

19. Evans DGR, Fentiman IS, McPherson K *et al*. Familial breast cancer. *British Medical Journal* 1994; **308**: 183–187.

20. Dupont WD & Page DL. Relative risk of breast cancer varies with time since diagnosis of atypical hyperplasia. *Human Pathology* 1989; **20**: 723–725.

21. Scolnick MH, Cannon-Albright LA, Goldgar DE *et al*. Inheritance of proliferative breast disease in breast cancer kindreds. *Science* 1990; **250**: 1715–1721.

22. Freedman AN, Seminara D, Gail MH *et al*. Cancer risk prediction models: a workshop on development, evaluation, and application. *Journal of the National Cancer Institute* 2005; **97**: 715–723.

23. Rockhill B, Spiegelman D, Byrne C *et al*. Validation of the Gail et al. model of breast cancer risk prediction and implications for chemoprevention. *Journal of the National Cancer Institute* 2001; **93**: 358–366.

24. Amir E, Evans DG, Shenton A *et al*. Evaluation of breast cancer risk assessment packages in the family history evaluation and screening programme. *Journal of Medical Genetics* 2003; **40**(11): 807–814.

25. Boyd NF, Lockwood GA, Martin LJ *et al*. Mammographic densities and breast cancer risk. *Cancer Epidemiology and Biomarkers Preview* 1998; **7**: 1133–1144.

26. Key TJ, Appleby PN, Reeves GK *et al.* Body mass index, serum sex hormones, and breast cancer risk in postmenopausal women. *Journal of the National Cancer Institute* 2003; **95**: 1218–1226.

27. Mitchell G, Antoniou AC, Warren R *et al.* Mammographic density and breast cancer risk in BRCA1 and BRCA2 mutation carriers. *Cancer Research* 2006; **66**(3): 1866–1872

28. Pharoah PD, Antoniou AC, Bobrow B *et al.* Polygenic susceptibility to breast cancer and implications for prevention. *Nature Genetics* 2002; **31**: 33–36.

29. Evans DGR, Binchy A, Eng C *et al.* Ten year follow up study of predictive testing for BRCA1 in five large BRCA1 linked families. *Clinical Genetics* 2008 (in press).

30. Easton DF, Ford D & Bishop DT. Breast and ovarian cancer incidence in BRCA1 mutation carriers. *American Journal of Human Genetics* 1994; **56**: 265–271.

31. Gayther SA, Mangion J & Russell P. Variations of risks of breast and ovarian cancer associated with different germline mutations of the BRCA2 gene. *Nature Genetics* 1997; **15**: 103–105.

32. Evans DGR, Donnai D, Ribeiro G *et al.* Ovarian cancer family and prophylactic choices. *Journal of Medical Genetics* 1992; **29**: 416–418.

33. Sutcliffe S, Pharoah PD, Easton DF *et al.* Ovarian and breast cancer risks to women in families with two or more cases of ovarian cancer. *International Journal of Cancer* 2000; **87**(1):110–117.

34. Steichen-Gersdorf E, Gallion HH, Ford D *et al.* Familial site specific ovarian cancer is linked to BRCA1 on 17q12-21. *American Journal of Human Genetics* 1994; **55**: 870–875.

35. Risch HA, McLaughlin JR, Cole DEC *et al.* Prevalence and penetrance of germline BRCA1 and BRCA2 mutations in a population series of 649 women with ovarian cancer. *American Journal of Human Genetics* 2001; **68**: 700–710.

36. Struewing J, Hartge P, Wacholder S *et al.* The risk of cancer associated with specific mutations of BRCA1 and BRCA2 among Ashkenazi Jews. *New England Journal of Medicine* 1997; **336**: 1401–1408.

37. Antoniou A, Pharoah PDP, Narod S *et al.* Average risks of breast and ovarian cancer associated with mutations in BRCA1 or BRCA2 detected in case series unselected for family history: a combined analysis of 22 studies. *American Journal of Human Genetics* 2003; **72**(5): 1117–1130.

38. Varley JM, Evans DGR & Birch JM. Li-Fraumeni syndrome – a molecular and clinical review. *British Journal of Cancer* 1997; **76**: 1–14.

39. Swift ML, Reitnauer PJ, Morrell D *et al.* Breast and other cancers in families with ataxia telangiectasia. *New England Journal of Medicine* 1987; **316**: 1289–1294.

40. Savitsky K, Bar-Shira A, Gilad S *et al.* A single ataxia telangectasia gene with a product similar to PI-3 kinase. *Science* 1995; **268**: 1749–1753.

41. Chenevix-Trench G, Spurdle AB, Gatei M *et al.* Dominant negative ATM mutations in breast cancer families. *Journal of the National Cancer Institute* 2002; **94**(3): 205–215.

42. Renwick A, Thompson D, Seal S *et al.* ATM mutations that cause ataxia-telangiectasia are breast cancer susceptibility alleles. *Nature Genetics* 2006; **38**(8): 873–875. Epub 2006 Jul 9.

43. Meijers-Heijboer H, van den Ouweland A, Klijn J *et al.* Low penetrance breast cancer susceptibility due to CHK2 1100delC in non-carriers of BRCA1 or BRCA2 mutations. *Nature Genetics* 2002; **31**(1): 55–59.

44. Seal S, Thompson D, Renwick A *et al.* Truncating mutations in the Fanconi anemia J gene, BRIP1, are low penetrance breast cancer susceptibility alleles. *Nature Genetics* 2006; **38**(11): 1239–1241.

45. Stacey SN, Sulem P, Johannsson OT *et al.* The BARD1 Cys557Ser variant and breast cancer risk in Iceland. *PLOS Medicine* 2006; **3**(7): e217.

46. Rahman N, Seal S, Thompson D *et al.* PALB2 which encodes a BRCA2-interacting protein is a breast cancer susceptibility gene. *Nature Genetics* 2006; E Pub ahead of print.

47. Easton DF, Pooley KA, Dunning AM *et al.* A genome-wide association study identifies multiple novel breast cancer susceptibility loci. *Nature* 2007; **447**(7148): 1087–1093.

48. Smith A, Moran A, Boyd MC *et al.* The trouble with phenocopies: are those testing negative for a family BRCA1/2 mutation really at population risk? *Journal of Medical Genetics* 2006; Nov 1; [Epub ahead of print].

49. Powles TJ, Eeles R, Ashley S *et al.* Interim analysis of the incidence of breast cancer in the Royal Marsden Hospital tamoxifen randomised chemoprevention trial. *Lancet* 1998; **352**: 98–101.

50. Fisher B, Constantino JP, Wickerham DL *et al.* Tamoxifen for prevention of breast cancer; report of the National Surgical Adjuvant Breast and Bowel Project PI study. *Journal of the National Cancer Institute* 1998; **90**: 1371–1388.

51. Veronesi U, Maisonneuve P, Costa A *et al.* Prevention of breast cancer with tamoxifen: preliminary findings from the Italian randomised trial among hysterectomised women. *Lancet* 1998; **352**: 93–97.

52. IBIS working party and principal investigators. First results from the International Breast Cancer Intervention Study (IBIS-1): a randomized prevention trial. *Lancet* 2002; **360**: 817–824.

53. Vogel VG, Constantinoi JP, Wicherham DL *et al.* Effects of tamoxifen vs raloxifene on the risk of developing invasive breast cancer and other disease outcomes: the NSABP Study of Tamoxifen and Raloxifene (STAR) P-2 trial. *Journal of the American Medical Association* 2006; **295**(23): 2727–2741.

54. Evans DGR, Lalloo F, Shenton A *et al.* Uptake of screening and prevention trials in women at very high risk of breast cancer. *Lancet* 2001; **358**: 889–890.

55. Rebbeck TR, Lynch HT, Neuhausen SL *et al.* Reduction in cancer risk after bilateral prophylactic oophorectomy in BRCA1 and BRCA2 mutation carriers. *New England Journal of Medicine* 2002; **346**: 1616–1622.

56. Tabar L, Faberberg G, Day NE *et al.* What is the optimum interval between mammographic screening examinations? An analysis based on the Swedish two county breast cancer screening trial. *British Journal of Cancer* 1987; **56:** 547–551.

57. Tabar L, Fagerberg G, Chen HH *et al.* Efficacy of breast cancer screening by age. *Cancer* 1995; **75:** 2507–2517.

58. Report of the coordinating group for breast cancer screening, Falun meeting, Falun, Sweden. Breast screening with mammography in women 40–49 years. *International Journal of Cancer* 1996; **68:** 693–699.

59. Lalloo F, Boggis CRM, Evans DGR *et al.* Screening by mammography women with a family history of breast cancer. *European Journal of Cancer* 1998; **34:** 937–940.

60. Moller P, Borg A, Evans DG *et al.* Survival in prospectively ascertained familial breast cancer: analysis of a series stratified by tumour characteristics, BRCA mutations and oophorectomy. *International Journal of Cancer* 2002; **101**(6): 555–559.

61. Maurice A, Evans DGR, Shenton A *et al.* The screening of women aged less than 50 years at increased risk of breast cancer by virtue of their family history. *European Journal of Cancer* 2006; **42**(10): 1385–1390.

62. Leach MO, Boggis CR, Dixon AK *et al.*; MARIBS study group. Screening with magnetic resonance imaging and mammography of a UK population at high familial risk of breast cancer: a prospective multicentre cohort study (MARIBS). *Lancet* 2005; **365**(9473): 1769–1778.

63. Law J. Cancers detected and induced in mammographic screening: new screening schedules and younger women with family history. *British Journal of Radiology* 1997; **70:** 62–69.

64. Moller P, Evans G, Maehle L *et al.* Use of cytology to diagnose hereditary breast cancer. *Disease Markers* 1999; **15:** 212–216.

65. McIntosh A, Shaw C, Evans G *et al.* Clinical guidelines and evidence review for the classification and care of women at risk of familial breast cancer, London: National Collaborating Centre for Primary Care/University of Sheffield. NICE guideline CG014. www.nice.org.uk 2004.

66. Goodnight JE, Quagliani JM & Morton DL. Failure of subcutaneous mastectomy to prevent the development of breast cancer. *Journal of Surgical Oncology* 1984; **26:** 198–201.

67. Hartmann LC, Schaid DJ, Woods JE *et al.* Efficacy of bilateral prophylactic mastectomy in women with a family history of breast cancer. *New England Journal of Medicine* 1999; **340:** 77–84.

68. Meijers-Heijboer EJ, van Geel B, van Putten WLJ *et al.* Breast cancer after prophylactic bilateral mastectomy in women with a BRCA1 or BRCA2 mutation. *New England Journal of Medicine* 2001; **345:** 159–164.

69. Rebbeck TR, Friebel T, Lynch HT *et al.* Bilateral prophylactic mastectomy reduces breast cancer risk in BRCA1 and BRCA2 mutation carriers: The PROSE Study Group. *Journal of Clinical Oncology* 2004; **22**(6): 1055–1062.

70. Hatcher MB, Falowfield L & A'Hern B. The psychosocial impact of bilateral prophylactic mastectomy: prospective study using questionnaires and semistructured interviews. *British Medical Journal* 2001; **322:** 1–7.

71. Lalloo F, Baildam A, Brain A *et al.* Preventative mastectomy for women at high risk of breast cancer. *European Journal of Surgical Oncology* 2000; **26:** 711–713.

72. Meijers-Heijboer EJ, Verhoog LC, Brekelmans CTM *et al.* Presymptomatic DNA testing and prophylactic surgery in families with a BRCA1 or BRCA2 mutation. *Lancet* 2000; **355:** 2015–2020.

73. Evans DGR, Eccles DM, Rahman N *et al.* A new scoring system for the chances of identifying a BRCA1/2 mutation, outperforms existing models including BRCAPRO. *Journal of Medical Genetics* 2004; **41**(6): 474–480.

74. Antoniou AC, Durocher F, Smith P *et al.* INHERIT BRCAs program members. BRCA1 and BRCA2 mutation predictions using the BOADICEA and BRCAPRO models and penetrance estimation in high-risk French-Canadian families. *Breast Cancer Research* 2006; **8**(1): R3.

75. Watson M, Murday V, Lloyd S *et al.* Genetic testing in breast/ovarian cancer (BRCA1) families. *Lancet* 1995; **346:** 583.

76. Lerman C, Narod S, Schulman K *et al.* BRCA1 testing in families with hereditary breast ovarian cancer. A prospective study of patient decision making and outcomes. *Journal of the American Medical Association* 1996; **275:** 1928–1929.

77. Holloway SM, Bernhard B, Campbell H *et al.* Uptake of testing for BRCA1/2 mutations in South East Scotland. *European Journal of Human Genetics* 2008; **16**(8): 906–912.

78. Lerman C, Daly M, Masny A *et al.* Attitudes about genetic testing for breast ovarian cancer susceptibility. *Journal of Clinical Oncology* 1994; **12:** 843–850.

79. Mohammed S, Barnes C, Watts S *et al.* Attitudes to predictive testing for BRCA1. *Journal of Medical Genetics* 1995; **32:** 140A.

80. Brooks L, Lennard F, Shenton A *et al.* BRCA1/2 predictive testing: a study of uptake in two centres. *European Journal of Human Genetics* 2004; **12**(8): 654–662.

81. Watson M, Foster C, Eeles R *et al.* Psychosocial impact of breast/ovarian (BRCA1/2) cancer-predictive genetic testing in a UK multi-centre clinical cohort. *British Journal of Cancer* 2004; **91**(10): 1787–1794.

82. Foster C, Watson M, Eeles R *et al.* Predictive genetic testing for BRCA1/2 in a UK clinical cohort: three year follow-up. *British Journal of Cancer* 2007; **96**(5): 718–724.

83. Lalloo F, Cochrane S, Bulman B *et al.* An evaluation of common breast cancer mutations within a population of Ashkenazi Jews. *Journal of Medical Genetics* 1998; **35:** 10–12.

Index